INTERPERSONAL RELATIONSHIPS

EIGHTH EDITION

PROFESSIONAL COMMUNICATION SKILLS FOR NURSES

Elizabeth C. Arnold, PhD, RN, PMHCNS-BC

Associate Professor, Retired University of Maryland
  School of Nursing Baltimore, Maryland

Family Nurse Psychotherapist Montgomery Village, Maryland

Kathleen Underman Boggs, PhD, FNP-CS

Family Nurse Practitioner, Associate Professor Emeritus College of Health and
  Human Services
University of North Carolina Charlotte, Charlotte, North Carolina

ELSEVIER

ELSEVIER

3251 Riverport Lane
St. Louis, Missouri 63043

INTERPERSONAL RELATIONSHIPS: PROFESSIONAL
COMMUNICATION SKILLS FOR NURSES, EIGHTH EDITION

ISBN: 978-0-323-54480-1

Notices

Previous editions copyrighted 2016, 2011, 2007, 2003, 1999, 1995, and 1989.

Library of Congress Control Number: 2018963457

Content Strategist: Yvonne Alexopoulos
Content Development Specialist: Diane Chatman and Luke Held
Publishing Services Manager: Deepthi Unni
Project Manager: Nayagi Athmanathan
Designer: Ryan Cook

Printed in the U.S.A.

Last digit is the print number: 9 8 7 6 5 4 3 2 1

Working together
to grow libraries in
developing countries

www.elsevier.com • www.bookaid.org

To the memory of my husband George Arnold, who believed in me and supported me unconditionally, to my parents, for their support and love, and to all the students I have had the privilege of teaching.
Elizabeth C. Arnold

For Michael, the love of my life.
Kathleen Underman Boggs

REVIEWERS AND CONTRIBUTORS

REVIEWERS

Karan S. Kverno, PhD, PMHCNS-BC, PMHNP-BC
Assistant Professor
Acute and Chronic Care
Johns Hopkins University School of Nursing
Baltimore, MD

Margaret Blanka Huml, RN, BSN, MN
Professor
Bachelor of Science in Nursing
Vancouver Island University
Nanaimo, British Columbia, Canada

Katharine A. Hungerford, RN, BScN, MEd
Professor of Nursing
Health Sciences
Lambton College of Applied Arts
Sarnia, Ontario, Canada

CONTRIBUTORS

Kim Siarkowski Amer, PhD, APRN
Associate professor
School of Nursing, Depaul University
Chicago, IL

Shari Kist, PhD, RN, CNE
Assistant Professor
Goldfarb School of Nursing
Barnes-Jewish College
St. Louis, MO

Pamela E. Marcus, MS, APRN
Associate Professor
Prince George's Community College
Largo, MD

Eileen O'Brien, PhD, RN
Undergraduate Program Director
    Psychology Department
University of Maryland
Baltimore County Campus
Baltimore, MD

ACKNOWLEDGEMENTS

We acknowledge our heartfelt appreciation for the contributions of the many professional nurses and other practitioners who helped us deepen and clarify our evolving thinking and understanding of communication over the past years.

We would like to thank Laura Holbrook, MSN, RN, consultant and educator in Health Team Communication, staff nurse in cardiology, Medical College of South Carolina for Contributing Chapter 26.

We are very grateful to the Elsevier editorial staff, particularly Tina Kaemmerer, Senior Content Development specialist, Diane Chatman, Content Development Specialist and Yvonne Alexopoulos, Senior Content Strategist. Their guidance, tangible support, and suggestions were invaluable in the content development of this 8th edition. Finally, we want to sincerely thank Nayagi Athmanathan and Karthikeyan Murthy, Senior Project Managers from Elsevier for their painstaking, precise copy-editing, and editorial support during the production process.

Elizabeth C. Arnold
Kathleen Underman Boggs

In 1989, Elsevier published the first edition of *Interpersonal Relationships: Communication Skills for Nurses*. It was originally developed at the University of Maryland School of Nursing to accompany a communication seminar course on interpersonal communication skills for nurses. Subsequent editions reinforced its salience as a key resource on nurse-patient relationships. This text has been twice recognized as an American Journal of Nursing book of the year (2004; 2007). Technology was in its infancy, and chronic disorders had not yet emerged as a primary focus of attention in focus health care. The latter is no longer the case.

The eighth edition is designed as a key interactive reference for nursing students and professional nurses. It has been updated and expanded to include new understandings of patient-centered communication and the support for self-management strategies needed in contemporary health care environments. New simulation exercises with reflective analysis discussions allow students to the pros and cons of various approaches and modern practice issues across clinical settings. Patient-centered relationships, self-management of chronic disorders, collaborative interprofessional communication, and team-based approaches are new content additions in the eighth edition. Just as the world has so has the scope of nursing practice, fueled by several intersecting factors. Nurses are educationally prepared to function at a higher level than ever before. They are expected to play a key role in promoting and supporting healthy behavior change.

The health care system possesses stronger diagnostic capabilities and better-targeted treatments for many acute health diseases. The nation's population is more culturally diverse at many different levels—psychosocial, educational, with multiple resource availability. This means that there are explanatory models for the same illness, and varied underlying principles about treatment.

Technology is an established part of virtually every health care endeavor. Our nation is part of a complex global community, increasingly interconnected through technology. Patients have more access to health information through the Internet, and this change means that patients are better able to self-manage their own health care. Attention has shifted from acute to chronic disorders as major causes of morbidity and mortality. By contrast with acute disorders, chronic conditions usually last a long time, sometimes a lifetime. Many people have to cope with more than one chronic condition, sometimes with competing care needs.

Currently, health care is as much a public health issue as it is a general health concern.

ABOUT THE CONTENT

Interpersonal Relationships: Communication Skills for Nurses consists of 26 chapters. The range of health care applications includes preventive health applications and can follow patients through the life cycle to include end-of-life communication and nursing interventions. The communication content supports health care applications across a broad service continuum of care that includes hospitals, long-term care, ambulatory and public health, rehabilitation, palliative and home care, and, more recently, preventive primary care health "homes."

Chapter topics in the eighth edition mirror the nation's shift from a health care system structured around medical disease to one based on an integrated holistic health approach to health care that begins with the patient's perception, values, concerns, and preferences. Contemporary health care relationships consider every health experience as a holistic *human experience*, which requires a fresh, new perspective and level of patient and family involvement. This belief is reflected throughout the text and explicitly in several appropriate chapters.

Although the text continues to draw evidence-based principles from nursing, medical science, technology, psychology, public health, and systems-based communication, the new contemporary health care landscape emphasizes a more personalized level of care, which honors the personal dignity, values, and preferences of patients in making significant health decisions and in implementing meaningful care choices in care. Patients are expected to actively engage in their own care and, in partnership with their care providers, to make meaningful care decisions related to achievement of mutually determined health goals. Updated communication skills, combined with patient-centered applications, create the therapeutic partnership that patients nowadays need to have to successfully self-manage long-term chronic disorders.

In 2010 an Institute of Medicine report on the Future of Nursing states: "nurses have a key role to play as collaborative team members, and leaders leading to a reformed, and better integrated patient-centered health care system." The eighth edition of *Interpersonal Relationships: Professional Communication Skills for Nurses* has been updated and revised to reflect the realities of this new and rapidly expanding health care landscape with an activated engagement of the patient and family participation in collaborative team-based health care relationships. Emphasis on safety in health care is stressed with a full chapter devoted to the importance of communication in making health care a quality, safe environment, immediately following the opening chapter on conceptual foundations of nursing practice.

The chapters on patient-centered relationship and communication have been updated to reflect the patient/family-centered focus incorporating patient preferences and values as the driver of care. The chapters on interprofessional collaboration and teamwork have been significantly reworked in line with the emerging team-based theme of different health care professional disciplines, working as a team as a preferred care model.

As the world has become better connected through technology, much more gets shared across clinical settings in real time. Nurses have a pivotal role in making use of e-health technologies at point of care and electronic documentation. Direct relationship centered communication between patients and a provider is further enhanced through secure patient portals.

The central phenomena of professional nursing practice take place within a collaborative interprofessional team of health care professionals with patients, providers, and families working together. This major paradigm shift in health care delivery from a disease-oriented to a person/family-centered model, which considers the patient as a person, is consistent with Institute of Medicine and other national reports.

The changes we have made in the 8th edition mirror a major paradigm shift in health care delivery from a "disease-focused" narrative to a more contemporary inclusive "patient-centered" preventive and health promotion emphasis in health care applications. The positioning of primary care as an essential component of health wellness is indicated in several chapters.

Greater attention in the text is directed to helping patients and families develop the healthy lifestyle and coping strategies needed to prevent or offset the impact of a marked increase in the incidence of chronic diseases. Such interventions are informed and proactive, as advocated by the Institute of Medicine, the World Health Framework for Action, and the Picker Institute.

The locus of health care delivery has shifted from the hospital to include community-based primary care delivery. Communication for continuity of care, across clinical settings, starting with health promotion and disease prevention, has become an essential component of care delivery. Shared decision making and therapeutic partnerships with patients require that nurses integrate patient preferences, values, motivations, and hopes with evidenced-based biomedical realities as the basis for shared decision making. A collaborative practice-ready workforce offering quality, safe health services strengthens the health care system and leads to improved health outcomes.

Computer technology has introduced a new dimension to health communication, allowing patients and clinical providers an immediate, transparent access to personal clinical records and offers secure portals for immediate discussion with providers. In this 8th edition, Chapter 25 has been retitled as Electronic Documentation, with relevant expanded content related to biomedical technologies documenting improved assessment, medication adherence, patient satisfaction, and sound decision making. New applications of use of technology at point of care are also discussed.

This edition has been revised and updated to meet the challenge of continuing to serve as a major communication resource for professional nurses in a time of significant changes in the national and global health care system. Some chapters have been retitled to better reflect the significance of these changes in the health care delivery system and to provide more up-to-date terminology. The simulation exercises in each chapter offer an additional opportunity for experiential understanding of concepts with appropriate reflective analysis related to each chapter. Although the text's content, exercises, and case examples continue to be written in terms of nurse-patient relationships, the interactional data are also applicable to clinical practice student relationships entered into by other health care disciplines.

Role clarity and the importance of well-defined, clear communication are crucial to ensuring the safety and quality of care delivery in interprofessional health care environments in which multiple inputs must be coordinated. To emphasize its importance, we have reordered this topic's chapter position to the beginning of the text so that it may serve as a foundational component of patient-centered communication. The chapter on patient relationships has been thoroughly revised and retitled to reflect the dimensions of patient-centered relationships in contemporary health care.

ABOUT THE CHAPTER ORGANIZATION

Each chapter incorporates a similar format to previous editions, consisting of chapter objectives, concepts, and an application section, connected by a relevant research study or meta-analysis of several studies relevant to the chapter topic. Suggested simulation exercises with critical analysis questions offer an interactive component to the student's study of text materials.

The chapters in the eighth edition (as previous editions) can be used as individual teaching modules. The text also can be used as a primary text or as a communication resource, integrated across the curriculum. Chapter text boxes and tables highlight important ideas in each chapter.

The eighth edition presents an updated synthesis of relationships in nursing and team-based health communication, with an emphasis on an integrated collaborative approach to patient- and family-centered professional relationships. Discussion questions for student reflective analysis are placed at the end of each chapter exercise.

The eighth edition is divided into six sections. As in previous editions, *Part I: Theoretical Foundations and Contemporary Dynamics in Patient-Centered Relationships and Communication,* introduces students to basic conceptual information needed for contemporary professional nursing practice. Chapter 1 traces the development of professional nursing, identifies its fundamental characteristics, and distinguishes between the science and art of nursing. The chapter introduces a theory-based systems approach to communication in contemporary nursing practice. Chapter 2 emphasizes communication concepts and strategies that nurses need to maintain a safe, quality health care environment. In Chapter 3, QSEN communication competencies, the nursing process, BSN essentials, and legal and ethical standards provide structural professional guides to action in health care communication. The process role of critical thinking and clinical judgment in providing safe, quality care is the focus of Chapter 4. *Part II: Essential Communication Competencies,* identifies the fundamental structure and characteristics of effective patient-centered communication skills and strategies. This section discusses selected professional approaches and communication strategies required for individual, intercultural, and group communication skill development.

The chapters in *Part III: Relationship Skills in Health Communication,* explore the nature of patient- and family-centered relationships in health care settings. The chapters discuss communication strategies nurses can use with individuals, groups, and families in health care settings. Applying therapeutic communication strategies in conflict situations and special attention to health promotion community strategies and health teaching complete the section.

The three chapters in *Part IV: Communication for Health Promotion and Disease Prevention,* emphasize the use of specialized health teaching and coaching strategies as communication tools to support patient understanding and self-management coping. **Part V, Responding to Special Needs**, focuses on the communication needs of special populations: children, older adults, patients with communication deficits, patients in palliative/end-of-life care, and with those experiencing a crisis.

Part V: Accommodating Patients with Special Communication Needs, professionals from different disciplines working together from different care perspectives as a health care team is recognized as a preferred model of contemporary care delivery. Chapters related to the concept of continuity of care across clinical settings and nursing applications in the use of electronic health records with accompanying taxonomies are discussed. This section also identifies major changes in managing health care data and digital transmission of vital health information. The role of data transfer as an increasingly important form of communication at point of care is highlighted in Chapter 26.

CHAPTER FEATURES

Each chapter begins with chapter objectives, followed by basic concepts, relevant clinical applications with updated references, and instructive case examples. *The Evidence-Based Practice* box offers a summary of research findings related to the chapter subject. This feature is intended to strengthen awareness of the link between research and practice. An exemplar related to *Ethical Dilemmas* is presented at the end of each chapter.

Simulation exercises, with opportunities for reflective analysis offer students an opportunity to practice, observe, and critically evaluate professional communication skills from a practice perspective in a safe learning environment.

Through active experiential involvement with relationship-based communication principles, students can develop confidence and skill in their capacity to engage in patient-centered communication across clinical settings. The comments and reflections of other students provide a wider, enriching perspective about the person-centered implications of communication in clinical practice.

This eighth edition continues to give voice to the centrality of patient-centered relational communication strategies as the basis for ensuring quality and safety in professional health care delivery. Health care has changed dramatically, with the expectation that patients will be actively involved in their care. Our hope is that the eighth edition will continue to serve as a primary reference resource for nurses seeking to hone their communication and relationship skills in both traditional clinical and nontraditional community-based health care settings.

As the single most consistent health care provider in many patients' lives, nurses have an awesome responsibility to provide communication that is professional, honest, empathetic, and knowledgeable in individual and group relationships. As nurses, we are answerable to our patients, our profession, and ourselves to communicate with all those involved with a patient's care in an authentic therapeutic manner and to advocate for the patient's health, care, and well-being within the larger sociopolitical community.

The opportunity to contribute to the evolving development of communication as a central tenet of professional nursing practice has been a privilege as well as a responsibility to our profession. We invite you as students, practicing nurses, and faculty to interact with the material in this text, learning from the content and experiential exercises but also seeking your own truth and understanding as interprofessional health care providers in furthering a positive influence on the health care crisis in the United States.

Elizabeth C. Arnold
Kathleen Underman Boggs

1

Historical Perspectives and Contemporary Dynamics

Elizabeth C. Arnold

OBJECTIVES

At the end of the chapter, the reader will be able to:

1. Discuss the historical evolution of professional nursing.
2. Describe the core components of nursing's metaparadigm.
3. Discuss the role of "ways of knowing," in patient-centered nursing care.
4. Compare and contrast linear and transactional models of communication.
5. Explain the use of systems thinking as a foundational construct in professional health care.
6. Discuss the role of health communication in interprofessional communication.

INTRODUCTION

This introductory chapter, provides the groundwork for understanding communication and relationship concepts presented in later chapters. The historical development of professional nursing, communication concepts, and systems thinking offer an evidence-based foundation for patient-centered communication, and interprofessional collaborative communication (IPC) as the preferred means for delivering safe, quality health care in contemporary care settings.

BASIC CONCEPTS

Foundations of Professional Nursing Practice

Historically, nursing is as old as humankind. Initially, women practiced nursing informally with care traditions passed down through the generations. Female family caregivers in the home with no formal education assumed primary nursing roles for the sick. There was a religious theme to caring for the sick. Deaconesses, appointed by the church, visited the sick in their homes. Nuns and monks staffed early hospitals, and cared for people who were unable to be cared for in their home (Egenes, 2017).

The "roots of professional nursing as a distinct occupation" began with Florence Nightingale's *Notes on Nursing* (1859) (Fig. 1.1). She established the first nursing school (St. Thomas's Hospital of London) in 1860. In doing so, Nightingale introduced the world to the functional roles of professional nursing. Her use of statistical data to document the need for hand washing to prevent infection during the Crimean War marks her as the profession's first nurse researcher. An early advocate for high-quality care, Nightingale viewed nursing as both a science and an art form (Alligood, 2014). Her solid defense of blending scientific evidence with caring about the humanity of the sick lives on, unblemished, in contemporary health care.

Evolution of Nursing as a Profession

As nursing care becomes more complex, *evidence-based practice knowledge* has replaced apprentice-type

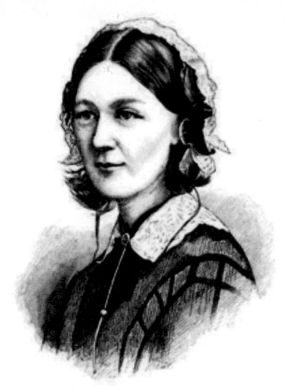

Fig. 1.1 Florence Nightingale is recognized as America's first professional nurse. (From Thinkstock)

training as the required foundation for professional nursing practice. Professional training for nurses also has expanded to include theory and basic sciences, general and liberal arts courses, and evidence-based clinical practice concepts. In 1923, Yale University became the first institution to provide a nursing curriculum based on educational considerations rather than on hospital needs. College level credits to support nursing practice, and clinical concepts related to nursing skill development, have become educational requirements for professional nursing.

During the late 1940s and in the 1950s, nursing scholars and their graduate students developed nursing theories to describe, explain, predict, and prescribe nursing phenomena. Nursing theory models continue to serve as organizing frameworks for research, education, and professional nursing practice. Alligood (2014) suggests however that nursing theory has moved past the conceptualization phase to a new "theory utilization era" concerned with theory applications in praxis.

Nursing Theory Development

Theory development is essential to maintaining the truth of any discipline (Reed & Shearer, 2007). Theory serves as a major source of clarifying nursing's unique body of knowledge. Theory concepts examine the phenomenon of professional nursing in *systematic ways*. They make visible the nature of the nursing domain, inform its clinical practice, and form a framework for research studies. D'Amour, Ferrada-Videla, Rodriguez, and Beaulieu (2005) define a **theoretical framework** "as a set of relationships that are understood to exist between various concepts" (p. 118).

Theoretical nursing models provide a foundation for generating hypotheses in research. They offer a common basis for education and act as a guide for nursing praxis. As the profession positions itself to play a key leadership role in a transformational health care system, there is a noticeable shift from theory development to a new era of theory applicability, and utilization in nursing praxis (Alligood, 2014).

Nursing's Metaparadigm: The Science of Nursing

Nursing's metaparadigm represents the most abstract form of nursing knowledge (Black, 2017). Four core constructs make up professional nursing's metaparadigm: *person, environment, health, and nursing*. Each of these four conceptual constructs has an internal consistency related to the knowledge structure of nursing, which is described in different ways across theoretical frameworks (Jarrin, 2012; Karnick, 2013; Marrs & Lowry, 2006).

CONCEPT OF PERSON

Knowledge of the "patient as a person" is the starting point in contemporary health care delivery (Zolnierek, 2013). *Person* is defined as the recipient of nursing care. The term "person" is applied to individuals, family units, the community, and selected target populations—for example, infants, elderly, and the mentally ill. For all individuals, mental, physical and social health are vital strands of life that are closely interwoven and deeply interdependent (p. 3) (World Health Organization [WHO], 2001, p. 17). Examples include gender, lifestyle, coping styles, habits, and cultural values, which are identified as "person" attributes.

Nurses have a legal responsibility to protect each patient's integrity and health rights to self-determination in health care. It is also an *ethical* professional responsibility, whether the person is a contributing member of society, a critically ill newborn, a comatose patient, or a seriously mentally ill individual (Shaller, 2007).

CONCEPT OF ENVIRONMENT

Environment describes the *context* in which health relationships take place (WHO, 2001). To consider the concept of "person" without considering the environmental factors acting as barriers or supports to health care participation is impracticable. Socioenvironmental factors represent the context that directly and indirectly influence a person's health perceptions and health behaviors. At the community level, poverty, education, religious and spiritual beliefs, type of community (rural or urban), family strengths and challenges, level of social support, health resource availability, and ease of care access are significant environmental determinants of health. Contextual factors are important in health promotion, disease prevention, and the capacity of individuals with chronic conditions to take major responsibility for self-management strategies. The importance of environment is underscored in a new American Nurses Association (ANA) Scope and Standard of Nursing Practice *(#17)*: "*The registered nurse integrates the principles of environmental health for nursing in all areas of practice*" (American Nurses Association [ANA], 2015).

CONCEPT OF HEALTH

The word **health** derives from the word *whole*. Health is a relative term, subject to personal interpretation. Culture, religious beliefs, and previous life experiences influence how a person perceives and interprets health and illness. For example, in some cultures, where poverty is a significant factor, having a robust body size is considered a sign of a healthy lifestyle. In a different culture, a similar body size would be considered a sign of an unhealthy lifestyle (Schiavo, 2014).

The WHO definition developed in 1948 describes **health** as "a state of complete physical, mental and social well-being, and not merely the absence of disease or infirmity". Present-day health concepts describe health on a continuum as stretching from birth to death (Masters, 2015). Better nutrition, an emphasis on hygiene, plus advances in diagnosis and treatment have reduced the incidence of acute diseases.

People are living much longer, but the incidence of chronic disorders associated with aging has also increased. The Centers for Disease Control and Prevention (CDC) reports that almost half the adult population has one or more *chronic* health conditions (Ward, 2015). Chronic diseases have overtaken acute disorders as a major cause of death and disability worldwide, accounting for 59% of deaths and 46% of the global burden of disease (Coleman et al., 2009, p. 75).

Contemporary health initiatives reflect an increasing shift in focus to healthy life style promotion, disease prevention, reducing health disparities, early risk assessments, and chronic disease self-care management strategies. "*Quality of life* includes both health and well-being". The term refers to an individual's subjective assessment of well-being (Mount, Boston, & Cohen, 2007). At the opposite end of well-being is the human experience of suffering and anguish, in large part, associated with health. Nordstrom et al. (2013) describe a healthy person as one who is able to "realize *his* or *her* vital goals, *not* vital goals in general" (p. 361). For example, an active 80-year-old woman can consider herself quite healthy, despite having osteoporosis and a controlled heart condition.

Paradigm Shift in Health Care Delivery

We are seeing dramatic changes in how professional nursing is practiced, and where health care is delivered. Until recent decades, care was delivered in acute-care settings, based on a disease-focused medical model. Many acute disorders that shortened people's lives have been eradicated, or are now viewed as manageable chronic conditions. Better diagnostic tools and effective treatments have given rise to improved medical outcomes and longevity. According to the CDC, nearly half of all adults suffer from one or more chronic disorders. Patients are charged with becoming active participants in partnership with their health care providers.

Beginning with the Institute of Medicine (IOM) Report, *Crossing the quality chasm: a new health system for the 21st century, in 2001*, there has been a radical shift to an emphasis on health care initiatives that advance the quality and safety of comprehensive health care. The Chronic Care Model is an integrated form of health care services, designed to provide safe quality health care across designated clinical settings. The model includes proactive health promotion and disease prevention care initiatives. Contemporary health care emphasizes health promotion and disease prevention, early intervention for chronic disorders, continuity of care, and activated patient participation as part of the health care team. Nurses play an important role in helping people of all ages engage in various health promotion and disease prevention activities needed to promote maximum personal health and wellbeing.

Exercise 1.1, The Meaning of Health, provides an opportunity to explore the multidimensional meaning of health.

EXERCISE 1.1   The Meaning of Health as a Nursing Concept

Purpose
To help students understand the dimensions of health as a nursing concept.

Procedure
1. Think of a person whom you think is healthy. In a short report (1–2 paragraphs), identify characteristics that led you to your choice of this person.
2. In small groups of three or four, read your stories to each other. As you listen to other students' stories, write down themes that you note.
3. Compare themes, paying attention to similarities and differences, and developing a group definition of health derived from the stories.

4. In a larger group, share your definitions of health and defining characteristics of a healthy person.

Reflective Analysis Discussion
1. Were you surprised by any of your thoughts about being healthy?
2. Did your peers define health in similar ways?
3. Based on the themes that emerged, how is health determined?
4. Is illness the opposite of being healthy?
5. In what ways, if any, did you find concepts of health to be culture or gender bound?
6. In what specific ways can you as a health care provider support the health of your patient?

CONCEPT OF NURSING

The International Council of Nurses (ICN) declares that nursing encompasses a continuum of health care services delivered by nurses, and that it is found across health care systems and in the community. This document states:

- Nursing encompasses autonomous and collaborative care of individuals of all ages, families, groups, and communities, sick or well and in all settings.
- Nursing includes the promotion of health, prevention of illness, and the care of ill, disabled, and dying people.
- Advocacy, promotion of a safe environment, research, participation in shaping health policy and in patient and health systems management, and education are also key nursing roles (International Council of Nurses [ICN], 2014).

The science of nursing (theory based, research, clinical guidelines) provides an essential focus and knowledge basis for professional nursing. Evidence-based nursing actions help patients achieve identified health goals through services ranging from health promotion, preventive care, and health education, to include direct care, rehabilitation, palliative care, research, and health teaching. *The patient is at the center of model, as its core concept.*

CONTEMPORARY NURSING

Nurses represent the largest group of health care professionals in the United States with over 3 million registered nurses (Institute of Medicine [IOM], 2010). The Pew Commission on Health Professionals has identified 21 professional competencies needed for professional nursing practice in the 21st century. These competencies are referenced in Box 1.1.

In 2012, the IOM (2012) charged professional nursing to take a leadership role in shaping a transformed health care system. Effective communication links with the competencies identified in Box 1.1 to make this goal possible.

NURSING: A PRACTICE DISCIPLINE

Professional nursing represents a practice discipline. Donaldson and Crowley (1978) characterized the nursing discipline as having a specialized perspective related to

"Principles and laws that govern the life processes, well-being, and optimum functioning of human beings, sick or well;

Patterning of human behavior in interaction with the environment in critical life situations; and

Processes by which positive changes in health status are affected". (p. 113)

Priority areas for national action, and a visible inclusion of a proactive preventive care and chronic-care focus in contemporary health care represent a broader, proactive approach to safe, quality health care (Fig. 1.2).

Professional nursing practice incorporates empirical concepts from the natural and biological sciences, while drawing from the social sciences of psychology, phenomenology, and sociology (McEwen & Wills, 2014). Contemporary nurses are expected to integrate evidence-based care

---

BOX 1.1   Pew Commission's Recommendations to Nursing Programs: 21 Nursing Competencies Needed for the Twenty-First Century

- Embrace a personal ethic of social responsibility and service.
- Exhibit ethical behavior in all professional activities.
- Provide evidence-based, clinically competent care.
- Incorporate the multiple determinants of health in clinical care.
- Apply knowledge of the new sciences.
- Demonstrate critical thinking, reflection, and problem-solving skills.
- Understand the role of primary care.
- Rigorously practice preventive health care.
- Integrate population-based care and services into practice.
- Improve access to health care for those with unmet health needs.
- Practice relationship-centered care with individuals and families.
- Provide culturally sensitive care to a diverse society.
- Partner with communities in health care decisions.
- Use communication and information technology effectively and appropriately.
- Work in interdisciplinary teams.
- Ensure care that balances individual, professional, system, and societal needs.
- Practice leadership.
- Take responsibility for quality of care and health outcomes at all levels.
- Contribute to continuous improvement of the health care system.
- Advocate for public policy that promotes and protects the health of the public.
- Continue to learn and help others learn.

From Bellack, J., & O'Neil, E. (2000). Recreating nursing practice for a new century: Recommendations and implications of the Pew Health Professions Commission's final report, *Nursing and Health Care Perspectives,* 21(1), 20.

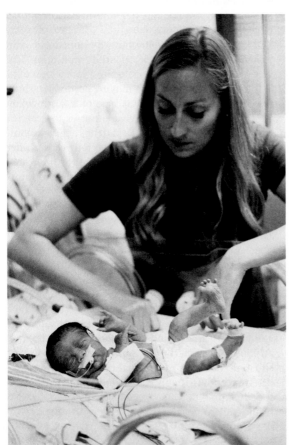

Fig. 1.2 Nurses care for patients and families at their most vulnerable in health situations. (Copyright © Yobro10/iStock/Thinkstock.)

principles into practice assessments, and to base their clinical judgments and care decisions on them (Epstein & Street, 2011; Smith & McCarthy, 2010). Professional nursing combines specialized knowledge and skills with prudent clinical judgment to meet patient, family, and community health care needs. Finkelman and Kenner (2009) differentiate between the science and art of nursing, stating that "**knowledge** represents the science of nursing, and **caring** represents the art of nursing" (p. 54). Both are needed to support the safety and quality of skilled care.

ART OF NURSING

Carnago and Mast (2015) argue that the use of factual data without a fuller knowledge and understanding of each individual patient situation can lead to lower safety and quality than perceiving the encounter as a whole. Professional nursing and health care practices are grounded in human interactions and relationships. The "art of nursing" references a blending of each nurse's intuitive thinking processes about the nature of health incident from the patient's perspective. The nurse's focus is on developing an individualized understanding of each patient as a unique human being. Perceptions are influenced by the nurse's life knowledge and professional experiences with other patients. Using this data takes into account the interactive factors that nurses must consider in order to blend their knowledge and skills with scientific understandings to provide safe, quality care.

Exercise 1.2, What Is Professional Nursing?, can help you look at your philosophy of nursing.

EXERCISE 1.2   What Is Professional Nursing?

Purpose

To help students develop an understanding of professional nursing.

Procedure

1. Interview a professional nurse who has been in practice for more than 12 months. Ask for descriptions of what he or she considers professional nursing to be today, in what ways he or she thinks nurses make a difference, and how the nurse feels the role might evolve within the next 10 years.
2. In small groups of three to five students, discuss and compare your findings.
3. Develop a group definition of professional nursing.

Reflective Discussion Analysis

1. What does nursing mean to you?
2. In what ways, if any, have your ideas about nursing changed now that you are actively involved in patient care as a nurse?
3. Is your understanding of nursing different from those of the nurse(s) you interviewed?
4. As a new nurse, how would you want to present yourself?

WAYS (PATTERNS OF KNOWING) IN NURSING

Nurses use "patterns of knowing" to bridge the interpersonal space between scientific understandings and patient-centered health experiences. It is this dimension of knowledge that helps nurses to individualize nursing and interprofessional care strategies (Zander, 2007). In a seminal work, Carper (1978) described *four patterns of knowing* embedded in nursing practice: empirical, personal, aesthetic, and ethical. Although described as individual patterns of knowing, in practice, nurses use these patterns as an integrated form of knowing about the patient. The patterns (ways) of knowing consist of:

- *Empirical ways of knowing:* knowledge that draws upon verifiable data from science. The process of empirical ways of knowing includes incorporating logical reasoning and problem solving. Nurses use empirical ways of knowing to provide scientific rationales when choosing and supporting appropriate nursing interventions. An evidenced-based research discussion or study is included related to the content of each chapter.
- *Personal ways of knowing:* knowledge that is "characterized as subjective, concrete, and existential" (Carper, 1978, p. 251). Personal knowing is relational. This pattern of knowing occurs when nurses connect with the "humanness" of a patient experience. Leenerts (2003) calls personal knowledge "a precondition for establishing a therapeutic relationship" (p. 158). Personal knowledge develops when nurses intuitively understand and connect with patients as unique human beings—because they share the experience of being human. Self-awareness allows nurses to self-check any biases that might prevent the development of an authentic personal connection with a patient, as well as to empathetically understand what is happening. Nurses may not always be able to define why they intuitively believe something is true, but they trust this knowledge. Because nurses learn to develop experiential knowledge of their own responses in previous clinical situations, this way of knowing can provide a better interpretation of difficult health situations.
- *Aesthetic ways of knowing* link the humanistic components of care with their scientific application. This way of knowing represents a deeper appreciation of the whole person or situation, a moving beyond the superficial to see the experience as part of a larger whole. Aesthetic ways of knowing enable nurses to experientially relate to the fear behind a patient's angry response, the courage of a patient with stage four cancer offering her suffering up for her classmates, or the pain of a father cutting off funds for a drug addicted son. By including aesthetic ways of knowing, the unseen parts of the story, allow everyone, including the patient, to learn new information.
- *Ethical ways of knowing* refer to principled care, which nurses experience when they confront the moral aspects of nursing care (Porter et al., 2011). Ethical ways of knowing refer to knowledge of what is right and wrong, attention to professional standards and codes in making moral choices, taking responsibility for one's actions, and protecting patient autonomy and rights. Carnago and Mast (2015) note, "To make an *ethical* decision, the nurse must consider the clinical situation, be aware of personal beliefs and values, and determine how to apply ethical and moral principles to the situation" (p. 389).

Chinn and Kramer (2015) recently introduced a **fifth pattern, Emancipatory ways of knowing.**

EXERCISE 1.3   Patterns of Knowing in Clinical Practice

Purpose

To help students understand how patterns of knowing can be used effectively in clinical practice.

Procedure

1. Break into smaller groups of three to four students. Identify a scribe for each student group.
2. Using the following case study, decide how you would use empirical, personal, ethical, and aesthetic patterns of knowing to see that Mrs. Jackson's holistic needs were addressed in the next 48 hours.

Case Study

Mrs. Jackson, an 86-year-old widow, was admitted to the hospital with a hip fracture. She has very poor eyesight because of macular degeneration and takes eye drops for the condition. Her husband died 5 years ago, and she subsequently moved into an assisted housing development. She had to give up driving because of her eyesight and

sold her car to another resident 5 months ago. Although her daughter lives in the area, Mrs. Jackson has little contact with her. This distresses her greatly, as she describes being very close with her until 8 years ago. She feels safe in her new environment but complains that she is very lonely and is not interested in joining activities. She has a male friend in the complex, but recently he has been showing less interest. Her surgery is scheduled for tomorrow, but she has not yet signed her consent form. She does not have advance directives.

Reflective Analysis Discussion

1. In a large group, have each student share their findings.
2. For each pattern of knowing, write the suggestions on the board.
3. Compare and contrast the findings of the different groups.
4. Discuss how the patterns of knowing add to an understanding of the patient in this case study.

- *Emancipatory ways of knowing:* Emancipatory ways of knowing include awareness of social problems and social justice issues as contributory determinants of health disparities. This pattern of knowing expands and supports the emergent goals of *Healthy People 2020*, with its focus on social determinants as a context for health care concerns. With improved knowledge of social, political, and economic determinants of health and well-being, nurses can serve as better advocates in helping patients individually, and the nation collectively, to identify and reduce the inequities in health care.

Exercise 1.3, Patterns of Knowing in Clinical Practice, provides practice with using patterns or ways of knowing in clinical practice.

CARING AS A CORE VALUE OF PROFESSIONAL NURSING

Caring is considered an *essential* functional construct in professional nursing practice, which defines the patient-centered relationship. Caring is an essential element in the development of interpersonal relationships in clinical settings (Wagner & Whaite, 2010). Think about your most important relationship in health care. What made it meaningful to you?

Exercise 1.4, A Caring Encounter.

Caring is the component of nursing care best remembered by patients, families, and nurses. Acts of caring are basically acts of kindness. Caring strengthens patient-centered knowledge and adds depth to other nursing competencies that nurses bring to the clinical situation (Rhodes, Morris, & Lazenby, 2011).

Professional caring is about the involvement of the nurse and patient in the encounter, and its meaning to the people involved. "Caring does not involve specific tasks. Instead it involves the creation of a sustained relationship with the other" (Crowe, 2000, p. 966). There are many forms of caring in clinical practice, some visible, others private and personal, known only to the persons experiencing feeling cared for. In a qualitative study, when graduate student nurses were asked to describe a professional caring incident in their practice, they identified the attributes of caring as (a) giving of self, (b) involved presence, (c) intuitive knowing and empathy, (d) supporting the patient's integrity, and (e) professional competence (Arnold, 1997).

FUNCTIONS OF COMMUNICATION IN HEALTH CARE SYSTEMS

More than any other variable, effective interpersonal communication supports the safety and quality in health care delivery (see Chapter 2).

EXERCISE 1.4 Comparing Linear and Transactional Models of Communication

Purpose

To help students see the difference between linear and circular models of communication.

Procedure

1. Role-play a scenario in which one person provides a scene that might occur in the clinical area using a linear model: sender, message, and receiver.
2. Role-play the same scenario using a circular model, framing questions that recognize the context of the message and its potential impact on the receiver, and provide feedback.

Discussion

1. Was there a difference in your level of comfort? If so, in what ways?
2. Was there any difference in the amount of information you had as a result of the communication? If so, in what ways?
3. What implications does this exercise have for your future nursing practice?

Definition

The term *communication* derives from the Latin, "communicare" meaning "to share" (Dima, Teodorescu, & Gifu, 2014). Communication connects people and ideas through words, nonverbal behaviors, and actions. People communicate as a key means to share information, ask questions, and to seek assistance. Words are used to persuade others, to take a position, and to create an understandable story. In fact, "communication represents the very essence of the human condition" (Hargie, 2011, p. 2). Human communication is unique. Only human beings have complex vocabularies and are capable of learning and using multiple language symbols to convey meaning.

Communication between health care providers and patients impacts the way care is delivered; it is as important as the care itself. Outcomes of effective interpersonal communication in health care relate to higher patient satisfaction and productive health changes. Patients are more likely to understand their health conditions through meaningful communication and to alert providers when something isn't working. Other specific ways interpersonal health communication impacts service quality is through:

- development of a workable treatment partnership;
- more effective diagnosis and earlier recognition of health changes;
- better understanding of the patient's condition;
- personalized compliance with therapeutic regimes;
- more efficient utilization of health services; and
- stronger, longer lasting positive outcomes.

Two-way communication provides the opportunity to share information, to be heard, and to be validated. Having the opportunity to provide input empowers patients and families to take a stronger position in contributing to their health care. The two communication models used most frequently are referred to as linear and transactional models (see Chapter 5 for details).

The **linear model** is the simplest communication model, consisting of sender, message, receiver, channels of communication, and context. Linear models focus only on the sending and receipt of messages, and do not necessarily consider communication as enabling the development of co-created meanings. They are useful in emergency health situations when time is of the essence to get immediate information.

Transactional models of communication are more complex. These models define interpersonal communication as a reciprocal interaction in which both sender and receiver influence each other's messages and responses as they converse. Each communicator constructs a mental picture of the other during the conversation, including perceptions about the other's attitude and potential reactions to the message. Previous experiences and exposure to concepts and ideas heighten recognition, and will influence the interpretation of the message. The outcome of transactional models represents a co-created set of collaborative meanings developed during the conversation. Exercise 1.4 provides a simulated exercise to demonstrate the difference between linear and transactional models of communication (Fig. 1.5).

Transactional models employ systems concepts. A human system (patient/patient/family and provider) receives information from the environment (*input*), internally processes it, and interprets its meaning (*throughput*). The result is new information or behavior (*output*). *Feedback loops* (from the receiver or the environment) provide information about the output as it relates to the data received and/or acted upon. Feedback either validates the received data or reflects a need to correct/modify its original input information. Thus transactional models draw attention to communication as having purpose and meaning-making attributes. Fig. 1.3 displays the process elements of transactional models.

EVIDENCE-BASED NURSING PRACTICE Evidence-based professional nursing practice serves as a critical foundation for nursing praxis, education, and research. The ICN (2014) defines *evidence-based nursing practice* as "a problem-solving approach to clinical decision making that incorporates a search for the best and latest evidence, clinical expertise and assessment, *and* patient preference values."

Integrating individual clinical expertise and judgment with objective evidence and collaborative interprofessional consultations is recognized as being critical to safe, quality professional nursing care. "It is a way of practicing owned by all nurses" (Taylor, Priefer, & Alt-White, 2016, p. 576). Fueled by professional communication, a strong evidence base represents a blending of the nurse's expertise with research findings and best practices guidelines. Nurses partner with patients to merge this data with patient preferences, value beliefs, and personal capacity to cope into jointly constructed action plans to resolve health issues. Ideally, professional nurses integrate their professional clinical expertise with "patterns of knowing" about their patients to customize research-based findings and clinical guidelines in providing skilled, patient-centered care. Sackett et al. (1996) makes the point: "External clinical evidence can inform, but can never replace, individual clinical expertise, and it is this expertise that decides whether the external evidence applies to the individual patient at all and, if so, how it should be integrated into the clinical decision" (p. 72). At the end of each chapter, we have included an evidence-based research study or suggestions for evidenced-based research to emphasize important praxis/research connections with each chapter's content.

Systems Theory Foundations

The WHO (2007) defines *a health care system* as "all organizations, people and actions whose primary intent is to promote, restore or maintain health" (p. 2). Systems theory provides a foundation for understanding the quality and safety of health care. It supports competency education for Nurses (quality and safety education for nurses (QSEN)) competencies (AACN, 2009), which is the central focus of Chapter 4, and is found in chapters throughout the text. The *knowledge, skills, and attitudes* (KSA) associated with QSEN competency-based nursing education build on evidence-based nursing practice information in both concepts and applications (Crownweldt, 2007).

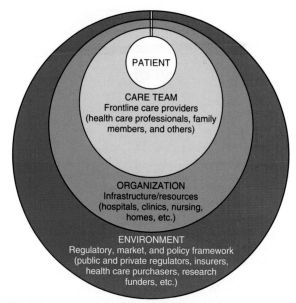

Fig. 1.3 Conceptual drawing of a four-level health care system, with the client (patient) as its core concept. (From National Academy of Engineering, Institute of Medicine, Committee on Engineering and the Health Care System; Reid, P. P., Compton, W. D., Grossman, J. H., et al. (eds). (2005). Building a better delivery system: a new engineering/health care partnership (p. 20). Washington, DC: National Academies Press. Retrieved from http://www.nap.edu/catalog/11378.html.)

Systems theory focuses on the interrelationships existing within a given system. It is a fundamental contributor to understanding the functional communication occurring within larger professional health organizations. Care transition guidelines and technology applications also reflect a systems approach to health care across clinical settings (Porter-O'Grady & Malloch, 2015; WHO, 2010). Systems' thinking is essential to understanding interprofessional team collaboration in health care (Clark, 2016; Dolansky & Moore, 2013).

Patients are considered essential team members in an interprofessional collaborative health care relationship. They are considered experts about the meaning of their presenting symptoms and illness course within a personalized life context. Team power and responsibility for care is shared with patients, with the patient holding the final say in all decisions (Mead & Bower, 2000).

Systems thinking helps you as a health professional understand *how* the interrelationships among different parts of your health care system contribute to its overall functioning at macro and micro levels. At a macro level, systems thinking reminds nurses to see how changes in one aspect of care provision can produce unexpected consequences for others in

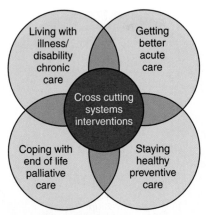

Fig. 1.4 Priority Areas for National Action. Four stages of life and health are described in the four circles, connected by the need for coordination across time and health care. (From Committee on Identifying Areas for Quality Improvement, Board on Health Care Services, Institute of Medicine; Adams, K., Corrigan, J. M. (eds.) (2003). *Priority areas for national action: Transforming health care quality. Washington, DC: National* Academies Press.)

the system. Systems thinking allows nurses to examine individual health care issues, and to consider how they link to larger health system care outcomes and national benchmarks. Health care systems represent integrated wholes, whose properties cannot be effectively reduced to a single unit (Porter-O'Grady & Malloch, 2015). These interacting parts work together to achieve important goals Fig. 1.4. Only by looking at the whole system can one fully appreciate its meaning of how its individual parts work together (Table 1.1).

Case Application

"Systems thinking moves a nurse from individualized care, turning a patient from side to side to avoid decubiti, to monitoring the pressure ulcer rate on the unit and comparing the unit rate to national benchmarks" (Phillips, Stalter, Dolansky, & Lopez, 2016, p. 16).

Interprofessional Education and Practice

The IOM Report (2010) advocates health team collaborative care as a key means of delivering patient-centered care delivery, particularly for management of chronic illness (Farrell, Payne, & Heye, 2015). A systems perspective can greatly enhance clinically team-based relational communication. Each health discipline has different training, agendas, and priorities, which must be integrated to achieve coordinated optimal health outcomes. Even professional vocabulary meanings can have various meanings among the different disciplines (Table 1.2). Principles of team-based health care include:

- Sharing goals
- Clear roles
- Mutual trust
- Effective communication
- Measurable processes and outcomes (IOM, 2012, p. 6)

How health providers use collaborative and networking skills to achieve clinical outcomes become a measure of systems-based team competence. According to Clark (2016), "the concept of TeamSTEPPS ... captures the full scope of systems thinking" (p. 87) (see Chapter 22).

DEVELOPING AN EVIDENCE-BASED PRACTICE

Background: This research article makes the case for greater integration and new pathways between big data science initiatives, and nursing as a means to improve patient care. "Big data is described as data of significant magnitude and level of imprecision that extends beyond traditional inquiry." Nurses can offer new opportunities by defining important questions and extending data sources from their practice experiences, applying data mining and modeling methods and addressing ethical, legal, and social implications (p. 48). These data offer a mapping of hidden insights and new knowledge that can be more fully accessed through big data methodologies.

Using Big Data to Inform Practice: This article highlights the need for big data initiatives and emerging exemplars to better inform nursing practice. An expanded body of data-driven information found in emerging big data initiatives provides a broader context for providing individualized care for patients.

Application to Your Clinical Practice: Big data enhances nursing's scientific potential in understanding the validity of, and designing tailored interventional strategies. See also Johns Hopkins Data Scientist Toolbox: https://www.coursera.org/course/datascitoolbox.

Brennan, P., & Bakken, S. (2015). Nursing needs big data and big data needs nursing. *Journal of Nursing Scholarship, 47*(5), 477–484.

APPLICATIONS

Paradigm Shifts in Health Care Delivery

For the purposes of this introductory chapter, we highlight some of the major paradigm shifts in health care applications that impact care delivery. Health care delivery has "moved from a 'one-professional: one patient' care model to a 'many professionals: one patient' model" (Baltaden et al., 2006, p. 549). The contemporary practice of health care is system based, with the locus of control for decision-making and clinical management of symptoms team shared with the patient and

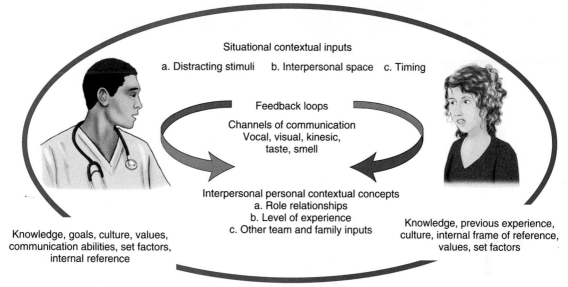

Fig. 1.5 Transactional model of communication.

TABLE 1.1	Criteria for Survival of the Nursing Profession Based on Evolutionary Principles
Criteria or Condition	**Evolutionary Principle**
Nursing needs to be relevant.	In nature, an organism will survive only if it occupies a niche, that is, performs a specific role that is needed in its environment.
Nursing must be accountable.	In every environment, there is a limited amount of resources. Organisms that are more efficient and use the available resources more effectively are much more likely to be selected by the environment.
Nursing needs to retain its uniqueness while functioning in a multidisciplinary setting.	In nature, an organism will survive only if it is unique. If it ceases to be so, it is in danger of losing its niche or role in the environment. In other words, it might lose out if the new species is slightly better adapted to the role, or if physically similar enough, it might even breed with that species and thus completely lose its identity. Successful organisms must also learn to coexist with many different species so that their role complements that of the other organisms.
Nursing needs to be visible.	In nature, organisms often are required to defend their niche and their territory usually by an outward display that allows other similar species to be aware of their presence. By being "visible," similar species can avoid direct conflict. In addition, visibility is also important for recognition by members of their own species, to allow for the formation of family and social units, based on cooperation and respect.
Nursing needs to have a global impact.	In nature, if a species is to survive, it must make its presence felt not just to its immediate neighbors but to all the members of its environment. Often, this results in a species adapting a unique presence, whether it is a color pattern, smell, or sound.
Nurses need to be innovators.	In evolution, the organisms that survive are, more often than not, innovators that have the flexibility to come up with new and different solutions to rapid changes in environmental conditions.
Nurses need to be both exceptionally competent and strive for excellence.	During evolution, when new niches open up, it is never possible for more than one species to occupy one niche. Only the best adapted and most competent among the competing organisms will survive; all others, even if only slightly less competent, will die.

From Bell (1997) as cited in Gottlieb, L. N., Gottlieb, B. (1998). Evolutionary principles can guide nursing's future development, *Journal of Advanced Nursing, 28*(5), 1099.

TABLE 1.2   National Reports With Goals, Relevant to Nursing's Role in the Transformation of the Health Care System

Institute of Medicine Report	Identified Goals
2000: *To err is human: building a safer health system*	• Establish a national focus to enhance knowledge base of safety. • Develop a public mandatory reporting system to identify and learn from errors. • Implement safety systems to ensure safe practices at the delivery level. • Raise performance standards and expectations for safety improvement.
2003: *Health professions education: a bridge to quality*	Competency in: • Delivering patient-centered care, • Working as part of interdisciplinary teams, • Practicing evidence-based medicine, • Focusing on quality improvement, and • Using information technology.
2009: *Redesigning continuing education in the health professions*	• Bring together health professionals from different disciplines in tailored learning environments. • Replace the current culture of continuing education (CE) with a new vision of professional development. • Establish a national interprofessional CE institute to foster improvements.
2010: *The future of nursing: leading change, advancing health*	• Practice at the full extent of their education and training. • Achievement of higher levels of education and training through an improved education system that promotes seamless academic progression. • Full partnership with physicians and other health professionals in redesigning health care in the United States. • Better data collection and improved information infrastructure regarding workforce planning and policy making. • Remove scope of practice barriers.
2010: *Healthy People 2020* (www.healthypeople.gov)	1. Attain high-quality, longer lives free of preventable disease, disability, injury, and premature death. 2. Achieve health equity, eliminate disparities, and improve the health of all groups. 3. Create social and physical environments that promote good health for all. 4. Promote quality of life, healthy development, and healthy behaviors across all life stages.

Data from Institute of Medicine (IOM). (2000). *To err is human: Building a safer health system*. Washington, DC: National Academies Press; IOM. (2003). *Health professions education: A bridge to quality*. Washington, DC: National Academies Press; IOM. (2009). *Redesigning continuing education in the health professions*. Washington, DC: National Academies Press; IOM. (2010). *The future of nursing: Leading change, advancing health*. Washington, DC: National Academies Press; IOM. (2012). The future of nursing: Accomplishments a year after the landmark report (editorial), *Journal of Nursing Scholarship, 44*(1), 1.

other members of the health care team (Frist, 2005). Health care thus becomes a *shared* reality. Recognizing the health care team as a microsystem composed of skilled interdependent team members, each representing a relevant discipline involved in the patient's care, creates a different work design.

Care processes are conceptualized as participatory management applications of self-management strategies aimed at controlling the symptoms of chronic disorders. At the center of this care paradigm is the patient. Instead of caring *for* their patients, nurses are charged with working *with* their patients

to develop and implement action plans that acknowledge the reality of the patient's health condition, while working to achieve desired clinical outcomes and personal well-being, everyone—healthcare professionals, patients and their families, researchers, payers, planners and educators—to make the changes that will lead to better patient outcomes (Baltaden and Davidoff, 2007, p. 2) Specific communication and interprofessional collaborative concepts related to community based continuity of care initiatives will be presented throughout subsequent chapters in this text.

Management of chronic health problems is linked to, but it is characteristically different from, care delivery for acute health problems. People with chronic health conditions will experience acute health episodes requiring prompt critical treatment. But many chronic problems are preventable, controllable, or resolvable with proactive health-promotion actions, and self-managed disease-prevention strategies. This paradigm shift "from an emphasis on individual disease conditions to population-level disease prevention and wellness promotion" reflects the reality of contemporary health care demands, including the multiple causes of illness and socioeconomic factors (Fawcett & Ellenbecker, 2015, p. 289).

Core components of today's health care system include an activated patient and the dual concepts of patient centeredness and patient empowerment. This broader shift in orientation has been strengthened through a decade of IOM reports calling for a transformed health care system, in which care is patient driven, and delivered within an interprofessional collaborative care framework.

In 2010, the IOM report on The Future of Nursing: Leading Change, Advancing Health, affirmed that "…nurses have great potential to lead innovative strategies" to improve health care (IOM, 2010, p. 4). This document states that:
- Nurses should practice to the full extent of their education and training.
- Nurses should achieve higher levels of education and training, through an improved education system that promotes seamless academic profession.
- Nurses should be full partners with physicians and other health professionals, in redesigning health care in the United States. (IOM, 2010).

The IOM Report (2010) states that "contemporary health care systems should focus on team collaboration". It is described as the most efficient means to deliver accessible, high-quality, patient-centered health care that addresses wellness and prevention of illness and adverse events, self-management of chronic illness, and interdependent clinical applications. *Interdependence* is a key element in a systems approach which underscores the ways in which various components interact with each other (Frenk et al., 2010, p. 1924). As providers from different professional health disciplines share responsibility with each other and selected patients, within and across clinical settings, the potential for fragmented or duplicative care is effectively diminished. Interprofessional collaboration is essential to the implementation of safe, quality care in a transformed health care system.

Summary

This chapter traces the development of nursing and health communication as a basic foundation for understanding concepts presented in later chapters. It identifies core concepts of nursing's metaparadigm, and discusses ways and patterns of knowing through which nurses integrate and apply relational knowledge to benefit patients and families in clinical settings.

The chapter discusses two evidence-based models of communication: linear and transactional. The process of communication is analyzed, and the contributions of communication theory to the study of developmental theories used by nurses as presented in this chapter helps nurses integrate scientific understandings with a personalized approach to individual patients.

Nursing is recognized as a critical professional body needed to transform the health care system according to the IOM's (2001) vision of a "high performance, patient centered health care system." A tidal wave of current and projected changes in the health care system creates the need for nurses to clearly "own" the essence of their discipline and to redefine their professional nursing role responsibilities embedded within a collaborative interprofessional patient-centered health care system. Contemporary professionalism supports team-based processes of multiple professions working together with cross-disciplinary responsibilities and accountability for achieving improved clinical outcomes (IOM, 2014).

ETHICAL DILEMMA

What Would You Do?

Craig Montegue is a difficult patient to care for. As his nurse, you find his constant arguments, poor hygiene, and the way he treats his family very upsetting. It is difficult for you to provide him with anything but the most basic care, and you just want to leave his room as quickly as possible. How could you use a patient-centered approach to understanding Craig? What are the ethical elements in this situation, and how would you address them in implementing care for Craig?

DISCUSSION QUESTIONS

1. In what specific ways is your nursing practice influenced by Carper's ways of knowing?
2. In what ways would you envision your leadership as a nurse being as important as your technical ability to deliver safe, quality care at the bedside?
3. How would you describe your role responsibilities as a nurse representative on an interprofessional care team?
4. What do you see as the major challenges faced by professional nurses today?

REFERENCES

AACN: The Essentials of Baccalaureate Education for Professional Nursing Practice, 2009. Retrieved from http://www.aacn.nche.edu/educationresources/BaccEssential-s08.pdf (Accessed 20.10.08).

Alligood, M. (2014). *Nursing Theory: Utilization and Application* (ed 5). Maryland Heights, MO: Mosby Elsevier.

American Nurses Association. (2015). *Scope and Standards of Nursing* (ed 3). Silver Spring, MD: American Nurses Association.

Arnold, E. (1997). Caring from the graduate student perspective. *International Journal for Human Caring, 1*(3), 32–42.

Baltaden, P., Ogrinc, G., & Bataldan, M. (2006). From one to many. *Journal of Interprofessional Care, 20*(5), 549–551.

Black, B. (2017). *Professional Nursing: Concepts and Challenges* (8th ed.). St. Louis, MO: Elsevier.

Carnago, L., & Mast, M. (2015). Using ways of knowing to guide emergencyo nursing practice. *Journal of Emergency Nursing, 41,* 387–390.

Carper, B. (1978). Fundamental patterns of knowing in nursing. *ANS. Advances in Nursing Science, 1,* 13–23.

Chinn, P., & Kramer, M. (2015). *Knowledge Development in Nursing: Theory and Process* (ed 9). St. Louis, MO: Mosby.

Clark, K. (2016). Systems thinking IPE/IPP, Team STEPPS and communicating: Are they interconnected? A look with a broad brush. *Nursing and Palliative Care, 1*(4), 85–88.

Coleman, K., Austin, B., Brach, C., & Wagner, E. (2009). Evidence on the chronic care model in the New Millenium. *Health Affairs, 28*(1), 75–85.

Cox, M., & Naylor, M. (Eds.). (2013). *Transforming patient care: aligning interprofessional education with clinical practice redesign. Proceedings of a conference sponsored by the Josiah Macy Jr. Foundation in January 2013.* New York: Josiah Macy Foundation.

Crownweldt, L., Sherwood, G., Barnsteiner, J., Disch, J., Johnson, J., et al. (2007). Quality and safety education for nurses. *Nursing Outlook, 55*(3), 122–131.

D'Amour, D., Ferrada-Videla, M., Rodriguez, L., & Beaulieu, M. (2005). The conceptual basis for interprofessional collaboration: Care concepts and theoretical frameworks. *Journal of Interprofessional Care, Supp. 1,* 116–131.

Dima, I. C., Teodorescu, M., & Gifu, D. (2014). New communication approaches vs. traditional communication. *International Letters of Social and Humanistic Sciences, 20,* 46–55.

Dolansky, M. A., & Moore, S. M. (2013). (September 30, 2013) "Quality and safety education for nurses (QSEN): The key is systems thinking". *Online Journal of Issues in Nursing, 18*(3).

Donaldson, S. K., & Crowley, D. M. (1978). The discipline of nursing. *Nursing Outlook, 26,* 113–120.

Egenes, K. (2017). History of nursing. In G. Roux, & J. Halstead (Eds.), *Issues and trends in nursing: Essential knowledge for today and tomorrow.* Sudbury, MA: Jones and Bartlett.

Epstein, R., & Street, R. (2011). The values and value of patient-centered care. *Annals of Family Medicine, 9*(2), 100–103.

Farrell, E., Payne, C., & Heye, M. (2015). Integrating interprofessional collaboration skills into the advanced practice registered socialization process. *Journal of Professional Nursing, 31,* 5–10.

Fawcett, J., & Ellenbecker, C. H. (2015). A proposed conceptual model of nursing and population health. *Nursing Outlook, 63*(3), 288–298.

Finkelman, A. W., & Kenner, C. (2009). *Teaching the IOM: Implications of the IOM Reports for Nursing Education.* Silver Spring, MD: American Nurses Association.

Frenk, J., Chen, L., Bhuta, Z., et al. (2010). Health professionals for a new century: Transforming education to strengthen health care systems. *Lancet, 376,* 1923–1958.

Frist, W. (2005). Health care in the 21st century. *The New England Journal of Medicine, 352,* 267–272.

Hargie, O. (2011). *Routledge. Skilled interpersonal communication: Research, theory and practice* (5th ed). New York: NY.

Institute of Medicine (IOM). (2001). *Crossing the Quality Chasm: A New Health System for the 21st Century.* Washington, D.C: National Academies Press.

Institute of Medicine (IOM). (2010). *The Future of Nursing: Leading Change, Advancing Health.* Washington, DC: National Academies Press.

Institute of Medicine (IOM). (2014). *Dying in America.*

Institute of Medicine (IOM). (2012). The future of nursing: Accomplishments a year after the landmark report (Editorial). *Journal of Nursing Scholarship, 44*(1), 1.

International Council of Nurses (ICN): *Definition of nursing.* Retrieved from http://www.icn.ch/about-icn/icn-definition-of-nursing/ (Accessed 30.06.14).

Jarrin, O. (2012). The integrality of situated caring. *Advances in Nursing Science, 35*(1), 14–24.

Karnick, P. (2013). The importance of defining theory in nursing: Is there a common denominator? *Nurs Science Q, 26*(1), 29–30.

Leenerts, M. H. (2003). Teaching personal knowledge as a way of knowing self in therapeutic relationship. *Nursing Outlook, 51*(4), 158–164.

Marrs, J., & Lowry, L. (2006). Nursing theory and practice: Connecting the dots. *Nursing Science Quarterly, 19*(1), 44–50.

Masters, K. (2015). *Nursing Theories: A framework for Professional Nursing* (ed 2). Burlingon MA: Jones and Bartlett Nursing.

McEwen, M., & Wills, E. (2014). *Theoretical Basis for Nursing* (ed 4). Philadelphia: Wolters Kluwer Health/Lippincott Williams & Wilkins.

Mead, N., & Bower, P. (2000). Patient-centredness: A conceptual framework and review of the empirical literature. *Social Science & Medicine, 51,* 1087–1110.

Mount, B., Boston, P., & Cohen, R. (2007). Healing connections: On moving from suffering to a sense of well-being. *Journal of Pain and Symptom Management, 33*(4), 372–388.

Nightingale, F. (1859). In Victor Skretkowicz (Ed.), *Commemorative edition notes on nursing, with historical commentary.* New York: Springer Publishing Company.

Nordstrom, K., Coff, C., Jonson, H., et al. (2013). Food and health: Individual, cultural, or scientific. *Genes & Nutrition, 8,* 857–863.

Phillips, J., Stalter, A., Dolansky, M., & Lopez, G. (2016). Fostering future leadership in quality and safety in health care through systems thinking. *Journal of Professional Nursing, 32*, 15–24.

Porter, S., O'Halloran, P., & Morrow, E. (2011). Bringing values back into evidenced based nursing: Role of patients in resisting empiricism. *ANS. Advances in Nursing Science, 34*(2), 106–118.

Porter-O'Grady, T., & Malloch, K. (2015). *Quantum Leadership Building Better Partnerships for Sustainable Health* (ed 4). Burlington MA: Jones & Bartlett Learning.

Reed, P., & Shearer, N. (2007). *Perspectives on Nursing Theory*. Philadelphia: Lippincott.

Rhodes, M., Morris, A., & Lazenby, R. (2011). Nursing at its best: Competent and caring. *Online Journal of Issues in Nursing, 16*(2), 10.

Sackett, D., Rosenberg, W., Gray, J., Haynes, R., & Richardson, W. (1996). Evidenced based medicine: What it is and what it isn't. *British Medical Journal, 312*(7023), 71–72.

Schiavo, R. (2014). *Health Communication: From Theory to Practice* (ed 2). San Francisco, CA: Jossey-Bass.

Shaller D: *Patient-Centered Care: What does it Take? 2007*, The Commonwealth Fund. Retrieved from http://www.commonwealthfund.org/publications/fund-reports/2007/oct/patient-centered-care--what-does-it-take (Accessed 18.12.16).

Smith, M., & McCarthy, M. P. (2010). Disciplinary knowledge in nursing education: Going beyond the blueprints. *Nursing Outlook, 58*, 44–51.

Taylor, M., Priefer, B., & Alt-White, A. (2016). Evidence-based practice: Embracing integration. *Nursing Outlook. (64)*, 275–282.

Wagner, D., & Whaite, B. (2010). An exploration of the nature of caring relationships in the writings of florence Nightingale. *Journal of Holistic Nursing, 4*, 225–234.

Ward, B., Shillier, J., & Goodman, R. (2015). Multiple chronic conditions among US adults: a 2012 update. *Preventing Chronic Disease, 11*, E62.

WHO (World Health Organization). (2001). *Mental Health, New Understanding, New Hope*. Geneva, Switzerland.

WHO. (2007). *A safer future: global public health security in the 21st century*. Geneva, Switzerland.

Zander, P. (2007). Ways of knowing in nursing: The historical evolution of a concept. *Journal of Theory Construction & Testing, 11*(1), 7–11.

Zolnierek, C. (2013). An integrative review of knowing the patient. *Journal of Nursing Scholarship, 46*(1), 3–10.

SUGGESTED READING

Batalden, P., & Davidoff, F. (2007). What is "quality improvement" and how can it transform health care. *Quality and Safety in Health Care, 16*(1), 2–3.

Bronstein, L. R. (2003). A model for interdisciplinary collaboration. *Social Work, 48*, 297–306.

Cherry, B., & Jacob, S. (2017). *Contemporary Nursing: Issues, Trends & Management* (ed 7). St. Louis, MO: Elsevier.

Clancy, T., Effken, J., & Pesut, D. (2008). Applications of complex systems theory in nursing education, research, and practice. *Nursing Outlook, 56*, 248–256.

Drenkard K: Patient centered care: QSEN competency definition. Retrieved from www.aacn.nche.edu/qsen/workshop -details/naples/KDPCC.pdf (Accessed 29.01.14).

Greene, S., Tuzzio, l, & Cherkin, D. (2012). A framework for making patient-centered care front and center. *The Permanente Journal, 16*(3), 49–53.

Huber, M., Knotterus, J. A., Green, L., et al. (2011). How should we define health? *BMJ: British Medical Journal, 343*, d4163.

Interprofessional Education Collaborative Expert Panel. (2011). *Core Competencies for Interprofessional Collaborative Practice: Report of an Expert Panel*. Washington, D.C: Interprofessional Education Collaborative.

Kirschenbaum, H., & Rogers, C. R. (2015). (ed 2). *(1902-87) International encyclopedia of the social and behavioral sciences* (vol. 20). . https://doi.org/1016/B978-0-08-097086.61113-3.

Kilgore, R., & Langford, R. (2010). Defragmenting care: Testing an intervention to increase the effectiveness of interdisciplinary health care teams. *Critical Care Nursing Clinics of North America, 22*, 271–278.

Lim, C., Berry, A., Hirsch, T., et al. (2016). "It just seems outside my health" How patients with chronic conditions perceive communication boundaries with providers. *Designing Interactive Systems*, 1172–1184.

Litwack, K. (2013). The future of nursing: You can't have knowledge you don't have. *Journal of Perianesthesia Nursing, 28*(3), 192–193.

MacDonald, M., Bally, J., Ferguson, L., Murray, B. L., & Fowler-Kerry, S. (2010). Knowledge of the professional role of others: A key interprofessional competency. *Nurse Education in Practice, 10*, 238–242.

Mackey, A., & Bassendowski, S. (2017). The history of evidence-based practice Nursing education and practice. *Journal of Professional Nursing, 33*, 51–55.

Malloch, K. (2014). Beyond transformational leadership to greater engagement: Inspiring innovation in complex organizations. *Nurse Leader, 12*(2), 60–63.

Martin, C., & Chanda, N. (2016). Mental health clinical simulation: Therapeutic communication. *Clinical Simulation in Nursing, 12*(6), 209–214.

McCrae. (2012). Whither nursing models? The value of nursing theory in the context of evidence-based practice and multidisciplinary health care. *Journal of Advanced Nursing, 68*(1), 222–229.

Melnyk, B. (2013). The future of evidence-based health care and worldviews: A worldwide vision and call for action to improve healthcare quality, reliability, and population health. *Worldviews on Evidence-Based Nursing, 10*(3), 127–128.

Melnyk, R. M., & Fineout-Overholt, E. (2011). *Evidence-Based Practice in Nursing & Health care* (ed 2). Philadelphia: Lippincott Williams & Wilkins.

Micheal, S., Candela, L., & Mitchell, S. (2002). Aesthetic knowing: Understanding the experience of chronic illness. *Nurse Educator, 27*, 25–27.

Mitchell, P., Wynia, M., Golden, R., et al. (2012). *Core Principles & Values of Effective Team-Based Health Care. Discussion Paper*. Washington, DC: Institute of Medicine. Retrieved from www.iom.edu/tbc.

Moody, L. (2005). E-health web portals: delivering holistic healthcare and making home the point of care. *Holistic Nursing Practice, 19*(4), 156–160.

National State Boards of Nursing: Evidence based practice for nursing. What is it, why should we do it, and how do we do it? *Nebraska Nursing News , 26*(3):14–17.

Pelletier, L., & Stichler, J. (2013). Action brief: Patient engagement and activation: A health reform imperative and improvement opportunity for nursing. *Nursing Outlook,* 51–54.

Pfaff, K., Baxter, P., Jack, S., & Ploeg, J. (2013). An integrative review of the factors influencing new graduate nurse engagement in interprofessional collaboration. *Journal of Advanced Nursing, 7*(1), 4–20.

Pilon, B., Ketel, C., Davidson, H., et al. (2015). Evidence-guided integration of interprofessional collaborative practice into nurse managed health centers. *Journal of Professional Nursing, 31*(4), 140–150.

Racine L. (2016). Theoretical nursing knowledge in the 21st century. *Advances in Nursing Science* APORIA *8*(2):25–27

Rogers, C. (1946). Significant aspects of patient-centered therapy. *The American psychologist, 1*, 415–422.

Scott, K., & McSherry, R. (2008). Evidence based nursing: Clarifying the concepts for nurses in practice. *Journal of Clinical Nursing, 18*(8), 1085–1095.

Smith, S., & Wilson, S. (2010). *New Directions in Interpersonal Communication.* Thousand Oaks, CA: Sage Publications.

U.S. Department of Health and Human Services (DHHS): 2010. *Healthy people* 2020. Retrieved from www.healthypeople.gov (Accessed 15.03.3).

U.S. Department of Health and Human Services (DHHS): 2010. *Healthy people 2020.* Retrieved from www.healthypeople.gov (Accessed 15.03.17).

Van der Lei, J. (2002). Information and communication technology in health care: Do we need feedback? *International Journal of Medical Informatics, 66*, 75–83.

Ward, B. W., Schiller, J. S., & Goodman, R. A. (2014). Multiple chronic conditions among US adults: A 2012 update. *Preventing Chronic Disease, 11*, E62.

Weiten, W., Lloyd, M., Dun, S., & Hammer, E. Y. (2009). *Psychology applied to modern life: adjustment in the 21st century.* Belmont CA: Wadsworth Cengage Learning.

WHO (World Health Organization). (2002). *Innovative care for chronic conditions: Building Blocks for Action.* Geneva Switzerland: Global Report: Noncommunicable Diseases and Mental Health.

WHO (World Health Organization). (2009). *Global standards for the initial education of professional nurses and midwives.* Geneva, Switzerland: WHO Press.

Zwarenstein, M., Goldman, J., & Reeves, S. (2009). Interprofessional collaboration: Effects of practice-based interventions on professional practice and healthcare outcomes. *The Cochrane Database of Systematic Reviews, 8*(3), 539–542 2009.

Clarity and Safety in Communication

Kim Siarkowski Amer

OBJECTIVES

At the end of the chapter, the reader will be able to:
1. Identify the role of communication in meeting safety goals.
2. Define the role of communication in a "culture of safety."
3. Describe why patient safety is a complex system issue and an individual function.
4. Analyze the relationship between open communication, error reporting, and a culture of safety.
5. Discuss advocacy for safe, high-quality care as a team member.
6. Create simulations to demonstrate use of standardized tools for clear communication affecting patient care, such as using situation, background, assessment, recommendation (SBAR) in a simulated conversation with a physician.

Communication is the key to safe health care. When health care workers communicate effectively, fewer errors occur and people are more satisfied. The majority of errors in health care are linked to a lack of proper communication. This lack of communication can be between nurses; among interdisciplinary teams, including physicians, physical and occupational therapists, dietitians, and pharmacists; or any member of the health care team. Since patient safety is the first priority in nursing care, effective communication should be incorporated in all of the components of planning so that nurses can provide the highest quality of care.

The ability to give safe and effective care is identified by the Quality and Safety Education for Nurses (QSEN) guidelines as an essential competency (QSEN, www.qsen.org/). Nurses and nursing students must be aware of the need for education regarding error prevention and the potential threats to safe care at multiple levels in the care system. Some examples of errors are wrong site surgery, equipment failure, incorrect labeling of specimens, falls, and medication errors. According to The Joint Commission (TJC), 60% to 70% of reported cases of errors (TJC, 2008) were the result of miscommunication.

GOAL

This chapter discusses communication strategies designed to promote a safe environment and focuses on commonly used **standardized tools** for clear communication. The tools for clear communication range from effective communication between nurses and physicians, such as using situation, background, assessment, recommendation (SBAR), to simple templates used when nurses finish the shift and report or "handoff" to the next nurse. Improving communication in health care has become an international priority, as recognized by the World Health Organization (WHO). The aim is to reduce patient mortality, decrease medical errors, and promote effective health care teamwork. A number of agencies and professional organizations are developing and updating guidelines for levels of communication that prevent errors and adverse patient outcomes. The goal is to increase the quality of care for and safety of our patients by embedding a "culture of safety" within all levels of health care. Since nurses play a critical role in patient safety, they need to be aware of best practices in communication. Globally, all nurses need to be responsible for making safety a priority (Kowalski & Anthony, 2017)

BASIC CONCEPTS

Safety Definition

Multiple health care organizations have issued definitions of safety. *Safety* is defined by the Institute of Medicine (IOM) as "prevention of harm to the patient" (National Academy of Sciences [NAS], 2017). The World Health Organization states that "**patient safety** is the prevention of errors and adverse effects to **patients** associated with health care" (www.euro.who.int/en/health-topics/Health-systems/patient-safety).

The nursing profession has always had safe practice as a major goal, as identified in the American Nurses Association (ANA) Code of Ethics for Nurses. The National Patient Safety Foundation (NPSF) has a more specific definition: "avoidance, prevention, amelioration of adverse outcomes or injuries stemming from the process of health care itself" (NPSF, n.d.). QSEN and the American Association of Colleges of Nursing offer a broader definition: safety is "the minimization of risk for harm to patients and to providers through both system effectiveness and individual performance" (Cronenwett et al., 2007).

Safety Incidences

In the United States, one in four hospitalized patients suffers some level of harm. Hospitals with higher satisfaction scores for physician-nurse communication on average have fewer safety events (Hospital Safety Score, 2016). Furthermore, almost as many errors are likely to occur in physicians' offices. When asked to identify which profession was responsible for patient safety, 90% to 96% of all professional disciplines surveyed said the nurse was responsible.

DEVELOPING AN EVIDENCE-BASED PRACTICE

The figures on preventable deaths from errors and miscommunication in health care have been revised upward globally despite the proven effectiveness of safety-promoting communication tools, such as checklists (TeamSTEPPS Webinar July 12, 2017).

The use of a checklist creates an expectation that organizations assess effective communication and safe practices during three perioperative periods: prior to administration of anesthesia, prior to skin incision, and prior to the patient leaving the operating room or procedural area. Through a Centers for Medicare and Medicaid Services (CMS)-designated website, organizations are expected to annually report whether or not a checklist was used for surgery. However, there is no penalty for not using a checklist (www.jointcommission.org).

The World Health Association and The Joint Commission are committed to encouraging the use of checklists prior to surgical procedures. Such checklists have been proven to dramatically reduce wrong site surgery and medication errors.

Application to Your Practice

Analyze patient report procedures, change of shift handoffs, and so on in your clinical area, and consider whether use of safety tools, such as checklists, would increase communication and improve patient safety.

Case Example: Decreased Central Line Catheter Infection in a Cohort Patient Study

In February 2017, a group of researchers explored the impact of a checklist and heightened awareness of nursing staff on central line infection rates. The cohort study had a dramatic difference.

Data are listed in the following table:

Variables	Test	Control	P
Male	57/82 (70%)	47/82 (57%)	0.093
Female	25/82 (30%)	35/82 (43%)	0.093
Age (years)	58.0 ± 20.5	57.0 ± 18.7	0.951
Infection Present	2/82 (2.50%)	31/82 (37.80%)	0.000
Maintenance (days)	10.0 ± 1.14	10.0 ± 18.2	0.235
Hospitalization time (days)	10.0 ± 1.14	10.0 ± 18.2	0.235
Mortality	32/82 (38.30%)	39/82 (47.60%)	0.232

Distribution of numbers, percentages, and values of the medians of patients in test and control groups and their P values are listed in the following table:

Variables	With Infection	No Infection	P	Beta
Test	2.50%	97.50%	.00	−0.442
Control	37.80%	62.20%	0.00	−0.442
Duration of CVC maintenance	22.0 ± 22.3	9.0 ± 9.6	0.00	0.385
Hospitalization time (days)	22.0 ± 22.3	9.0 ± 9.6	0.00	0.385

The test group had 2.5% infections versus the control group that had 37.8%, a finding that is dramatically statistically significant. A major part of the study was positive communication and the implementation of the checklist in the experimental group. A working group of multiple health professionals and regular meetings enhanced the collaboration and communication for the study.

Gameiro, A. J. R., Focaccia, R., da Silva, G. M., Souza, C. V., & Scorcine, C. R. O. (2017). A cohort study on nurse-led checklist intervention to reduce catheter-related bloodstream infection in an intensive care unit. *Journal of Intensive and Critical Care, 3,* 1.

Principles Related to the Occurrence of Unsafe Events

Miscommunication

Much has changed in health care practice since the landmark 1999 IOM study that found that preventable health care errors were responsible for almost 98,000 deaths each year in the United States. The series of IOM reports, as described in Chapter 1, instigated a major effort to make patient safety a national priority. Yet, hospitalized patients still suffer harm. Failure to communicate or inaccurate communication results in an inability to detect and correct errors (Hospital Safety Score, 2016).

Multiple studies have pinpointed miscommunication as a major causative agent in sentinel events, that is, errors resulting in unnecessary death and serious injury. According to The Joint Commission International, miscommunication is the root cause in nearly 70% of reported sentinel events. The curricula for the health professions include interdisciplinary team communication and present the benefits of rounding and professional handoffs.

Case Example: Student Nurse Lakesha

Student nurse Lakesha after handoff to the nurse (staff RN): "I am assigned to give the meds today. I'll be giving them with my instructor." However, she meant all the oral meds for the team, since her instructor assigned these to her, but not the intravenous (IV) medications. Fortunately, her instructor was there to clarify the message. This is an excellent example of inadequate communication potentially doing harm to the patient. If the IV medications were not given for 8 hours, there could have been serious consequences. When policy says to report near misses along with errors, does your agency track near misses by students?

Errors Are Usually System Problems

Most Errors Are Preventable

It is estimated that 70% of reported errors are preventable. "Preventable" means the error occurs because of confused orders, poor communication of expectations, or a failure to communicate potential risks, such as allergies to medications, infection control, or fall risk (Kear & Ulrich, 2015). Fatigue is repeatedly cited as a factor contributing to errors. The most common cause of error is incomplete communication during the very many "handoffs" transferring responsibility for patient care to another care provider, another unit, or agency. It is estimated that in 1 day, a patient may experience up to eight handoffs. The use of a consistent blueprint, or handoff sheet or tool, is an excellent way to ensure comprehensive and safer handoffs (Anderson, Malone, Shanahan, & Manning, 2015; Smeulers et al., 2016). Just like the use of checklists for central line insertion decrease infections, the use of a consistent handoff tool prevents errors of omission and optimizes nursing care. Errors have a high financial cost, in addition to the human cost, exceeding $29 billion per year just in the United States (AHRQ, n.d.[a]).

GENERAL SAFETY COMMUNICATION GUIDELINES FOR ORGANIZATIONS

Unlike other countries, such as Great Britain, in the United States there is no one national database for reporting unsafe care, making data less readily accessible. The Centers for Medicare and Medicaid Services (CMS) does require reporting for patients who have Medicare. Other US government agencies (e.g., Agency for Healthcare Research and Quality [AHRQ]) and professional nursing groups (e.g., AACN, ANA, QSEN) have made recommendations for clear communication strategies to provide safer care that affect both your communication with other nurses and with other health team members. The AACN (2006a) recommends using research- and evidence-based safety communication strategies as a basis for your clinical practice. The Leapfrog group has been consistently rating hospital safety through standard indicators, and the most recent report shows some improvement in indicators, such as a 21% decline in hospital infections (Leapfrog Group, 2017).

BARRIERS TO SAFE, EFFECTIVE COMMUNICATION IN THE HEALTH CARE SYSTEM

Risk and Resistance Models for Chronic Illness and Health Care

Safe and effective care is determined by multiple factors. The risk and resistance model (Fig. 2.1, Pelsi & Amer, 2017) was designed to illustrate the complex interactions that influence child adaptation to chronic illness. A similar model (Fig. 2.2) illustrates the risk and resistance factors for safe and effective care. In Fig. 2.1, the patient, the child with chronic illness, is the center of Amer's risk and resistance model. The resistance or supportive variables are in the points of the star and include social support, self-perception, developmental level, age and economic status,

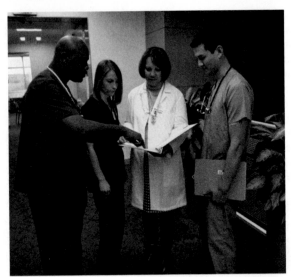

Fig. 2.1 Stress of Illness. Clear communication creates safer patient care. (Adapted from Carey M, Buchan H, Sanson-Fisher R: The cycle of change: implementing best-evidence clinical practice, Int J Qual Healthc 21(1):37-43, 2009; Cronenwett L, Sherwood G, Barnsteiner J, et al: Quality and safety education for nurses, Nurs Outlook 55(3):122-131, 2007.)

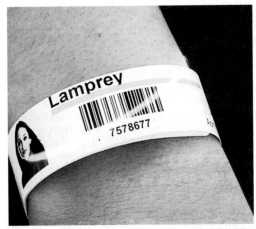

Fig. 2.2 Risk and Resistance Factors for Safe and Effective Care. Nurse scans patient's name band for accurate identification.

knowledge of disease, and length of illness; the broader family variables are included in the larger frame. Implicit is the assumption that a chronic illness is a stressor and the coping strategies (CS) are essential for positive adaptation. Conversely, the same variables can present a risk for the child. For example, a child with a chaotic family, a history of depression, lack of economic resources, and lack of knowledge about the disease is at a much higher risk for not adapting to the illness.

Fig. 2.2 illustrates the risk and resistance factors that affect safe and effective nursing care. At the center is patient safety versus patient risk. The factors that affect the patient risk or offer protection from risk include teamwork, staffing, handoffs, nurse education level, knowledge of standards, and knowledge of risks to patients. In addition, a lower risk to the patient is present when the nurse is an expert in the use of informatics, including the electronic health record (EHR), medication reconciliation, and having access to all patient records. When viewing the concept of safety and effective nursing care, such a model provides a quick glimpse of the multiple factors to consider. Communication is the thread that is part of the multiple factors. For example, teamwork needs to be led by excellent communicators. EHRs are only useful if those who document communicate well in written form.

Fragmentation

The structure of health care organizations are complex. Health care systems can form large multistate entities, often a result of an amalgamation of a number of previously unaffiliated agencies and practices. This organizational complex amalgam of differing philosophy can impede communication. Fragmentation of systems operations or disparate basic policies can be a barrier to safer care. To prevent fragmentation and gaps in communication, evidenced-based practices must be reinforced and implemented at a systemwide level. Although most hospitals and agencies have a policy on error reports, they may lack a systemwide department for processing safety information. An exemplar to be emulated is that of Kaiser Permanente, which implemented a national patient safety plan in 2000. The standard reporting procedures are streamlined, and the aggregate data can be easily retrieved.

Handoffs or transfers of patient care. Miscommunication errors most often occur during a handoff procedure, when one staff member transfers responsibility for care to another staff member. More than half of all incidences of reported serious miscommunications occurred during *patient handoff and transfer,* when those assuming responsibility for the patient (coming on duty) are given a verbal, face-to-face synopsis of the patient's current condition by those who had been caring for the patient and are now going off duty (Smeulers et al., 2016).

Patient care responsibility is transitioned or handed off to the next shift of nurses or when the patient is transferred to another unit. Transition times are high risk for incomplete communication and consequently result in more errors. This has been attributed to frequent interruptions, inconsistent report format, and omission of key information (Cornell & Gervis, 2013). Some agencies have adopted standardized handoff communication tools, including the use of handheld devices (Anderson, Malone, Shanahan, & Manning, 2015). The most ideal clinical handoff is between two nurses in the patient's room with access to the EHR. Discussing the care of the patient with the patient's input is ideal. The use of simple summary aids, such as a whiteboard with critical information, such as "patient likes to be called Emma" and ALLERGIC TO SULFA. The most important part of the handoff is taking the time to adhere to the essential elements, including a thorough review of the assessment and planning of the patient's care.

Underreporting of Errors in a Punitive Climate

Many health care providers express concern about reporting errors or near miss incidents. If we are to create a culture of safety, the system needs to be redesigned to be nonpunitive. A culture of safety is characterized by installing a strong, nonpunitive reporting system; supporting care providers after adverse events; and developing a method to inform and compensate patients who are harmed. Other disciplines have better models for safety. One example is aviation's successful crew resource management (CRM) practice model, which has been used as a template. One necessary step is to require the reporting of near misses so new, safer protocols can be created. Each time an error or near miss occurs, the team members get together and discuss in a nonjudgmental way to determine improved processes to help decrease future errors. *We need to establish a nonpunitive climate. We need to create*

this new climate of safety in which agencies, policies, and employees maintain a vigilant, proactive attitude toward adverse events. Recognizing that human error occurs, everyone's focus needs to be on correcting system flaws to avoid future adverse events, rather than finding the one to blame.

Fatigue

Errors are more likely to occur during long shifts with little rest or nutrition. The risk of error nearly doubles when nurses work more than 12 consecutive hours. Specifically, the last two hours of the shift are when nurses are the most fatigued (Amer, 2013). When a nurse neglects to take a break or refuel with water and a snack, productivity and safety suffer. The effect of fatigue in the final hours of a 12-hour shift is important for all nurses to recognize so structures can be created to minimize fatigue.

INNOVATIONS THAT FOSTER SAFETY

Communication problems and communication solution strategies identified as "best practices" for creating a culture of safety are summarized in Table 2.1. Beyond individual changes to create safer climates for our patients, we need to advocate for organizational system changes. Leadership is needed to incorporate the three C's that promote safer clinical practice:

1. Communication clarity
2. Collaboration
3. Cooperation

TABLE 2.1   Safe Communication: Problems and Recommended Best Practices

Communication Problem	Best Practice Communication Solution
Health care system complexity	Agency establishes safety as a priority. Agency policies adopt procedures to promote transparency and accountability.
Hierarchical status difference with decreased willingness to communicate	Team training such as TeamSTEPPS. Clarify duties of each team member.
Distraction or preoccupation	Policy that isolates you from interruptions (signal to others not to interrupt, such as wearing vest when administering meds). Team members maintain safety awareness as a priority. Control high levels of ambient noise/alarm fatigue. Establish policy to limit interruptions during crucial times.
Heavy workload	Held accountable for evidence-based practice. Support from administration and colleagues. Team members share common safety goals, which each person sees as his or her responsibility.

Continued

TABLE 2.1 Safe Communication: Problems and Recommended Best Practices—cont'd	
Communication Problem	**Best Practice Communication Solution**
Stress and practice pressures due to lack of time, leading to use of shortcuts and poor communication	Adherence to safety protocols, especially in med administration. Team huddles, meetings, bedside rounds.
Staff fail to say what they mean; fail to speak up about safety concerns (lack of assertiveness)	All staff receive continuing education that emphasizes safety promotion, communication, and assertiveness training. Use of time-outs.
Attitude of not believing in usefulness of practice guidelines	Ease of access and increased availability of evidence-based practice guidelines specifically relevant to your patient. Value electronic decision-support apps. Participate in team meetings, conference calls, and opportunities to share successes.
Education silos in which each discipline has own jargon and assumptions	Use of standardized communication tools. Team training. Each team member is encouraged to give input.
Cultural differences or language issues	Cultural-sensitivity education, especially relevant to adapting communication strategies.
Miscommunication	Adapt communication, and verify receipt of message. Use standardized communication. Participate in simulations and critical event training scenarios to foster clear, efficient communication. Read back and record verbal orders immediately. With patients, use teach-backs or "show me" techniques. Solicit questions.
Avoidance of confrontation and communication with the conflict person	Use conflict-resolution skills. Practices open communication. Be assertive in confronting the problem.
Cognitive difficulty obtaining, processing, or understanding Lack of training	Continuing education units about effective communication skills. Avoidance of factors interfering with decision making such as, fatigue. Seek continuing education units, in-service.
Resistance from patient or family to following guidelines for safe, effective care	Team recognizes that safe outcomes require work and communicates that this must involve patient and family. Bedside rounds, briefings, and involving patient in daily care-plan goal setting.

TeamSTEPPS, Team Strategies and Tools to Enhance Performance and Patient Safety.
Adapted from Leonard M, Graham S, Bonacum D: The human factor: the critical importance of effective teamwork and communication in providing safe care, *Qual SafSafe Health Care* 13(Suppl 1):i85-i90, 2004.

Create a Culture of Safety

Agencies are working toward promoting a culture of safety in many ways (PSNet, Safety Culture, PrimerID=5). A major focus is to improve the **clarity of communication.** This occurs through the use of standardized communication tools and team training. This is evidenced by more than 6000 recent articles and the assessment and intervention tools available from AHRQ's PSNet (http://psnet.ahrq.gov/).

Leadership is essential to change to a just culture model, in which the organization creates a balance between accountability of individuals and the institutional system (Ring & Fairchild, 2013). Establishment of an organizational culture of safety requires us to acknowledge the complexity of any health care system. Strong leaders can change the focus to safety practices as a shared value. Creating a safe environment requires us to communicate openly, to be vigilant, to be willing to speak up, and to be held accountable.

Create a Team Culture of Collaboration and Cooperation

Creating effective health teams means getting all team members to value teamwork more than individual autonomy. Team *collaborative communication strategies* involve shared responsibility for maintaining open communication and engaging in mutual problem solving, decision making, and coordination of care. Teamwork failures, including poor communication and failures in physician supervision, have been implicated in two-thirds of harmful errors to patients (Amer, 2013; Singh, Thomas, Peterson, & Studdert, 2007). Creating a safe environment requires all team members to communicate openly, to be vigilant and accountable, and to express concerns and alert team members to unsafe situations.

Create a Nonpunitive Culture

Establishing a **just culture** system creates expectations of a work environment in which staff can speak up and express concerns and alert team members to unsafe situations. A just culture does not mean eliminating individual accountability, but rather puts greater emphasis on an analysis of the problems that contribute to adverse events in a system (Rideout, 2013).

Establishing open communication about errors is an important aspect of just culture. Most state boards of nursing require nurses to report unsafe practice by coworkers, but many nurses have mixed feelings about reporting a colleague, especially to a state agency. Physicians also have reservations about reporting problems. Barriers to reporting include fear, threat to self-esteem, threat to professional livelihood, and lack of timely feedback and support. Ethical incentives to reporting are protection of the patient and professional protection.

In a nonpunitive reporting environment, staff are encouraged to report errors, mistakes, and near misses. They work in a climate in which they feel comfortable making such reports. In safety literature, compiling a database that includes near-miss situations that could have resulted in injury is important information in preventing future errors. A complete error-reporting process should include timely feedback to the person reporting. Administrators should assume errors will occur and put in place a plan for "recovery" that has well-rehearsed procedures for responding to adverse events.

Best Practice: Communicating Clearly for Quality Care

AHRQ, medical and nursing organizations, and health care delivery organizations have undertaken initiatives designed to foster "**best practice**" safer patient care by designing evidence-based protocols for care. *Use "best practices" by increasing use of evidence-based "best practice" versus "usual practice."* The AHRQ funds research to identify the most effective methods of promoting clear communication among health team members and agencies and the most effective treatments. This information is used to develop and distribute protocols for best practice, including formats of standard communication techniques. We need more studies of interventions to promote best communication between nurses and physicians with documented outcomes for patients.

Developing an evidence-based best practice requires closing the gap between best evidence and the way communication occurs in your current practice (see Fig. 2.1). Apply information from evidence-based best practice databanks for safe practice. The process for development of practice guidelines, protocols, situation checklists, and so on is not transparent or easy. Solutions include gathering more evidence on which to base our practice. When is the "evidence" sufficiently strong to warrant adoption of a standardized form of communication about care? Many best practice protocols are available on free web sites, such as AHRQ's (www.ahrq.gov), or proprietary sites, such as Mosby's Nursing Consult.

EHRs improve the safety of patient care and empower providers to have better-quality care delivery and more accountability for preventive care and compliance with standard care protocols. EHRs aid in decision support, for example, providing data for the physician about the number of patients who need mammograms. EHRs are discussed in Chapter 25.

Standardized Communication as an Initiative for Safer Care

We are restructuring our health care system to make patient care safer. The consensus is that this requires improving communication. Good nurse-physician collaborative communication has empirically been associated with a lower risk for negative patient outcomes and greater satisfaction (Amer, 2013). The renewed focus on improving patient safety is resulting in the standardization of many health care practices. **Standardization of communication** is an effective tool to avoid incomplete or misleading messages. Standardization needs to be institutionalized at the system level and implemented consistently at the staff level. Safe communication about patient care needs to be clear, unambiguous, timely, accurate, complete, open, and understood by the recipient to reduce errors.

Patient Safety Outcomes

Standardized tools for clear communication prevent harm to patients. Standardization is best practice. Regulatory agencies have begun mandating the use of standardized communication tools in certain areas of practice. The more consistent the language that is used, the more optimal the outcome.

Nurse-Specific Initiatives

Nurses are often the "last line of defense" against error. Nurses are in a position to prevent, intercept, or correct errors. To prevent errors, nurses need to be clearly communicating to other members of the health team. Your clarity of communication can prevent safety risks, such as medication errors, patient injuries from falls, clinical outcomes related to patient nonadherence to the treatment plan, and high rehospitalization rates. Poor communication can compromise patient safety. One sample case might be that of Nurse Kay in the following example.

Case Example: Kay

Ms. Kay, RN, a newly hired staff nurse, has eight patients assigned to her on a surgical unit. She calls the resident for additional pain medication for a patient. Dr. Andrews, a first-year resident on a 3-month thoracic surgery rotation, has responsibility for more than 80 patients this weekend when he is on call. Many of these he has never seen. In the phone call, Ms. Kay uses nursing diagnoses to describe the patient and is irritated when Dr. Andrews does not seem to recognize the patient, nor understand her. What could Kay do to improve the situation?

Interruptions interfere with a nurse's ability to perform a task safely, yet interruptions have become an almost continual occurrence. These interruptions are tied to an increased risk of errors (PSNet, Nursing and Patient Safety, PrimerID=22). Nonverbal strategies to signal others to avoid distracting communication have been suggested, such as wearing an orange vest when preparing and administering medications.

Medication Process

A particular focus for error reduction is during the entire medication process, ranging from ordering to administration. The definition of *an adverse medication event* is harm to a patient as a result of exposure to a drug, which occurs in at least 5% of all hospitalized patients (PSNet, Handoffs and Signouts, PrimerID=9). We have expanded the definition to include near misses. For example, a nurse prepares an ordered med but recognizes that the ordered dose far exceeds safe parameters. While some medication errors stem from lack of knowledge about the drug, side effects, incompatibility, and other factors

---

involved in ordering or compounding, the majority of errors occur during the nurse's actions in administering the medication. TJC (2007) concluded that drug errors occur when communication is unclear or when a nurse fails to follow the rules for verification: right med, right patient, right dose, and right time.

APPLICATIONS

Communication interventions shown to improve safe communication are listed in Table 2.1. These are best practices. For example, when there is conflicting information or a concern about a potential safety breach, nurses use the "two challenge rule." The nurse states his or her concern twice. This is theoretically enough cause to stop the action for a reassessment.

A discussion of the **standardized tools** used to promote safe interdisciplinary and nursing communication will be the main focus of our application section. Quality and safety education competencies have been developed for all nurses by national nurse leaders, which emphasize safety (QSEN, 2017). The mantra for safe communication should be simplify, clarify, verify.

Attitude

The NAS (IOM) has urged organizations to create an environment in which safety is a top priority. Strive to develop an attitude in which safety is always a priority. Our prime goal is to improve communication about a patient's condition among all the people providing care to that patient. Errors occur when we assume someone else has addressed a situation.

Patient Safety Outcome

Once nurses understand the use of clinical guidelines and evidence-based practice procedures and become comfortable accessing this information, they see that they are providing a higher quality of care, improving their decision-making skills, and avoiding errors, resulting in safer care for their patients. They have fewer error incident reports, fewer patient falls, fewer medication events, less delay in treatment for patients, and fewer wound infections, among other outcomes (Saintsing, Gibson, & Pennington, 2011).

TOOLS FOR SAFER CARE

Skills Acquisition Through Simulation

Skill acquisition is described as "a gradual transition from rigid adherence to rules, to an intuitive mode of reasoning that relies heavily on deep tacit understanding" (Peña, 2010, p. 3).

Communication and practice skills are developed and refined through clinical situation simulations. The students learn in a safe low-stakes simulation lab. The simulations can be low fidelity with model patients or high fidelity with computerized human patient simulators. The students can practice their communication, critical thinking, and clinical judgment skills. Since the instructor is present with several students in the lab, there is a more dynamic experience than the one-on-one in clinical settings. Students should feel free to attempt assessments, get feedback, and improve over time.

Ideally, the simulations should have an interdisciplinary cast of characters. The simulation allows practice without the risk of potentially devastating outcomes in an actual patient care situation.

Simulation laboratories are integrated into most nursing programs and hospitals. You can view sample scenarios on the Internet (even on sites such as YouTube). Practicing clinical assessments and interventions can help build the students' confidence and increase their communication and clinical decision-making skills (Hooper, Shaw, and Zamzam, 2015). In summary, simulations are designed to increase cognitive decision-making skills, increase technical proficiency, and enhance teamwork, including efficient communication skills.

Patient Safety Outcome

More research is needed about the impact of practice simulations on nursing communications that affect actual patient safety. Certainly strong evidence shows increased skill proficiency increases patient safety.

Introduction to Use of Standardized Communication Tools

Use of Checklists

A checklist is defined as a specific, structured list of actions to be performed in a specific clinical setting whose contents are based on evidence (PSNet, Checklists, PrimerID=14). The user's goal is to follow each step in the process. Following a checklist ensures that key steps will not be omitted or important information missed due to *fatigue, pressure, distraction,* or other factors. A checklist is a cognitive guide to accurate task completion or to complete the communication of information. If every step on the list is completed, the possibility of miscommunication or slips leading to error are greatly reduced. Some examples include the WHO's *Surgical Safety Checklist.* Since it was introduced in 2008, use of the WHO checklist has nearly doubled the adherence to surgical standards of care. Another example is the Association of Perioperative Registered Nurses' (AORN) *Comprehensive Surgical Checklist* (Denholm, 2013). This list combines WHO suggestions and TJC guidelines to produce a color-coded list.

Surgical suites and emergent care sites are places that use time-out checklists; these stop everyone in their tasks to verify correctness. Staff verbally run down completion of the list to avoid wrong patient, wrong procedure/surgery, and wrong site. TJC, with its universal protocol, does not mandate a specific checklist, just requires that one be used. In 2012, CMS issued requirements to use checklists. AORN has advocated use of a preoperative checklist for years.

Unit checklists are used when, for example, the floor nurse uses a preoperative checklist to verify that everything has been completed before sending the patient to the surgical suite, but then this list is again checked when the patient arrives, but before the actual surgery. Such system redundancies are used to prevent errors. But they have limited and specific uses and do not address underlying communication problems. No standardized protocol exists for checklist development, so use of expert panels with multiple pilot testing is recommended. One example found in most agency preoperative areas is a checklist where standard items are marked as having been done and available in the patient's record or chart. For example, laboratory results are documented regarding blood type, clotting time, and so forth. Adoption of assertion checklists empowers any team member to speak up when they become aware of missing information.

Patient Safety Outcomes

Evidence shows that the use of checklists improves communication and patient safety, especially in areas managing rapid change, such as preoperative areas, emergency departments, and anesthesiology. According to Amer (2013) use of a simple checklist saved more than 1500 lives in a recent 18-month test period. A study by Semel et al. (2010) found that if a hospital has a baseline major complication rate following surgery of more than 3%, the use of a checklist would generate cost savings once it prevented five major complications. However, some nurses in surgical areas have complained that lists are redundant, take too much time, or are not used by all surgeons.

Use of Situation, Background, Assessment, Recommendation

The **SBAR** method uses a standardized verbal communication tool with a structured format to create a common language between nurses and physicians and others on the health team. It is especially useful when brief, clear communication is needed in acute situations, such as emergent declines in patient status or during handoffs. See Table 2.2 for the SBAR format.

TABLE 2.2	**SBAR Structured Communication Format**	
S	Situation	Identify yourself; identify the patient and the problem. In 10 s, state what is going on. This may include patient's date of birth, hospital ID number, verification that consent forms are present, etc.
B	Background	State relevant context and brief history. Review the chart if possible before speaking or telephoning the physician. Relate the patient's background, including patient's diagnosis, problem list, allergies, relevant vital signs, medications that have been administered, and laboratory results, etc.
A	Assessment	State your conclusion, what you think is wrong. List your opinion about the patient's current status. Examples would be patient's level of pain, medical complications, level of consciousness, problem with intake and output, or your estimate of blood loss, etc.
R	Recommendation or request	State your informed suggestion for the continued care of this patient. Propose an action. What do you need? In what time frame does it need to be completed? Always include an opportunity for questions. Some sources recommend that any new verbal orders now be repeated for feedback clarity. If no decision is forthcoming, reassert your request.

Adapted from personal interviews: Bonacum, D. (2009). CSP, CPHQ, CPHRM, Vice President, Safety Management, Kaiser Foundation Health Plan, Inc., February 25; Fleischmann, J. A. (2008). *Medical vice president of Franciscan Skemp.* LaCrosse, WS: Mayo HealthCare System.

SBAR is designed to convey only the most critical information by eliminating excessive language. It eliminates the authority gradient, flattening the traditional physician-to-nurse hierarchy, making it possible for staff to say what they think is going on. This improves communication and creates collaboration. This concise format has gained wide adoption in the United States and Great Britain. SBAR is used as a situational briefing, so the team is "on the same page." It is used across all types of agencies, groups, and even in e-mails. SBAR simplifies verbal communication between nurses and physicians because content is presented in an expected format. Some hospitals use laminated SBAR guidelines at the telephones for nurses to use when calling physicians about changes in patient status and requests for new orders. Documenting the new order is the only part of SBAR that gets recorded. Refer to Box 2.1 for an example. Then practice your use of SBAR format in Simulation Exercises 2.1, 2.2, and 2.3.

Patient Safety Outcomes

Evidence-based reports show that patient adverse events have decreased through the use of SBAR, including decreases in unexpected deaths. Practicing the use of standardized communication formats by student nurses has been found to improve their ability to effectively communicate with physicians about emergent changes in a patient's condition, and its use has been shown to help develop a mental schema that facilitates rapid decision making by nurses (Vardaman et al., 2012). This format sets expectation about what will be communicated to other members of the health care team.

BOX 2.1 Situation, Background, Assessment, Recommendation Example

Clinical Example of Use of SBAR Format for Communicating With Patient's Physician

S Situation "Dr. Preston, this is Wendy Obi, evening nurse on 4G at St. Simeon Hospital, calling about Mr. Lakewood, who's having trouble breathing."

B Background "Kyle Lakewood, DOB 7/1/60, a 53-year-old man with chronic lung disease, admitted 12/25, who has been sliding downhill × 2 h. Now he's acutely worse: his vital signs are heart rate 92 bpm, respiratory rate 40 breaths/min with gasping, blood pressure 138/94 mm Hg, oxygenation down to 72%."

A Assessment "I don't hear any breath sounds in his right chest. I think he has a pneumothorax."

R Recommendation "I need you to see him right now. I think he needs a chest tube."

Adapted from Leonard, M., Graham, S., & Bonacum, D. (2004). The human factor: The critical importance of effective teamwork and communication in providing safe care. *Quality and Safety in Health Care, 13*(Suppl 1), i85–i90.

TJC, the Institute for Health Care Improvement, and AACN all support the use of SBAR as a desirable structured communication format. (TJC requires hospitals to develop a standardized handoff format.) Thus, we consider the SBAR tool as a best-practice protocol. In addition to using SBAR when there is a change in a patient's health status, this communication format is used at shift change

---

SIMULATION EXERCISE 2.1   Using Standardized Communication Formats

Purpose

To practice the situation, background, assessment, recommendation (SBAR) technique.

Case Study

Mrs. Robin, date of birth January 5, 1950, is a preoperative patient of Dr. Hu's. She is scheduled for an abdominal hysterectomy at 9 a.m. She has been NPO (fasting) since midnight. She is allergic to penicillin. The night nurse reported that she got little sleep and expressed a great deal of anxiety about this surgery immediately after her surgeon and anesthesiologist examined her at the time of admission. Preoperative medication consisting of

atropine was administered at 8:40 instead of 8:30 as per order. Abdominal skin was scrubbed with Betadine per order, and an intravenous (IV) drip of 1 L 0.45 saline was started at 7 a.m. in her left forearm. She has a history of chronic obstructive pulmonary disease, controlled with an albuterol inhaler, but has not used this since admission yesterday.

Directions

In triads, organize this information into the SBAR format. Student no. 1 is giving the report. Student no. 2 role-plays the nurse receiving the report. Student no. 3 acts as the observer and evaluates the accuracy of the report.

SIMULATION EXERCISE 2.2   Telephone Simulation: Conversation Between Nurse and Physician About a Critically Ill Patient

Purpose

To increase your telephone communication technique using structured formats.

Procedure

Read the case, and then simulate making a phone call to the physician on call. It is midnight.

Case

Ms. Babs Pointer, date of birth January 14, 1942, is 6-h post-op for knee reconstruction, complaining of pain and

thirst. Her leg swelling has increased 4 cm in circumference, lower leg has notable ecchymosis spreading rapidly. Temperature 99°F; respiratory rate 20 breaths/min; pedal pulse absent.

Discussion/Written Paper

Record your conversation for later analysis. In your analysis, write up an evaluation of this communication for accurate use of situation, background, assessment, recommendation (SBAR) format, effectiveness, and clarity.

SIMULATION EXERCISE 2.3   Situation, Background, Assessment, Recommendation for Change of Shift Simulation

Purpose

To practice use of situation, background, assessment, recommendation (SBAR) procedure.

Procedure

In post conference, have Student A be the day-shift nurse reporting to Student B, who is acting as the evening nurse. Practice reporting on their assigned patients'

conditions, or simulate four or five postoperative patients' status. Use the SBAR format.

Discussion

Have the entire post-conference group of students critique the advantages and disadvantages of using this type of communication.

---

between nurse colleagues and between nurses and physicians during rounds, transfers, and handoffs from one care setting or unit to another. Some suggest that agencies conduct annual SBAR-competency validations.

A distinct advantage of using SBAR or other standardized communication tools between physicians and nurses is that it decreases professional differences

in communication styles. In a study by Compton et al. (2012), 78% of physicians surveyed stated they receive enough information to make clinical decisions. Several authors speculate that use of SBAR leads to creation of cognitive schemata in staff. Use of this structured format enables less-experienced nurses to give as complete a report as experienced nurses.

Use of the electronic SBAR format when transferring patients to another unit or during change of shift report has been shown to enhance the amount, consistency, and comprehensiveness of information conveyed, yet to not take any longer than a traditional shift report (Cornell & Gervis, 2013).

Crew Resource Management-Based Tools

CRM is another communication tool similar to SBAR, which was adapted from the field of aviation. This tool provides rules of conduct for communication, especially during handoff care transitions. Just prior to an event, such as surgery, all members of the team stop and summarize what is happening. Each team member has an obligation to voice safety concerns.

Briefing. In team situations, such as in the operating room, the team may use another sort of standardized format: a briefing. The leader (the surgeon, in this case) presents a brief overview of the procedure about to happen, identifies roles and responsibilities, plans for the unexpected, and increases each team member's awareness of the situation. The leader asks anyone who sees a potential problem to speak up. In this manner, the leader "gives permission" for every team member to speak up. This can include the patient also, as many patients will not speak unless specifically invited to do so. A debriefing is usually led by someone other than the leader. It occurs toward the end of a procedure and is a recap or summary as to what went well or what might be changed. This is similar to the feedback nurses ask patients to do after they have presented some educational health teaching, which verifies that the patient understood the material.

Debriefing. Debriefing occurs after a surgery or critical incident. It is a callback or review during which each team member has an opportunity to voice problems that arose, identify what went well, and suggest changes that can be made.

Patient Safety Outcomes

Mortality rates have decreased using this tool in the surgical area. Staff identify adverse events that were avoided due to the information communicated during the briefing (Bagian, 2010). Use of structured handoff tools increases perceptions of adequate communication (Jukkala, James, Autrey, Azuero, & Miltner, 2012).

TEAM TRAINING MODELS

Teamwork is described in Chapters 23 and 24 on continuity of the physician-nurse communication.

The majority of reported errors have been found to stem from poor teamwork and poor communication. An effective team has clear, accurate communication understood by all. All team members work together to promote a climate of patient safety. To improve interdisciplinary health team collaboration and communication, it is recommended that physicians and nurses jointly share communication training and team-building sessions to develop an "us" rather than "them" work philosophy. When clashes occur, differences need to be settled. Specific conflict-resolution techniques are discussed in Chapter 23.

Ideally, the health care team would provide the patient with more resources, allow for greater flexibility, promote a "learning from each other" climate, and promote collective creativity in problem solving. Use of standardized communication tools fosters collaborative practice by creating shared communication expectations. Obstacles to effective teamwork include a lack of time, a culture of autonomy, heavy workloads, and the different terminologies and communication styles held by each discipline. Building in redundancy cuts errors but takes extra time, which can be irritating.

TeamSTEPPS Model

One prominent safety model is Team Strategies and Tools to Enhance Performance and Patient Safety (TeamSTEPPS). This program emphasizes improving patient outcomes by improving communication using evidence-based techniques. Communication skills include briefing and debriefing, conveying respect, clarifying team leadership, cross-monitoring, situational monitoring feedback, assertion in a climate valuing everyone's input, and use of standard communication formats, such as SBAR and the Comprehensive Unit-based Safety Program (CUSP) (TeamSTEPPS National Conference, 2017). Creating a team culture means each member is committed to:

- open communication with frequent, timely feedback;
- protecting others from work overload; and
- asking for and offering assistance.

AHRQ's CUSP was designed to implement teamwork and communication. It is a multifaceted strategy to help create a culture of safety; urging health care workers to use communication tools. CUSP incorporates team training with strategies to translate research into staff's evidence-based practice.

TeamSTEPPS With "I PASS the BATON."

Regarding handoffs, AHRQ's TeamSTEPPS program recommends that all team members use the "I PASS the BATON" mnemonic during any transition by staff in patient care. Table 2.3 explains this communication strategy.

TABLE 2.3 PASS the BATON

I	Introduction	Introduce yourself and your role.
P	Patient	State patient's name, identifiers, age, sex, location.
A	Assessment	Present chief complaint, vital signs, symptoms, diagnosis
S	Situation	Current status, level of certainty, recent changes, response to treatment
S	Safety concerns	Critical laboratory reports, allergies, alerts (e.g., falls)
B	Background	Comorbidities, previous episodes, current medications, family history
A	Actions	State what actions were taken and why.
T	Timing	Level of urgency, explicit timing and priorities
O	Ownership	State who is responsible.
N	Next	State the plan: what will happen next, any anticipated changes.

Developed by the US Department of Defense: Department of Defense Patient Safety Program. (2005). *Healthcare communications toolkit to improve transitions in care.* Falls Church, VA: TRICARE Management Activity.

Veterans Administration Clinical Team Training Program

The Department of Veterans Affairs has developed a multidisciplinary program for building teams. Based on principles from aviation's CRM, it is an entire program infused with techniques and standardized care strategies to improve open communication. One example is the concept of "assertive inquiry," modeled on aviation CRM, under which any member of the crew is empowered to speak up if they have a safety concern.

PATIENT SAFETY OUTCOMES OF TEAM TRAINING PROGRAMS

Multiple studies tend to demonstrate increased satisfaction, primarily from nurses, when team communication strategies are implemented. In a review of findings from multiple studies, Weaver found moderate support that improvements in patient safety are associated with CUSP.

Nursing Teamwork

The traditional patient report from one nurse handing over care to another nurse needs to be accurate, specific, and clear and allow time for questions to foster a culture of patient safety. Team training is one tool used to increase collaboration between physicians and nurses. The use of teams is a concept that has been around for years within the medical and nursing professions. For example, medicine has used medical rounds to share information among physicians. Nursing has end-of-shift reports, when responsibility is handed over to the next group of nurses. Using SBAR or any other standardized communication format for reports, especially if these reports are at the bedside, results in a safer environment for your patients, includes patients as active team members, and has been shown not to increase report duration (Woods et al., 2008).

Interdisciplinary Rounds and Team Meetings

Contemporary health care teams use "interdisciplinary rounds" to increase communication among the whole team—physicians, pharmacists, therapists, nurses, and dieticians. This strategy may increase communication and positively affect patient outcome. For example, daily discharge multidisciplinary rounds have been correlated with decreased length of hospital stay. Magnet hospitals in Illinois use hourly rounding by the nurse and nurse assistant to ensure patient status is assessed.

Interdisciplinary "team" meetings can be held daily or weekly to explore common goals, concerns, and options; smooth problems before they escalate into conflicts; or provide support. Lower on the scale are *clinical teaching rounds,* where once a week, a physician teaches nurses, with the goal of encouraging physician communication with the nursing staff.

A **huddle** is a brief, informal gathering of the team to decide on a course of action. Huddles reinforce the existing plan of care or inform team members of changes to the plan. A team huddle can be called by any team member.

Callouts and **time-outs** allow staff to stop and review. As mentioned earlier, TJC mandates that staff working in surgery have a time-out in which all team members review the details of the surgery about to take place to prevent wrong patient, wrong site surgeries.

Standardized Handoff Tools

Many formats are available to foster complete, organized transfer of information, including electronic handoff checklists. In addition to the checklists already described, TJC released SHARE, a targeted solutions tool.

S = Standardize crucial content: give patient's history, key current data

H = Hardwire your system: develop or use standardized tools, checklists

A = Allow opportunities for questions: use critical thinking, share data with entire team

R = Reinforce: common goal, member accountability

E = Educate: team training on use of standardized handoffs with real-time feedback

Patient Safety Outcomes

Strategies to improve interdisciplinary communication break down barriers, increase staff satisfaction (Rosenthal, 2013), decrease night pager calls to residents, and hopefully help to improve the quality of care.

Technology-Oriented Solutions Create a Climate of Patient Safety

Health information technologies (HITs) are a key tool for increasing safety and a means to decrease health care costs and increase quality of care. HITs, text messaging, and dedicated smart phones are some of the technological innovations discussed in Chapters 25 and 26, as are clinical decision support systems, electronic clinical pathways and care plans, and computerized registries or national databanks that monitor treatment.

Electronic transmission of prescriptions involves sending medication orders directly to the patient's pharmacy in the community. This can help decrease errors caused by misinterpretation of handwritten scripts.

Radiofrequency identification (RFID), which puts a computer chip in identity cards or even into some people, is an emerging technology that allows you to locate a certain nurse, identify a patient, or even locate an individual medication. RFID may be able to be incorporated into the nurse's handheld computer.

Prevention of misidentification of the patient is an obvious error-prevention strategy. Before administering medication, the nurse needs to verify patient allergies, use another nurse to verify accuracy for certain stock medications, and reverify the patient's identity. TJC's best practice recommendation is to check the patient's name band and then ask the patient to verbally confirm his or her name and give a second identifier, such as date of birth.

Use of technology, such as *bar-coded name bands,* offers protection against misidentification (AHRQ, n.d.[b]). Some bar-coded name bands include the patient's picture, along with the patient's name, date of birth, and bar code for verification of patient identity.

Whiteboards have long been used at the central nursing station to list the census and the staff assigned to care, in delivery suites to list labor status, and in surgical suites to track procedures and staff. Now we have electronic whiteboards, and patients are invited to add to the information displayed on them.

Patient Safety Outcomes

Many agencies, including the Veterans Administration (VA) hospital system, have used bar codes for years. When a new medication is ordered by a physician, it is transmitted to the pharmacy, where it is labeled with the same bar code as is on the patient's name band. The nurse administering that medication must first verify both codes by scanning with the battery-operated bar-code reader, just as a grocery store employee scans merchandise. In the VA, this resulted in a 24% decrease in medication administration errors (Wright & Katz, 2005). In a similar fashion, bar-coded labels on laboratory specimens prevent mix-ups.

OTHER SPECIFIC NURSING EFFORTS

Following Safety Policies

Implementing unit-based safety programs, such as CUSP, and following policy helps decrease errors and improve the efficiency of care. Measures to improve efficiency may also increase the time you have for communication with patients. Examples of safety redundant processes are the two identifiers required before administering a procedure or medicine or the use of the two-challenge rule.

Work-arounds are shortcuts. Nurses under pressure of time constraints have sometimes developed shortcuts commonly known as work-arounds. These are nonapproved methods to expedite one's work. An example is printing an extra set of bar codes for all your patients who are scheduled to receive medication at 10 a.m. and scanning them all at once rather than scanning each patient's bar-code name band in his or her room.

Patient Safety Outcomes

Deviating from safety protocols inherently introduces risks. While in the short term, some time may be saved, in the long run, mistakes cost millions of dollars each year, harm patients, and put you at risk for liability or malpractice suits.

Transforming Care at the Bedside

Begun in 2003, Transforming Care at the Bedside (**TCAB**; pronounced *tee-cab*) is an Institute for Healthcare Improvement initiative funded by the Robert Wood Johnson Foundation to improve patient safety and the quality of hospital bedside care by empowering nurses at the bedside to make system changes (Amer, 2013; Robert Wood Johnson Foundation, 2008).

This program has four core concepts to improve care:

1. Create a climate of safe, reliable patient care. Uses practices, such as brainstorming and retreats for staff nurses, to develop better practice and better communication ideas. One example is nurses initiate presentation of the patient's status to physicians at morning rounds using a standard format. Another strategy is to empower staff nurses to make decisions.
2. Establish unit-based vital teams. Interdisciplinary, supportive care teams foster a sense of increased professionalism for bedside nurses. This, together with better nurse-physician communication, should positively affect patient outcomes.
3. Develop patient-centered care. This ensures continuity of care and respects family and patient choices.
4. Provide value-added care. This eliminates inefficiencies, for example, by placing high-use supplies in drawers in each patient's room.

Patient Safety Outcomes

Evaluation in more than 60 project hospitals showed that units using this method cut their mortality rate by 25% and reduced nosocomial infections significantly. Nurse-physician collaboration and communication was improved, with both physicians and nurses voicing increased satisfaction. Nurses said that overall they felt empowered (Amer, 2013; Stefancyk, 2008a, 2008b).

Patient-Provider Collaborations

Communicating with patients about the need for them to participate in their care planning was the goal set in 2009 by TJC. Goal 13 states, "Encourage patients' active involvement in their own care as a patient safety strategy," which includes having patients and families report their safety concerns. Patients and their families should be specifically invited to be an integral part of the care process. Another strategy is to provide more opportunities for communication.

Emphasize to Patients That They Are Valued Members of the Health Team

Let your patient know he or she is expected to actively participate in his or her care. Safe care is a top goal shared by patient and care provider. Empowering your patient to be a collaborator in his or her own care enhances error prevention. Emphasize this provider-patient partnership, and increase open communication through bedside rounds, bedside change of shift handoffs, and patient access to their own records. In building the relationship, to establish rapport, participants follow the mnemonic PEARLS (*p*artnership; *e*mpathy; *a*pology, such as "sorry you had to wait"; *r*espect; *l*egitimize or validate your patient's feelings and concerns with comments, such as "many people have similar concerns"; *s*upport).

Use Written Materials

In one hospital system, pamphlets are given to patients upon admission, instructing them to become partners in their care. A nurse comes into the patient's room at a certain time each day, sits, and makes eye contact. Together, nurse and patient make a list of today's goals, which are written on a whiteboard in the patient's room (Runy, 2008). As a part of safety and communication, awareness of language barriers can be signaled to everyone entering the room by posting a logo on the chart, in the room, or on the bed. Use of interpreters and information materials written in the patient's primary language may also reduce safety risks.

Assess Patient's Level of Health Literacy

As mentioned, it is important to make verbal and written information as simple as possible. As a nurse, you need to assess the health literacy level of each patient. Provide privacy to avoid embarrassment. Obtain feedback or teachbacks to determine the patient's understanding of the information you have provided: simplify, clarify, verify!

Patient Safety Outcomes

We need more data regarding patient involvement effects on safety. The evidence does show increases in patient satisfaction after changing to a model of bedside report (Radtke, 2013). AHRQ advises patients to speak up if they have a question or concern, to ask about test results rather than to assume that "no news is good news." Placing information, such as fall prevention posters in the room of an at-risk patient, have been reported by agencies to reduce the number of falls.

SUMMARY

Major efforts to transform the health care system are ongoing. We maximize patient safety by minimizing the risk for errors made by all health care workers. Because miscommunication has been documented to be one of the most significant factors in error occurrence, this chapter focused on communication solutions. It described some individual and system solutions that should help all nurses practice more safely and effectively.

ETHICAL DILEMMA: What Would You Do?

You are a new nurse working for hospice, providing in-home care for Ms. Wendy, a 34-year-old with recurrent spinal cancer. At a multidisciplinary care-planning conference 2 months ago, Dr. Chi, the oncologist, and Dr. Spenski, the family physician, hospice staff, and Ms. Wendy agreed to admit her when her condition deteriorated to the point that she would require ventilator assistance. Today, however, when you arrive at her home, she states a desire to forego further hospitalization. Her family physician is a personal friend and agrees to increase her morphine to handle her increased pain, even though you feel that such a large dose will further compromise her respiratory status.

1. What are the possibilities for miscommunication?
2. What steps would you take to get the health care team "on the same page"?

DISCUSSION QUESTIONS

1. Examine Table 2.1, and give one example you have seen for each of the best-practice communication solutions provided.

2. Use the SBAR exercises given. What was the easiest part? Or the hardest? Many schools actually have students telephone physicians and role-play a scenario. Have you had to do that yet?

REFERENCES

Agency for Healthcare Research and Quality (AHRQ). www.ahrq.gov/.

AHRQ [a]. National healthcare quality report. 2005. www.ahrq.gov.

AHRQ [b]. Medical errors: the scope of the problem: an epidemic of errors. Author. www.ahrq.gov/.

AHRQ's PSNet [patient safety network], n.d. https://psnet.ahrq.gov/primers/primer/22/Nursing-and-Patient-Safety/ Accessed 9/27/18.

Amer, K. S. (2013). *Quality and safety for transformational nursing: care competencies.* Boston: Pearson Publishing.

Anderson, J., Malone, L., Shanahan, K., & Manning, J. (2015). Nursing bedside clinical handover—an integrated review of issues and tools. *Journal of Clinical Nursing, 24,* 662–671.

Bagin, J. P. (2010). Medical team communication training before, during and after surgery improves patient outcomes. *JAMA, 304*(5), 1693–1700.

Compton, J., Copeland, K., Flanders, S., Cassity, C., Spetman, M., Xiao, Y., & Kennerly, D. (2012). Implementing SBAR across a large multihospital health system. *Joint Commission Journal on Quality and Patient Safety, 38*(6), 261–268.

Cornell, P., & Gervis, M. T. (2013). Improving shift report focus and consistency with the situation, background, assessment, recommendation protocol. *The Journal of Nursing Administration, 43*(7/8), 422–428.

Cronenwett, L., Sherwood, G., Barnsteiner, J., Disch, J., Johnson, J., Mitchell, P., et al. (2007). Quality and safety education for nurses. *Nursing Outlook, 55*(3), 122–131.

Denholm, B. (2013). Time-out checklist. *AORN, 98*(1), 87–90.

Five years after the launch of the leapfrog hospital safety grade, patient safety improves, but crucial work remains, *Leapfrog Group.* http://www.hospitalsafetygrade.org/about-us/newsroom/display/527797. April 2017.

Behaviors that undermine a culture of safety. Sentinel Event Alert Issue 40. http://www.jointcommission.org/sentinelevent-alert-issue-40-behaviors-that-undermine-a-culture-of-safety/. Accessed 9/27/18.

Gameiro, A. J. R., Focaccia, R., da Silva, G. M., Souza, C. V., & Scorcine, C. R. O. (2017). A cohort study on nurse-led checklist intervention to reduce catheter-related bloodstream infection in an intensive care unit. *Journal of Intensive and Critical Care, 3,* 1.

Hospital Safety Score. (2016). Latest hospital safety scores show incremental progress in patient safety. New Letter Grades Shift, U.S. State Rankings. www.hospitalsafetyscore.org/latest-hospital-safety-scores-show-incremental-progress.

Institute of Medicine (IOM). (1999). *To err is human: building a safer health system.* Washington, DC: The National Academies Press.

Joint Commision, The (TJC). 2007. Preventing medication errors. In RA Porche (ed.), *Frontline of defense: the role of nurses in preventing sentinel events* (2nd ed). Oakbrook Terrace, Il.

Jukkala, A. M., James, D., Autrey, P., Azuero, A., & Miltner, R. (2012). Developing a standardized tool to improve nurse communication during shift report. *Journal of Nursing Care Quality, 27*(3), 240–246.

Kear, T., & Ulrich, B. (2015). Patient safety and patient safety culture in nephrology nurse practice settings: Issues, solutions and best practices. *Nephrology Nursing Journal, 42*(2), 113–122.

Kowalski, S. L., & Anthony, M. (2017). Nursing's evolving role in patient safety. *American Journal of Nursing, 117,* 34–38.

Leonard, M., & Bonacum, D. (2008). *SBAR application and critical success factors of implementation. Kaiser permanente health care system presentation.* Rochester, MN: Pulmonary and Critical Care Medicine, Mayo Healthcare System.

National Academies of Sciences (NAS). (2017). Health & medicine division [formerly IOM]. www.nationalacademies.org/hmd/.

National Patient Safety Foundation (NPSF). (n.d.). www.npsf.org/. Accessed 9/27/18.

Pelsi, N., & Amer, K. (2017). Alternative interventions for children coping with chronic conditions: a critical review of the literature. *DePaul Discoveries*, *6*(1), Article 2. https://via.library.depaul.edu/depaul-disc/vol6/iss1/2.

Peña, A. (2010). The Dreyfus model of clinical problem-solving skills acquisition: a critical perspective. *Medical Education Online*, *15*(1), 4846. https://doi.org/10.3402/ meo.v15i0.4846. https://doi.org/10.3402/meo.v15i0.4846.

Quality and Safety Education for Nurses (QSEN). (2017). www.qsen.org/.

Radtke, K. (2013). Improving patient satisfaction with nursing communication using bedside shift report. *Clinical Nurse Specialist*, *27*(1), 19–25.

Rideout, D. (2013). "Just Culture" encourages error reporting, improves patient safety. *OR Manger*, *29*(7), 1.

Ring, L., & Fairchild, R. M. (2013). Leadership and patient safety: A review of the literature. *Journal of Nursing Regulation*, *4*(1), 52–56.

Robert Wood Johnson Foundation. (2008). The Transforming Care At the Bedside (TCAB) Toolkit. http://www.rwjf.org/en/research-publications/find-rwjf-research/2008/06/the-transforming-care-at-the-bedside-tcab-toolkit.html.

Rosenthal, L. (2013). Enhancing communication between nightshift RNs and hospitalists. *The Journal of Nursing Administration*, *43*(2), 59–61.

Runy, L. A. (2008). The nurse and patient safety. *Hospitals & Health Networks*, *82*(11), 1.

Saintsing, D., Gibson, L. M., & Pennington, A. W. (2011). The novice nurse and clinical decision-making: How to avoid errors. *Journal of Nursing Management*, *19*, 354–359.

Semel, M. E., Resch, S., Haynes, A. B., Funk, L. M., Bader, A., Berry, W. R., et al. (2010). Adopting a surgical safety checklist could save money and improve the quality of care in U.S. hospitals. *Health Affairs (Project Hope)*, *29*, 1593–1599.

Singh, H., Thomas, E., Peterson, L., & Studdert, D. M. (2007). Medical errors involving trainees. *Archives of internal medicine*, *167*(19), 2030–2036.

Smeulers, M., Dolman, C. D., Atema, D., van Dieren, S., Maaskant, J. M., & Vermeulen, H. (2016). Safe and effective nursing shift handover with NURSEPASS: An interrupted time series. *Applied Nursing Research*, *32*, 199–205.

Stefancyk, A. L. (2008a). Transforming care at the bedside: Transforming care at Mass General. *American Journal of Nursing*, *108*(9), 71–72.

TeamSTEPPS National Conference. (June, 2017). Cleveland, Ohio.

The Joint Commission International With Robert Wood Johnson Foundation. *The Future of Nursing*. Author, 2010. www.nap.edu/catalog.php?record_id=12956/ 7/1/14. The Joint Commission International, WHO Solutions. www.jointcommissioninternational.org/24839/.

Vardaman, J. M., Cornell, P., Gondo, M. B., Amis, J. M., Townsend-Gervis, M., & Thetford, C. (2012). Beyond communication: The role of standardized protocols in a changing health care environment. *Health Care Management Review*, *37*(1), 88–97.

Woods, D. M., Holl, J. L., Angst, D., Echiverri, S. C., Johnson, D., Soglin, D. F., et al. (2008). Improving clinical communication and patient safety: Clinician-recommended solutions. *Journal for Healthcare Quality*, *30*(5), 4354.

Wright, A. A., & Katz, I. T. (2005). Bar coding and patient safety. *New England Journal of Medicine*, *353*(4), 329–331.

3

Professional Guides for Nursing Communication

Kathleen Underman Boggs

OBJECTIVES

At the end of the chapter, the reader will be able to:

1. Describe the impact on nursing communication of standards and guidelines for care and communication issued by multiple organizations.
2. Discuss competencies expected of the newly graduated nurse as listed by Quality and Safety Education for Nurses (QSEN) and other organizations, specifically as they affect communication.
3. Discuss legal and ethical standards in nursing practice relevant to communication, including social media.
4. Construct examples of communications that meet patient privacy legal requirements, such as the American Health Insurance Portability and Accountability Act (HIPAA).
5. Translate empirical knowledge into clinical practice by applying Evidence Based Practice (EBP) information to construct a case study.

This chapter introduces the student to standards and guidelines that influence nursing care, with the focus on communication in both academia and clinical practice. It provides a brief overview of communication as a component of the nursing process. Globally, standards mandate that nurses provide care with compassion and respect for the inherent dignity, worth, and uniqueness of every individual (Fig. 3.1).

BASIC CONCEPTS

Standards as Guides to Communication in Clinical Nursing

As nurses we are guided by standards, policies, ethical codes, and laws. Factors external to the nursing profession, such as technology innovations, research reports, and government mandates, are driving major changes in the way nurses communicate. As described in Chapter 1, our focus is not only on laws but also on guidelines from professional organizations affecting communications in our practice.

In an ideal work environment, we nurses demonstrate professional conduct by using established evidence-based "best practices" to provide safe, high-quality care for our patients. In an ideal work environment, we have excellent communication with our patients, their families, and with all members of the interdisciplinary health care team. Effective communication is essential to workplace efficiency and effective delivery of care.

Effective Communication Concepts

Effective communication is defined as *a two-way exchange of information* among patients and health providers ensuring that the expectations and responsibilities of all are clearly understood. It is an active process for all involved. Two-way communication provides feedback, which enables understanding by both senders and receivers. It is *timely, accurate, and usable.* Messages are processed by all parties until the information is clearly understood by all and integrated into care. A number of international, national, and professional organizations have issued standards, guidelines, and recommendations impacting the way nurses communicate. Strong emphasis is placed on decreasing miscommunication at high-risk times by using standardized communication tools. Let's consider a general summary of these recommendations for effective, safe communication by looking at 7 "Cs":

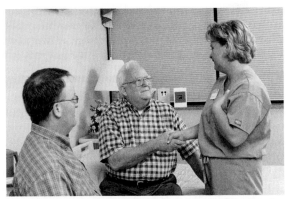

Fig. 3.1 The nurse in all professional relationships, practices with compassion and respect for the inherent dignity, worth, and uniqueness of every individual. (Harris K. Nursing practice implications of the year of ethics. AWHONN, 19(2), 1, 2015.)

- **Correct**/accurate (The Joint Commission [Joint Commission], 2011; International Council of Nurses [ICN], 2012; Institute of Medicine [Institute of Medicine], 2001, 2010; World Health Organization [WHO])
- **Clear** (Aspden, Wolcott, Bootman, & Cronenwett 2007; TeamSTEPPS, Agency for Healthcare Research and Quality [AHRQ], n.d.; Joint Commission, 2011)
- **Concise, Concrete, Complete** (AHRQ, www.ahrq.gov; American Association of Colleges of Nursing [AACN], 2006; Aspden et al. 2007; Joint Commission, R3 Report, n.d.; Joint Commission, 2011)
- **Confidential** [ICN, 2012; Institute of Medicine/RWJ, 2010]
- **Contemporary**/Timely [Joint Commission, 2011; ICN, 2012]

Communication problems occur when there are failures in one or more categories: the system, the transmission, or in the reception. The Joint Commission attributes 60% of sentinel events to miscommunication (TJC R3 Report, n.d.). The IOM, now the National Academy of Medicine Division of the National Academies of Science, Engineering and Medicine, cites poor communication as a causative factor in 70% of health care errors. Current reports continue to show the strong relationship between poor communication and errors (Institute for Healthcare Improvement, 2017).

- **System failures** occur when the necessary channels of communication are absent or not functioning.
- **Transmission failures** occur when the channels exist but the message is never sent or is not clearly sent.
- **Reception failures** occur when channels exist and necessary information is sent, but the recipient misinterprets the message.

Outcomes

IOM stresses clarity of communication throughout their "Crossing the Quality Chasm" series of reports (Aspden et al., 2007). Why are nurses interested in using communication standards to modify and clarify their own communication? Ideally because we are motivated to provide the best, safest possible care. Outcomes for failure to adhere to established nursing practice and professional performance standards range from harm to patients all the way to professional and legal ramifications, potentially including a negative civil judgment against a professional nurse. Consider the case of Kay Smite.

Case Example: Graduate Nurse Kay

Immediately following graduation from her nursing program, Kay Smite, GN, takes an entry position on a busy surgical unit in a small-sized general hospital. With no orientation she is assigned to work evening shift, with one registered nurse and two aides. During her second week when the registered nurse calls in ill, Kay is told by the evening supervisor that she is "charge nurse" this evening, and a float nurse will be sent as soon as possible to help with the workload. A surgeon arrives and rapidly gives verbal instructions to limit his pre-op craniotomy patient's head hair shaving to the incision site only, tomorrow when the preparation procedure is done in the operating suite. As a student, Kay never spoke to a physician. He writes an order stating "patient will be shaved according to head nurse's instructions." He asks Kay to call the operating room to relay these instructions, which she does. Nothing is in the record describing the area to be shaved. When the day shift arrives in the surgical suite, the telephone message from Kay is not passed on. Mr. Smith's head is completely shaved, and he threatens a lawsuit.

1. What standards of communication were violated?
2. What do you think is wrong with this entire work environment?
3. What would you change in this unfortunate but true situation?

The Agency **for Healthcare Research and Quality** in the US Department of Health and Human Services has taken a leading role in health care in the United States to improve safety. As part of their Congressional mandate, AHRQ funds research compiles evidence to develop and publish "best practices" evidenced-based care protocols. For years they operated TeamSTEPPS safety and communication training programs, an operation now continued by the American Hospital Association. An amazing number of resources are available on the internet (www.ahrq.gov/).

PROFESSIONAL NURSING ORGANIZATIONS ISSUING HEALTH CARE COMMUNICATION GUIDELINES

Professional standards of practice serve the dual purpose of providing a standardized benchmark for evaluating the quality of their nursing care and offering the consumer a common means of understanding nursing as a professional service relationship. In this way, standards are used to communicate with the public as to what can be expected from professional nurses. Globally, professional practice organizations are issuing practice standards for nursing care that specify clear, comprehensive communication as a requirement. Examples include The Australian Practice Standards for Specialist Critical Care Nurses (Gill, Kendrick, Davies, & Greenwood, 2016); the Colleges of Nurses of Ontario or the Registered Nurses' association of Ontario, Canada; the Practice Guidelines of Great Britain; the American Nurses Association (ANA) (2010).

Curriculum for Quality and Safety in Communication

Clear communication is a premier competency deemed essential for nurses (Clark et al., 2016). Application of standards of professional communication necessitates use of critical thinking and problem-solving skills in all aspects of care (described in Chapter 4). Box 3.1 lists ANA Standards specifically related to Communication.

The American Association of Colleges of Nursing

The AACN makes recommendations for nursing curricula. For example, they suggest nursing students learn application of evidence-based clinical practices. An example of a specific communication recommendation is learning standard protocol for "handing off" communication when one nurse turns over care of the patient to another. Another is mastering open communication and interdisciplinary cooperation techniques especially for working in health care teams, while another is using technology to assist communications (AACN, 2006; Reeves et al., 2017). The State Boards of Nursing allow up to 50% of clinical experience to occur in simulation labs, so students can practice skills, including effective, safe communication.

Quality and Safety in Nursing Education

American nursing leaders established the QSEN national initiative with the goal of promoting high quality, safe care for all levels of patients across all sites (Cooper, 2017). Altmiller and Dolanski (2017) and others say QSEN has become a national initiative in both academia and clinical nursing. To accomplish this they want to transform nursing education by building on IOM's recommendations to identify essential competencies for nurses and teach these within nursing curricula (Cronenwett et al., 2007). For undergraduates, QSEN identifies six areas of nursing competency as well as the knowledge, skills, and attitudes (KSA) associated with each competency (Barnsteiner et al., 2013, 2017). QSEN's web site provides training, resources, and consultants to translate QSEN competencies into teaching strategies. In each of the six competencies, QSEN specifies the *knowledge*, *skills*, and *attitudes* that are the learning objectives for each competency, such as the following examples:

- **Patient-centered care.** This competency is defined as empowering the patient/family to be a full partner in providing compassionate, coordinated care. In the KSAs, under "**knowledge,**" you are expected to integrate multiple dimensions of care, including communication, to involve the patient and family. In terms of "**skills,**" you are expected to elicit patient values and preferences during your initial interview and care plan development and to communicate their preferences to other members of the health care team. In terms of "**attitudes,**" you are to value expressions of patient values, as well as their expertise regarding their own health status. In meeting the QSEN competency of providing

---

> ## BOX 3.1 ANA Standards of Nursing Practice: #11 Communication
>
> - Assesses communication format preferences of health care consumers, families, and colleagues.
> - Assesses his or her own communication skills in encounters with health care consumers, families, and colleagues.
> - Seeks continuous improvement of communication and conflict resolution skills.
> - Conveys information to health care consumers, families, the interprofessional team, and others in communication formats that promote accuracy.
> - Questions the rationale supporting decisions when they do not appear to be in the best interest of the patient.
> - Discloses observations or concerns related to hazards and errors in care or the practice environment to the appropriate level.
> - Maintains communication with other providers to minimize risks associated with transfers and transitions in care delivery.
> - Contributes his or her own professional perspective in discussions with the interprofessional team.
>
> American Nurses Association. (2010). *Nursing scope and standards of practice* (p. 54). Silver Spring, MD: ANA.

patient-centered care, do you communicate with your patients to engage them in planning care?

- **Teamwork and collaboration.** With this competency, you are able to function effectively within nursing and on interprofessional teams, to foster open communication, mutual respect, and shared decision making to achieve quality care. A partial example of expected knowledge objectives for this competency might be that you know the various roles and scope of practice for team members and are able to analyze differences in communication style preferences for patient, family, and for other members of the health care team. In terms of "skill," you are expected to be able to adapt your own style of communicating and to initiate actions to resolve any conflicts. In terms of "attitudes," your behavior shows that you value teamwork and different styles of communication (www.QSEN.org/). As a student, are you having experiences in which you practice directly communicating with physicians?

As you can see in Table 3.1, *communication is a major component* of QSEN's six competencies. The QSEN web site gives you access to the case study of Lewis Blackman, a healthy, active 15-year-old, who died unnecessarily following elective surgery (www.qsen.org/videos/the-lewis-blackman-story). This case details a series of miscommunications and lack of intervention by staff nurses and physicians. In addition to the inaction on the part of nurses, fragmentation of the care system and the barrier of the physician-nurse power hierarchy are implicated. When members of the health care team are not empowered to speak up and participate, a major threat to patient safety occurs. Blackman's mother, Helen Haskell, states that it is her belief that "Lewis' death could have been averted by a knowledgeable, assertive nurse." Effectively working as part of a health care team

---

TABLE 3.1 QSEN's Six Prelicensure Competencies, Definitions, and Selected Communication Examples

Competency	Definition	Partial Examples[a]
1. Patient-centered care (Arnold and Boggs discussed in every chapter)	Focus on fully partnering with patient to provide care that incorporates his or her values and preferences to give safe, caring, compassionate effective care. To do so requires us to communicate preferences to other health team members	(K) Integrate understanding of arts, sciences, including communication, to apply nursing process. (S) Use communication skills in intake clinical interview to ask about patient preferences, to develop care plan, to communicate these to others. Use communication tools. (A) Value patient expertise and input
2. Teamwork and collaboration (Arnold and Boggs discussed in Chapters 2, 3, 6, 22, 23, and 24)	For teamwork we need mutual respect, open communication, and shared decision making with all team members	(K) Know scope of practice. Analyze differences in communication styles. (S) Adapt own style to the needs of the team in the current situation. Communicate openly, share in decision making, resolve potential conflicts. (A) Respect contributions of every team member
3. Evidence-based practice (EBP) (Arnold and Boggs discussed in Chapters 1, 2, 3, and 23, with examples and application to practice in every chapter)	Incorporate the best practices based on newest evidence with our clinical expertise to deliver optimal care	(K) Identify sources of EBP. Differentiate quality of evidence. (S) Use EBPs, after analyzing research findings and care protocols relevant to our patient's diagnosis; communicate these to others. (A) Value research, appreciate need to seek EBP information
4. Quality improvement (Arnold and Boggs discussed in Chapters 2 and 25)	Collect data on common outcome measures of our care to compare with accepted outcomes (benchmarks)	(K) Identify differences between our agency practices and "best practices." (S) Use communication tools to make patient care explicit. (A) Value own and others contributions

Continued

TABLE 3.1 QSEN's Six Prelicensure Competencies, Definitions, and Selected Communication Examples—cont'd

Competency	Definition	Partial Examples[a]
5. Safety (Arnold and Boggs incorporated throughout with focused discussion in Chapters 2 and 25)	Minimize risk of harm, analyzing root causes of error, moving from a blame culture to a just culture should increase communication, prevent future problems; result is safer care	(K) Analyze safety processes in own workplace. (S) Speak up proactively (about potential safety violations) and report near misses. (A) Appreciate how variation from established protocols creates risk
6. Informatics (Arnold and Boggs discussed in Chapters 2, 25, and 26)	Use technology to effectively communicate and manage patient care, make decisions, and access evidence-based treatment information	(K) Contrast benefits and limitations of different communication technologies. (S) Use electronic skills to access available databases to design an effective, evidence-based care plan. (A) Protect confidentiality

[a]K = knowledge; S = skill; A = attitude.
QSEN, Quality and Safety Education for Nurses.

requires open communication, mutual respect, and shared decision making with the patient and family included.

Additional QSEN competencies are defined for graduate nursing education (Disch & Barnsteiner, 2012).

These and other QSEN competencies will be discussed throughout this book, as related to communication. For more information and descriptions of the KSA attached to each competency, refer to www.QSEN.com. A drawback is the lack of adequate evaluation of achievement of these competencies (Dolansky, Schexnayder, Patrician, & Sales, 2017).

Other models are also available that identify core competencies expected of nurses. All of them stress excellent communication, coordination, and collaborative skills. For example, Lenburg's Competency Outcomes Performance Assessment Model includes oral skills, writing skills, and electronic skills (Amer, 2013).

CODES CONTAINING ETHICAL STANDARDS

Ethics is a critical part of everyday nursing practice (National Nursing Summit, 2015). Nurses have an ethical accountability to the patients they serve that extends beyond their legal responsibility in everyday nursing situations. Nurses have consistently been rated very highly in public opinion polls for honest and ethical behavior (Lowe, 2015). The process for applying ethical decision making will be described in Chapter 4.

Ethical Codes

All legitimate professions have standards of conduct. A Code of Ethics for Nurses provides a broad conceptual framework outlining the principled behaviors and value beliefs expected of professional nurses in delivering health care to individuals, families, and communities. Embodied in ethical codes are Nursing's core values as illustrated in Fig. 3.2. Written Codes are found in most nations. An International Code of Ethics was adopted by ICN in 1953 and revised in 2012. This code identifies four fundamental nursing responsibilities as being to promote health, prevent illness, restore health, and alleviate suffering. Moreover, the code says each nurse has the responsibility to maintain a clinical practice that promotes ethical behavior, while sustaining collaborative, respectful relationships with coworkers. Among many elements of the code, those addressing communication state we need to ensure that each patient receives accurate, sufficient communication in a timely manner and to maintain confidentiality.

Professional nurses, regardless of setting, are expected to follow ethical guidelines in their practice. As listed in Box 3.2, American Nurses Association Code of Ethics for Nurses (with interpretive statements) (ANA, 2015) establishes principled guidelines designed to protect the integrity of patients related to their care, health, safety, and rights. It provides guidelines for your ethical practice and decision making to protect patient rights, to provide a mechanism for professional accountability, and to educate about sound ethical conduct (Olson, 2016).

Ethical standards of behavior require a clear understanding of the multidimensional aspects of an ethical dilemma, including intangible human factors that make each situation unique (e.g., personal and cultural values or resources). Chapter 4 discusses nurses and ethics in more depth, while Simulation Exercise 3.1 provides an opportunity to consider the many elements in an ethical nursing dilemma. When an ethical dilemma cannot be resolved

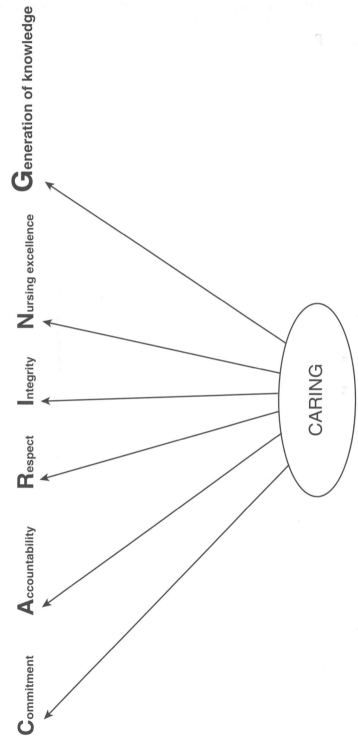

Fig. 3.2 Communication in the nursing process. (From Harris K. Nursing practice implications of the year of ethics. *AWHONN*, 19(2), 1, 2015.) Modified from Potter PA, Perry AG, Stockert PA, et al. Fundamentals of nursing, ed 8, St. Louis, 20173, Mosby.

BOX 3.2 American Nurses Association Code of Ethics for Nurses

1. The nurse, in all professional relationships, practices with compassion and respect for the inherent dignity, worth, and uniqueness of every individual, unrestricted by considerations of social or economic status, personal attributes, or the nature of health problems.
2. The nurse's primary commitment is to the patient, whether an individual, family, group, or community.
3. The nurse promotes, advocates for, and strives to protect the health, safety, and rights of the patient.
4. The nurse is responsible and accountable for individual nursing practice and determines the appropriate delegation of tasks consistent with the nurse's obligation to provide optimum patient care.
5. The nurse owes the same duties to self as to others, including the responsibility to preserve integrity and safety, to maintain competence, and to continue personal and professional growth.
6. The nurse participates in establishing, maintaining, and improving health care environments and conditions of employment conducive to the provision of quality health care and consistent with the values of the profession through individual and collective action.
7. The nurse participates in the advancement of the profession through contributions to practice, education, administration, and knowledge development.
8. The nurse collaborates with other health professionals and the public in promoting community, national, and international efforts to meet health needs.
9. The profession of nursing, as represented by associations and their members, is responsible for articulating nursing values, for maintaining the integrity of the profession and its practice, and for shaping social policy.

SIMULATION EXERCISE 3.1 Applying the Code of Ethics for Nurses to Professional and Clinical Situations

Purpose
To help students identify applications of the Code of Ethics for Nurses.

Procedure
Break into small groups of four or five students and role-play the following clinical scenarios:

1. Barbara Kohn is a 75-year-old woman who lives with her son and daughter-in-law. She reveals to you that her daughter-in-law keeps her locked in her room when she has to go out because she does not want her to get in trouble. She asks you not to say anything as that will only get her into trouble.
2. The nursing supervisor asks you to "float" to another unit that will require some types of tasks that you believe you do not have the knowledge or skills to perform. When you explain your problem, she tells you that she understands, but the unit is short staffed and she really needs you to do this.
3. Bill Jackson is an elderly patient who suffered a stroke and is uncommunicative. He is not expected to live. The health care team is considering placement of a feeding tube based on his wife's wishes. Mrs. Jackson agrees that he probably will not survive but wants the feeding tube just in case the doctors are wrong.
4. Dr. Holle criticizes a nurse in front of a patient, Mrs. DiTupper, and her family.

Reflective Analysis and Discussion
Share each ethical dilemma with the group and collaboratively come up with a resolution that the group agrees on, using the nurse's code of ethics to work through the situations.

1. Describe some of the challenges your group encountered in resolving different scenarios.
2. Select a situation that offers the most challenge ethically and explain your choice.
3. Justify any problems in which the code of ethics was not helpful.
4. Create a scenario depicting you utilizing the knowledge gained from this exercise in your nursing practice.

---

through interpersonal negotiation, an ethics committee composed of biomedical experts reviews the case and makes recommendations. Of particular importance to the nurse-patient relationship are ethical directives related to the nurse's primary commitment to:

- Patient welfare
- Patient autonomy
- Recognition individual is unique and worthy of respect
- Truth telling and advocacy

LEGAL STANDARDS

As stressed in the IOM/Robert Wood Johnson Foundation (RWJ) report, nurses must be accountable for their own contributions to delivery of high-quality care (2010). As professional nurses, we are held legally accountable for all aspects of the nursing care we provide to patients and families, including documentation and referral. Of special relevance to communication within the nurse-patient relationship are issues of confidentially, informed consent, and professional liability.

Classifications of Laws in Health Care

Statutory Laws

These are legislated laws, drafted and enacted at various government levels. In the United States, Medicare and Medicaid amendments to the Social Security Act are examples of federal statutory laws, while state Nurse Practice Acts are examples of statutory laws.

Civil laws. These are developed through court decisions, which are created through precedents, rather than written statutes. Most infractions for malpractice and negligence are covered by civil law and are referred to as torts. A tort is defined as a private civil action that causes personal injuries to a private party. Deliberate intent is not present. Four elements are necessary to qualify for a claim of malpractice or negligence.

- The professional duty was owed to patient (professional relationship).
- A breach of duty occurred in which the nurse failed to conform to an accepted standard of care.
- Causality in which a failure to act by professional standards was a proximate cause of the resulting injury.
- Actual damage or injuries resulted from breach of duty.

As nurses, we are legally bound by the principles of civil tort law to provide the care that any reasonably prudent nurse would provide in a similar situation. If taken to court, this standard would be the benchmark against which our actions would be judged.

Criminal law. These laws are applicable to cases in which there is intentional misconduct or a serious violation of professional standards of care. The most common nurse violation of criminal law is failure to renew a professional nursing license, which means that a nurse is practicing nursing without a license.

Malpractice and Legal Liability in Nurse–Patient Relationships

In the nurse-patient relationship, the nurse is responsible for maintaining the professional conduct of the relationship. Examples of unprofessional conduct include:

- Breaching patient confidentiality

- Verbally or physically abusing a patient
- Assuming nursing responsibility for actions without having sufficient preparation
- Delegating care to unlicensed personnel, which could result in injury
- Following a doctor's order that would result in patient harm
- Failing to assess, report, or document changes in patient health status
- Falsifying records
- Failing to obtain informed consent
- Failure to question a physician's orders, if they are not clear
- Failure to provide required health teaching
- Failure to provide for patient safety (e.g., not putting the side rails up on a patient with a stroke)

Effective and frequent communication with patients and other providers is one of the best ways to avoid or minimize the possibility of harm leading to legal liability.

Documentation as a Legal Record

As described in Chapter 25, nurses are responsible for the accurate and timely documentation of nursing assessments, the care given, and the outcome responses. This documentation represents a permanent record of health care experiences. In the eyes of the law, failure to document in written form any of these elements means the actions were not taken.

APPLICATIONS

As illustrated in Fig. 3.2, Communication in the Nursing Process, communication standards and skills are an integral component of the knowledge, experience, skills, and attitudes encompassed in using the nursing process to deliver care. As we emphasized, standards for clear, complete communication are specified in professional codes and guidelines. Nursing students need opportunities to practice effectively communicating before entering the workforce. Throughout this book, emphasis is placed on the importance of guiding your practice through application of both professional standards and EBPs in your nursing care. Discussing case studies and exercises offers opportunities to hone communication skills.

EVIDENCE-BASED PRACTICE

EBP is a conscious choice to use the most current research to provide "best care." Translating knowledge into practice using findings from multiple empirical studies to help solve clinical problems is universally advocated (Al-Mowani, Al-Barmawi, Al-Hadid, & Aljabery, 2016). As discussed in Chapter 1, **EBP** guidelines are clinical behaviors compiled from the best current research evidence available and the expertise of clinicians. IOM's *The Future of Nursing* report (2010) specifies that nursing education provides opportunities for students to develop competency in the use of EBP and collaborative teamwork to ensure the delivery of safe, patient-centered care across settings internationally (Leung, Trevena, & Waters, 2016). Saunders, Vehvilainen-Julkenen, and Stevens' (2016) findings show student use of EBP results in increased use in later clinical practice. Internationally EBP has various names. For example, in Canada it may be termed "knowledge translation," while in Great Britain it may be "evidence-based nursing."

Use of EBPs is a QSEN competency. Each nurse is expected to be able to integrate "best current evidence" with clinical expertise and patient/family preferences and values to deliver optimum care (Barnsteiner et al., 2013; Sales, 2017). In developing this skill, you learn to determine which data are scientifically valid and useful in guiding your practice. By consulting EBP guidelines, your ability to make specific clinical decisions about care for your patient is enhanced, so you can give the highest quality care. Do you have a clinical question? Many sources are available to you; for example, guidelines from agencies such as AHRQ or specialty nursing organizations (www.guideline.gov/index.aspx).

Assets Which Support Use of Evidence-Based Practice Information

Accessibility of Information

Taking ownership of improving your practice means continuing to increase your awareness of what credible evidence is available. Repeated study findings show staff nurses are unaware of evidence that could improve their care. Barnsteiner (2017) says that 75% of the time nurses get their information from their experience and only 58% of the time

from a policy. It is true that much of nursing and medicine is not yet based on evidence. When a policy or guideline is not yet available, you can access specific journal research articles using any of several databases such as CINAHL (QSEN module on EBP). Careful critical thinking is needed when relying on just one study's findings. As Disch points out, even when we have available best evidence, sometimes we choose not to apply it. She gives the example that oral care is often not done, even though strong evidence exists that oral care reduces ventilator-associated pneumonia. The "Best Evidence for Best Practice" motto encourages us to use EBP samples provided in this book to stimulate discussion and to encourage seeking out findings you can apply in your clinical practice.

Workload Time Constraints

With higher patient acuity and decreased resources to complete assigned tasks, staff nurses are challenged to find time to seek out evidence (Jun, Kovner, & Stimpfel, 2016). Yet maintaining competency depends on valuing this clinical inquiry (Leung et al., 2016).

Leadership

Exposure to leaders who value EBP and membership on a health team valuing getting current evidence to set clear goals and using recommended interventions helps (White & Spruce, 2015).

Organizational Culture

A culture respecting "Best Practice" must be created. Administrators who build consensus toward use of EBP are likely to have nurses who value and use clinical practice guidelines. Clear interprofessional communication is an important component (Jun et al., 2016).

DEVELOPING AN EVIDENCE-BASED PRACTICE
Evidence-based practice is built on finding, analyzing, and applying empirical findings that will help solve patient-care problems. Acceptance of new care techniques is based on analysis of multiple findings. For teaching purposes the authors often present findings from just one study. So let's consider a study from South Africa. See if you can find other sources to validate these study findings. This study was designed to answer the question "How do students use social media in the clinical environment?" Nyangeni, DeRand, and VanRooyen (2015) used a qualitative, descriptive design to analyze semi-structured interviews from a convenience sample of 12 undergraduate student nurses. Interviews were coded separately by two researchers to identify common themes. Following a method by Tesch, analysis continued until no new themes emerged.

Findings: Analysis revealed two main themes with many subthemes. First, students showed lack of aware-

ness of responsible use of social media, violating patient's rights to privacy, posting pictures of medical procedures on social media without informed consent being sought, even though students knew that this information remains in circulation long after they have deleted it from their network site. Authors found a sort of competition among students to be the first to post titillating information sometimes just to entertain their friends. A second major theme involved a blurring of boundaries between personal and professional roles, with posting of pictures of themselves with their patients just as they would do with their friends. Narrative comments included the information that they had seen staff nurses doing this!

Application to Your Clinical Practice
Why did students have cell phones with them in clinical areas? Were privacy issues not covered in school in a way that made an impact on behavior? Examine the quality of this

research. Are these findings valid? Authors such as Sinclair, McLoughlin, and Warne (2015) write that social media platforms are very useful to students both for learning and for support. In fact empirical data show student use of social media helps stress coping (Warshawski, Barnoy, & Itzhaki, 2017). With constant advances in social media, the blurring of boundaries between personal and professional roles is happening in many professions. Try Googling your name and find how many pictures of you appear. Reflect on whether posts of patients could lead to harm? Apply guidelines in Table 3.2 to your practice. How can sites be used for learning?

Many web sites provide you with information for competency in procedures and with lists of Nursing Outcomes Classification and Nursing Interventions Classification categories and codes.

For fun, check out the sites available to you from the AHRQ, n.d, including their hyperlinks to YouTube, for videos that you can use in teaching young patients (www.youtube.com/user/AHRQHealthTV/). Just click on "prevention is the key to a healthy life" or other topics.

TABLE 3.2   Online Guidelines for Nurses Using Social Media

Principles	Actions
Posts are bound by confidentiality and privacy laws, such as Health Insurance Portability and Accountability Act	Refrain from posting identifiable patient information. This absolutely applies to photos or videos. It applies even if you do not show their face.
Professional ethical standards need to be followed	Separate personal from professional information. Use two separate sites? Observe professional boundaries. Do not cross into social friendships.
Social media sites are public forums. Legal liability laws apply. Clicking on "restricted access" does not qualify as a private site	Any disparaging comments are considered "cyber bullying" Use privacy settings. Understand that colleagues, employers, and even patients may read your posts.
Libel laws and nursing ethical codes apply to online information. Regulatory agencies such as State Boards act on complaints	Social media is permanent and universal. For example, Tweets may be retweeted. Civil, criminal, and professional penalties may apply.

Nursing Process

The **nursing process** consists of five progressive phases: assessment, problem identification and diagnosis, outcome identification and planning, implementation, and evaluation. Fig. 3.2 illustrates how this process is central to patient care. As a dynamic, systematic clinical management tool, it functions as a primary means of directing the sequence, planning, implementation, and evaluation of nursing care to achieve specific health goals. Continual and timely communication is a component of each step in the nursing process. Specifically communication plays a role in:

- Establishing and maintaining a therapeutic relationship
- Helping the patient to promote, maintain, or restore health, or to achieve a peaceful death
- Facilitating patient management of difficult health care issues through communication
- Providing quality nursing care in a safe and efficient manner

The nursing process is closely aligned with meeting professional nursing standards in providing total care. Table 3.3 illustrates the relationship. The nursing process begins with your first encounter with a patient and family,

and ends with discharge or referral. Although there is an ordered sequence of nursing activities, each phase is flexible, flowing into and overlapping with other phases of the nursing process. For example, in providing a designated nursing intervention, you might discover a more complex need than what was originally assessed. This could require a modification in the nursing diagnosis, the identified outcome, the intervention, or the need for a referral.

You employ communication skills in each step. From introducing yourself and explaining the purpose during initial assessment all the way through, traditionally nurses have used Gordon's Functional Health Patterns in their assessment. Refer to Box 3.3. Refer to any nursing fundamentals textbook for a full discussion.

Prioritize

Traditionally nurses also have used Maslow's Hierarchy of Needs (see Chapter 1) to prioritize goals and objectives. Examples of nursing problems associated with each level of Maslow's hierarchy are included in Table 3.4. Priority attention should be given to the most immediate, life-threatening problems. Use communication skills

TABLE 3.3 Relationship of the Nursing Process to Professional Nursing Standards in the Nurse–Patient Relationship

Nursing Process: Assessment	Related Nursing Standard
Collects data/information from: • Patient history/interview • Own observations; physical examination • The family • Past records/tests • Other members of health team	The nurse collects data throughout the nursing process related to patient strengths, limitations, available resources, and changes in the patient's condition
Analyzes data	The nurse organizes cluster behaviors and makes inferences based on subjective and objective data, combined with personal and scientific nursing knowledge
Verifies data	The nurse verifies data and inferences with patient to ensure validity
Nursing Process: Diagnosis	
Identifies health care needs/problems and formulates biopsychosocial statements	The nurse develops a comprehensive biopsychosocial statement that captures the essence of the patient's health care needs/problems (see Box 3.3, Gordon's Functional Health Patterns). The nurse validates the accuracy of the statement with the patient and family; this statement becomes the basis for nursing diagnoses
Establishes nursing diagnosis Nurse uses NANDA-approved diagnoses and codes	The nurse develops relevant nursing diagnoses. Prioritizes them based on most immediate needs in the current health care situation (see Table 3.3, Identifying Nursing Problems Associated with Maslow's Hierarchy of Needs)
Nursing Process: Outcome Identification and Planning	
Identifies expected outcomes (for each NANDA diagnosis, there are several NOC suggested outcomes)	The nurse and patient mutually and realistically develop expected outcomes based on patient needs, strengths, and resources
Specifies short-term goals	The nurse and patient mutually and realistically develop expected outcomes based on patient needs, strengths, and resources
Nursing Process: Implementation	
Takes appropriate nursing action interventions. Nursing interventions alter patient's status/symptoms	The nurse encourages, supports, and validates the patient in taking agreed-on action to achieve goals and expected outcomes through integrated, therapeutic nursing interventions and communication strategies
Nursing Process: Evaluation	
Evaluates goal achievement. Expected outcome is stated and nurse is quickly able to identify patient's current status	The nurse and patient mutually evaluate attainment of expected outcomes and survey each step of the nursing process for appropriateness, effectiveness, adequacy, and time efficiency. Modifies the plan if evaluation shows expected outcome not achieved

NANDA, North American Nursing Diagnosis Association; *NOC,* Nursing Outcomes Classification.

BOX 3.3 Gordon's Functional Health Patterns

1. Health perception–health management pattern
2. Nutritional–metabolic pattern
3. Elimination pattern
4. Activity-exercise pattern
5. Sleep-rest pattern
6. Cognitive-perceptual pattern
7. Self-perception–self-concept pattern
8. Role-relationship pattern
9. Sexuality-reproductive pattern
10. Coping–stress-tolerance pattern
11. Value-belief pattern

to validate these priorities with your patient and health team. Try Simulation Exercise 3.2 to practice considering cultural, age, and gender-related themes when using the nursing process with different types of patients.

Use communication skills to collaborate with health team members and with patient and family members as you implement the nursing process. Your communication skills help you collaborate with your patient to provide safe quality care.

TABLE 3.4 **Identifying Nursing Problems Associated With Maslow's Hierarchy of Needs**	
Psychological survival needs	Circulation, food, intake/output, physical comfort, rest
Safety and security needs	Domestic abuse, fear, anxiety, environmental hazards, housing
Love and belonging	Lack of social support, loss of significant person or pet, grief
Self-esteem needs	Loss of a job, inability to perform normal activities, change in position or expectations
Self-actualization	Inability to achieve personal goals

After using your communication skills to obtain feedback from your patient, contrasting actual progress with expected outcomes, analyze factors that might have effected goal achievement. Communicate with team members to modify interventions as needed.

ISSUES IN APPLICATION OF ETHICAL AND LEGAL GUIDELINES

Moral Distress

Moral distress occurs when an agency attempts to require you to act contrary to your personal values or in a way you know is ethically inappropriate (American Association of Critical Care Nurses [AACCN], 2008). ANA (2015) describes their Code of Ethics as "nonnegotiable, encompassing all nursing activities and may supersede specific policies of institutions." If you are unable to provide care, you are obligated to ensure that the patient will have care from another well-qualified nurse. ANA supports the rights of patients to self-determination. As a nurse you have an ethical obligation to support them in their choices.

Protecting the Patient's Privacy

ANA supports a patient's right to privacy, which is to have control over personal identifiable health information, whereas confidentiality refers to your obligation not to divulge anything said in a nurse-patient relationship.

SIMULATION EXERCISE 3.2 Using the Nursing Process as a Framework in Clinical Situations

Purpose
To help develop skills in considering cultural, age, and gender role issues in assessing each patient's situation and developing relevant nursing diagnoses.

Procedure
1. In small groups of three to four students, role play how you might assess and incorporate differences in patient/family values, knowledge, beliefs, and cultural background in delivery of care for each of the following. Indicate what other types of information you would need to make a complete assessment.
2. Identify and prioritize nursing diagnoses for each to ensure patient-centered care.
   - Michael Sterns was in a skiing accident. He is suffering from multiple internal injuries, including head injury. His parents have been notified and are flying in to be with him.
   - Lo Sun Chen is a young Chinese woman admitted

for abdominal surgery. She has been in this country for only 8 weeks and speaks very little English.
   - Maris LaFonte is a 17-year-old unmarried woman admitted for the delivery of her first child. She has had no prenatal care.
   - Stella Watkins is an 85-year-old woman admitted to a nursing home after suffering a broken hip.

Analytical Reflection and Discussion
1. The needs of each can be different based on age, gender role, or cultural background. Explain how you account for these differences.
2. Describe any common themes in the types of information each group decided it needed to make a complete assessment.
3. Construct a scenario demonstrating your use of the knowledge gained from this exercise to show how you apply information in your clinical practice.

Institutional policies and federal law provide specific guidelines that all health care providers are required to follow. The patient's right to have personal control over personal information is upheld through legal regulations. The Code of Ethics of ANA (2015) specifically addresses the nurse's responsibility to safeguard the patient's right to privacy.

Health Insurance Portability and Accountability Act Regulatory Compliance

In the United States, federal legislation, known as the HIPAA of 1996, went into effect in 2003 to protect patient privacy. The goals of HIPAA regulations are to assure that individual's information is protected while allowing the flow of information needed to provide quality care. A nurse is obligated to protect confidential information, unless required by law to disclose that information. Healthcare providers must provide patients with a written notice of their privacy practices and procedures. Agencies are audited for compliance. The key elements of the HIPAA privacy regulations are presented in Box 3.4.

HIPAA privacy rules govern the use and disbursement of individually identifiable health information, and give individuals the right to determine and restrict access to their health information. Patients have the right to access their medical records, request copies, and/or request amendments to health information contained in the record. The Fair Health Information Practices Act of 1997 stipulates civil and criminal penalties for not allowing patients to review their medical records. HIPAA regulations protect the confidentiality, accuracy, and availability of all electronic protected information, whether created, received, or transmitted. Strict maintenance of written records in a protected, private environment is required. Other potential issues of concern about privacy involve cell phones, picture taking, the use of handheld devices, the use of fax machines, Internet user ID and passwords, and the use of electronic monitoring devices.

Health care providers must get written authorization before disclosing personal medical information. Written authorization is not required in situations concerning the public's health, criminal and legal matters, quality assurance, and aggregate record reviews for accreditation. Information can be shared among health care providers. The Office of Civil Rights enforces HIPAA regulations. Agencies and providers face severe penalties for violations, with improper disclosure of medical information punishable by fines or imprisonment. Study the policies in your area to determine to whom and under what conditions personal health information can be released. More information can be obtained through the web site (www.hhs.gov/hipaa/for-professionals/privacy/laws-regulations). Accessed 9/24/18.

BOX 3.4 Overview of Federal HIPAA Guidelines Protecting Patient Confidentiality

- All medical records and other individually identifiable health information used or disclosed in any form, whether electronically, on paper, or orally, are covered by HIPAA regulations.
- Providers and health plans are required to give patients a clear written explanation of how their health information may be used and disclosed.
- Patients are able to see and get copies of their own records and request amendments.
- Health care providers are required to obtain consent before sharing their information for treatment, payment, and health care operations. Patients have the right to request restrictions on the uses and disclosures of their information.
- People have the right to file a formal complaint with a covered provider or health plan, or with the US Department of Health and Human Services (DHHS), about violations of Health Insurance Portability and Accountability Act (HIPAA) regulations.
- Health information may not be used for purposes not related to health care (e.g., disclosures to employers to make personnel decisions) without explicit authorization.
- Disclosure of information is limited to the minimum necessary for the purpose of the disclosure.
- Written privacy procedures must be in place to cover anyone who has access to protected information related to how information will be used and disclosed.
- Training must be provided to employees about the use of HIPAA privacy procedures.
- Health plans, providers, and clearinghouses that violate these standards will be subject to civil liability, and if knowingly violating patient privacy for personal advantage, can be subject to criminal liability.
- Use and disclosure is permitted for treatment, payment, and health care operations activities; for notification; for public health for preventing or controlling disease to lessen an imminent threat; or in cases of abuse, disclosure is permitted to government authorities.

Adapted from Health Insurance Portability and Accountability Act (HIPAA) Guidelines: www.hss.gov/ocr/privacy.

The Joint Commission Privacy Regulations

In the United States, TJC requires agencies to have written privacy policies, to orient the staff to these policies, and to demonstrate staff awareness of their privacy policy (Joint Commission, 2017).

Ethical Responsibility to Protect Patient Privacy in Clinical Situations

In addition to legally mandated informational privacy, informal protection of the patient's right to control the access of others to one's person in clinical situations is an ethical responsibility. Simple strategies that nurses can use to protect the patient's right to privacy in clinical situations include:

- Providing privacy for the patient and family when disturbing matters are to be discussed
- Explaining procedures to patients before implementing them
- Entering another person's personal space with warning (e.g., knocking or calling the patient's name) and, preferably, waiting for permission to enter
- Providing an identified space for personal belongings
- Encouraging the inclusion of personal and familiar objects on the nightstand
- Decreasing direct eye contact during hands-on care
- Minimizing body exposure to what is absolutely necessary for care
- Using only the necessary number of people during any procedure
- Using touch appropriately

Confidentiality

Protecting the privacy of patient information and confidentiality are related, but separate concepts. **Confidentiality** is defined as providing *only* the information needed to provide care for the patient to other health professionals who are directly involved in their care. The assurance of confidentiality reflects ethical principles such as autonomy and beneficence (Alderman, 2017). These are discussed in Chapter 4. This information on a "need to know" basis should be made clear to each patient as they enter the clinical setting. Other than these individuals, the nurse must have the patient's written permission to share their private communication, unless the withholding of information would result in harm to them or to someone else, or in cases where abuse is suspected. Confidential information about the patient cannot be shared with the family or other interested parties without the patient or designated legal surrogate's written permission. Shared confidential information, unrelated to identified health care needs, should not be communicated or charted in the patient's medical record.

Confidentiality within the nurse-patient relationship involves the nurse's legal responsibility to guard against invasion of the patient's privacy related to the following:

- Releasing information to unauthorized parties
- Unwanted visitations in the hospital
- Discussing patient problems in public places or with people not directly involved in their care or on any social media platform

- Taking pictures without consent or using the photographs without the patient's permission
- Performing procedures, such as testing for human immunodeficiency virus, without permission
- Publishing data about a patient in any way that makes them identifiable without their permission

Professional Sharing of Confidential Information

Nursing reports and interdisciplinary team case conferences are acceptable forums for the discussion of health-related communications shared by patients or families. Other venues include change-of-shift reports, one-on-one conversations with other health professionals about specific care issues, and patient-approved consultations with their families. Select agencies, such as insurance companies, can also access information during audits. Discussion of patient care should take place in a private room with the door closed. Only relevant information specifically related to assessment or treatment should be shared. Discussing private information casually with other health professionals, such as in the lunch room or on social media, is an abuse of confidentiality. The ethical responsibility to maintain patient confidentiality continues even after discharge.

Mandatory Reporting

Disclosure should be limited (ANA, 2001). However, under certain circumstances you are required to report patient personal health information. Certain communicable or sexually transmitted diseases, child and elder abuse, and the potential for serious harm to another individual are considered exceptions to the sharing of confidential information. Legally required mandatory disclosures may differ slightly across states or provinces. In general, nurses are required to report all notifiable infectious diseases and abuse to appropriate state and local reporting agencies. This duty to report supersedes the patient's right to confidentiality or privileged communication with a health provider. Relevant data should be released only to the appropriate agency and handled as confidential information. The information provided must be the minimum amount needed to accomplish the purposes of disclosure, and the patient should be informed about what information will be disclosed, to whom, and for what reason(s).

Informed Consent

Informed consent is defined as giving care acquiescence knowing the purpose, the extent of the risks and benefits, and the possible alternatives of treatment (AHRQ, n.d.). Ethical principles, such as autonomy (self-determination) and beneficence, are the basis for **informed consent.** In today's health care market, legal decision making requires that you educate patients about their care. Informed consent is a patient safety issue and a patient-centered care issue, but primarily it is a legal right protected by common law and case law. It is a focused communication process in which you provide all relevant information related to a procedure or treatment, offering full opportunity for discussion, questions, and expressions of concern, before asking the patient or health care agent to sign a legal consent form. EBP indicates that you use more than one method for educating each patient about the procedure (Mahjoub & Rutledge, 2011). Unless there is a life-threatening emergency, all patients have the right to decide about whether to consent. Internationally, part of the ICN Code of Ethics says that nurses ensure that the individual receives accurate, sufficient, and timely information in a culturally appropriate manner on which to base consent for care and related treatment, supporting their right to choose or refuse treatments (ICN, 2012). Box 3.5 lists elements that must be part of an informed consent for it to be legal.

Allowing a patient to sign a consent form without fully understanding the meaning invalidates the legality of consent. Ending the conversation leading to the actual signing of the consent form should always include the question, "Is there anything else that you think might be helpful in making your decision?" This type of dialogue gives the patient permission to ask a question or address concerns.

Nurses are accountable for verifying the competency of a patient to give consent. Only legally competent adults can give legal consent; adults who are mentally retarded, developmentally disabled, or cognitively impaired cannot give legal consent. Evaluation of competency is made on an individual basis (e.g., in the case of emancipated adolescents no longer under their parent's control, brain-injured patients, or those with early dementia) to determine the extent to which they understand what they are signing.

BOX 3.5 Elements of a Legally Valid Informed Consent

- Is a patient-based decision
- Is signed voluntarily, without coercion
- Patient has full knowledge of purpose, risks, benefits
- Nurse has verified patient is competent to make decision
- Patient has knowledge of possible alternative procedures
- Patient knows they have the right to refuse or discontinue care
- If risk is involved, a written consent form is signed (and witnessed) except in emergencies

---

Surrogates. Legislation globally stipulates that a legal guardian or personal health care agent can provide consent for the medical treatment of adults who lack the capacity to consent on their own behalf. In most cases, legal guardians or parents must give legal consent for minor children, who are defined as those younger than 18, unless the youth is legally considered an emancipated minor.

Duration. There is no recommended duration of consent unless it is stipulated in the document, so a form could address repeated procedures. But a new consent form should be signed if the patient's condition changes. Many agencies require that the signature on a consent form be witnessed.

Malpractice. One legal definition is professional nursing standard measured negligence: performing duties or omitting to do what a prudent nurse would do in the same situation in this community, which causes some injury or harm to the patient (Ballard et al., 2016; Smith, 2016). The reasons for rising rates on claims against nurses include failure to communicate risk issues to other staff, as well as fatigue, medication error, etc. (Brown, 2016). All nurses are advised to carry their own malpractice insurance even if their employer has coverage. Remember to document everything about changes in patient condition, including who was notified and what outcome followed this notification.

Use of Social Media

Postings on social media platforms are an everyday happening for many. Powerful sites, such as Facebook, Twitter, LinkedIn, Myspace, Snapchat, etc., use the Internet to connect relationships, transforming the way people interact.

Advances

Social media is transforming traditional nurse-patient interactions. By allowing us to communicate with hundreds of people simultaneously we potentially have the power to provide health care information and support. We do need to differentiate between general open-to-all social sites, even with privacy settings, and secure restricted sites such as those created by care agencies for internal professional staff use. "A post is forever" is a useful mantra.

Privacy Cautions

TJC has acknowledged instant messaging has a place, but so far they have not given approval for using e-messaging for physician orders, or for conveying other data. Governmental agency privacy regulations apply to you in your off-duty time as well as during clinical time. Students cannot, at any time, reveal private health information. This includes posting any pictures taken in a clinical facility or during a home health care visit. Read about Cassie in the case study.

Case Example

Cassie takes great pleasure in the semester-long home visit assignment caring for Clyde, age 4, who has severe cerebral palsy. She feels this is a great learning experience and that she is contributing to Clyde's progress. Today she uses her smart phone to snap a really cute pic of him enjoying his first ice cream cone and shares it with her friends, later posting it on her Facebook page.

According to the National Council of State Boards of Nursing (NCSBN), nurses breach patient privacy when they post enough to allow recognition of a patient, or when they post degrading information (NCSBN, 2011).

Consequences for violations can be severe. Student nurses have been dismissed from their schools; State boards have censured, fined, or even revoked the license to practice. Violations of privacy laws also carry a risk of civil law suits and sanctions such as fines for the individual. The misuse of electronic communication also has consequences for educational programs, placing in jeopardy the school's relationship with a community agency they rely on for clinical experiences.

Blurring Between Professional Role and Personal Life

People have become accustomed to posting so much on social media sites that they sometimes don't stop to think about whether a posting violates patient privacy laws or ethical nurse conduct. We need to differentiate between our personal posts and our professional duty to protect patient privacy and confidentially, and to avoid potential harm to patients, coworkers, or employers. As Westrick (2016) comments, we need to use extreme caution when discussing any patient-related experience. Refer to ANA's "Six tips for nurses using Social Media" (www.nurseworld.org), part of their "Social Networking Principles Toolkit" (2011). Table 3.2 lists social media use guidelines compiled from multiple organizations to help you reflect on this issue. Articles note the difficulty beginning nursing students have in translating a cautionary lecture about social media use into behavior. Recommendations include using senior students as peer teachers, feeling that their experiences with social media problems will have greater credibility and relevance (Marnocha, Marnocha, Cleveland, Limberg, & Wnuk, 2017).

SUMMARY

This chapter addresses major factors effecting current nursing communication. Standards issued by various agencies and organizations guide nurses in their communications with and about patients. Standards provide a measurement benchmark, which is used to assess nursing competency as they apply evidence-based practice and clinical guidelines. Ethical and legal aspects of nursing communication, especially HIPAA privacy regulations, have been described. The ANA Standards for Communication and ANA's Code of Ethics for Nurses provide important guides to the choice of communication. The nursing process serves as a clinical management framework, and communication is woven into each of the steps. All phases are patient-centered, where the patient is an active participant and decision maker. The importance of maintaining the patient's privacy and confidentiality have been stressed, especially with regard to posts on social media platforms.

> **ETHICAL DILEMMA: What Would You Do?**
> As a student nurse, you observe a staff nurse making a medication error, but you are not able to intervene. She is visibly upset by her error. The patient was not actually harmed by the medication error, but the nurse hesitates to report the error. What would you do?

DISCUSSION QUESTIONS

1. Identify three ways to communicate effectively with each member of your patient's health care team.

2. Assemble some examples of nurses choosing not to follow written standards for communication, and then critique these examples.

REFERENCES

Agency for Healthcare and Quality (AHRQ). Teaching module: making informed consent an informed choice. www.ahrq.gov/sites/default/files/ wysiwyg/professionals/systems/hospitals/implementation-guide-making-informed-consent-informed-choice.pdf/. n.d.

Alderman, E. M. (2014). Confidentiality in pediatric and adolescent gynecology: When we can, when we can't, and when we're challenged. *Journal of Pediatric & Adolescent Gynecology, 30*(2), 176–183.

Al-Mowani, M., Al-Barmawi, Al-Hadid, L., & Aljabery, A. (2016). Developing a tool that explores factors influencing the adoption of evidence-based principles in nursing practice in Jordan. *Applied Nursing Research, 32*, 122–127.

Altmiller, G., & Dolanski, M. A. (2017). Quality and safety education for nurses. *Nurse Educator, 42*(5S), S1–S2.

Amer, K. S. (2013). *Quality and safety for transformational nursing: Core competencies.* Boston: Pearson Inc, Personal communication, 2017.

American Association of Colleges of Nursing (AACN). (2006). Hallmarks of quality and safety. *Journal of Professional Nursing, 22*(6), 329–330.

American Association of Critical Care Nurses (AACCN). (2008). *Public policy statement: Moral distress.* http://www.aacn.org/wd/practice/docs/moral-distress.pdf. Accessed 9/19/18.

American Nurses Association (ANA). (2015). Code of ethics. www.nursingworld.org.

American Nurses Association (ANA). (2010). *Nursing: Scope and standards of practice* (ed 2). Silver Spring, MD: Author. www.nursingworld.org/practice-policy/nursing_excellence/ethicsfor nurses/code-of-ethics. Accessed 9/19/18.

ANA Social Networking privacy toolkit,: ANAs Principles for Social Networking and the Nurse: Guidance for Registered Nurses. Silver Spring, Md., (2011). www.nursingworld.org/.

Aspden, P., Wolcott, J., Bootman, J. L., & Cronenwett, L. R. (2007). *Committee on identifying and preventing medication errors: Preventing medication errors: Quality chasm series.* Washington, DC: National Academies Press. www.nap.edu.

Ballard, K., Haagenson, D., Christiansen, L., Damgaard, G., Halstead, J. A., Jason, R. R., et al. (2016). Scope of nursing practice decision-making framework. *Journal of Nursing Regulation, 7*(3), 19–21.

Barnsteiner, J. (May, 2017). Opening remarks. QSEN National Conference. Chicago, Il.

Barnsteiner, J., Disch, J., Johnson, J., McGuinn, K., Chappell, K., & Swartwout, E. (2013). Diffusing QSEN competencies across Schools of Nursing: The AACN/RWJF faculty development institutes. *Journal of Professional Nursing, 29*(2), 1–8.

Brown, G. (2016). Averting malpractice issues in today's nursing practice. *ABNF*, 25–27 (Spring).

Canadian Nurses Association: The code of ethics for registered nurses. Author: Alberta, Canada. http://www.cna-aiic.ca/en. Accessed 9/19/18

Clark, M., Raffray, M., Hendricks, K., & Gagnon, A. J. (2016). Global and public health core competencies for nursing education: a systematic review of essential competencies. *Nurse Education Today, 40*, 173–180.

College of Nurses, Ontario: Entry into practice: Competencies for Ontario registered nurses. www.cno.org/Global/docs/prac/41070_refusing.pdf (practice guidelines: communication).

Cooper, E. (2017). Quality and Safety Education for Nurses implementation: Is it sustainable. *Nurse Educator, 42*(5), S8–S11.

Cronenwett, L., Sherwood, G., Barnsteiner, J., et al. (2007). Quality and safety education for nurses. *Nursing Outlook, 55*(6), 122–131.

Disch, J., & Barnsteiner, J. (2012). Second generation QSEN. *Nursing Clinics of North America, 47*(3), 323–416.

Dolansky, M. A., & Schexnayder, J. (2017). Patrician PA Sales A: New approaches to integrating Quality and Safety education for Nurses: competencies in nursing education. *Nurse Educator, 42*(55), S12–S17.

Gill, F. J., Kendrick, T., Davies, H., & Greenwood, M. (2016). A two phase study to revise the Australian Practice Standards for specialist critical care nurses. *Australian Critical Care*, e1–e9. www.elsevier.com/locate/aucc.

Health Insurance Portability and Accountability Act (HIPAA). (1996). U.S. department of health and human services (DHHS). *Summary of the HIPAA privacy rule.* Accessed 10/17/13 http://www.hhs.gov/ocr/privacy/.

Institute for Healthcare Improvement. (2017). New survey looks at patient experiences with medical error. www.ihi.org/about/news/Documents/IHIPressRelease-Patient-Safety-Survey-Sept28-17.pdf.

Institute of Medicine (IOM) www.nationalacademies.org/HMD

IOM: Crossing the quality chasm: a new health system for the 21st century. (2001). Washington, DC: National Academy Press.

IOM. (2010). *The future of nursing.* Washington, DC: National Academies Press.

IOM/RWJ Report. 2010

International Council of Nurses (ICN). (2012). *The ICN Code of Ethics for Nurses, revised.* www.ICN.ch/about-ICN/code-of-ethics-for-nurses/.

Joint Commission, The (TJC).

TJC. TJC, R3 Report, n.d. pc.02.01.21. www.jointcommission.org/ [search for R3 report]

TJC.. (2017). *Comprehensive accreditation manual for hospitals.* Chicago: Author.

TJC. National Patient Safety Goals. 2011. www.patient safety.gov/

Jun, J., Kovner, C. T., & Stimpfel, A. W. (2016). Barriers and facilitators of nurses' use of clinical practice guidelines: An integrative review. *International Journal of Nursing Studies, 60*, 54–68.

Leung, K., Trevena, L., & Waters, D. (2016). Development of a competency framework for evidence-based practice in nursing. *Nurse Education Today, 39*, 189–196.

Lowe, N. K. (2015). Nursing, nurses and ethics [editorial]. *JOGNN, 44*, 339–340.

Mahjoub, R., & Rutledge, D. N. (2011). Perceptions of informed consent for care practices: Hospitalized patients and nurses. *Applied Nursing Research, 24*(4), 1–6.

Marnocha, S., Marnocha, M., Cleveland, R., Limberg, C. Y., & Wnuk, J. (2017). A peer-delivered educational intervention to improve nursing student cyberprofessionalism. *Nurse Educator, 42*(5), 245–249.

National Council of State Boards of Nursing (NCSBN), n.d. www.ncsbn.org/ Accessed 9/19/18.

National Nursing Summit. (2015). Executive Summary: A blueprint for 21st century nursing ethics. *Nursing Outlook, 63*(4), 379–383. www.bioethicsinstitute.org/nursing-ethics-summit-report.

Nyangeni, T., Du Rand, S., & Van Rooyen, D. (2015). Perceptions of nursing students regarding responsible use of social media in the Eastern Cape. *Curationis* 38(2), Art.#1496, 9 pages, http//dx.doi.org/10.4102/curations. v38i2.1496.

Olson, L. L. (2016). The ANA Code of Ethics for Nurses with interpretive statements: Resource for nursing regulation. *Journal of Nursing Regulation, 7*(2), 9–20.

Quality and Safety for Nurses (QSEN), n.d. www.qsen.org/ competencies/ Accessed 9/19/18.

Quality and Safety Education Quality and Safety Education for Nurses (QSEN) Institute: Lewis Blackman Story. www.qsen.org/.

Reeves, S. A., Denault, D., Huntington, J. T., Ogrinc, G., Southard, D. R., & Vebell, R. (2017). Learning to overcome hierarchical pressures to achieve safer patient care. *Nurse Educator, 42*(5S), S27–S31.

Sales A. *QSEN National Conference, presentation.* (May 29, 2017). Chicago.

Saunders, H., Vehvilainen-Julkenen, K., & Stevens, K. R. (2016). Effectiveness of an educational intervention to strengthen nurses' readiness for evidence based practice: a single-blind randomized controlled study. *Applied Nursing Research, 31*, 175–185.

Sinclair, W., McLoughlin, M., & Warne, T. (2015). To Twitter to Woo: harnessing the power of social media in nurse education to enhance the student's experience. *Nurse Education in Practice, 15*, 507–511.

Smith, J. (2016). Medical malpractice: Nursing issues. *Encyclopedia of Forensic & Legal Medicine, 3*, 451–454.

Warshawski, S., Barnoy, S., & Itzhaki, M. (2017). Factors associated with nursing students' resilience: Communication skills course, use of social media, and satisfaction with clinical placement. *Journal of Professional Nursing, 33*(2), 153–161.

Westrick, S. J. (2016). Nursing students' use of electronic and social media: Law, ethics, and E-professionalism. *Nursing Education Perspectives, 37*(1), 16–22.

White, S., & Spruce, L. (2015). Perioperative nursing leaders implement clinical practice guidelines using Iowa Model of Evidence Based Practice. *AORN Journal, 102*(1), 50–59.

World Health Organization. www.WHO.int.

4

Clinical Judgment: Critical Thinking and Ethical Decision Making

Kathleen Underman Boggs

OBJECTIVES

At the end of the chapter, the reader will be able to:

1. Define patient-centered care communication terms related to thinking, ethical reasoning, and critical thinking.
2. Discuss three principles of ethics underlying bioethical reasoning and apply within the nurse-patient relationship.
3. Describe the 10 steps of critical thinking.
4. Analyze and apply the critical thinking process used in making clinical decisions.
5. Demonstrate ability to analyze, synthesize, and evaluate a complex simulated case situation to make a clinical judgment.
6. Utilize evidenced-based practice competency by discussing the application of findings from research to clinical practice.

This chapter examines the principles of ethical decision making and the process for critical thinking. Both are essential foundational knowledge for you to make effective nursing clinical judgments and to deliver safe, competent care (Kaya, Senyuva, & Brodur, 2017). In addition to developing technical nursing skills, your ability to use critical thinking and ethical reasoning skills and to communicate these will be a determining factor in your competency as a nurse (Trobec & Starcic, 2015). Successfully developing these abilities contributes to success on the NCLEX-RN licensure examination (Romeo, 2010). Ethical responsibility is a big aspect of nursing care. It is a much wider concept than legal responsibility, engaging not only your patients but also your entire community (Tschudin, 2013). Making ethical decisions requires that you understand the process. In this book, the focus is on the current literature in bioethics as held in Western society. In addition to basic content presented in this chapter, an ethical dilemma is included in each subsequent chapter to help you begin applying your reasoning process.

Critical thinking is a learned skill that teaches you how to use a systematic process to make your clinical decisions. In the past, expert nurses accumulated this skill with on-the-job experience, through trial and error. But this essential nursing skill can be learned with continual practice and conscientious applications while in school. The Applications section of this chapter specifically walks you through the reasoning process in applying the 10 steps of critical thinking. Simulation exercises in each chapter help you practice applying these skills.

BASIC CONCEPTS

Types of Thinking

There are many ways of thinking (Fig. 4.1). Students often attempt to use total recall by simply memorizing a bunch of facts (e.g., memorizing the cranial nerves by using a **mnemonic** such as "On Old Olympus' Towering Tops. . ."). At other times, we rely on developing habits by repetition, such as practicing cardiopulmonary resuscitation (CPR) techniques. More structured methods of thinking, such as **inquiry**, have been developed in disciplines related to nursing. For example, you are probably familiar with **the scientific method**. As used in research, this is a logical, linear method of systematically gaining new information, often by setting up an experiment to test an idea. The nursing process uses a method of systematic steps: assessment before planning, planning before intervention, and evaluation.

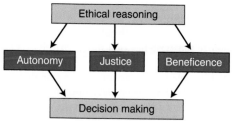

Fig. 4.1 Guiding ethical principles that assist in decision making.

This chapter focuses on the most important concepts that help you develop your clinical judgment abilities.

ETHICAL REASONING

As Trobec and Starcic (2015) say, quality nursing care, in part, depends on nursing values and ethics. Nurses report patient well-being and dignity to be an important value related to giving care. They report feeling distress when forced to act contrary to what they believe is their patient's best interests (Gronlund, Soderberg, Zingmarken, Sandlund, & Darlquist, 2015). Yet we nurses often face moral dilemmas while giving care. Most nurses report facing ethical dilemmas at least on a weekly basis. As care becomes even more complex we will be confronted even more often (Sinclair, Pappas, & Marshall, 2016). The three most commonly reported issues involve patient choice, quality of life, and end-of-life decisions. As a nurse you will frequently have to act in value-laden situations. For example, you may have patients who request abortions or who want "do not resuscitate" (DNR; "no code") orders. Willingness to comply with ethical and professional standards is a hallmark of a professional.

Many professions have difficulty applying ethical principles to clinical care situations. When tested, health care professionals, including physicians and nurses, respond correctly to ethical dilemma questions less than half of the time. Is being ethically correct less than half the time acceptable? Practice in applying ethical principles is important. Although most health care agencies now have ethics committees that often are the primary party involved in resolving difficult ethical dilemmas, you, the nurse, will be called on to make ethical decisions.

As nurses, we need to have a clear understanding of the ethics of the nursing profession. Many nursing organizations have formally published ethical codes to promote ethical care and protect patient rights. Examples include, the Federation of European Countries or the American Nurses Association (ANA, 2015). Refer to ANA's Code of Ethics listed in Chapter 3.

Case Example

During an influenza pandemic, Ada Kelly, RN, is reassigned to work on an unfamiliar pulmonary intensive care unit. Patients there have a severe form of infectious flu with respiratory complications and are receiving mechanical ventilation. She worries that if she refuses to care for these assignments, she could lose her job or even her license. But she also fears carrying this infection home to her two preschool children.

This case highlights conflicting duties: employer/patient versus self/family. According to the ANA, nurses are obligated to care for all patients, but there are limits to the personal risk of harm a nurse can be expected to accept. It is her *moral duty* if patients are at significant risk for harm that her care can prevent. This situation becomes a *moral option* only if there are alternative sources of care (i.e., other nurses available).

Ethical Theories and Decision-Making Models

Ethical theories provide the bedrock from which we derive the principles that guide our decision making. There is no one "right" answer to an ethical dilemma: The decision may vary depending on which theory the involved people subscribe to. The following section briefly describes the most common models currently used in bioethics. They are, for the most part, representative of a Western European and Judeo-Christian viewpoint. As we become a more culturally diverse society, other equally viable viewpoints may become acculturated. This discussion focuses on three decision-making models: utilitarian/goal-based, duty-based, and rights-based models.

The **utilitarian/goal-based model** says that the "rightness" or "wrongness" of an action is always a function of its consequences. Rightness is the extent to which performing or omitting an action will contribute to the overall good of the patient. Good is defined as maximum welfare or happiness. The rights of patients and the duties of a nurse are determined by what will achieve maximum welfare. When a conflict in outcome occurs, the correct action is the one that will result in the greatest good for the majority. An example of a decision made according to the goal-based model is forced mandatory institutionalization of someone with tuberculosis who refuses to take medicine to protect other members of the community. The patient's hospitalization produces the greatest balance of good over harm for the majority. Thus, "goodness" of an action is determined solely by its outcome.

The **dentological** or **duty-based model** is person centered. It incorporates Immanuel Kant's deontological philosophy, which holds that the "rightness" of an action is determined by other factors in addition to its outcome. Respect for every person's inherent dignity is a consideration. For example, a straightforward implication would be that a physician (or nurse) may never lie to a patient. Do you agree? Decisions based on this duty-based model have a religious–social foundation. Rightness is determined by moral worth, regardless of the circumstances or the individual involved. In making decisions or implementing actions, the nurse cannot violate the basic duties and rights of individuals. Decisions about what is in the best interests of the patient require consensus among all parties involved. Examples are the medical code "do no harm" and the nursing duty to "help save lives."

The **human rights-based model** is based on the belief that each patient has basic rights. Our duties as health care providers arise from these basic rights. For example, a patient has the right to refuse care. Conflict occurs when the provider's duty is not in the best interests of the patient. The patient has the right to life and the nurse has the duty to save lives, but what if the quality of life is intolerable and there is no hope for a positive outcome? Such a case might occur when a neonatal nurse cares for an infant with anencephaly (born without brain tissue in the cerebrum) in whom even the least invasive treatment would be extremely painful and would never provide any quality of life.

Ethical dilemmas arise when an actual or potential conflict occurs regarding principles, duties, or rights. Of course, many ethical or moral concepts held by Western society have been codified into law. Laws may vary by country and region, but a moral principle should be universally applied. Moral principles are shared by most members of a group, such as physicians or nurses, and represent the professional values of the group. Conflict arises when a nurse's professional values differ from the law. Conflict may also arise when you have not come to terms with situations in which your personal values differ from the profession's values. One example is doctor-assisted suicide (euthanasia).

Case Example

Francine belongs to the "Socrates Society" whose members believe they have the right of self-termination. *Legally,* at the turn of the 21st century, such an act was legal in Oregon but illegal in Michigan. *Professionally,* the ANA Code of Ethics guides you to do no harm. *Personally,* you believe euthanasia is morally wrong. Can you assist Francine who is now too weak to reach for her suicide pill?

Bioethical Principles

To practice nursing in an ethical manner, you must be able to recognize the existence of a **moral problem**. Once you recognize a situation that puts your patient in jeopardy, you must be able to take action. Three essential, guiding, ethical principles have been developed from the theories cited earlier. The three principles that can assist us in decision making are autonomy, beneficence (nonmaleficence), and justice (Fig. 4.2).

Autonomy Versus Medical Paternalism. Autonomy is the patient's right to self-determination. In the medical context, respect for autonomy is a fundamental ethical principle. It is the basis for the concept of informed consent, which means your patient makes a rational, informed decision without coercion. In the past, nurses and physicians often made decisions for patients based on what they thought was best for them. This *paternalism* sometimes discounted the wishes of patients and their families. The ethical concept of autonomy has emerged strongly as a right in Western countries. Aspects involving the individual's right to participate in medical decisions about his own care have become law in many places.

This moral principle of autonomy means that each patient has the right to decide about his or her health care. Patients who are empowered to make such decisions are more likely to comply with the treatment plan. Internal factors, such as pain, may interfere with a patient's ability to choose. External factors, such as coercion by a care provider, may also interfere. As a nurse, you and your employer must legally obtain the patient's permission for all treatment procedures. In the United States, under the Patient Self-Determination Act of 1991, all patients of agencies receiving Medicaid funds must receive written information about their rights to make decisions about their medical care. Nurses, as well as physicians, must provide them with all the relevant and accurate information they need to make an "informed" decision whether they agree to treatments. Nursing codes, such as the ANA Code, state that it is the nurse's responsibility to assist patients to make these decisions, as discussed in Chapter 3 (see section "Informed Consent").

Many of the nursing theories incorporate concepts about autonomy and empowering the patient to be responsible for self-care, so you may find this easy to accept as part of your nursing role. However, what happens if the patient's right to autonomy puts others at risk? Whose rights take precedence?

The concept of autonomy also has been applied to the way we practice nursing, but our professional autonomy has some limitations. For example, the American

Medical Association's Principles of Medical Ethics says a physician can choose whom to serve, except in an emergency; however, the picture is a little different in nursing practice. According to the ANA Committee on Ethics, nurses are ethically obligated to treat patients seeking their care. A nurse has autonomy in caring for a patient, but this is somewhat limited because legally nurses must also follow physician orders and be subject to physician authority. Before the nurse or physician can override a patient's right to autonomy, he or she must be able to present a strong case for their point of view based on either or both of the following principles: beneficence and justice.

Autonomy Case Example

Ms. Dorothy Newt, 72 years of age, refuses physician-assisted suicide after being diagnosed with Alzheimer disease. She also refuses entry into a long-term care facility, deciding instead to rely on her aged, disabled spouse to provide her total care as she deteriorates physically and mentally. As her home health nurse, you find he is unable to provide the needed care and ask her physician to transfer her to an extended-care facility.

Beneficence and Nonmaleficence

Beneficence implies that a decision results in the greatest good or produces the least harm to the patient. This is based on the Hippocratic Oath and its concept of "do no harm." Avoiding actions that bring harm to another person is known as *nonmaleficence.* An example is the Christian belief of "do not kill," which has been codified into law but has many exceptions (e.g., soldiers sent to war are expected to kill the enemy).

In health care, beneficence is the underlying principle for Nursing Codes of Ethics, saying that the good of your patient is your primary responsibility. Nursing theorists have incorporated this into the nursing role, so you may find this easy to accept. Helping others may be why you chose to become a nurse. In nursing, you not only have the obligation to avoid harming your patients, but you also are expected to advocate for their best interests.

Beneficence is challenged in many clinical situations (e.g., requests for abortion or euthanasia). Currently, some of the most difficult ethical dilemmas involve situations where decisions may be made to withhold treatment. For example, decisions are made to justify such violations of beneficence in the guise of permitting merciful death. Is there a moral difference between actively causing death or in withholding treatment, when the outcome for the patient is the same death? There are clear legal differences. In many places, a health care worker who intentionally acts to cause a patient's death is legally liable.

Other challenges to beneficence occur when the involved parties hold different viewpoints about what is best for the patient. Consider a case in which the family of an elderly, poststroke, comatose, ventilator-dependent patient wants all forms of treatment continued, but the health care team does not believe it will benefit the patient. The initial step toward resolution may be holding a family conference and really listening to the viewpoints of family members, asking them whether their relative ever expressed wishes verbally or in writing in the form of an advance directive or living will. Maintaining a trusting, open, mutually respectful communication may help avoid an adversarial situation.

Beneficence Case Example

Mr. Harper, 62 years of age, is admitted with end-organ failure. You are expected to assess for any pain that he has and treat it. Do you seek a palliative order even though his liver cannot process drugs? It is estimated that more than 50% of conscious patients spend their last week of life in moderate to severe pain. Who is advocating for them?

Justice

Justice is actually a legal term; however, in ethics, it refers to being fair or impartial. A related concept is equality (e.g., the just distribution of goods or resources, sometimes called *social justice* or *distributive justice*). Within the health care arena, this distributive justice concept might be applied to scarce treatment resources. As new and more expensive technologies that can prolong life become available, who has a right to them? Who should pay for them? If resources are scarce, how do we decide who gets them? Should a limited resource be spread out equally to everyone? Or should it be allocated based on who has the greatest need?

Unnecessary Treatment. Decisions made based on the principle of justice may also involve the concept of unnecessary treatment. Are all operations that are performed truly necessary? Why do some patients receive antibiotics for viral infections, when we know they do not kill viruses? Are unnecessary diagnostic tests ever ordered solely to document that a patient does not have condition X, just in case there is a malpractice lawsuit?

Social Worth. Another justice concept to consider in making decisions is that of social worth. Are all people equal? Are some more deserving than others? If Dan is 7 years old instead of 77 years old, and the expensive medicine would cure his condition, should these factors affect the decision to give him the medicine? If there is only one liver available for transplant today, and there are two equally viable potential recipients—Larry, age 54 years, whose alcoholism destroyed his own liver; or Kay, age 32 years, whose liver was destroyed by hepatitis she got while on a life-saving mission abroad—who should get the liver?

Veracity. Truthfulness is the bedrock of trust. And trust is an essential component of the professional nurse-patient relationship. Not only is there a moral injunction against lying, but it is also destructive to any professional relationship. Generally, nurses would agree that a nurse should never lie to a patient. However, there is controversy about withholding information. We need clarity about truth telling. There will be times when we need to exercise some judgment about to whom to disclose information. We have an obligation to protect potentially vulnerable patients from information that would cause emotional distress. Although it is never acceptable to lie, nurses have evaded answering questions by saying, "You need to ask your physician about that." Can you suggest another response?

Justice Case Example

Lee, age 18 years, is admitted to the emergency department (ED) bleeding from a chest wound. His blood pressure is falling, shock is imminent. Tomas, Sue, and Mary were registered ahead of Lee, but do not have life-threatening complaints. ED's triage protocol says care for the least stable patient is a priority. Is this a "just distribution" of ED resources?

Steps in Ethical Decision Making

The process of moral reasoning and making ethical decisions has been broken down into steps. These steps are only a part of the larger model for critical thinking. If you are the moral agent making this decision, you must be skillful enough to implement the actions in a morally correct way.

In deciding how to spend your limited time with these patients, do you base your decision entirely on how much good you can do for each one? Under distributive justice, what should happen when the needs of these four conflict? You could base your decision on the principle of beneficence and do the greatest good for the most patients, but this is a very subjective judgment. In using ethical decision-making processes, nurses must be able to tolerate ambiguity and uncertainty. One of the most difficult aspects for the novice nurse to accept is that there often is no one "right" answer; rather, usually several options may be selected, depending on the person or situation.

Ethical Decision-Making Case Example

You are assigned to four critical patients on your unit. Mrs. Rae, 83 years of age, is unconscious, dying, and needs suctioning every 10 minutes. Mr. Jones, 47 years of age, has been admitted for observation for severe bloody stools. Mr. Hernandez, 52 years of age, has newly diagnosed diabetes and is receiving intravenous (IV) drip insulin; he requires monitoring of vital signs every 15 minutes. Mr. Martin, 35 years of age, is suicidal and has been told today he has inoperable cancer. Would one of them benefit more from nursing care than the others?

CRITICAL THINKING

Critical thinking is the basis of all our clinical reasoning, problem solving, and decision making. Critical thinking is a complex, analytical method of thinking, in which you purposefully use specific thinking skills to make clinical decisions. You are able to reflect on your own thinking process to make effective interventions that improve your patient's outcome. Although no consensus has been reached on a critical thinking definition in the nursing arena, we generally define critical thinking as the purposeful use of a specific cognitive framework to identify and analyze problems. Critical thinking enables us to recognize emergent situations, make clear, objective, clinical decisions, and intervene appropriately to give safe, effective care. It encompasses the steps of the nursing process, but possibly in a more circular loop than we usually envision the nursing process. By thinking critically, we can modify our care based on responses to these nursing interventions.

Characteristics of a Critical Thinker in Making Clinical Decisions

PROCESS. Critical thinkers are skilled at using inquiry methods. They approach problem solutions in a systematic, organized, and goal-directed way when making clinical decisions. They continually use past knowledge, communication skills, new information, and observations to make these clinical judgments. Table 4.1 summarizes the characteristics of a critical thinker.

ACT. Expert nurses recognize that priorities change continually, requiring constant assessment and alternative interventions. When the authors analyzed the decision-making process of expert nurses, they all used the critical thinking steps described in this chapter when they made their clinical judgments, even though they were not always able to verbally state the components of their thinking processes. Expert nurses organized each input of patient information

TABLE 4.1	**Characteristics of a Critical Thinker**
KNOWLEDGE [thought processes]	• Be reflective and anticipate consequences • Combine existing knowledge and standards with new information (transformation) • Incorporate creative thinking • Recognize when information is missing and seek new input • Discard irrelevant information (discrimination) • Effectively interpret existing data • Consider alternative solutions
SKILLS	• Think in an orderly way, using logical reasoning in complex problem situations • Diligently persevere in seeking relevant information • Recognize deviations from expected patterns • Revise actions based on new input • Evaluate solutions and outcomes
ATTITUDE	• Be inquisitive, desire to seek the truth • Seek to develop analytical thinking • Maintain open-mindedness and flexibility

and quickly distinguished relevant from irrelevant information. They seemed to categorize each new fact into a problem format, obtaining supplementary data and arriving at a decision about diagnosis and intervention. Often, they commented about comparing this new information with prior knowledge, sometimes from academic sources and "best practice protocols" but most often from information gained from other nurses. They constantly scan for new information, and constantly reassess their patient's situation. This is not linear. New input is always being added. This contrasts with novice nurses who tend to think in a linear way, collect lots of facts but not logically organize them, and fail to make as many connections with past knowledge. Novice nurses' assessments are more generalized and less focused, and they tend to jump too quickly to a diagnosis without recognizing the need to obtain more facts.

REFLECT. Critical thinking is more than just a *cognitive process* of following steps. It also has an *affective component*—the willingness to engage in self-reflective inquiry. Most nurse educators say this sense of inquiry is crucial (Carter, Creedy, & Sidebotham, 2016). As you learn to

be a critical thinker, you improve and clarify your thinking process skills, reflect on this process, and learn from the situation so that you are more accurately able to solve problems based on available evidence (Johnsen, Fossum, Vivekananda-Schmidt, Fruhling, & Slettebo, 2016). An attitude of openness to new learning is essential. Although cognitive thinking skills can be taught, you also need to be willing to consciously choose to apply this process.

Barriers to Thinking Critically and Reasoning Ethically

Attitudes and Habits

Barriers that decrease a nurse's ability to think critically, including attitudes such as "my way is better," interfere with our ability to empower patients to make their own decisions. Our thinking habits can also impede communication with patients or families making complex bioethical choices. Examples include becoming accustomed to acknowledging "only one right answer" or selecting only one option. Behaviors that act as barriers include automatically responding defensively when challenged, resisting changes, and desiring to conform to expectations. Cognitive barriers, such as thinking in stereotypes, also interfere with our ability to treat a patient as an individual.

Cognitive Dissonance

Cognitive dissonance refers to the mental discomfort you feel when there is a discrepancy between what you already believe and some new information that does not go along with your view. In this book, we use the term to refer to the holding of two or more conflicting values at the same time.

Personal Values Versus Professional Values

We all have a *personal value system* developed over a lifetime that has been extensively shaped by our family, our religious beliefs, and our years of life experiences. Our values change as we mature in our ability to think critically, logically, and morally. Strongly held values become a part of self-concept. Our education as nurses helps us acquire a *professional value system*. In nursing school, as you advance through your clinical experiences, you begin to take on some of the values of the nursing profession (Box 4.1). You are acquiring these values as you learn the nursing role. The process of this role socialization is discussed in Chapter 22. For example, maintaining patient confidentiality is a professional value, with both a legal and a moral requirement. We must take care that we do not allow our personal values to obstruct care for a patient who holds differing values.

Values Clarification and the Nursing Process

The nursing process offers many opportunities to incorporate *values clarification* into your care. During the

BOX 4.1   Five Core Values of Professional Nursing

Five *core values of professional nursing* have been identified by the American Association of Colleges of Nursing:

- Human dignity
- Integrity
- Autonomy
- Altruism
- Social justice

assessment phase, you can obtain an assessment of the *patient's values* with regard to the health system. For example, you interview Mr. Smith for the first time and learn that he has obstructive pulmonary disease and is having difficulty breathing, but he insists on smoking. Is it appropriate to intervene? In this example, you know that smoking is detrimental to a person's health and you, as a nurse, find the value of health in conflict with his value of smoking. It is important to understand your patient's values. When your values differ, you attempt to care for this patient within his or her reality. In this example, Mr. Smith has the right to make decisions that are not always congruent with those of health care providers.

When identifying specific nursing diagnoses, it is important that your diagnoses are not biased. Examples of value conflicts might be spiritual distress related to a conflict between spiritual beliefs and prescribed health treatments, or ineffective family coping related to restricted visiting hours for a family in which full family participation is a cultural value. In the planning phase, it is important to identify and understand the patient's value system as the foundation for developing the most appropriate interventions. Plans of care that support rather than discount the patient's health care beliefs are more likely to be received favorably. Your interventions include values clarification as a guideline for care. You help patients examine alternatives. During the evaluation phase, examine how well the nursing and patient goals were met while keeping within the guidelines of the patient's value system.

To summarize, in case of conflict (with own personal ethical convictions), nurses must put aside their own moral convictions to provide necessary assistance in a case of emergency when there is imminent risk to a patient's life. Ethical reasoning and critical thinking skills are essential competencies for making clinical judgments, in an increasingly complex health care system. To apply critical thinking to a clinical decision we need to base our intervention on the best evidence available. Developing higher levels of critical thinking is a learned ability (Van Graan, 2016).

DEVELOPING AN EVIDENCE-BASED PRACTICE   The purpose of this study was to compare the impact of two teaching methods on ethical reasoning. Active online learning outcomes were compared with classroom teaching outcomes for 436 Slovenian nursing students. Pre- and posttests measured the comprehension and application to real life ethical problems.

Results: After initial lectures, students developed their abilities through active engagement in group work, role-play, and discussion either online or in the classroom. No differences were found between groups. Both methods resulted in the development of ethical competencies, communication competencies, interpersonal skills, critical thinking, and collaboration. Online students reported they missed face-to-face contact, which reveals much via nonverbal communication.

Application to practice: This type of active learning has also been shown to help students develop their critical thinking skills needed for clinical reasoning (Costello, 2017). In this study's active learning environment, students cited the importance of collaboration and communication in developing their own learning. If we apply this to patient learning, it suggests a need to actively engage patients in their learning process.

Clinical decision: We need to base our intervention on *the best evidence* available to provide quality care. As health care becomes increasingly complex, and care shifts from hospital to home, nurses need to use high levels of thinking (Johnsen et al., 2016). Your ability to use the critical thinking process in making tough clinical decisions is a learned ability (Van Graan, Williams, & Koen, 2016).

Skills can be learned by participating in simulated patient case situations. According to Nelson (2017) and others, accepted teaching-learning methods for assessing critical thinking include use of case studies, questioning, reflective journalism, portfolios, concept maps, and problem-based learning

From Trobec, I., & Starcic, A. I. (2015). Developing nursing ethical competencies online versus in the traditional classroom. *Nursing Ethics, 22*(3), 352–366.

APPLICATIONS

Accrediting agencies for nursing curriculum require the inclusion of content on critical thinking. Accepted methods for accessing your critical thinking abilities include case study analysis, questioning, reflective journaling, patient simulations, portfolios, concept mapping, and problem-based learning.

EXERCISE 4.1 Autonomy

Purpose

To stimulate class discussion about the moral principle of autonomy.

Procedure

In small groups, read the three case examples in this chapter and discuss whether the patient has the autonomous right to refuse treatment if it affects the life of another person.

Reflective Analysis

Prepare your argument for an in-class discussion.

EXERCISE 4.2 Beneficence

Purpose

To stimulate discussion about the moral principle of beneficence.

Procedure

Read the following case example and prepare for discussion:

Dawn, a staff nurse, answers the telephone and receives a verbal order from Dr. Smith. Ms. Patton was admitted this morning with ventricular arrhythmia. Dr. Smith orders Dawn to administer a potent diuretic, furosemide (Lasix) 80 mg, IV, STAT. This is such a large dose that she has to order it up from pharmacy.

As described in the text, you are legally obliged to carry out a doctor's orders unless they threaten the welfare of your patient. How often do nurses question orders? What would happen to a nurse who questioned orders too often? In a research study using this case simulation, nearly 95% of the time the nurses participating in the study attempted to implement this potentially lethal medication order before being stopped by the researcher!

Reflective Analysis

1. What principles are involved?
2. What would you do if you were this staff nurse?

EXERCISE 4.3 Justice

Purpose

To encourage discussion about the concept of justice.

Procedure

Consider that in order to contain costs, several years ago the state of Oregon attempted to legislate restrictions on what Medicaid would pay for. A young boy needed a standard treatment of bone marrow transplant for his childhood leukemia. He died when the state refused to pay for his treatment.

Read the following case example and in a small group answer the discussion questions:

Mr. Diaz, aged 74 years, has led an active life and continues to be the sole support for his wife and disabled daughter. He pays for health care with Medicare government insurance. The doctors think his cancer may respond to a very expensive new drug, which is not paid for under his coverage.

Discussion

1. Does everyone have a basic right to health care, as well as to life and liberty?
2. Does an insurance company have a right to restrict access to care?

SOLVING ETHICAL DILEMMAS AS PART OF CLINICAL DECISION MAKING

Nurses indicate a need for more information about dealing with the ethical dilemmas they encounter, yet most say they receive little education in doing so. Exercises 4.1 (autonomy), 4.2 (beneficence), and 4.3 (justice) give you this opportunity.

The ethical issues that nurses commonly face today can be placed in three general categories: moral uncertainty, moral or ethical dilemmas, and moral distress. *Moral uncertainty* occurs when a nurse is uncertain as to which moral rules (i.e., values, beliefs, or ethical principles) apply to a given situation. For example, should a terminally ill patient who is in and out of a coma and chooses not to eat or drink anything be required to have IV therapy for hydration purposes? Does giving IV therapy constitute giving the patient extraordinary measures to prolong life? Is it more comfortable or less comfortable for the dying person to maintain a high hydration level? When there is no clear definition of the problem, moral uncertainty develops, because the nurse is unable to identify the situation as a moral problem or to define specific moral rules that apply. Strategies that might be useful in dealing with moral uncertainty include using the values clarification process, developing a specific philosophy of nursing, and acquiring knowledge about ethical principles.

Ethical or moral dilemmas arise when two or more moral issues are in conflict. An ethical dilemma is a problem in which there are two or more conflicting but equally right answers. Organ harvesting of a severely brain-damaged infant is an example of an ethical dilemma. Removal of organs from one infant may save the lives of several other infants. However, even though the brain-damaged child is definitely going to die, is it right to remove organs before the child's death? It is important for the nurse to understand that, in many ethical dilemmas, there is often no single "right" solution. Some decisions may be "more right" than others, but often what one nurse decides is best differs significantly from what another nurse would decide.

The third common kind of ethical problem seen in nursing today is *moral distress.* Moral distress results when the nurse knows what is "right" but is bound to do otherwise because of legal or institutional constraints. When such situations arise (e.g., a terminally ill patient who does not have a "do not resuscitate" medical order and therefore resuscitation attempts must be made), nurses may experience inner turmoil (American Association of Colleges of Nursing [AACN], 2008).

Nurses have reported that three of their most commonly encountered ethics problems have to do with resuscitation decisions for dying patients lacking clear code orders; patients and families who want more aggressive treatment; and colleagues who discuss patients inappropriately.

Because values underlie all ethical decision making, nurses must understand their own values thoroughly before making an ethical decision. Instead of responding in an emotional manner on the spur of the moment (as people often do when faced with an ethical dilemma), the nurse who uses the values clarification process can respond rationally. It is not an easy task to have sufficient knowledge of oneself, of the situation, and of legal and moral constraints to be able to implement ethical decision making quickly. Expert nurses still struggle and still have uncertainties (Gronlund et al., 2015). Taking time to examine situations can help you develop skills in dealing with ethical dilemmas in nursing, and the exercises in this book will give you a chance to practice. Each chapter in this book has included at least one ethical dilemma, so you can discuss what you would do.

As nurses, we advocate for our patient's best interests. To do so, we avoid a "paternalistic" imposing of what we think is in their best interests, instead listening and eliciting their preferences, to work collaboratively with the health care team in developing an ethical patient-centered plan of care. Issues most frequently necessitating ethical decisions occur at the beginning of life and at the close of life.

Finally, reflect on your own ethical practice. How important is it for your client to be able to always count on you? Consider the following journal entry (Milton, 2002):

> I ask for information, share my needs, to no avail. You come and go…
> "Could you find out for me?" "Sure, I'll check on it."
> [But] check on it never comes…

> Who can I trust? I thought you'd be here for me…
> You weren't. What can I do?
> Betrayal permeates…

PROFESSIONAL VALUES ACQUISITION

Professional values or ethics consist of the values held in common by the members of a profession. Professional values are formally stated in professional codes. One example already mentioned is the ANA Code of Ethics for Nurses. Often, professional values are transmitted by tradition in nursing classes and clinical experiences. They are modeled by expert nurses and assimilated as part of the role socialization process during your years as a student and new graduate. Professional values acquisition should perhaps be the result of conscious choice by a nursing student.

APPLYING CRITICAL THINKING TO THE CLINICAL DECISION-MAKING PROCESS

This section discusses a procedure for developing critical thinking skills as applied to solving clinical problems. Different examples illustrate the reasoning process developed by several disciplines. Unfortunately, each discipline has its own vocabulary. Table 4.2 shows that we are talking about concepts with which you are already familiar. It also contrasts terms used in education, nursing, and philosophy to specify 10 steps to help you develop your critical thinking skills. For example, the nurse performs a "patient assessment," which in education is referred to as "collecting information" or in philosophy may be called "identifying claims."

The process of critical thinking is systematic, organized, and goal directed. As critical thinkers, nurses are able to explore all aspects of a complex clinical situation. This is a learned process. Among many teaching-learning techniques helping you develop critical thinking skills, most are included in this book: reflective journaling, concept maps, role-playing, guided small group discussion, and case study discussion. An extensive case application follows. During your learning phase, the critical thinking skills are divided into 10 specific steps. Each step includes a discussion of application to the clinical case example provided.

To help you understand how to apply critical thinking steps, read the following case and then see how each of the steps can be used in making clinical decisions. Components of this case are applied to illustrate the steps and to stimulate discussion in the critical thinking process; many more points may be raised. From the outset, understand that, although these are listed as steps, they do not occur in a rigid, linear way in real life. The model is best thought of as a circular model. New data are constantly being sought and added to the process.

TABLE 4.2 Reasoning Process

Generic Reasoning Process	Diagnostic Reasoning in the Nursing Process	Ethical Reasoning	Critical Thinking Skill
Collect and interpret information	Gordon's functional patterns of health assessment	Identify ethical problem (parties, claim, basis)	1. Clarify concepts 2. Identify own, patient, and professional values and differentiate
Identify problem	Statement of nursing diagnosis	Consider ethical dilemma: • State the problem • Collect additional information • Develop alternatives for analysis	1. Integrate data and identify missing data 2. Collect new data 3. Identify problem 4. Apply criteria 5. Look at alternatives 6. Examine skeptically 7. Check for change in context
Plan for problem solving	Prioritization of problems/interventions	Prioritized claims	1. Make decision, select best action plan, and act to implement
Implement plan	Nursing action	Take moral action	
Evaluate	Outcome evaluation	Moral evaluation of outcome and reflect on the process used	Evaluate the outcome and reflect on the process

Case Example

Day 1—Mrs. Vlios, a 72-year-old widowed teacher, has been admitted to your unit. Her daughter, Sara, lives 2 hours away from her mother, but she arrives soon after admission. According to Sara, her mother lived an active life before admission, taking care of herself in an apartment in a senior citizens' housing development. Sara noticed that for about 3 weeks now, telephone conversations with her mother did not make sense or she seemed to have a hard time concentrating, although her pronunciation was clear. The admitting diagnosis is dehydration and dementia, rule out Alzheimer disease, organic brain syndrome, and depression. An IV drip of 1000 mL dextrose/0.45 normal saline is ordered at 50 drops/hour. Mrs. Vlios's history is unremarkable except for a recent 10-pound weight loss. She has no allergies and is known to take acetaminophen regularly for minor pain.

Day 2—When Sara visits her mom's apartment to bring grooming items to the hospital, she finds the refrigerator and food pantry empty. A neighbor tells her that Mrs. Vlios was seen roaming the halls aimlessly 2 days ago and could not remember whether she had eaten. As Mrs. Vlios's nurse, you notice that she is oriented today (to time and person). A soft diet is ordered, and her urinary output is now normal.

Day 5—In the morning report, the night nurse states that Mrs. Vlios was hallucinating and restraints were applied. A nasogastric tube was ordered to suction out stomach contents because of repeated vomiting. Dr. Green tells Sara and her brother, Todos, that their mother's prognosis is guarded; she has acquired a serious systemic infection, is semi-comatose, is not taking nourishment, and needs antibiotics and hyperalimentation. Sara reminds the doctor that her mother signed a living will in which she stated she refuses all treatment except IVs to keep her alive. Todos is upset, yelling at Sara that he wants the doctor to do everything possible to keep their mother alive.

Step 1: Clarify Concepts

The first step in making a clinical judgment is to identify whether a problem actually exists. Poor decision makers often skip this step. To figure out whether there is a problem, you need to think about what to observe and what basic information to gather. If it is an ethical dilemma, you not only need to identify the existence of the moral problem, but also you need to identify all the interested parties who have a stake in the decision. Figuring out exactly what the problem or issue is may not be as easy as it sounds.

Look for Clues

Are there hidden meanings to the words being spoken? Are there nonverbal clues?

Identify Assumptions

What assumptions are being made?

Case Discussion

This case is designed to present both physiological and ethical dilemmas. In clarifying the problem, address both domains.

- Physiological concerns: Based on the diagnosis, the initial treatment goal was to restore homeostasis. By day 5, is it clear whether Mrs. Vlios's condition is reversible?
- Ethical concerns: When is a decision made to initiate treatment or to abide by the advance directive and respect Mrs. Vlios's wishes regarding no treatment?
- What are the wishes of the family? What happens when there is no consensus?
- Assumptions: Is the diagnosis correct? Does she have dementia? Or was her confusion a result of dehydration and a strange hospital environment?

Step 2: Identify Your Own Values

Values clarification helps you identify and prioritize your values. It also serves as a base for helping patients identify the values they hold as important. Unless you are able to identify your patient's values and can appreciate the validity of those values, you run the risk for imposing your own values. It is not necessary for your values and your patient's values to coincide; this is an unrealistic expectation. However, whenever possible, the patient's values should be taken into consideration during every aspect of nursing care. Discussion of the case of Mrs. Vlios presented in this section may help you with the clarification process.

Having just completed the exercises given earlier should help your understanding of your own personal values and the professional values of nursing. Now apply this information to this case.

Case Discussion

Identify the values of each person involved:

- Family: Mrs. Vlios signed an advance directive. Sara wants it adhered to; Todos wants it ignored. Why? (Missing information: Are there religious beliefs? Is

there unclear communication? Is there guilt about previous troubles in the relationship?)
- Personal values: What are yours?
- Professional values: Nurses are advocates for their patients; beneficence implies nonmaleficence ("do no harm"), but does autonomy mean the right to refuse treatment? What is the agency's policy? What are the legal considerations? Practice refining your professional values acquisition by completing the values exercises in this chapter.

In summary, you need to identify which values are involved in a situation or which moral principles can be cited to support each of the positions advocated by the involved individuals.

Step 3: Integrate Data and Identify Missing Data

Think about knowledge gained in prior courses and during clinical experiences. Try to make connections between different subject areas and clinical nursing practice.

- Identify what data are needed. Obtain all possible information and gather facts or evidence (evaluate whether data are true, relevant, and sufficient). Situations are often complicated. It is important to figure out what information is significant to this situation. Synthesize prior information you already have with similarities in the current situation. Conflicting data may indicate a need to search for more information.
- Compare existing information with past knowledge. Has this patient complained of difficulty thinking before? Does she have a history of dementia?
- Look for gaps in the information. Actively work to recognize whether there is missing information. Was Mrs. Vlios previously taking medications to prevent depression? For a nurse, this is an important part of critical thinking.
- Collect information systematically. Use an organized framework to obtain information. Nurses often obtain a history by asking questions about each body system. They could just as systematically ask about basic needs.
- Organize your information. Clustering information into relevant categories is helpful. For example, gathering all the facts about a patient's breathing may help focus your attention on whether they are having a respiratory problem. In your assessment, you note the rate and character of respirations, the color of nails and lips, the use of accessory muscles, and the grunting noises. At the same time, you exclude information about bowel sounds or deep tendon reflexes as not being immediately relevant to this patient's respiratory status. Categorizing information also helps you notice

whether there are missing data. A second strategy that will help you organize information is to look for patterns. It has been indicated that experienced nurses intuitively note recurrent meaningful aspects of a clinical situation.

Case Discussion

Rely on prior didactic knowledge or clinical experience. Cluster the data. What was Mrs. Vlios's status immediately before hospitalization? What was her status at the time of hospitalization? What information is missing? What additional data do you need?

- Physiology: Consider pathophysiological knowledge about the effects of hypovolemia and electrolyte imbalances on the systems such as the brain, kidneys, and vascular system. What is her temperature? What are her laboratory values? What is her 24-hour intake and output? Is she still dehydrated?
- Psychological/cognitive: How does hospitalization affect older adults? How do restraints affect them?
- Social/economic: Was weight loss a result of dehydration? Why was she without food? Could it be due to economic factors or mental problems?
- Legal: What constitutes a binding advance directive in the state in which Mrs. Vlios lives? Is a living will valid in her state, or does the law require a health power of attorney? Are these documents on file at the hospital?

Step 4: Obtain New Data

Critical thinking is not a linear process. Expert nurses often modify interventions based on the response to the event, or change in the patient's physical condition. Constantly consider whether you need more information. Establish an attitude of inquiry and obtain more information as needed. Ask questions; search for evidence; and check reference books, journals, the ethics sources on the Internet, or written professional or agency protocols.

Evaluate conflicting information. There may be time constraints. If a patient has suspected "respiratory problems," you may need to set priorities. Obtain data that are most useful or are easily available. It would be useful to know oxygenation levels, but you may not have time to order laboratory tests. But perhaps there is a device on the unit or in the room that can measure oxygen saturation.

Sometimes you may need to change your approach to improve your chances of obtaining information. For example, when the charge nurse caring for Mrs. Vlios used an authoritarian tone to try to get the sister and brother to provide more information about possible drug overdose, they did not respond. However, when the charge nurse changed his approach, exhibiting empathy, the daughter

volunteered that on several occasions her mother had forgotten what pills she had taken.

Case Discussion

List sources from which you can obtain missing information. Physiological data such as temperature or laboratory test results can be obtained quickly; however, some of the ethical information may take longer to consider.

Step 5: Identify the Significant Problem

- Analyze existing information: Examine all the information you have. Identify all the possible positions.
- Make inferences: What might be going on? What are the possible diagnoses? Develop a working diagnosis.
- Prioritize: Which problem is most urgently in need of your intervention? What are the appropriate interventions?

Case Discussion

A significant physiological concern is sepsis, regardless of whether it is an iatrogenic (hospital-acquired) infection or one resulting from immobility and debilitation. A significant ethical concern is the conflict among family members and the patient (as expressed through her living will). At what point do spiritual concerns take priority over a worsening physical concern?

Step 6: Examine Skeptically

Thinking about a situation may involve weighing positive and negative factors, and differentiating facts that are credible from opinions that are biased or not grounded in true facts.

- Keep an open mind.
- Challenge your own assumptions.
- Consider whether any of your assumptions are unwarranted. Does the available evidence really support your assumption?
- Discriminate between facts and inferences. Your inferences need to be logical and plausible, based on the available facts.
- Are there any problems that you have not considered?

In trying to evaluate a situation, consciously raising questions becomes an important part of thinking critically. At times there will be alternative explanations or different lines of reasoning that are equally valid. The challenge is to examine your own and others' perspectives for important ideas, complicating factors, other plausible interpretations, and new insights. Some nurses believe that examining information skeptically is part of each step in the critical thinking process rather than a step by itself.

Case Discussion

Challenge assumptions about the cause of Mrs. Vlios's condition. For example, did you eliminate the possibility that she had a head injury caused by a fall? Could she have liver failure as a result of acetaminophen overdosing? Have all the possibilities been explored? Challenge your assumptions about outcome: Are they influenced by expected probable versus possible outcomes for this client? If she, indeed, has irreversible dementia, what will the quality of her life be if she recovers from her physical problems?

Step 7: Apply Criteria

In evaluating a situation, think about appropriate responses.

- Assess standards for "best practices" related to your patient's situation.
- Laws: There may be a law that can be applied to guide your actions and decisions. For example, by law, certain diseases must be reported to the state. If you suspect physical abuse, there is a state statute that requires professionals to report abuse to the Department of Social Services.
- Legal precedents: There may have been similar cases or situations that were dealt with in a court of law. Legal decisions do guide health care practices. In end-of-life decisions, when there is no legally binding health care power of attorney, the most frequent hierarchy is the spouse, then the adult children, then the parents.
- Protocols: There may be standard protocols for managing certain situations. Your agency may have standing orders for caring for Mrs. Vlios if she develops respiratory distress, such as administering oxygen per face mask at 5 L/min.

Case Discussion

Many criteria could be used to examine this case, including the Nurse Practice Act in the area of jurisdiction; the professional organization code of ethics or general ethical principles of beneficence and autonomy; the hospital's written protocols and policies; state laws regarding living wills; and prior court decisions about living wills. Remember that advance directives are designed to take effect only when individuals become unable to make their own wishes known.

Step 8: Generate Options and Look at Alternatives

- Evaluate the major alternative points of view.
- Involve experienced peers as soon as you can to assist you in making your decision.
- Use clues from others to help you "put the picture together."
- Can you identify all the arguments—pros and cons—to explain this situation? Almost all situations will have strong counterarguments or competing hypotheses.

Case Discussion

The important concept is that neither the physician nor the nurse should handle this alone; rather, others should

be involved (e.g., the hospital bioethics committee, the ombudsman client representative, the family's spiritual counselor, and other medical experts such as a gerontologist, psychologist, and nursing clinical specialist).

Step 9: Consider Whether Factors Change if the Context Changes

Consider whether your decision would be different if there were a change in circumstances. For example, a change in their age, in the site of the situation, or in their culture may affect your decision. A competent nurse prioritizes the aspects of a situation that are most relevant and can modify her actions based on the patient's responses. A competent nurse anticipates consequences.

Case Discussion

If you knew the outcome from the beginning, would your decisions be the same? What if you knew Mrs. Vlios had a terminal cancer? What if Mrs. Vlios had remained in her senior housing project and you were the home health nurse? What if Mrs. Vlios had remained alert during her hospitalization and refused IVs, hyperalimentation, nasogastric tubes, and so on? What if the family and Mrs. Vlios were in agreement about no treatment? Would you make more assertive interventions to save her life if she were 7 years old, or a 35-year-old mother of five young children?

Step 10: Evaluate and Make the Intervention

After analyzing available information in this systematic way, you need to make a judgment or decision. An important part of your decision is your ability to communicate it coherently to others and to reflect on health status outcomes.

- Justify your conclusion.
- Evaluate outcomes.
- Test out your decision or conclusion by implementing appropriate actions.

As a critical thinker, you need to be able to accept that there may be multiple solutions that can be equally acceptable. In other situations, you may need to make a decision even when there is incomplete knowledge. Be able to cite your rationale or present your arguments to others for your decision choice and interventions. Revise interventions as necessary.

Clinical Decision Making

While we have yet to arrive at a universal consensus for understanding clinical decision making, many articles cite components of models developed by Levett-Jones et al. (2010), Tanner (2006), Hunter and Arthur (2016), and others. Making clinical decisions is complex. As illustrated in Fig. 4.2, we could perhaps think of decision making

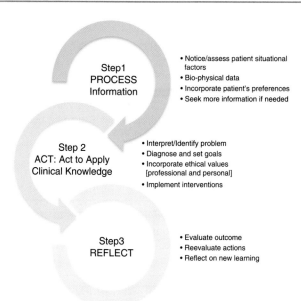

Step 1
PROCESS
Information
- Notice/assess patient situational factors
- Bio-physical data
- Incorporate patient's preferences
- Seek more information if needed

Step 2
ACT: Act to Apply
Clinical Knowledge
- Interpret/Identify problem
- Diagnose and set goals
- Incorporate ethical values [professional and personal]
- Implement interventions

Step 3
REFLECT
- Evaluate outcome
- Reevaluate actions
- Reflect on new learning

Fig. 4.2 The clinical decision-making process.

and intervention as striving to achieve P.A.R. We need to Process, Act, and Reflect in order to provide safe, competent, nursing care.

PROCESS. As a nurse, you are faced with processing copious amounts of information quickly in using our critical thinking skills; we assess patient status and notice factors that characterize our patient's current situation. We incorporate our existing clinical knowledge to help us understand what is happening. This includes processing information from our assessment, from biophysical data, from our knowledge of patient preferences and our understanding of current circumstances.

ACT. Applying our clinical knowledge to identify problems, incorporate ethical values, and set goals, we make appropriate interventions. We recognize the need to continually gather and analyze new information.

REFLECT. After you implement interventions, we examine outcomes. Was your assessment correct? Did you obtain enough information? Did the benefits to the patient and family outweigh the harm that may have occurred? In retrospect, do you know you made the correct decision? Did you anticipate possibilities and complications correctly? Did you communicate with the health team in a timely manner? This kind of self-examination can foster self-correction and learning. Reflecting on one's own thinking is the hallmark of a critical thinker. This self-reflection facilitates our learning.

This is a cyclical nursing care process in which constant reevaluation and reflection on one's actions and subsequent outcomes becomes new input (Lee, Bae, & Seo, 2016).

While the example of Mrs. Vlios described a hospitalized situation, it is even more essential that nurses in the community be able to apply critical thinking to clinical decision making so they may implement safer, evidence-based high-quality care in independent situations. Recognizing and treating deteriorations might prevent hospitalization (Johnsen et al., 2016).

Summarizing the Learning Process

Learning these steps in critical thinking results from repeated application. In addition to using peer discussions of the case studies, recording role-playing of simulated patient situations using standardized patient models or computer-generated problems gives opportunity for practice. A new graduate nurse must, at a minimum, be able to identify essential clinical data, know

---

EXERCISE 4.4   Your Analysis of an Expert's Critical Thinking: Interview of Expert Nurse's Case

Purpose
To develop awareness of critical thinking in the clinical judgment process.

Procedure
Find an experienced nurse in your community and record him or her describing a real patient case. You can use a smart phone to record an interview that takes only a few minutes. During the interview, have the expert describe an actual case in which there was a significant change in the patient's health status. Have the expert describe the interventions and thinking process that took place during this situation. Ask what nursing knowledge, laboratory data, or experience helped the nurse make his or her decision. You can work with a partner. Remember to protect confidentiality by omitting all names and other identifiers.

Reflective Analysis
Analyze the recording using an outline of the 10 steps in critical thinking. Discussion should first include citation examples of each step noted during their review of the recorded interview, followed by application of the broad principles. Discussion of steps missed by the interviewed expert can be enlightening, as long as care is taken to avoid any criticism of the guest "expert."

when to initiate interventions, know why a particular intervention is relevant, and differentiate between problems that need immediate intervention versus problems that can wait for action. Repeated practice in applying critical thinking can help a new graduate fit into the expectations of employers. In addition to lab situations, learning can occur through the analysis of interviews with experienced nurses about their decision making, as described in Exercise 4.4.

Try responding to the Gonzales case example.

> **Case Example**
> Mr. Gonzales has terminal cancer. His family defers to the attending physician, who prescribes aggressive rescue treatment. The hospice nurse is an expert in the expressed and unexpressed needs of terminal clients. She advocates for a conservative and supportive plan of care. A logical case could be built for each position.

SUMMARY

Ethical reasoning and critical thinking are systematic, comprehensive processes to aide you in making clinical decisions. An important concept is to forget the idea that there is only one right answer in discussing ethical dilemmas. Accept that there may be several equally correct solutions depending on each individual's point of view.

Critical thinking is not a linear process. Analysis of the thinking processes of expert nurses reveals that they continually scan new data and simultaneously apply these steps in clinical decision making. They monitor the effectiveness of their interventions in achieving desired outcomes for their patient. A nurse's moral reasoning and critical thinking abilities often have a profound effect on the quality of care given, which affects health outcomes. Functioning as a competent nurse requires that you have knowledge of medical and nursing content, "best practice" guidelines, an accumulation of clinical experiences, and an ability to think critically.

Almost daily, we confront ethical dilemmas and complicated clinical situations that require expertise as a decision maker. We can follow the 10 steps of the thinking process described in this chapter to help us respond to such situations. Developing clinical judgment is a learned process, one which requires repeated application.

> **ETHICAL DILEMMA: WHAT WOULD YOU DO?** The Moyers family has power of attorney over hospitalized, terminally ill Gail Midge, aged 42 years. They are consistently at her bedside and refuse to allow you and other nurses to administer pain medication ordered by Mrs. M's physician, since they fear it will overdose her, causing her death. Gail often moans, cries with pain, and begs you for pain meds. The family threatens a lawsuit if she is given anything and then dies. What would you do?
>
> Based on a case reported by Pavlish, Brown-Sullivan, Herish, Shirk, and Rounkle (2011, p. 390). The nurse in this case considered conflicting variables from each point of view and assumed responsibility for initiating action, calling the palliative care team and the ethics consultation team.

REFLECTIVE ANALYSIS AND DISCUSSION QUESTIONS

1. Consider the Quality and Safety Education for Nurses competency of patient-centered care and the concept of autonomy; apply this to a case QSEN (LEVEL 2). When does a patient have the right to refuse treatment?
2. Use standards to analyze the characteristics of a **critical thinker** listed in Table 4.1 (LEVEL 3). How did you develop these? Were they innate or when did you acquire them?
3. Construct an example showing when a nurse has an ethical obligation (LEVEL 4). By choosing to become a nurse, do you assume an **ethical** obligation to treat any patient assigned to you? When are there exceptions?

REFERENCES

American Association of Colleges of Nursing (AACN). (2008). *Moral distress statement.* www.aacn.org/WD/practice/DOCS/moral_distress.pdf.

American Nurses Association [ANA]. (2015). *Code of ethics for nurses with interpretive statements.* Silver Spring, MD.: Author.

Carter, A. G., Creedy, D. K., & Sidebotham, M. (2016). Efficacy of teaching methods used to develop critical thinking in nursing and midwifery undergraduate students: A systematic review of the literature. *Nurse Education Today, 40,* 209–218.

Costello, M. (2017). The benefits of active learning: Applying Brunner's discovery theory to the classroom: Teaching clinical decision-making to senior nursing students. *Teaching and Learning in Nursing, 12,* 212–213. https://doi.org/10/1016/j.teln.2017.02.005.

Gronlund, C. E. C. F., Soderberg, A. I. S., Zingmarken, K. M., Sandlund, S. M., & Darlquist, V. (2015). Ethically difficult situations in hemodialysis care-nurses' narratives. *Nursing Ethics*, *26*(6), 711–722.

Hunter, S., & Arthur, C. (2016). Clinical reasoning of nursing students on clinical placement: Clinical educators' perceptions. *Nurse Education in Practice*, *18*, 73–79.

Johnsen, H. M., Fossum, M., Vivekananda-Schmidt, P., Fruhling, A., & Slettebo, A. (2016). Teaching clinical reasoning and decision-making skills to nursing students: Design, development, and usability evaluation of a serious game. *International Journal of Medical Informatics*, *94*, 39–48.

Kaya, H., Senyuva, E., & Brodur, G. (2017). Developing critical thinking disposition and emotional intelligence of nursing students: A longitudinal research. *Nurse Education Today*, *48*, 72–77.

Lee, J., Lee, Y. J., Bae, J., & Seo, M. (2016). Registered nurses' clinical reasoning skills and reasoning process: A think-aloud study. *Nurse Education Today*, *46*, 75–80.

Levett-Jones, T., Hoffman, K., Dempsey, J., et al. (2010). The 'five rights' of clinical reasoning: An educational model to enhance nursing students' ability to identify and manage clinically 'at risk' patients. *Nurse Education Today*, *30*, 515–520.

Milton, C. (2002). Ethical implications for acting faithfully in nurse-person relationships. *Nursing Science Quarterly*, *15*, 21–24.

Nelson, A. E. (2017). Methods faculty use to facilitate nursing students' critical thinking. *Teaching and Learning in Nursing*, *12*, 62–66.

Pavlish, C., Brown-Sullivan, K., Herish, M., Shirk, & Rounkle, A. (2011). Nursing priorities, actions, and regrets for ethical situations in clinical practice. *Journal of Nursing Scholarship*, *43*(4), 385–395.

Quality and Safety Education for Nurses (QSEN) Competencies: (n.d.) www.qsen.org/competencies. Accessed 9/20/18.

Romeo, E. M. (2010). Quantitative research on CT and predicting nursing students' NCLEX-RN performance. *The Journal of Nursing Education*, *49*(7), 378–386.

Sinclair, J., Pappas, E., & Marshall, B. (2016). Nursing students' experiences of ethical issues in clinical practice: A New Zealand study. *Nurse Education in Practice*, *17*, 1–7.

Tanner, C. A. (2006). Thinking like a nurse: a research-based model of clinical judgment in nursing. *The Journal of Nursing Education*, *45*, 204–211.

Trobeck, I., & Starcic, A. I. (2015). Developing ethical competencies online versus in the traditional classroom. *Nurs Ethics*, *22*(3), 352–366.

Tschudin, V. (2013). Two decades of nursing ethics: Some thoughts on changes. *Nurs Ethics*, *20*(2), 123–125.

Van Graan, A. C., Williams, M. J. S., & Koen, M. P. (2016). Professional nurses' understanding of clinical judgment: a contextual inquiry. *Health SA Gesondheid*, *21*, 280–293.

5

Developing Patient-Centered Communication Skills

Elizabeth C. Arnold

OBJECTIVES

At the end of the chapter, the reader will be able to:

1. Discuss the concept of health communication.
2. Describe the elements of patient-centered communication.
3. Apply communication strategies and skills in patient-centered relationships.
4. Discuss active listening responses used in therapeutic communication.
5. Discuss the use of verbal responses as a communication strategy.
6. Describe other forms of communication used in nurse-patient relationships.

INTRODUCTION

Nurses communicate on many different levels—with patients, families, other professional disciplines, and with a variety of external care providers involved with a patient's care. Although professional communication uses many of the same strategies as social communication, professional communication represents a specialized form of communication. It always has goals and a health-related purpose. Chapter 5 focuses on patient-centered communication skills, and describes communication strategies that nurses can use to inform, support, educate, and empower people to effectively self-manage their health-related issues.

Communicating as a professional nurse can be a challenge. Relational *and* informational aspects do not exist in the words themselves, but rather in their potential interpretations by the communicators engaged in the dialogue. Consequently, professional communication is carefully thought out, and always considerate of how the recipient might respond to it. Keep in mind that effective communication represents a *combination* of relationship building, information sharing, and decision making in

communication, all of which are needed to achieve critically important clinical outcomes.

Professional conversations differ from social conversations. Nurses must learn to be equally skilled communicating with professional audiences and with knowing how to translate technical and medical material into understandable information for patients and family members. They need to competently communicate with physicians and other health professional colleagues, using professional technical or medical language. Talking with patients requires a different skill set that bridges technical dialogue needed for health and social care with socially understandable exchange of ideas. Professional conversations have health-related expectations, and legal/ethical boundaries about what can and cannot be shared with others. Chapter 5 focuses on the development of communication skills in health care circumstances.

Schiavo (2013) notes, "Being sick is among one of the most vulnerable times in people's lives, especially in the case of severe, chronic, or life threatening diseases" (p. 116). Patients respond best when they believe their care providers are placing full attention on their concerns as a high priority. Incorporation of patient preferences and values in their care provides evidence that this characteristic lies at the heart of patient-centered care. Other indicators involve accurate clinical assessments, full informed consent, shared decision making, and effective health teaching geared to patient needs and preferences. Ongoing collaborative conversations between patient/families, and their health care providers have a direct impact on the quality and safety of clinical care, the achievement of meaningful clinical outcomes, and patient satisfaction. Patients and families are expected to be active partners, with designated health care providers, in their health care to whatever extent is possible (Errasti-Ibarrondo et al., 2015). Frequent consultation with other team professionals involved in a patient's care helps ensure continuity of care. This, in turn, acts to promote personal health efficacy, and to strengthen trust in the partnership required for self-management of chronic disorders. The importance of patient involvement is further emphasized by its inclusion as a measurable indicator of pay-for-performance reimbursement. Compliance with treatment and patient/family satisfaction are considered critical outcomes intimately tied to communication.

BASIC CONCEPTS

Definitions

Communication refers to each transmission of information, whether intentional or not. Nonverbal behaviors, written communication, tone of voice, and words are forms of communication. The concept takes into consideration the values, words and ideas, emotions, and body language of sender, receiver, and context. Increasingly people use media and other technology to communicate messages formally and informally.

Each message is intended to convey intended meaning, to exchange or strengthen ideas and feelings, and to share significant life experiences. Accompanying the message are nonverbal qualifiers in the form of gestures, body movements, eye contact, and personal or cultural symbols.

Functions of Professional Communication in Health Care Systems

More than any other variable, effective interpersonal communication skills support safety and quality in health care delivery (see Chapter 2). Professional communication skills connect virtually all concepts and activities related to human health and well-being. Today's nurses should be equipped with a strong understanding of human

> ### BOX 5.1 Basic Assumptions of Communication Theory
>
> - All behavior is communication, and it is impossible to not communicate.
> - Every communication has content and a relationship (metacommunication) aspect.
> - We know about ourselves and others primarily through communication.
> - Faulty communication results in flawed feeling and acting.
> - Feedback is the only way we know that our perceptions about meanings are valid.
> - Silence is a form of communication.
> - All parts of a communication system are interrelated and affect one another.
> - People communicate through words (digital communication) and through nonverbal behaviors and analog-verbal modalities; both forms are needed to interpret a message appropriately.

Bavelas, J.,& Jackson, D. (1967). Some tentative axioms of communication. In *Pragmatics of human communication—a study of interactional patterns, pathologies and paradoxes* (pp. 29–52). New York: W. W. Norton.

bio-psychosocial functioning, medical and nursing management of diverse health disorders, health-related ethical/legal issues, end-of-life care, and team collaboration, among others.

Professional communication is defined as a complex interactive process, used in clinical settings to help patients achieve health-related goals (Street & Mazor, 2017). The outcomes of effective interpersonal communication in health care relate to patient satisfaction, productive health changes, patient safety, and better service quality. Patients are more likely to understand their health conditions through meaningful communication, and to alert providers when something is not working. Other specific ways that professional health communication impacts service quality is through:

- development of workable medical partnerships;
- increased patient satisfaction;
- more effective diagnosis, and earlier recognition of health changes;
- better understanding of the patient's condition;
- personalized meaningful adherence to recognized therapeutic regimes;
- more efficient utilization of health services; and
- stronger, longer lasting positive outcomes.

Box 5.1 identifies professional communication as a performance standard for nurses.

Communication Models

Chapter 5 builds on basic concepts of linear and transactional communication. The application section describes the use of active listening responses, verbal communication strategies, and other communication techniques that nurses and other health professionals consciously used to facilitate patient- and family-centered health care. Communication concepts and strategies presented in the chapter provide a practical methodology for connecting with patients and families to improve health outcomes.

Linear Model

The *linear model* is the simplest communication model, which consists of sender, message, receiver, channels of communication, and context. Linear models focus only on the sending and receipt of messages. They do not necessarily consider communication as enabling the development of co-created meanings. Linear models are communication constructs, used in emergency health situations when time is of the essence to get immediate information.

Transactional Model

Transactional models are more complex. These models define communication as a reciprocal interaction process in which sender and receiver influence each other's messages and responses simultaneously as they converse. Each communicator constructs a mental picture of the other during the conversation, including perceptions about the other's attitude, and potential reactions to the message. Previous exposure to conversational concepts and ideas heighten the recognition and nature of the message interpretation. The outcome represents a new co-created set of collaborative meanings.

Transactional models employ systems concepts in which a human system (patient/patient/family) receives information from the environment *(input)*, internally processes it, and interprets its meaning *(throughput)*. The result is new information or behavior referred to as *output*. *Feedback loops* (from the receiver, or the environment) provide information about the output as it relates to the data received, and/or acted upon. This feedback either validates the received data, or reflects a need to correct/modify original input information. Thus, transactional models draw attention to communication as being relational, and having purpose and meaning-making attributes. Fig. 5.1 displays the elements of transactional models.

PROFESSIONAL COMMUNICATION SKILLS

Therapeutic communication, a term introduced by Jurgen Ruesch in 1961, refers to a dynamic interactive process entered into by health care providers, with

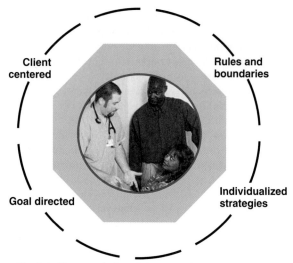

Fig. 5.1 Characteristics of therapeutic communication.

their patients and significant others, for the purpose of achieving identified health-related goals (Ruesch, 1961). Therapeutic communication occurs in a variety of ways: through words, facial expressions, body language, e-mail, writing, and behaviors. Nurses and patients conduct treatment activities, collaborate with those involved in the patient's care, exchange information and make shared decisions about all aspects of care with patients and families. What makes communication 'therapeutic' is its purpose, its active engagement of the patient as a full partner in a health related interactive process, and inclusion of relevant patient values and goals. emphasized throughout the dialogue. Additionally, the message is carefully crafted to take the patient's values, culture, developmental level, interest, and general health condition into account and, the patient is encouraged and to take shared responsibility for treatment outcomes (Rosenberg & Gallo-Silver, 2011).

Each therapeutic conversation is unique because the people holding them are different. Each brings different professional insights, personal strengths, and weaknesses to the discussion (Caughan & Long, 2000a, 2000b). At first glance, it may appear that therapeutic communication doesn't require extra or specialized study. This is not true. In therapeutic conversation, health care providers must maintain a skilled mindfulness, which allows them to consider each patient's unique situation, while simultaneously monitoring their own personal responses and reactions and other corroborative evidence. This is what Peplau (1960) meant by the nurse being a "participant observer" in therapeutic relationships.

Patient-Centered Communication Skills

Patient-centered communication skills in health care provide the lifeblood of clinical tasks such as obtaining a clinical history, explaining a diagnosis, and providing competent nursing care with related health teaching. Communication competency offers a primary means for establishing a trusting collaborative relationship with patients and families. Communication is embedded within all professional relationships.

The quality of health care relationships strongly affects the outcome of the health encounter (Van Dalen, 2013; Watzlawick, Beavin, & Jackson, 1967). Interpersonal communication skills influence the completeness of diagnostic information, the quality of shared decision making, and the level of patient motivation to achieve constructive clinical outcomes. "Positive" clinical experiences involve human communication encounters in which a patient's human needs and values are respected, and the humanity of the clinician is transparent. Interestingly, the human connection sometimes influences a person's health care impression of a care experience as much, if not more, than the level of provider competence. With "negative" clinical encounters, patients experience disconnects with the knowledge and interpersonal care the patient or family expects from the provider, in part because of the way the information gets presented. It becomes an uncomfortable, rather than a productive, encounter. Poor communication is implicated as a key factor in clinical safety errors, and malpractice allegations (Gluyas, 2015).

CHARACTERISTICS OF PATIENT-CENTERED COMMUNICATION

Honesty, clarity, and empathy are fundamental ingredients of effective therapeutic conversations. In clinical practice *empathy* refers to being emotionally attuned to a patient's perspective of a situation, as well as to its reality (see Chapter 11). Referred to as the patient's *frame of reference or world view,* a patient's "perception" of an illness may differ significantly from the nurse's frame of reference. Therapeutic communication helps to link the different perspectives into a workable common ground for discussion, and the development of constructive goals and actions. Reflective responses based on the nurse's knowledge and integration with ways of knowing are designed to encourage further dialogue.

Defined Interpersonal Boundaries

Professional conversations have *defined interpersonal boundaries,* related to their purpose, discussion topics, focus, sharing of thoughts and feelings, time, and prescribed settings (see also Chapter 10). Unlike social conversations, in which each participant spontaneously expresses thoughts and feelings, professional conversations focus on patient and family health care needs. Interactions are patient centered, and the associated dialogue is health related. Only the patient is expected to consistently reveal personal information related to his or her health situation.

Health-Related Purpose

Professional conversations take place within a defined health care format, and terminate when the health-related purpose is achieved, or the patient is discharged. Characteristics of professional conversations include:
- Specific rules and boundaries, related to function and privacy
- Defined therapeutic goals
- Patient centered
- Individualized strategies related to health-related goals

All patient conversations are subject to federal guidelines and professional standards regarding confidentiality and protected patient information.

Nonverbal Communication Supports

Behavioral signals, found in the tone of voice, inflections and intonations, facial expression (particularly the eyes), and body language, accompany verbal messages. This is true for both nurse and patient. As nurses, we sometimes forget that our patients are assessing us at the same time we are observing them.

In face-to-face interactions, nurses have a rich range of visual and vocal cues, which provide additional data about the patient, if read correctly. Knowledge of patient habits, beliefs, preferences, cultural behaviors, and attitudes can support or contradict the spoken words. Facial expressions, body postures and movements, agitation, or blushing often suggest what the patient may be feeling about the verbal message. However, these cues may be easily misinterpreted, so asking for clarifying feedback to ensure that all parties are looking at a situation from a similar perspective is essential.

ACTIVE LISTENING

Active listening is a dynamically focused interpersonal process in which a nurse hears a patient's message, decodes its meaning, asks questions for clarification, and provides feedback to the patient. It is a transactional process that integrates the verbal and nonverbal components of a message. Nurses demonstrate active listening through their body language, asking open-ended questions, and careful observational listening prompts. Leaning slightly forward with the upper part of your body, maintaining eye contact, restating patient concerns, nodding, and summarizing conceptually are important communication connectors.

The goal of active listening is to understand what the patient is trying to communicate through his or her story.

Active listening requires full attention to understanding the patient's perspective without making any judgments. Using the listening responses presented later in the chapter increases understanding.

Box 5.2 shows the ANA standards for professional performance which are used as guides in professional communication. As you ask clarifying questions, and share your own thinking responses about what you are seeing or hearing, you can develop a more in-depth understanding of the health care situation from the patient's perspective.

Included with each verbal message are important nonverbal instructions (*metacommunication*) about how to interpret the message (see Chapter 6). If a nurse sits down in a relaxed position with full attention and good eye contact and actively listens, these verbal and nonverbal activities indicate interest and commitment. The same verbal message, delivered while looking at the clock or your watch, provides a nonverbal message that the patient does not have your full attention.

Sometimes, the emotional nonverbal component of a message differs from the verbal message. Nurses need to be sensitive to what is left out of the message, as well as to what is included. This too is important information to explore and consider. If you notice nonverbal behaviors that seem to contradict words, it is appropriate to call the patient's attention to the discrepancy with a simple statement, such as, "I notice that you seem a little subdued when we talked about… Is something going on that we should talk about?"

Verbal Responses

Verbal responses refer to the spoken words in a professional conversation. Words are a meaning-making basic tool that enables health care providers and patients to organize data about their health problems, explore different options, resolve issues, make common meaning of their experiences, and dialogue with each other. Unlike the written word, verbal dialogue cannot be erased, although words can be explained or modified.

The meaning of words resides in the person who uses them, not in the words themselves. When languages or word meanings differ, their significance changes. Nurses should pay close attention to the patient's language style formats (Kettunen, Poskiparta, & Liimatainen, 2001) and mirror them, when possible.

Choice of words matters. Terminology should be clear, complete, concrete, and easily understandable to the listener. Words should neither overstate nor understate the situation. Since both words and nonverbal behaviors are subject to misinterpretation, nurses need to check in with their patients to ensure the accuracy of their perceptions. For example, "I'd just like to check in with you to make sure that I understand. Are you saying that… ?"

Factors That Influence Communication
Personal Factors

Developing a common understanding of the dialogue, which occurs between nurses and patients, is a critical outcome of professional communication. Personal and environmental factors influence communication availability and readiness. For example, eye contact, full attention on the patient coupled with genuine respect and clear, concise messages encourage patient participation. Words that respect a person's culture, spiritual beliefs, and educational level are more likely to capture the patient's attention. Factors that affect the accurate transmission of communicated messages are found in Fig. 5.2.

People communicate nonverbally through body language, eye contact, and level of attention. The nurse should consciously use body language, gestures, and minimal verbal cues to encourage further communication. Physical cues are used to support or refute the meaning of words.

Obstacles to Effective Communication Within the Patient

Barriers to effective communication can occur within patients when they are:
- Preoccupied with pain, physical discomfort, worry, or contradictory personal beliefs

- Unable to understand the nurse's use of language, terminology, or frame of reference
- Struggling with a personal emotionally laden topic,
- Feeling defensive, insecure, or judged
- Confused by the complexity of the message—too many issues, tangential comments
- Deprived of privacy, especially if the topic is a sensitive one
- Have sensory or cognitive deficits that limit or compromise the receiving of accurate messages

Obstacles Within the Nurse

Barriers within the nurse occur when the nurse is not fully engaged with the patient for one or more of the following reasons:
- Preoccupation with personal agendas
- Being in a hurry to complete physical care
- Making assumptions about patient motivations
- Cultural stereotypes
- Defensiveness, or personal insecurity about being able to help the patient

- Thinking ahead to the next question
- Intense patient emotion or aggressiveness
- Weak language that does not add value to the conversation

Exercise 5.1 is designed to help students identify difficult communication issues in nursing practice.

Self-Awareness

Nurses have an ethical and professional responsibility to resolve personal issues so that countertransference feelings do not affect communication. Patient-centered communication requires greater self-awareness. Before you begin, think about the goals you want to achieve with your patient. Remember to include areas of importance and concern to the patient. Self-awareness of personal vulnerabilities and prejudices allow nurses to maintain the authenticity, patience, neutrality, and understanding needed for therapeutic exploration of patient issues. Make sure that your nonverbal behaviors support rather than contradict your words; by staying flexible you will get further than if you only use focused questioning as conversational prompts.

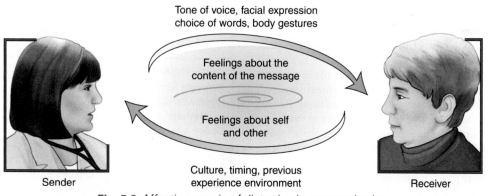

FACTORS THAT INFLUENCE COMMUNICATION.

Tone of voice, facial expression choice of words, body gestures

Feelings about the content of the message

Feelings about self and other

Culture, timing, previous experience environment

Sender   Receiver

Fig. 5.2 Affective margin of distortion in communication.

EXERCISE 5.1   Simulation Exercise: Complicated Communication Issues With Patients

Purpose: To help students identify common complicated communication issues with patients.

Procedure
In groups of three to four students:
1. In round-robin fashion, each student should share an "elevator version" of a nursing experience that illustrates a challenging communication encounter you have had, or witnessed in a nurse-patient encounter.
2. Identify what components made the conversation difficult.

3. If you had the conversation, what might you do differently?

Reflective Discussion Analysis
1. Were there any common themes that your group found in the identified communication challenges?
2. Explore the insights you gained from doing this exercise.
3. How could you use what you learned from doing this exercise in your future nursing practice?

Environmental Factors

Privacy, space, and timing affect therapeutic conversations. Patients need privacy free from interruption and environmental noise for meaningful dialogue to take place. "Noise" refers to any distraction, which interferes with being able to pay full attention to the discussion. It can be physical in the form of environmental distractions, even being tired. Semantic noise can occur in the form of cross-cultural language differences or psychological noise associated with mental illness. For example, TV or music can be distracting.

People require different amounts of personal space for conversational ease (Hall, 1959). Therapeutic conversations typically take place within a social distance (3–4 feet is optimal). Culture, personal preference, nature of the relationship, and the topic will influence personal space needs. DeVito (2016) identifies four types of distance ranges typically associated with usual communication in the United States.

1. Close intimate relationships range from touch to 18 inches.
2. Personal distance ranges from 18 inches to 4 feet.
3. Social distance ranges from 4 to 12 feet.
4. Public distance ranges from 12 feet to more than 25 feet. (pp. 152–153)

Patients experiencing anxiety usually need more physical space, whereas those experiencing a sudden physical injury, or undergoing a painful procedure appreciate having the nurse in closer proximity. Sitting at eye level with bedridden patients is helpful.

Timing is important. Planning communication for periods when the patient is able to participate physically and emotionally is time-efficient and respectful of the patient's needs. Give your patients enough time to absorb material, to share their impressions, and to ask questions. Patient behavior can cue the nurse about emotional readiness and available energy. The presence of pain or variations in energy levels, anger, or anxiety will require extra time to inquire about the change in the patient's behavior and its meaning, before proceeding with the health care dialogue.

Communication as a Shared Partnership

Patient-centered care and collaborative partnerships in current health care deliverables require a broader span of collaborative communication skills to accomplish the active partnership needed for managing chronic disorders. Patients expect to be listened to and involved in their own care. But they also need support to do so. Epstein and Street (2007) identify six core, overlapping functions of patient-centered communication needed to achieve beneficial health outcomes:

- "Fostering healing relationships"
- Exchanging information
- Responding to emotions
- Managing uncertainty
- Making decisions
- Enabling patient self-management (p. 17)

Patient-centered communication is an interactive reciprocal exchange of ideas in which nurses try to understand what it is like to be this person in this situation with this illness. Each patient and family has its unique set of values, patterns of behavior, and preferences that must be taken into account. How patients communicate with the nurse varies, based on culture and social background factors. Their readiness to learn, personal ways of relating to others, physical and emotional conditions, life experiences, and place in the life cycle are related factors in planning and implementing contemporary care through therapeutic conversations.

Patient-centered conversations include discussions needed for collaborative decision making and for teaching patients self-management skills. Talking about complex personal health problems with a trained health professional allows patients and families to hear themselves, as they put health concerns into words. Feedback provided by the health professional ideally helps patients to realistically sort out their priorities and to determine the actions they want to take to effectively cope with their health circumstances.

APPLICATIONS

Effective communication is an art, as well as a professional competency. It is not only what you say, but also how you say it. Certain personality traits and attitudes—for example, a good sense of humor, a nonjudgmental respectful

---

DEVELOPING AN EVIDENCE-BASED PRACTICE

Purpose: To investigate which communication factors correlate with the constructs of positive therapeutic alliance.

Method: Assessment of communication factors included interaction styles, verbal, and nonverbal factors, while factors associated with the therapeutic alliance included collaboration, affective bond, agreement, trust, and empathy. Participants included health clinicians and patients in primary, secondary, and tertiary care settings. Over 3000 papers were identified from the initial search of seven online data bases. Twelve studies met the inclusion criteria, which yielded 67 communication related to interaction styles, and verbal and nonverbal factors.

Findings: Interaction factors related to the provision of emotional support, and asking questions and listening to what patients have to say showed the greatest strength.

Application to Your Practice: Using patient-centered interaction styles with careful listening, and encouraging patient involvement with a focus on emotional issues can enhance the therapeutic alliance.

Pinto, R. Z., Ferreira, M., Oliveira, V., Franco, M., Adams, R., Maher, C., et al. (2012). Patient-centred communication is associated with positive therapeutic alliance: a systematic review. *Journal of Physiotherapy, 58*, 77–87.

attitude, and maintaining a calm, thoughtful manner throughout the communication process—are intangible characteristics of conversational ease.

Engaging the Patient

A patient-centered communication process starts with the first encounter. Your initial presentation of yourself will influence the communication that follows. Each patient should have your full attention. This means clearing your own mind of any preconceived notions, biases, and even your own thoughts. Entering the patient's space with an open, welcoming facial expression, respectful tone, and direct eye contact, declares your interest and intent to know this person. Your posture immediately gives a message to the patient, either inviting trust, or conveying disinterest. Whether you are sitting or standing, your posture should be relaxed, facing the patient and leaning slightly forward. Shaking the patient's hand with an open facial expression and a smile signals to the patient that he or she is the most important person in your orbit for the moment.

Introductions are important, especially if many health professionals are involved in the patient's care (Van Servellen, 2009). Introduce yourself, and identify the patient by name before beginning the conversation. When more people than just the patient, (family or other health team members) are involved in a discussion, expand the introductions. Center your attention on the patient, but do not ignore other participants. You can include family members with eye contact, physical cues, and so forth throughout the conversation.

Eye contact is an important inclusive gesture. Ask for the patient's name first, followed by the names of others and their relationship to the patient. It is better to be more formal than informal until you get to know the patient better.

Building Rapport

Begin with asking routine questions about the reason for admission, and other common information. Routine questions help to put the patient and family at ease. However, when you ask the patient to tell you about his/her health concerns and what prompted him/her to seek help at this time, keep this part of the conversation open. Allow the patient to tell you about his or her personal situation from a personal perspective, with few interruptions. Sequence questions going from easy general to more complex questions.

Keep in mind that patients will vary in their ability to effectively communicate their feelings, preferences, and concerns (Epstein & Street, 2007). Personal characteristics, culture, previous life and health experiences, and education level, create differences. Considering these factors allows you to phrase questions, and to interpret answers in more meaningful ways.

Being attentively present, providing relevant information, and actively listening to patient concerns help to build rapport. Patients who feel safe, accepted, and validated by their health care providers find it easier to collaborate with them. Although rapport building begins with the initial encounter, it continues as a thread throughout the nurse-patient relationship. Remember that patients are looking to you not only for competence, but also for sincerity and genuine interest in them as individuals. Exercise 5.1 provides an opportunity to practice an initial patient-centered interview.

Developing a Shared Partnership

The idea of health care as a shared partnership in which the patient is an equal stakeholder and treatment partner in ensuring quality health care is relatively new. Building a shared, workable partnership alliance requires:

- Empathetic objectivity, which allows you to experience patients as they are, not the way you would like them to be.
- A "here and now" focus on the current issues and concerns important to the patient.
- Demonstration of respect, and asking questions about cultural and social differences that can influence treatment.
- Authentic interest in the patient and a confident manner that communicates competence.
- The capability to consider competing goals, and alternative ways to meet them.

Finding Common Ground

Patient-centered communication strategies allow patient and nurse to find common ground related to the patient's explanations of problems, their priorities, and their treatment goals. Before you can participate in the development of a shared approach to a problem, you have to give your full attention to what you are hearing from your patient.

The aspects of care that are most important to a patient and family, and what helps or hinders their capability to self-manage their health problems, is critical information. Look for themes revealing fears, feelings, and level of engagement. Patients also need to understand the full range of therapeutic choices available to them in treating and self-managing their illness. This is critical information, particularly for situations requiring informed consent. Exercise 5.2 is designed to increase the student's understanding of communication strategies in building rapport.

Observing Nonverbal Cues

Burgoon, Guerrero, and Floyd (2009) note that up to 65% of interpersonal communication is nonverbal. Patients cannot always put their concerns into words. Some are not even aware of what is worrying them or what to do about their concerns. Others experience powerful emotions that make verbalizing personal concerns difficult.

Watch for nonverbal cues from the patient. There are different "channels" of nonverbal communication (e.g., facial expressions, vocal tones, gestures and body positions, body movements, touch, and personal space). Take note of

---

BOX 5.3   Physical Behavioral Cues

Emblems: Gestures or body motions having a common verbal interpretation (e.g., handshaking, baby waving bye-bye, sign language).

Illustrators: Actions that accompany and emphasize the meaning of the verbal message (e.g., smiling, a stern facial expression, pounding the fist on a table).

Affect Displays: Facial presentation of emotional affect. Affect displays have a larger range of meaning and act to support or contradict the meaning of the verbal message. (Nurses need to validate accuracy of perception with the patient.)

Regulators: Nonverbal gestures, such as nodding, facial expression, hand gestures to stop conversation or, to reinforce, or modify what is being said in the course of the conversation.

Adaptors: Patient specific, repetitive, nonverbal actions that are part of a patient's usual response to emotional issues. Examples include nervous foot tapping, blushing, hair twirling.

Physical Characteristics: Nonverbal information about the patient observed about the outward appearance of the person (e.g., body odor, physical appearance [dirty hair, unshaven]).

Adapted from Blondis, M., & Jackson, B. (1982). *Nonverbal communication with patients: back to the human touch* (pp. 9–10), (2nd ed.). New York: Wiley.

---

whether cues such as the patient's facial expression, body movements, posture, and breathing rate support or contradict the meaning of the spoken message.

Changes in body language and nonverbal cues can indicate discomfort with the discussion. The patient who declares that he is ready for surgery and seems calm may be sending a different message through the tense muscles the nurse accidentally touches. The differences between words and body language cues can suggest that the patient may be worried about the surgery. Environmental cues, such as a half-eaten lunch or noncompliance with treatment, can provide other nonverbal evidence that a patient is in distress. When this happens, you can comment on your perception: "I'm wondering what you are feeling right now, about what I am saying," or, "I noticed when I mentioned _____, your expression changed" (Weiten et al., 2009). Like verbal communication, nonverbal behaviors and signals are culture bound so they may mean different things in different cultures (see also Chapter 7; Samovar, Porter, & McDaniel, 2009). Exercise 5.3 provides practice with asking open-ended questions to facilitate information sharing.

Active Listening

Active listening is defined as an *intentional* form of listening. It involves more than simply hearing words. The importance of listening in health care communication cannot be overestimated. When a person is ill, listening require extra effort. It also involves noting feelings and looking for underlying themes. The goal is mutual understanding of facts and emotions. Active listening contributes to fewer incidents of misunderstanding, more accurate comprehensive data, and stronger health relationships (Straka, 1997).

Listening responses in a patient-centered health environment ask about *all* relevant patient health concerns. They take into account the patient's values, preferences,

---

EXERCISE 5.2   Simulation Exercise: Active Listening

Purpose: To develop skill in active listening and an awareness of the elements involved.

Procedure

1. Students break up into pairs. Each will take a turn reflecting on and describing an important experience they have had in their lives. The person who shares should describe the details, emotions, and outcomes of his or her experience. During the interaction, the listening partner should use listening responses such as clarification, paraphrasing, reflection, and focusing, as well as attending cues, eye contact, and alert body posture to carry the conversation forward.

2. After the sharing partner finishes his or her story, the listening partner indicates understanding by: (a) stating in his or her own words what the sharing partner said; and (b) summarizing perceptions of the sharing partner's feelings associated with the story and asking for validation. If the sharing partner agrees, then the listening partner can be sure he or she correctly utilized active listening skills.

Reflective Discussion Analysis

In the large group, have pairs of students share their discoveries about active listening. As a class, discuss aspects of nursing behavior that will foster active listening in patient interactions.

and expectations related to treatment goals, priorities, and attitudes about treatment suggestions. Open-ended questions, such as the ones identified below, are core clinical questions:

- "What is important to you now?"
- "What do you see as the next step?"
- "What are you hoping will happen with this treatment?"

Listening responses can be integrated with asking for validation of patient preferences, for example, asking the patient, "How does the idea of _____ sound to you?" or "How easy will it be for you to learn to use your crutches?" Each of these questions, and others along the same line can encourage a patient to explore potential concerns, expand on an idea, or voice confusion. This information is essential to achieve a shared understanding and realistic clinical expectations.

A patient-centered interview begins with encouraging patients to tell their story in an authentic way (Platt & Gaspar, 2001). Open-ended questions are a major means of helping patients tell their story, of obtaining relevant information, and of reducing misunderstandings. There are different ways of asking questions. Questions fall into three categories: open-ended, closed-ended, and circular.

Open-Ended Questions

Open-ended questions are defined as questions that are open to interpretation, and cannot be answered by "yes, or no," or a one-word response. They allow patients to express their problems or health needs in their own words. Open-ended questions usually begin with words such as "what," "how," or "can you describe for me…," etc. They provide a broader context for each patient's unique health concerns and are likely to yield more complete information. Open-ended questions invite patients to think and reflect on their situation. They help connect relevant elements of the patient's experience (e.g., relationships, impact of the illness on self or others, environmental barriers, and potential resources or concerns).

Open-ended questions are used to elicit the patient's thoughts and perspectives without influencing the direction of an acceptable response. For example:

"Can you tell me what brought you to the clinic (hospital) today?"

"What has it been like for you since the accident?"

"Where would you like to begin today?"

"How can I help you?"

Ending the dialogue with a general open-ended question, such as "Is there anything else concerning you right now?" or "Is there anything we have overlooked today?" can provide relevant information that might otherwise be overlooked. Exercise 5.4 provides an opportunity to practice the use of open-ended questions.

Focused Questions

Focused questions require more than a yes or no answer, but they place limitations on the topic to be addressed. They are useful in emergencies and in other situations when immediate concise information is required. Focused questions can clarify the timing and sequence of symptoms, and concentrate on details about a patient's health concerns. For example, they can include when symptoms began, what other symptoms the patient is having, and what a patient has done to date to resolve the problem.

Patients with limited verbal skills sometimes respond better to focused questions because they require less interpretation. Examples of focused questions include:

"Can you tell me more about the pain in your arm?"

EXERCISE 5.3   Simulation Exercise: Using Patient-Centered Communication Role-Play

Purpose: To use patient-centered communication strategies in an assessment interview.

Procedure

1. Develop a one-paragraph scenario of a patient situation that you are familiar with before class.
2. Pair off as patient and nurse.
3. Conduct an initial patient-centered 15-min assessment interview using one of the scenarios, with the author of the paragraph taking the role of the nurse and the other student taking the patient role.
4. Reverse roles and repeat with the second student's scenario.

Reflective Discussion Analysis

1. In what ways were patient-centered communication strategies used in this role-play?
2. How awkward was it for you in the nursing role to incorporate queries about the patient's preferences, values, and so on?
3. What parts of the interview experience were of greatest value to you when you assumed the patient role?
4. If you were conducting an assessment interview with a patient in the future, what modifications might you make?
5. How could you use what you learned from doing this exercise in future nurse-patient interviews?

EXERCISE 5.4   Simulation Exercise: Observing for Nonverbal Cues

Purpose: To develop skill in interpreting nonverbal cues.

Procedure
1. Watch a dramatic movie (that you haven't seen before) with the sound off for 5–15 min.
2. As you watch the movie, write down the emotions you see expressed, the associated nonverbal behavior, and your interpretations of the meaning and the other person's response.

Reflective Discussion Analysis
In a large group, share your observations and interpretations of the scenes watched. Discussion should focus on the variations in the interpretations of the nonverbal language. Discuss ways in which the nurse can use observations of nonverbal language with a patient in a therapeutic manner to gain a better understanding of the patient. Time permitting, the movie segment could be shown again, this time with the sound. Discuss any variations in the interpretations without sound versus with verbal dialogue. Discuss the importance of validation of nonverbal cues.

"Can you give me a specific example of what you mean by… ?"
"When did your stomach pain begin?"

Focused questions help patients to organize data and to prioritize immediate concerns; for example, you might ask a question at the end of the conversation such as, "Of the concerns we talked about today, which has been the most difficult for you?"

Circular questions are a form of focused questions that look at how other people within the patient's support circle respond to a patient's health issues. These questions are designed to identify differences in the impact of an illness on individual family members, and to explore changes in relationships brought about by the health circumstances. For example, "When your dad says he doesn't want hospice care because he is a fighter, what is that like for you?"

Closed-Ended Questions

Closed-ended questions are defined as narrowly focused questions, for which a single answer, for example, "yes," "no," or a simple phrase answer serves as a valid response. They are useful in emergency situations when the goal is to obtain information quickly, and the context or patient's emotional reactions are of secondary importance because of the seriousness of the immediate situation. Examples of closed-ended questions include:
"Does the pain radiate down your left shoulder and arm?"
"When was your last meal?"

What the Nurse Listens for: Themes

Behind the actual words exist themes. *Themes* refer to the underlying message, present, but not identified in the patient's words. Listening for themes requires observing and understanding what the patient is not saying, as well as what the person actually reveals through words.

Identifying the underlying themes in a therapeutic conversation can relieve anxiety and provide direction for individualized nursing interventions. For example, the patient may say to the nurse, "I'm worried about my surgery tomorrow." This is one way of framing the problem. If the same patient presents his concern as, "I'm not sure I will make it through the surgery tomorrow," the underlying theme of the communication changes from a generalized worry to a more personal theme of survival. Alternatively, a patient might say, "I don't know whether my husband should stay tomorrow when I have my surgery. It is going to be a long procedure, and he gets so worried." The theme (focus) here expresses a concern about her relationship with her husband. In each communication, the patient expresses a distinct theme of concern related to a statement, but the emphasis in each requires a different response.

Emotional objectivity in making sense of patient themes is essential. *"Emotional" objectivity* refers to seeing what an experience is like for another person, not how it fits or relates to other experiences, not what causes it, why it exists, or what purposes it serves. It is an attempt to see attitudes and concepts, beliefs, and values of an individual as they are to him at the moment he expresses them—not what they were or will become (Moustakas, 1974, p. 78). Exercise 5.4 provides practice in listening for themes.

ACTIVE LISTENING RESPONSES

Active listening responses are essential components of patient-centered communication. They show the patient that the nurse is fully present as a professional partner in helping the patient understand a change in health status and the best ways to cope with it (Keller & Baker, 2000). Through active listening, a new level of understanding can develop; potential or actual problems can be reframed and resolved with the development of collaborative shared goals. The minimal verbal cues, clarification, restatement, paraphrasing, reflection, summarization, silence, and touch are examples of skilled listening responses that nurses can use to guide therapeutic interventions (Table 5.1).

Listening Responses
Minimal Cues and Leads
Nonverbal signals are transmitted through body action, (smiling, nodding, and leaning forward, encourage patients to continue their story). Short phrases such as "Go on" or "And then?" or "Can you say more about… ?" are useful verbal prompts. Exercise 5.5 provides an opportunity to practice minimal cues and verbal prompts in patient-centered communication.

Clarification
Clarification is defined as a brief question or a request for validation. It is used to better understand a patient's message; for example, "You stated earlier that you were concerned about your blood pressure. Tell me more about what concerns you." The tone of voice used with a clarification response should be neutral, not accusatory or demanding. Failure to ask for clarification when part of the communication is poorly understood means that you might act on incomplete or inaccurate information. You can practice this response in Exercise 5.6 and 5.7.

Restatement
Restatement is an active listening strategy used to broaden a patient's perspective or when the nurse needs to provide a sharper focus on a specific part of the message. For example, you might say, "Let me see if I have this right…" (followed

TABLE 5.1	Active Listening Responses
Listening Response	**Example**
Minimal cues and leads	Body actions: smiling, nodding, leaning forward
	Words: "mm," "uh-huh," "oh really," "go on"
Clarification	"Could you describe what happened in sequence?" "I'm not sure I understand what you mean. Can you give me an example?"
Restatement	"Are you saying that… (repeat patient's words)?" "You mean… (repeat patient's words)?"
Paraphrasing	Patient: "I can't take this anymore. The chemo is worse than the cancer. I just want to die."
	Nurse: "It sounds as though you are saying you have had enough."
Reflection	"It sounds as though you feel guilty because you weren't home at the time of the accident." "You sound really frustrated because the treatment is taking longer than you thought it would."
Summarizing	"Before moving on, I would like to go over with you what I think we've accomplished thus far."
Silence	Briefly disconnecting but continuing to use attending behaviors after an important idea, thought, or feeling
Touch	Gently rubbing a person's arm during a painful procedure

---

EXERCISE 5.5   Simulation Exercise: Asking Open-Ended Questions

Purpose: To develop skill in the use of open-ended questions to facilitate information sharing.

Procedure
1. Break up into pairs. Role-play a situation in which one student takes the role of the facilitator and the other the sharer. (If you work in the clinical area, you may want to choose a clinical situation.)
2. As a pair, select a topic. The facilitator begins asking open-ended questions.
3. Dialogue for 5–10 min on the topic.
4. In pairs, discuss perceptions of the dialogue and determine what questions were comfortable and

open-ended. The student facilitator should reflect on the comfort level experienced with asking each question. The sharing student should reflect on the efficacy of the listening responses in helping to move the conversation toward his or her perspective.

Reflective Discussion Analysis
As a class, each pair should contribute examples of open-ended questions that facilitated the sharing of information. Compile these examples on the board. Formulate a collaborative summation of what an open-ended question is, and how it is used. Discuss how open-ended questions can be used sensitively with uncomfortable topics.

EXERCISE 5.6   Simulation Exercise: Listening for Themes

Purpose: To help students identify underlying themes in messages.

Procedure
1. Divide into groups of three to five students.
2. Take turns telling a short story about yourself—about growing up, important people or events in your life, or significant accomplishments (e.g., getting your first job).
3. As each student presents a story, listen carefully to asking questions for clarification, if needed. Write them down so you will not be tempted to change them as you hear the other stories. Notice nonverbal behaviors accompanying the verbal message. Are they consistent with the verbal message of the sharer?
4. When the story is completed, each person in the group shares his or her observations with the sharer.

5. After all students have shared their observations, validate their accuracy with the sharer.

Reflective Discussion Analysis
1. Were the underlying themes recorded by the group consistent with the sharer's understanding of his or her communication?
2. As others related their interpretations of significant words or phrases, did you change your mind about the nature of the underlying theme?
3. Were student interpretations of pertinent information relatively similar or significantly different?
4. If they were different, what implications do you think such differences have for nurse-patient relationships in nursing practice?
5. What did you learn from doing this exercise?

EXERCISE 5.7   Simulation Exercise: Minimal Cues and Leads

Purpose: To practice and evaluate the efficacy of minimal cues and leads.

Procedure
1. Initiate a conversation with someone outside of class and attempt to tell the person about something with which you are familiar for 5–10 min.
2. Make note of all the cues that the person puts forth that either promote or inhibit conversation.
3. Now try this with another person and write down the different cues and leads you observe as you are speaking and your emotional response to them (e.g., what most encouraged you to continue speaking).

Reflective Discussion Analysis
As a class, share your experience and observations. Different cues and responses will be compiled on the board.

Discuss the impact of different cues and leads on your comfort and willingness to share about yourself. What cues and leads promoted communication? What cues and leads inhibited sharing?

Variation
This exercise can be practiced with a clinical problem simulation in which one student takes the role of the professional helper and the other takes the role of patient. Perform the same scenario with and without the use of minimum encouragers. What were the differences when encouragers were not used? Was the communication as lively? How did it feel to you when telling your story when this strategy was used by the helping person?

EXERCISE 5.8   Simulation Exercise: Using Clarification

Purpose: To develop skill in the use of clarification.

Procedure
1. Write a paragraph related to a clinical experience you have had.
2. Place all the student paragraphs together and then pick one (not your own).
3. Develop clarification questions you might ask about the selected clinical experience.

Reflective Discussion Analysis
Share with the class your chosen paragraph and the clarification questions you developed. Discuss how effective the questions are in clarifying information. Other students can suggest additional clarification.

EXERCISE 5.9   Simulation Exercise: Role-Play Practice With Paraphrasing and Reflection

Purpose: To practice the use of paraphrasing and reflection as listening responses.

Procedure

1. The class forms into groups of three students each. One student takes the role of patient, one the role of nurse, and one the role of observer.
2. The patient shares with the nurse a recent health problem he or she encountered, and describes the details of the situation and the emotions experienced. The nurse responds, using paraphrasing and reflection in a dialogue that lasts at least 5 min. The observer records the statements made by the helper. At the end of the dialogue, the patient writes his or her perception of how the helper's statements affected the conversation, including what comments were most helpful. The helper writes a short summary of the listening

responses he or she used, with comments on how successful they were.

Discussion

1. Share your summary and discuss the differences in using the techniques from the helper, patient, and observer perspectives.
2. Discuss how these differences related to influencing the flow of dialogue, helping the patient feel heard, and the impact on the helper's understanding of the patient from both the patient and the helper positions.
3. Identify places in the dialogue where one form of questioning might be preferable to another.
4. How could you use this exercise to understand your patient's concerns?
5. Were you surprised by any of the summaries?

---

by a restatement of the patient's words) (Coulehan et al., 2001). Restatement is effective when a patient overgeneralizes, or seems stuck in a repetitive line of thinking. When sparingly implemented in a questioning manner, a restatement strategy focuses the patient's attention on the possibility of an inaccurate or global assertion.

Paraphrasing

Paraphrasing is a listening response used to check whether the nurse's translation of the patient's words represent an accurate interpretation of the message. The strategy involves the nurse *taking* the patient's original message and transforming it into his or her own words, without losing the meaning. A paraphrase should be shorter and more specific than the patient's initial statement so that the focus is on the core elements of the original statement. Your objective in using paraphrasing as an active listening response is to find a common understanding of issues important to your patients. Paraphrasing allows you to summarize or streamline a message, and/or highlight key points of the longer message.

Reflection

Reflection is an active listening response that focuses on the emotional part of a message. It offers nurses a way to empathetically mirror their sense of how a patient may be emotionally experiencing their health situation. There are several ways to use reflection, for example:

- Reflection on vocal tone: "You seem to have some anger and frustration in your voice as you describe your accident" or "You sound happy when you talk about your grandson."

- Reflection example, linking feelings with content: "It sounds like you feel _____ because _____."

- Linking current feelings with past experiences: "It seems as if this experience reminds you of feelings you had with other health care providers, when you didn't feel understood."

A reflective listening response should be a simple observational comment, expressed tentatively, not an exhaustive comment about the patient's emotional reaction. It offers an opportunity for the patient to validate or to change the narrative. When reflecting on an emotional observation, students sometimes feel they are putting words into the patient's mouth when they "choose" an emotion from their perception of a patient's message. This would be true if you were choosing an emotion out of thin air, but not when you empathetically mirror what you are hearing from the patient. You can simply present potential or observable be the underlying feelings present in the patient's narrative, without interpreting its meaning. Exercise 5.8 provides practice in using paraphrasing and reflection as listening responses.

Summarization

Summarization is an active listening skill used to review content and process. Summarization pulls several ideas and feelings together, either from one interaction or from a series of interactions, into a few brief sentences. This would be followed by a comment seeking validation, such as "Tell me if my understanding of this agrees with yours." A summary statement can also be useful as a bridge to changing the topic or focus of the conversation. The summarization

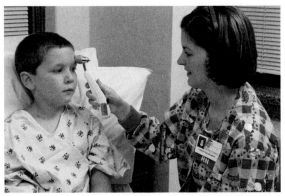

Fig. 5.3 Whether you are sitting or standing, your posture should be relaxed, with the upper part of your body inclined slightly toward the client.

should be completed before the end of the conversation, but with enough time before you leave the room, for validation or questions. Exercise 5.9 is designed to provide insight into the use of summarization as a listening response.

Silence

Silence, delivered as a brief pause, is a powerful listening response. Intentional pauses can allow the patient to think. A short pause lets the nurse step back momentarily and process what has been heard, before responding. Silence can be used to emphasize important points that you want the patient to reflect on. By pausing briefly after presenting a key idea and before proceeding to the next topic, it encourages a patient to reflect on what has just been discussed (Fig. 5.3).

When a patient falls silent, it can mean many things: something has touched the patient, the patient is angry, or does not know how to respond, or the patient is thinking about *how* to respond. A verbal comment to check on the meaning of the message is helpful.

Not all listening responses are helpful. Nurses need to recognize when their responses are interfering with objectivity or are inviting premature closure. Table 5.2 provides definitions of negative listening responses that block communication.

MIRRORING COMMUNICATION PATTERNS

Communication patterns provide a different type of information. Being respectful of the patient's communication pattern involves accepting the patient's communication style as a part of who the person is, without expecting that person to be different (see also Chapter 6). Some patients exaggerate information; others characteristically leave out highly relevant details. Some talk a lot, using dramatic language and multiple examples; others say very little and have

TABLE 5.2 Negative Listening Responses		
Category of Response	**Explanation of Category**	**Examples**
False reassurance	Using pseudocomforting phrases in an attempt to offer reassurance	"It will be okay." "Everything will work out."
Giving advice	Making a decision for a patient; offering personal opinions; telling a patient what to do (using phrases such as "ought to," "should")	"If I were you, I would…" "I feel you should…"
False inferences	Making an unsubstantiated assumption about what a patient means; interpreting the patient's behavior without asking for validation; jumping to conclusions	"What you really mean is you don't like your physician." "Subconsciously, you are blaming your husband for the accident."
Moralizing	Expressing your own values about what is right and wrong, especially on a topic that concerns the patient	"Abortion is wrong." "It is wrong to refuse to have the operation."
Value judgments	Conveying your approval or disapproval about the patient's behavior or about what the patient has said using words such as "good," "bad," or "nice"	"I'm glad you decided to…" "That really wasn't a nice way to behave." "She's a good patient."

to be encouraged to provide details. The rule of thumb is to start where the patient is, and to mirror the patient's communication style.

Evaluation of the patient's present overall pattern of interaction with others includes strengths and limitations, family communication dynamics, and developmental and educational levels. Culture, role, ways of handling conflict, and ways of dealing with emotions also reflect and influence communication patterns. For example, AJ is a patient with chronic mental illness. She frequently interrupts and presents with a loud, ebullient opinion on most things. This is AJ's communication pattern. To engage successfully with her, you would need to listen, while accepting her way of communicating as a part of who she is, without being judgmental, joining in with arguing the validity of her position, or getting lost in detail. Remember that patients who are anxious often use a controlling form of communication, and are preoccupied with their own version of events. They may have difficulty listening to or assimilating information. Taking a little extra time to establish rapport and gently set limits on what is open for discussion can help patients like AJ remain focused in conversations.

VERBAL COMMUNICATION AND RESPONSES

Active listening, and verbal responses are inseparable from each other. Each informs and reinforces the other. Exercise 5.3 presents a summary of the therapeutic interviewing skills presented in this chapter as they apply to the phases of the nurse-patient relationship. With shorter time frames for patient contact, nurses need to verbally connect with patients, beginning with the first encounter. As the relationship develops, it is important to make room for questions to ensure that care remains patient centered. You can use a simple lead, such as, "I'm wondering what questions you might have about what we have been discussing."

If this question is a nonstarter, you could follow up with a short statement, for example, "One question I am frequently asked is…."

Most patients are not looking for brilliant answers from the nurse. Rather, they seek feedback and want caring support that suggests a compassionate understanding of their particular dilemma. No matter what level of communication exists in the relationship, the same needs— "hear me," "touch me," "respond to me," "feel my pain and experience my joys with me"—are fundamental themes. These are the themes addressed by patient-centered communication.

Words help patients assess the healthy elements of their personality (their strengths) and enables them to use these elements in coping with their current health problems. Nurses use verbal responses to teach, encourage, support, provide, and gather/validate provided information in guiding a patient toward goal achievement. Nurses should offer guidance, but no judgment.

Verbal response strategies include mirroring, focusing, metaphors, humor, reframing, feedback, and

> ### BOX 5.4 Guidelines to Effective Verbal Communication Strategies
>
> - Define unfamiliar terms and concepts.
> - Match content and delivery with each client's developmental and educational level, experiential frame of reference, and learning readiness.
> - Keep messages clear, concrete, honest, and simple to understand.
> - Put ideas in a logical sequence of related material.
> - Relate new ideas to familiar ones when presenting new information.
> - Repeat main ideas.
> - Reinforce key points with vocal emphasis and pauses.
> - Keep language as simple as possible; use vocabulary familiar to the client.
> - Focus only on essential elements; present one idea at a time.
> - Use as many sensory communication channels as possible for key ideas.
> - Make sure that nonverbal behaviors support verbal messages.
> - Seek feedback to validate accurate reception of information.

validation, all of which are designed to strengthen the coping abilities of the patient, alone or in relationship with others. Nurses use observation, validation, and patterns of knowing to gauge the effectiveness of verbal interventions. On the basis of the patient's reaction, the nurse may decide to use simpler language, or to try a different strategy in collaboratively working with a patient. Another strategy is to make a simple statement, like "Let me think about that a little bit and get back to you." Obviously, it is important to return to the topic later if you use this strategy.

When making verbal responses or providing information, do not overload the patient with too many ideas, or details. If you find you are doing most of the talking, you need to back up and use listening responses to elicit the patient's perspective. It is important to give the patient honest feedback, and to do so while letting the patient modify the direction in a win–win situation that is negotiated with shared goals to whatever extent is possible.

People can absorb only so much information at one time, particularly if they are tired, fearful, or discouraged. Introducing new ideas *one at a time* allows the patient to more easily process data. Repeating key ideas and reinforcing information with concrete examples facilitates understanding and provides an additional opportunity for the patient to ask questions. Paying attention to nonverbal response cues from the patient that support understanding or that reflect a need for further attention is an important dimension of successful communication.

Matching Responses

Responses that encourage a patient to explore feelings about limitations or strengths at a slightly deeper but related level of conversation are likely to meet with more success.

Verbal responses should neither expand nor diminish the meaning of the patient's remarks. Notice the differences in the nature of the following responses to a patient.

Case Example

Patient: "I feel so discouraged. No matter how hard I try, I still can't walk without pain on the two parallel bars."

Nurse: "You want to give up because you don't think you will be able to walk again."

At this point, it is unclear that the patient wants to give up, so the nurse's comment expands on the patient's meaning without having sufficient data to support it. Although it is possible that this is what the patient means, it is not the only possibility. The more important dilemma for the patient may be whether his or her efforts have any purpose. The next response focuses only on the negative aspects of the patient's communication and ignores the patient's comment about his or her efforts.

Nurse: "So you think you won't be able to walk independently again."

In the final response example below, the nurse addresses both parts of the patient's message and makes the appropriate connection. The nurse's statement invites the patient to validate the nurse's perception.

Nurse: "It sounds to me as if you don't feel your efforts are helping you regain control over your walking."

Using Plain Language

Plain language refers to the use of clear-cut, simple easy to understand words to convey ideas, particularly those that are more abstract. It is important to speak with a general spirit of inquiry and concern for the patient that stimulates trust. Verbal messages should address core issues in a comprehensible, concise manner, taking into account the

---

BOX 5.5   What the Nurse Listens For

- Content themes.
- Communication patterns.
- Discrepancies in message content, body language, and verbalization.
- Feelings, revealed in a person's voice, body movements, and facial expressions.
- What is not being said, as well as what is being said.
- The patient's preferred representational system (auditory, visual, tactile).
- The nurse's own inner responses and personal ways of knowing.
- The effect communication produces in others involved with the patient.

BOX 5.6   Guidelines to Effective Verbal Communication in the Nurse-Patient Relationship

- Use plain language.
- Simplify unfamiliar terms and concepts to improve comprehension.
- Validate the understanding of word meanings.
- Match content and delivery with the patient's developmental, and literacy level.
- Keep in mind the patient's experiential frame of reference, learning readiness, and general medical condition.
- Keep messages clear, concrete, honest, and simple to understand.
- Put ideas in a logical sequence of related material.
- Relate new ideas to familiar ones when presenting new information.
- Repeat key ideas.
- Keep language as simple as possible; use vocabulary familiar to the patient.
- Focus only on essential elements; present one idea at a time.
- Use as many sensory communication channels as possible for key ideas.
- Make sure that nonverbal behaviors support verbal messages.
- Seek frequent feedback to validate accurate reception of information.

---

guidelines for effective verbal expressions, listed in Boxes 5.4 and 5.5.

Before responding or giving information, consider your patient' receptivity. Consider the level of anxiety and potential culture or language issues—both your own and that of your patient. Remember your frame of reference may be quite different from theirs.

Avoid using jargon, or clinical language that patients may have trouble understanding. Unless patients and/or families can associate new ideas with familiar words and ideas, the nurse might as well be talking in a different language. Patients and families may not tell the nurse that they do not understand for fear of offending the nurse, or of revealing personal deficits or their personal anxiety.

Start with finding out what the patient already knows, or believes about his or her health situation. Giving information that fails to take into account a patient's previous experiences, or assumes that they have knowledge they do not possess, tends to fall on deaf ears. Frequent validation with the patient related to content helps reduce this problem.

Focusing

In today's health care delivery system, nurses must make every second count. It is important for nurses and patients to select the most pressing or relevant health care topics for discussion.

Sensitivity to patient need and preferences should be factors to take into consideration. You should not force a patient to focus on an issue that he or she is not yet willing to discuss unless it is an emergency situation. You can always go back to a topic when the patient is more receptive. For example, you might say, "I can understand that this is a difficult topic for you, but I am here for you if you would like to discuss [identified topic] later."

Presenting Reality

Presenting reality to a patient who is misinterpreting it can be helpful as long as the patient does not perceive that the nurse is criticizing the patient's perception of reality. A simple statement, such as "I know that you feel strongly about _____, but I don't see it that way," is an effective way for the nurse to express a different interpretation of the situation. Another strategy is to put into words the underlying feeling that is being implied but is not stated.

Giving Feedback

Feedback is a message a nurse gives to the patient in response to a question, verbal message, or observed behavior. Feedback can focus on the content, the relationship between people and events, the feelings generated by the message, or parts of the communication that are not clear. Feedback should be specific and directed to the behavior. It should not be an analysis of the patient's motivations.

Verbal feedback provides the receiver's understanding of the sender's message and personal reaction to it. Effective feedback offers a neutral mirror, which allows a patient to view a problem or behavior from a different perspective. Feedback is most relevant when it only addresses the topics under discussion, and does not go beyond the data presented by the patient. Effective feedback is clear, honest, and reflective. Feedback supported with realistic examples is believable, whereas feedback without documentation to support it can lack credibility.

Case Example

An obese mother in the hospital was feeding her newborn infant 4 ounces of formula every 4 hours. She was concerned that her child vomited a considerable amount of the undigested formula after each feeding. Initially, the nursing student gave the mother instructions about feeding the infant no more than 2 ounces at each feeding in the first few days of life, but the mother's behavior persisted, and so did that of her infant. The nursing student began to ask questions and discovered that the patient's mother had fed her 4 ounces right from birth with no problem, and she considered this the norm. This additional information helped the nurse work with the patient in seeing the uniqueness of her child and understanding what the infant was telling her through his behavior. The patient began to feel comfortable and confident in feeding her infant a smaller amount of formula consistent with his needs.

Effective feedback is specific rather than general. Telling a patient he or she is shy or easily intimidated is less helpful than providing a behavioral example, "I noticed when the anesthesiologist was in here that you didn't ask her any of the questions you had about your anesthesia tomorrow. Do you want to look at what you might want to know so you can get the information you need?" With this response, the nurse provides precise information about an observed behavior, and offers a potential solution. The patient is more likely to respond with validation, or correction, and the nurse can provide specific guidance.

Feedback can be about the nurse's observations of nonverbal behaviors; for example, "You seem (angry, upset, confused, pleased, sad, etc.) when..." Request for feedback can be framed as a question, requiring the patient to elaborate; for example, "I want to be sure that we have the same understanding of what we have talked about. Can you tell me in your own words what we discussed?"

Not all feedback is equally relevant, nor is it always accepted. A benchmark for deciding whether feedback is appropriate is to ask yourself, "Does this feedback advance the goals of the relationship?" and "Does it consider the individualized needs of the patient?" If the answer to either question is "no," then while the feedback may be accurate, it may be inappropriate in the current context. Most people find "why" questions difficult to answer. In general, avoid asking "why" questions to patients as an initial questioning strategy. Motivation typically is multi-determined, so often it is more difficult to answer. Asking "how" or "what" questions are usually focused and more easily answered.

Timing is a critical element. Feedback given as soon as possible after a behavior in need of change is observed is most effective. Other factors (e.g., a patient's readiness to hear feedback, privacy, and the availability of support from others) contribute to effectiveness. Providing feedback about behaviors over which the patient has little control only increases the personalized feelings of low self-esteem, and leads to frustration. Feedback should be to the point and empathetic.

People also give nonverbal feedback. Expressions such as surprise, boredom, anxiety, or hostility send a message about how the listener is responding internally to the message. When you receive nonverbal messages suggesting uncertainty, concern, or inattention, it is important to ask for validation.

Validation

Validation is a special form of feedback, which is used to ensure that both participants have the same basic understanding of messages. Word meanings lie within people, not in the words themselves. The meaning of the same word has cultural and contextual implications that can be different for each communicator. Simply asking patients whether they understand what was said is not an adequate method of validating message content. Instead, you might ask, "How do you feel about what I just said?" or "I'm curious what your thoughts are about what I just told you." If the patient does not have any response, you can suggest that the patient can respond later, "Many people do find they have reactions or questions about [the issue] after they have had a chance to think about it. I would be glad to discuss this further." Validation can provide new information that helps the nurse frame comments that are more responsive to the patient's need.

OTHER FORMS OF COMMUNICATION

Touch

Touch, the first of our senses to develop, and the last to leave, is a nurturing form of communication and validation. Intentional comforting touch benefits the nurse as well as the patient (Connor & Howett, 2009). Touch is a powerful listening response used when words would break a mood or when verbalization would fail to convey the empathy or depth of feeling between nurse and patient. A hand placed on a frightened mother's shoulder or a squeeze of the hand can speak far more eloquently than words in times of deep emotion. Touch stimulates comfort, security, and a sense of feeling valued (Herrington & Chioda, 2014; Sundin & Jansson, 2003). Patients in pain, those who feel diminished because of altered appearance, lonely and dying patients, and those experiencing sensory deprivation or feeling confused respond positively to the nurse who is unafraid to enter their world and touch them. Children and the elderly are comforted by touch (Fig. 5.4).

How you touch a patient in providing everyday nursing care is a form of communication. For example, gentle massage of a painful area helps patients relax. Holding the hand of a patient with dementia can reduce agitation. Gently rubbing a patient's forehead or stroking the head is comforting to very ill patients.

Case Example

It was Jovan's third birthday. There was a party of adults (his mother and father, his grandparents, his great-uncle and great-aunt, and me, his aunt), because Jovan was the only child in the family. While we were sitting and chatting, Jovan was running around and playing. At a moment of complete silence, Jovan's great-uncle asked him solemnly: "Jovan, who do you love the best?" Jovan replied, "Nobody!" Then Jovan ran to me and whispered in my ear: "You are Nobody!" (Majanovic-Shane, 1996, p. 11).

Case Example

Brendan's grandfather has dementia. He is in the hospital, which terrifies him. When Brendan visits him, he sits quietly beside the bed at eye level, and gently massages his hand. The confused, wild look in his eyes disappears as he listens to his grandson recall special moments he shared with his granddad and he peacefully closes his eyes.

Patients vary in their comfort with touch. Touch is used as a common form of communication in some cultures, whereas in others, it is reserved for religious purposes, or is seldom used as a form of communication (Samovar et al., 2009). Before touching a patient, assess the patient's receptiveness to touch. If the patient is paranoid, out of touch with reality, verbally inappropriate, or mistrustful, touch generally is contraindicated as a listening response.

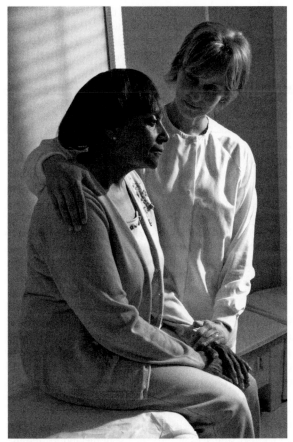

Fig. 5.4 Touch is an important form of communication, particularly when patients are stressed. (Copyright © Thinkstock Images/Stockbyte/Thinkstock.)

SPECIALIZED COMMUNICATION STRATEGIES

Metaphors

Familiar images promote understanding. Metaphors represent an unrelated figure of speech that can help patients and families process difficult, new, or abstract information by comparing it with more familiar images from ordinary life experience. Landau, Arndt, and Cameron (2018) suggest that a metaphor example can be more persuasive than a medical explanation. For example, chronic lung disease as "emphysema is like having lungs similar to 'swiss cheese'," and the airways in asthma are like "different sized drainpipes that can get clogged up and need to be unclogged" (Arroliga et al., 2002). A familiar concrete image can help a patient connect with an abstract medical diagnosis that is harder to comprehend. Data supported by a metaphoric explanation can be more persuasive than a literal explanation. The choice of metaphor is important. For example, Periyakoil (2008)

suggests that using war or sports metaphors with patients experiencing advanced metastatic cancer can result in an unintended impact when the patient can no longer fight the valiant battle or win the game by playing according to prescribed moves.

Humor

Humor is a powerful patient-centered communication technique when used for a specific therapeutic purpose. Humor recognizes the incongruities in a situation, or an absurdity present in human nature or conduct (Random House Dictionary, 2009). Humor lightens the mood and puts a tense situation in perspective. A good laugh can bond communicators together in a shared conversation in ways that might not happen otherwise. Humor works best when rapport is well established, and a level of trust exists between the nurse and patient (McGhee, 1998). A humorous comment should fit the situation, not dominate it. When using humor, it is best to focus on an idea, event, or situation, or something other than the patient's personal characteristics.

Humor and laughter have healing purposes. Laughter generates energy and activates β-endorphins, a neurotransmitter that creates natural highs and reduces stress hormones (Hassed, 2001). The surprise element in humor can cut through an overly intense situation and put it into perspective.

The following factors contribute to the successful use of humor:
- Knowledge of the patient's response pattern
- An overly intense situation
- Timing
- Situation lending itself to an imaginative or paradoxical solution
- Gearing the humor dynamics to the patient's developmental level and interests
- Focus on the humor in a situation or change in circumstance rather than a patient's personal characteristics.

Case Example

Karen, the mother of 4-year-old Megan, had just returned from a long shopping trip in which she had purchased several packages of paper towels. While she was in another room, Megan took everything out of four kitchen drawers, put them on the floor, and put the paper towels in the drawers. Her mother expressed her anger to Megan in no uncertain terms. As she was leaving the kitchen, she heard Megan say to herself, "Well, I guess she didn't like that idea." Karen's anger was permanently interrupted by her daughter's innocent humorous remark.

USING TECHNOLOGY IN PATIENT-CENTERED RELATIONSHIPS

The many uses of technology in communication are detailed in Chapters 25 and 26. Increasingly, nurses are incorporating technology to communicate in digital encounters with patients and families (Collins, 2014). Although technology can never replace face-to-face time with patients, voice mail, e-mail, and telehealth virtual home visits help connect patients with care providers and provide critical information.

Currently, technology is used as a form of communication to support face-to-face communication. For example, routine laboratory results, appointment scheduling, and links to information on the Web can be transmitted through technology. Present-day technology allows people to use the Internet as a communication means to share common experiences with others who have a disease condition, to consult with experts about symptoms and treatment, and to learn up-to-date information about their condition. Nurses can help patients assess the value of web health information.

The electronic nurse-patient relationship begins when the nurse comes online or begins speaking to the patient on the phone. From that point forward, the nurse needs to follow defined standards of nursing care using communication principles identified in this chapter. At the end of each telehealth encounter, nurses need to provide their patients with clear directions and contact information should additional assistance be required. Confidentiality and protection of identifiable patient information is an essential component of telehealth conversations.

Telephone communication is an essential communication link. Periodic informational telephone calls enhance family involvement in the long-term care of patients. Over time, some families lose interest, or find it too painful to continue active commitment. Interest and support from the nurse reminds families that they are not simply interchangeable parts in their loved one's life; their input is important.

SUMMARY

This chapter discusses basic therapeutic communication strategies that nurses can use with patients across clinical settings. Nurses use active listening responses, such as paraphrasing, reflection, clarification, silence, summarization, and touch, to elicit complete information. Observation is a primary source of information, but all nonverbal behaviors need to be validated with patients for accuracy.

Open-ended questions give the nurse the most information, because they allow patients to express ideas and feelings as they are experiencing them. Focused or closed-ended questions are more appropriate in emergency clinical situations, when precise information is needed quickly.

Nurses use verbal communication strategies that fit the patient's communication patterns in terms of level, meaning, and language to help patients meet treatment goals (Box 5.6). Other strategies include the use of metaphors, reframing, humor, confirming responses, feedback, and validation. Feedback provides a patient with needed information.

DEVELOPING AN EVIDENCE-BASED PRACTICE
The **purpose** of this research was to answer the question: "what exactly is patient-centered communication?" (p. 2131).

Method: This research project was designed to examine and critique different approaches to patient-centered communication related to the conceptualization of patient-centered communication and measurement approach. The research focused on seven different measures of patient-centered communication.

Results: Measures differed relating to whether the measures yielded information about behavior or how well the behavior was performed; whether it focused on the patient or clinician, or interaction as a whole. The article presented a multidimensional framework for developing patient-centered communication measures, but recommended development of a better understanding of the specific domains of patient-centered communication.

Application to Your Clinical Practice: As a profession, nurses need to contribute to the evidence-based development of patient-centered communication based on continued dialogue with patients and other professional colleagues. The measures is not simply that the patient talks more than the clinician or shows interest in the patient's concerns!

Street, R. L. (2017). The many disguises of patient-centered communication: problems of conceptualization and measurement. *Patient Education and Counseling*, 100, 2131–2134.

Case Example

Patient: "I don't know about taking this medicine the doctor is putting me on. I've never had to take medication before, and now I have to take it twice a day."

Nurse: "It sounds like you don't know what to expect from taking the medication."

Case Example: Asking for validation can present a fuller explanation.

Mr. Brown (to nurse taking his blood pressure): "I can't stand that medicine. It doesn't sit well." (He grimaces and holds his stomach.)

Nurse: "Are you saying that your medication for lowering your blood pressure upsets your stomach?"

Mr. Brown: "No, I just don't like the taste of it."

Sometimes validation is observational rather than expressed through words.

Case Example: Inviting active patient participation in mutually developed self management strategies.

Jane Smith has been coming to the clinic to lose weight. At first she was quite successful, losing 2 pounds per week. This week she has gained 3 pounds. The nurse validates the weight change with the patient and asks for input.

Nurse: "Jane, over the past 6 weeks you have lost 2 pounds per week, but this week you gained 3 pounds. There seems to be a problem here. Let's discuss what might have happened and how you can get back on track with your goal of losing weight."

Case Example: Touch is particularly useful with patients who are not in a position to have a verbal discussion.

"I found out that if I held Sam's hand he would lie perfectly still and even drift off to sleep. When I sat with him, holding his hand, his blood pressure and heart rate would go down to normal and his intracranial pressure would stay below 10. When I tried to calm him with words, there was no response—he [had] a blood pressure of 160/90!" (Chesla, 1996, p. 202).

ETHICAL DILEMMA: What Would You Do?

You have had a wonderful relationship with a patient and the patient's family. They have revealed issues they had never talked about before and raised questions that extended beyond the health care situation that they did not have the time to finish. You are about to end your rotation. What do you see as your professional and ethical responsibility to this patient and family?

REFERENCES

American Nurses Association (ANA). (2007). *Scope and standards of practice* (ed 3). Silver Spring, MD: American Nurses Association.

Arroliga, A., Newman, S., Longworth, D., & Stoller, J. K. (2002). Metaphorical medicine: Using metaphors to enhance communication with patients who have pulmonary disease. *Annals to Internal Medicine, 137*(5 Part 1), 376–379.

Burgoon, J., Guerrero, L. K., & Floyd, K. (2009). *Nonverbal Communication*. Boston, MA: Allyn and Bacon.

Caughan, G., & Long, A. (2000a). Communication is the essence of nursing care: 1. Breaking bad news. *British Journal of Nursing, 9*(14), 931–938.

Caughan, G., & Long, A. (2000b). Communication is the essence of nursing care: 2. Ethical foundations. *British Journal of Nursing, 9*(15), 979–984.

Chesla, C. (1996). Reconciling technologic and family care in critical-care nursing. *Image Journal of Nursing Scholarship, 28*(3), 199–203.

Collins, R. (2014). Best practices for integrating technology into nurse communication processes technology can close communication gaps that separate nurses from patient and families. *American Nurse Today, 9*(11).

Connor, A., & Howett, M. (2009). A conceptual model of intentional comfort touch. *Journal of Holistic Nursing, 27*(2), 127–135.

Coulehan, J. L., Platt, F. W., Egener, B., Frankel, R., Lin, C. T., Lown, B., et al. (2001). Let me see if I have this right…: Words that help build empathy. *Annals of Internal Medicine, 135*, 221–227.

Definition of Humor. (2009). *Random House dictionary*. New York: Random House, Inc. dictionary.com.

DeVito, J. (2016). *The Interpersonal communication Book* (ed 14). Edinburg Gate Essex: Pearson Education Limited.

Epstein, R. M., & Street, R. L. (2007). *Patient-centered communication in cancer care: promoting healing and reducing suffering*. Bethesda, MD: National Cancer Institute, NIH Publication No, 07–6225.

Errasti-Ibarrondo, B., Perez, M., Carrasco, J., Lama, M., Zaragoza, A., & Arantzamendi, M. (2015). Essential elements of the relationship between the nurse and the person with advanced and terminal cancer: a meta-ethnography. *Nursing Outlook, 63*(3), 255–268.

Gluyas, H. (2015). Effective communication and teamwork promotes patient safety. *Nursing Standard*, *29*(49), 50–57.

Hall, E. (1959). *The silent language*. New York: Doubleday.

Hassed, C. (2001). How humour keeps you well. *Australian Family Physician*, *30*(1), 25–28.

Herrington, C., & Chioda, L. (2014). Human touch effectively and safely reduces pain in the newborn intensive care unit. *Pain Management Nursing*, *15*(1), 107–115.

Keller, V., & Baker, L. (2000). Communicate with CARE. *RN*, *63*(1), 32–33.

Kettunen, T., Poskiparta, M., & Liimatainen, L. (2001). Empowering counseling—a case study: Nurse-patient encounter in a hospital. *Health Education Research*, *16*, 227–238.

Majanovic-Shane, A. (1996). Metaphor: A propositional comment and an invitation to intimacy. In: *Paper presented at the Second Conference for Sociocultural Research, Geneva Switzerland*.

McGhee, P. (1998). Rx laughter. *RN*, *61*(7), 50–53.

Moustakas, C. (1974). *Finding yourself: finding others*. Englewood Cliffs, NJ: Prentice Hall.

Peplau, H. (1960). Talking with patients. *American Journal of Nursing*, *60*(7), 964–966.

Peplau, H. (1960). Peplau's theory of interpersonal relations. *Nursing Science Quarterly*, *10*(4), 162–167.

Periyakoil, V. (2008). Using metaphors in medicine. *Journal of Palliative Medicine*, *11*(6), 842–844.

Platt, F., & Gaspar, D. L. (2001). Tell me about yourself"; the patient-centered interview. *Annals of Internal Medicine*, *134*(11), 1079–1085.

Rosenberg, S., & Gallo-Silver, L. (2011). Therapeutic communication skills and student nurses in the clinical setting. *Teaching and Learning in Nursing*, *6*, 2–8.

Ruesch, J. (1961). *Therapeutic communication*. New York: Norton.

Samovar, L., Porter, R., & Roy, C. (2017). *Communication between cultures* (9th ed.). Boston, MA: Cenage Learning.

Schiavo, R. (2013). *Health communication: from theory to practice* (2nd ed.). New York: Jossey Bass.

Straka, D. A. (1997). Are you listening—have you heard? *Advanced Practice Nursing Quarterly*, *3*(2), 80–81.

Street, R., & Mazor, K. (2017). Clinician-patient communication measures: drilling down into assumption, approaches, and analyses. *Patient Education and Counseling*, *100*, 1612–1618.

Sundin, K., & Jansson, L. (2003). "Understanding and being understood" as a creative caring phenomenon: In care of patients with stroke and aphasia. *Journal of Clinical Nursing*, *12*, 107–116.

Van Dalen, J. (2013). Communication skills in context: Trends and perspectives. *Patient Education and Counseling*, *92*, 292–295.

Van Servellen, G. (2009). Talking the talk to improve your skills. *Nursing*, *39*(12), 22–23.

Watzlawick, P., Beavin, J. H., & Jackson, D. D. (1967). *Pragmatics of human communication*. New York: WW Norton & Company.

SUGGESTED READING

Epstein, E., & Peters, E. (2009). Beyond information: Exploring patient preferences. *JAMA*, *302*, 195–197.

Kagan, P. (2008). Feeling listened to: A lived experience of human becoming. *Nursing Science Quarterly*, *21*(1), 59–67.

Street, G., & Makoul, N. K. (2008). How does communication heal? Pathways linking clinician-patient communication to health outcomes. *Patient Education and Counselling*, *74*, 295–301.

VanDulmen, S. (2017). Listen, when words don't come easy. *Patient Education and Counseling*, *100*, 1975–1978.

6

Variation in Communication Styles

Kathleen Underman Boggs

OBJECTIVES

At the end of this chapter, the reader will be able to:

1. Describe the component systems of communication, describing congruence between verbal and nonverbal messages.
2. Reflect on how communication style influences the nurse-patient relationship.
3. Discuss how metacommunication messages may affect patient responses.
4. Cite examples of body cues that convey nonverbal messages.
5. Apply findings of research studies for evidence-based clinical practice.

Every individual has different preferred methods for giving and receiving communication. These vary depending of the particular individual and specific situation. This chapter explores styles of communication that serve as a basis for building a relationship to provide safe, effective patient-centered care. Patient-centered communication is an underlying component of all six of the prelicensure competencies identified in the Quality and Safety Education for Nurses (QSEN) project. Communication style is defined as a set of specific speech-related characteristics cueing another as to how to interpret a message. You can and should learn to modify your communication style in your clinical practice (White et al., 2016). For patients, effective communication has been shown to produce better health outcomes, greater satisfaction, and increased understanding, shorter hospital stays, and decreased costs (Kee, Khoo, Lim, & Koh, 2017). Style is defined as the manner in which one communicates. It is important to learn as much as possible about your own communication style. Some of us tend to be more assertive, more forceful, and even dominant in our relationships, imposing our desires on others, whereas others seek more of an equal partnership, bargaining or negotiating in a give-and-take fashion. At the other end of the personal style spectrum, some individuals tend to withdraw or even put all of the other person's desires ahead of their own needs.

In developing a style suitable to professional nurse-patient or nurse-team-patient relationships, we modify our personal style to fit our professional role. As learners, students are monitored in the clinical setting as we demonstrate expected communication styles that convey warmth, trustworthiness, and respectful assertiveness and use our newly acquired therapeutic communication skills Fig. 6.1.

Verbal style includes pitch, tone, and frequency. Nonverbal style includes facial expression, gestures, body posture and movement, eye contact, distance from the other person, and so on. These nonverbal behaviors are clues patients give us to help us understand their words. Sharpening our observational skills helps us gather data needed for nursing assessments and interventions. Both of us, patient and nurse, enter this new relationship with our own specific styles of communication.

Some individuals depend on a mostly verbal style to convey their meaning, whereas others rely on nonverbal strategies to send the message. Warren (2015) estimates that at least 90% of messages are conveyed not with words but via verbal pitch and nonverbal cues. Some communicators emphasize giving information; others have as a priority the conveying of interpersonal sensitivity. Longer nurse-patient relationships allow each person to better understand the other's communication style.

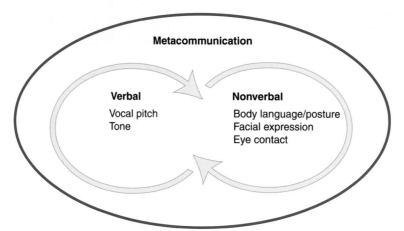

Fig. 6.1 Factors in Communication Styles.

BASIC CONCEPTS

Metacommunication

Communication is a combination of verbal and nonverbal behaviors integrated for the purpose of sharing information. Within the nurse-patient relationship, any exchange of information between two individuals also carries messages about how to interpret the communication.

Metacommunication is a broad term used to describe all of the factors that influence how the message is perceived. It is a message about how to interpret what is going on. Metacommunicated messages may be hidden within verbalizations or be conveyed as **nonverbal** gestures and expressions. Some studies report greater compliance to requests when they are accompanied by a metacommunication message asking for a response to the appropriateness of the request. Sydney's case should clarify this concept.

Case Example: Student Nurse Sydney

Student (smiling, making eye contact, and using warm tone): Hi, I am Sydney. We nursing students are trying to encourage community awareness in promoting environmental health and are looking for people to hand out fliers. Would you be willing?
(Metacommunication): I realize that this is a strange request, seeing that you do not know who I am, but I would really appreciate your help. I am a nice person. In this metacommunicated message about how to interpret meaning, the student nurse used both verbal and nonverbal cues. She conveyed a verbal message of caring; making appropriate, encouraging responses; and sending a nonverbal message by maintaining direct eye contact, presenting a smooth face without frowning, and using a relaxed and fluid body posture without fidgeting.

In a professional relationship, verbal and nonverbal components of communication are intimately related. A student studying American Sign Language for the deaf was surprised that it was not sufficient merely to make the sign for "smile" but that she had to actually show a smile at the same time. This congruence helped to convey her message. You can communicate your acceptance, interest, and respect nonverbally. What style can we use to most positively affect our patients' health practices? A comprehensive review shows that we have inadequate information about this.

VERBAL COMMUNICATION

Words are symbols used by people to think about ideas and to communicate with others. Choice of words is influenced by many factors (e.g., your age, race, socioeconomic group, educational background, and gender) and by the situation in which the communication is taking place.

The interpretation of the meaning of words may vary according to the individual's background and experiences. It is dangerous to assume that words have the same meaning for all persons who hear them. Language is useful only to the extent that it accurately reflects the experience it is designed to portray. Consider, for example, the difficulty an American would have in communicating with a person who speaks only Vietnamese, or the dilemma of the young child with a limited vocabulary who is trying to tell you where it hurts. One's voice can be a therapeutic part of treatment, as with Mrs. Garcia.

Case Example: Mrs. Garcia

For weeks, while giving care to Mrs. Garcia, a 42-year-old unconscious woman, her nurse used soothing touch and conversation. She also encouraged Mr. Garcia to do the same. When the woman later regained consciousness, she told the nurse that she recognized her voice.

Meaning

There are two levels of meaning in language: denotation and connotation. Both are affected by one's culture. **Denotation** refers to the generalized meaning assigned to a word; **connotation** points to a more personalized meaning of the word or phrase. For example, most people would agree that a dog is a four-legged creature, domesticated, with a characteristic vocalization referred to as a bark. This would be the denotative, or explicit, meaning of the word. When the word is used in a more personalized way, it reveals the connotative level of meaning. "What a dog" and "His bark is worse than his bite" are phrases some people use to describe personal characteristics of human beings rather than animals. We need to be aware that many messages convey only a part of the intended meaning. Do not assume that the meaning of a message is the same for the sender and the receiver until mutual understanding is verified. To be sure you are getting your message across, ask for feedback.

VERBAL STYLE FACTORS THAT INFLUENCE NURSE-TO-PATIENT PROFESSIONAL COMMUNICATION

The following six **verbal** styles of communication are summarized in Table 6.1, Fig. 6.2:

1. *Moderate pitch and tone in vocalization.* The oral delivery of a verbal message, expressed through tone of voice, inflection, sighing, and so on, is referred to as **paralanguage.** It is important to understand this component of communication because it affects how the verbal message is likely to be interpreted. For example, you might say, "I would like to hear more about what you are feeling" in a voice that sounds rushed, high-pitched, or harsh. Or you might make this same statement in a soft, unhurried voice that expresses genuine interest. In the first instance, the message is likely to be misinterpreted by the patient, despite your good intentions. Your caring intent is more apparent to the patient in the second instance. Voice inflection (pitch and tone), loudness, and rate of speaking either support or contradict the content of the verbal message. Varying your pitch helps others perceive you more positively (Ahmadian, Azarshahi, & Paulhus, 2017). Ideas may be conveyed merely by

TABLE 6.1 Styles That Influence Professional Communications in Nurse-Patient Relationships	
Verbal	**Nonverbal**
Moderates pitch and tone	Allows therapeutic silences; listens
Varies vocalizations	Uses congruent nonverbal behaviors
Encourages involvement	Uses facilitative body language
Validates worth	Uses touch appropriately
Advocates for patient as necessary	Proxemics—respects patient's space
Appropriately provides needed information: briefly and clearly, avoiding slang	Attends to nonverbal cues

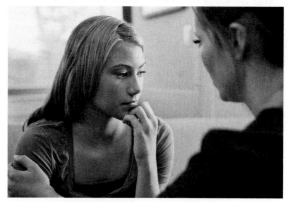

Fig. 6.2 Nurse talks with depressed teen. Copyright © monkeybusinessimages/iStock/Thinkstock.

emphasizing different portions of your statement. When the tone of voice does not fit the words, the message is less easily understood and is less likely to be believed. Some, especially when upset, communicate in an emotional rather than intellectual manner. A message conveyed in a firm, steady tone is more reassuring than one conveyed in a loud, emotional, abrasive, or uncertain manner. In contrast, if you speak in a flat, monotone voice when you are upset, as though the matter were of no consequence, you confuse your patient, making an appropriate response difficult.

2. *Vary vocalizations.* In some cultures sounds are punctuated, whereas in others sounds have a lyrical or singsong quality. We need to orient ourselves to the characteristic voice tones associated with other cultures.
3. *Encourage involvement.* Professional styles of communication have changed over time. We now partner with our patients in promoting their optimal health. We expect and encourage them to assume responsibility for their own health. Consequently provider-patient communication has changed. Paternalistic, "I'll tell you what to do" styles are no longer acceptable. Reflect on Ms. Kelly's case to see how patient becomes partner.
4. *Validate patient's worth.* Styles that convey caring send a message of individual worth that sustains the relationship. For example, some prefer providers who use a "warm" communication style to show

---

Case Example

Nurse practitioner Kay Boggs, FNP, sitting in the exam room with Ms. Kelly, is typing into the Electronic Health Record on her tablet. She says "You are still 40 pounds overweight, but are making progress losing!" She shares the screen to show a basal metabolic weight graph contrasting Ms. Kelly's body mass with the norm. Is this paternalistic? Or is this potentially a way of engaging her patient in a weight-loss discussion? Initial studies show that when providers gazed at computer screens instead of maintaining eye contact with their patients, the patients became detached. Recently the *Journal of the American Medical Association* and other publications have suggested sharing pertinent screen images with patients as a strategy for getting them to be more involved (Asan, Young, Chewing, & Montague, 2015).

---

caring, give information, and talk about their own feelings. Confirming responses validate the intrinsic worth of the person. These are responses that affirm the right of the individual to be treated with respect. They also affirm autonomy (i.e., the patient's right, ultimately, to make his or her own decisions). Disconfirming responses, in contrast, disregard the validity of patients' feelings by either ignoring them or by imposing a value judgment. Such responses take the form of changing the topic, offering reassurance without supporting evidence, or presuming to know what patients mean without verifying the message with them. More experienced nurses use more confirming communication. These communication skills are learned.

2. *Advocate for the patient when necessary.* Our personalities affect our style of social communication; some of us are naturally shy. But in our professional relationships we must often assume an assertive style of communicating with other health providers or agencies to obtain the best care or services for our patient.
3. *Provide needed information appropriately.* Providing accurate information in a timely manner in understandable amounts is discussed throughout this book. In our social conversations there is often a rhythm: "You talk, I listen," then "I get to talk, you listen." However, in professional communications, the content is more goal-focused. Self-disclosure from the nurse must be limited. It is not appropriate to tell a patient your problems.

NONVERBAL COMMUNICATION

Most of our person-to-person communication is **nonverbal**. All our words are accompanied by nonverbal cues that offer meaning about how to interpret the message. Think of the most interesting lecturer you ever had. Did this person lecture by making eye contact? By using hand gestures? By moving among the students? By conveying enthusiasm?

The function of nonverbal communication is to give us cues about what is being communicated. We give meaning about the purpose or context of our message nonverbally; this can increase the accuracy and efficiency of its impact on the listener. Some of these nonverbal cues are conveyed by tone of voice, facial expression, and body gestures or movement. Skilled use of nonverbal communication through therapeutic silences, use of congruent nonverbal behaviors, body language, touch, proxemics, and attention to nonverbal cues such as facial expression can build rapport. Emotional meanings are communicated through body language Fig. 6.3.

Aspects of Nonverbal Style That Influence Nurse-Patient Professional Communication

We must be aware of the ways in which our nonverbal messages are conveyed. The position of your hands, the look on your face, and the movement of your body all give cues regarding your meaning. It is important to use attending behaviors, such as leaning forward slightly, to convey to the patient that his or her conversation is worth listening to. Think of the last time an interviewer kept fidgeting in his seat, glanced frequently at his wall clock, or shuffled his papers while you were speaking. How did this make you feel? What nonverbal message was being conveyed?

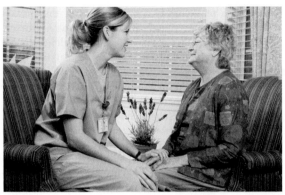

Fig. 6.3 Emotional meanings are communicated through body language, particularly facial expression.

Table 6.1 summarizes the following six nonverbal behaviors of a competent nurse:

1. *Allow silences.* In our social communications, the norm is a question-response sequence. The goal is to have no overlap and no gap between turns (Sicoli, Stivers, Enfield, & Levinson, 2015). We often become uncomfortable if conversation lags. There is a tendency to rush in to fill the void. But in our professional nurse-patient communication, we use silence therapeutically, allowing needed time to think about things.

2. *Use congruent nonverbal behaviors.* Nonverbal behavior should be congruent with the message and should reinforce it. If you knock on your instructor's office door to seek help, do you believe her when she says she would love to talk if you see her grimace and roll her eyes at her secretary? In another example, if you smile while telling your nurse-manager that your assignment is too much to handle, the seriousness of your message will be negated. Try to give nonverbal cues that are congruent with the message you are verbally communicating. When nonverbal cues are incongruent with the verbal information, messages are likely to be misinterpreted. When your verbal message is inconsistent with the nonverbal expression of the message, the nonverbal expressions assume prominence and are generally perceived as more trustworthy than the verbal content. You need to comment on any incongruence to help your patient. For example, when you enter a room to ask Mr. Sala if he is having any postoperative pain, he may say "No," but he grimaces and clutches his incision. After you comment on the incongruent message, he may admit that he is having some discomfort. Can you think of a clinical situation in which you changed the meaning of a verbal message by giving nonverbal "don't believe what I say" cues?

3. *Use facilitative body language. Kinesics* is an important component of nonverbal communication. Commonly referred to as **body language**, it is defined as involving the conscious or unconscious body positioning or actions of the communicator. Words direct the content of a message, whereas emotions accentuate and clarify the meaning of the words. Some nonverbal behaviors, such as tilting your head or facing your patient at an angle, promote communication. Lang (2016) urges us to pay attention to our body position, commenting that turning away conveys nervousness. He suggests viewing Amy Cuddy's TED talk.

   • **Posture.** Leaning forward slightly communicates interest and encourages your patient to keep the conversation going. Keep your arms uncrossed with palms open, knees uncrossed, and body loose, not tight and tense. Turning away indicates lack of interest, whereas directly and closely facing the patient, crossing your arms and staring unblinkingly, or jabbing your finger in the air suggests aggression.

   • **Facial expression.** Six common facial expressions (surprise, sadness, anger, happiness/joy, disgust/contempt, and fear) represent global, generalized interpretations of emotions common to all cultures. Facial expression either reinforces or modifies the message the listener hears. The power of the facial expression far outweighs the power of the actual words. So try to maintain an open, friendly expression without being boisterously cheerful. Avoid furrowing your forehead or assuming a distracted or bored expression.

   • **Eye contact.** Making direct eye contact, but not staring, generally conveys a positive message. Most patients interpret direct eye contact as an indication of your interest in what they have to say, although there are cultural differences.

   • **Gestures.** Some gestures, such as affirmative head nodding, help to facilitate conversation by showing interest and attention. The use of open-handed gestures can also facilitate communication. Avoid folding your arms across your chest or fidgeting. Hargestam, Hultin, Brulin, and Jacobsson (2016) showed that team leaders use gestures to reinforce verbal directions to team members, thus speeding up intervention in a crisis situation.

4. *Touch.* Touching is one of the most powerful ways you have of communicating nonverbally. Within a professional relationship, affective touch can convey caring, empathy, comfort, and reassurance. When a nurse touches patients, this contact can be perceived by the patient as either an expression of caring or negatively as a threat. Care must be taken to abide by the

patient's cultural proscriptions about the use of touch. The literature cites variations across cultures, such as the proscription some Muslim and Orthodox Jewish men follow against touching women other than family members. They might be uncomfortable shaking the hand of a female health care provider. In another example, some Native Americans use touch in healing, so that casual touching may be taboo. The vast majority of patients report feeling comforted when a professional health provider touches them (Atenstaedt, 2012). The "best" type of touch cited by patients is holding one of their hands (Kozlowska & Doboszynska, 2012). All nurses giving direct care use touch to assess and to assist. We touch to help our patient walk, roll over in bed, and so on. However, just as you would be careful about invading someone's personal space, you must be careful about when and where on the body you touch your patients. Your use of touch can elicit misunderstanding if it is perceived as invasive or inappropriate. Gender and culture determine perceptions about being touched. Therapeutic touch is discussed in Chapter 5.

5. *Proxemics.* We can use physical space to improve our interactions. **Proxemics** refers to the perception of what is a proper distance to be maintained between oneself and others. The way in which we use space communicates messages. You've heard the phrase "Get out of my face," used when someone stands too close; such closeness is often interpreted as an attempt to intimidate.
    - Each culture prescribes expectations for appropriate distance depending on the context of the communication. For example, the Nonverbal Expectancy Violations Model defines "proper" social distance for an interpersonal relationship as 1.5 to 4 feet in Western cultures. Americans, Canadians, and other Westerners tend to become uncomfortable if someone stands closer than 3 feet. The interaction's purpose determines the appropriate space, so that appropriate distance in space for intimate interaction would be zero distance, with increased space needed for personal distance, social distance, and public distance. In almost all cultures, zero distance is shunned except for loving or caring interactions. In giving physical care, nurses enter this "intimate" space. Caution is needed when you are at this closer distance, lest your actions be misinterpreted, since violating personal space can be threatening.

6. Attend to Nonverbal Body Cues
    - *Posture.* Often, the emotional component of a message can be indirectly interpreted by observing body language. Rhythm of movement and body stance may convey a message about the speaker. For example, when patients speak while directly facing you, this conveys more confidence than if they turn their bodies away from you at an angle. A slumped, head-down posture and slow movements might give you an impression of lassitude or low self-esteem, whereas an erect posture and decisive movement suggest confidence. Rapid, diffuse, agitated body movements may indicate anxiety. Forceful body movements may symbolize anger. When someone bows her head or slumps her body after receiving bad news, it conveys sadness. Can you think of other cues that body posture might give you?
    - *Facial expression.* Facial characteristics such as frowning or smiling add to the verbal message conveyed. Almost instinctively, we use facial expression as a barometer of another person's feelings, motivations, approachability, and mood. From infancy, we respond to the expressive qualities of another's face, often without even being aware of it. Therefore assessing facial expression together with other nonverbal cues may reveal vital information that will affect the nurse-patient relationship. For example, a worried facial expression and lip biting may suggest anxiety. Absence of a smile in greeting or grimacing may convey a message about how ill your patient feels.
    - *Eye contact.* Research suggests that individuals who make direct eye contact while talking or listening create a sense of confidence and credibility, whereas downward glances or averted eyes signal submission, weakness, or shame. In addition to conveying confidence, maintaining direct eye contact communicates honesty. Failure to maintain eye contact, known as *gaze aversion,* is perceived as a nonverbal cue meaning that the person is lying to you. If your patient's eyes wander around during a conversation, you may wonder if he is being honest. Even young children are more likely to attribute lying to those who avert their gaze.
    - *Gestures.* Movements of extremities may give cues. Making a fist can convey how angry someone is, just as the use of stabbing, abrupt hand gestures may suggest distress, whereas hugging one's arms closely (self-embracing gestures) may suggest fear.

Assessing the extent to which nonverbal cues communicate emotions can help you to communicate better. Studies repeatedly show that the failure to acknowledge nonverbal cues is often associated with inefficient communication by the health provider.

It is best if we verify our assessment of the meaning of observed nonverbal behaviors. Body cues, although suggestive, are imprecise. When communication is limited by the state of a person's health, pay even closer attention to nonverbal cues. Your patient's pain, for example, can be assessed through facial expression even when he or she is only partially conscious. What would you say to Mr. Geeze?

Case Example: Mr. Geeze

Mr. Geeze smiles but narrows his eyes and glares at the nurse. An appropriate comment for the nurse to make might be, "I notice you are smiling, but you say that you would like to kill me for mentioning your fever to the doctor. It seems that you might be angry with me."

Use of an incompatible communication style or failing to validate what patients are communicating nonverbally can adversely affect the level of support you can offer, leaving your patient feeling anxious or even hopeless. In this situation the patient may reject your well-meaning advice (Hawthorn, 2015).

COMMUNICATION ACCOMMODATION THEORY

Howard Giles (n.d.) theorized that people adapt or adjust their speech, vocal patterns (diction, tone, rate of speaking), dialect, word choice, and gestures to accommodate others. This theory suggests that it is desirable to adjust one's speech to our conversational partners to help facilitate our interaction, increase our acceptance, and improve trust and rapport. This is known as *convergence*. Convergence is thought to increase the effectiveness of your communication.

Accommodation can occur unconsciously or can be a conscious choice. For example, when you are speaking to a child, you might deliberately assume a more assertive, commanding style to get the child to obey. Choice of a distinctly different style is known as *divergence*. Conversely, you might choose convergence when you want to teach something about a disease condition. You might attempt to match your patient's speed and speech cadence. You definitely adapt or accommodate by choosing to match your vocabulary in an effort to be better understood. In general, if the person choosing to use convergence has more power in the relationship, he or she may be perceived as patronizing. This theory assumes that people are communicating in a rational manner. During a conflict, people can become

unreasonable or irrational; this would not a time to choose the use of an accommodation style.

EFFECTS OF SOCIOCULTURAL FACTORS ON COMMUNICATION

Communication is also affected by such style factors as cultural background, age cohort, gender, ethnicity, social class, and location. Of course, not everyone communicates in the manner described. These are broad generalizations as described in the literature.

Culture

We must communicate in a culturally competent manner. Although there is clear evidence that effective communication is related to better patient health outcomes, greater satisfaction, and better compliance, there is less evidence showing how cultural competency directly affects health outcomes. As in the following case, communication problems may be cultural. You must develop an awareness of the values of specific cultures to adapt your style. Chapter 7 deals in depth with concepts of intercultural communication.

Case Example: Ms. Sui

The Australian health system developed "bridging" orientation programs for foreign nurse graduates to help them develop communication styles effective in dealing with Australian patients (Philip, Manias, & Woodward-Kron, 2015). Mary Sui is a newly arrived, newly employed nurse in Sydney. According to her supervisor, Ms. Sui has excellent technical nursing skills, but she is reluctant to engage in social chit-chat or use humor to establish rapport as well as to engage with team members (perhaps due to perceptions about hierarchies in her native culture). Even though she speaks English, she only reluctantly communicates with patients (perhaps due to uncertainty in a new health environment), and she seems to lack experience of using self-reflection in examining mistakes. She is advised to enroll in a cultural orientation program, which can help nurses from culturally and linguistically diverse areas transition into their new staff nurse positions.

Age Cohort and Generational Diversity

The members of today's nursing workforce now span four generations. As might be expected, members of different generations hold differing views regarding work motivation, personal values, and attitudes toward their work; they also have differing communication styles and preferences. Differences exist in people's communication styles when they are interacting with authority figures. Differences also occur in learning styles and commitment to the organization (QSEN, n.d.). If ignored, generational differences can become a source of conflict in the workplace.

Each age cohort, born approximately every 20 years, has some communication style characteristics in common, which differentiate each group from prior generations. Communication Accommodation Theory, as described earlier, has been used to explore intergenerational communication problems. In considering the generation gap, beliefs about communication and goals for interactions differ among cohorts. For example, accommodation theory has been used to explore ageism, the negative evaluation of the elderly by those who are younger. In society, youth may deliberately choose divergence, purposely amplifying differences as by talking more rapidly, using slang, or emphasizing difference in values. In health care settings, studies of the generation gap and ageism stereotypes have found miscommunication outcomes in intergenerational interactions between providers and patients. How well would you respond to a patronizing style?

Some nurses might prefer digital communication via secure texting on cell phones, whereas others might prefer face-to-face communication.

Younger nurses and physicians, raised in the digital age, may rely on the Internet and social medial for information, social interaction, and communication. The nursing literature suggests that agencies and supervisors need to determine a person's preferred method of communication. People learn and communicate best if they are engaged in their preferred style.

Gender

Communication patterns are integrated into gender roles, which are defined by an individual's culture. In communication studies, gender differences have been shown to be greatest in terms of the use and interpretation of nonverbal cues. This may reflect gender differences in intellectual style as well as culturally reinforced standards of acceptable role-related behaviors. Of course there are wide variations within the same gender.

We are now questioning whether traditional ideas about male and female differences in communication are as prevalent as previously thought. Is there really a major difference in communication according to gender?

What is factual and what is a stereotype? More health care communication studies need to be done before we will really know. Because traditional thinking about

gender-related differences in communication content and process in both nonverbal and verbal communication are being revised, consider what you read critically.

Traditionally, women in most cultures were said to tend to avoid conflict and to want to smooth over differences. They were said to demonstrate more effective use of nonverbal communication and to be better decoders of nonverbal meaning. Feminine communication was thought to be more person-centered, warmer, and more sincere. Studies show that women tend to use more facial expressiveness, to smile more often, to maintain eye contact, to touch more often, and to nod more often. Women have a greater range of vocal pitch and also tend to use different informal patterns of vocalization than men. They use more tones signifying surprise, cheerfulness, and unexpectedness. Women tend to view conversation as a connection to others.

Traditionally, men in Western cultures were thought to communicate in a more task-oriented, direct fashion, to demonstrate greater aggressiveness, and to boast about their accomplishments. They have also been viewed as more likely to express disagreement. Studies show that men prefer a greater interpersonal distance between themselves and others and that they use gestures more often. Men are more likely to maintain eye contact in a negative encounter, although overall they maintain less direct eye contact; they also use less verbal communication than women in interpersonal relationships. Men are more likely to initiate an interaction, talk more, interrupt more freely, talk louder, disagree more, use hostile verbs, and talk more about issues.

Gender Differences in Communication in Health Care Settings

The effects of gender on communication have long been discussed in the literature. But do these differences actually affect performance? It has been suggested that more effective communication occurs when provider and patient are of the same gender, although this was not found to be true in some studies. In professional health care settings, women have been noted to use more active listening, using encouraging responses such as "Uh-huh," "Yeah," and "I see," and to use more supportive words.

Location

Patients in urban areas have reported poorer communication by their health care providers. One factor that might affect these results is that rural patients tend to be cared for by the same providers. In a clinic or other busy location, lack of privacy certainly affects the style as well as the content of communications.

DEVELOPING AN EVIDENCE-BASED PRACTICE Communication skill development is needed to address differences in language and culture in the nurse-patient relationship so as to avoid unsafe, unsatisfactory care. A number of recent studies link intercultural communication with skill development (Crawford, Candlin, & Roger, 2017; Sharpe & Hemsley, 2016). Effective communication skills can be taught, as demonstrated by Claramita, Tuah, Riskione, Prabandari, and Effendy (2016).This study compared communication skills of nursing students undergoing a training class and using a guide with a control group of students not using it. The University of Gadjah Mada guide is specifically oriented to Southeast Asian cultures, which emphasize mutual understanding, strong kinship ties, strong nonverbal behavior, and the use of traditional medicine. This guide has four phases:

The "ready phase," in which the nurse gains information about the patient's cultural values, gender values, and family involvement in decision making.

The "greet phase," in which the nurse establishes rapport and builds trust.

The "invite phase," in which the nurse explores the patient's physical complaints and feelings.

The "discuss phase," in which two-way communication continues.

Results

The group undergoing the cultural training session and using the guide demonstrated improved communication skills and dialogue and increased patient satisfaction when tested with standardized (simulated) patients. The researchers also noted that this training advanced the nurse's role as patient advocate.

Application to Your Clinical Practice

Using this model and the exercises in this book, you can prepare for interaction by increasing your awareness of your patients' cultural values, instigating the interaction by building rapport in a culturally sensitive way, using therapeutic skills such as active listening, demonstrating respect, focusing on patient concerns, and offering assistance in the form of teaching or advocacy depending on each patient's needs. In the last "discuss phase," you might best use the "informed" style of communication advocated by Moss, Reiter, Rimer, and Brewer (2016), in which you offer factual information to your patients while emphasizing to them that all health care decisions are theirs to make. In this way you will avoid a paternalistic communication style that implies, "I know what you should do."

APPLICATIONS

Knowing Your Own Communication Style

The style of communication you use can influence your patients' behaviors and their ability to reach their health goals. An aggressive communication style from a health care provider tends to create hostility or antipathy, whereas the use of an assertive, empathic style while seeking to make a point may lead to best outcomes. Users of a passive communication style are basically not active in helping patients to achieve their goals, whereas users of a more persuasive style wait to listen to before trying to make their points.

Patients report being dissatisfied with poor communication more than with other aspects of their care. Simulation exercises in prior chapters should give you the basic skills you need in your nurse-patient relationships, but remember that you bring your own communication style with you, as does your patient. Because we differ widely in our personal communication styles, it is important for you to identify your style and to know how to modify it for certain patients. Try Simulation Exercise 6.1 for a quick profile of your personal communication style. How does your affective style come across?

Do patients view you as empathic, caring, and reassuring? Experienced nurses adapt their innate social style so that their professional communications fit the patient and the situation. You too must modify your style to be sure that it is compatible with your patients' needs. Think about the potential for incompatibility in the following Michaels case.

Case Example: Mr. Michaels

Nurse (in a firm tone): Mr. Michaels, it's time to take your medicine.

Mr. Michaels (in a complaining tone): You are so bossy!

Empathic communication is crucial to your nursing care and may improve a patient's health outcome. Recognize how others perceive you. Consider all the nonverbal factors that affect their perceptions of you, such as gender, manner of dress, appearance, skin tone, hairstyle, age, role as a student, gestures, and mannerisms. Simulation Exercise 6.2 may increase your awareness of gender bias.

The initial step in identifying your own style may be to compare your style with those of others. Ask yourself, "What makes someone perceive a nurse either as authoritarian or as accepting and caring?" The Simulation Exercise 6.3 video may help you to compare your style with those of others.

Develop an awareness of alternative styles that you can comfortably assume if the occasion warrants. For example, Watts et al. (2017) suggests assessing whether changing your style to speak more slowly, using more nonverbal communication, and involving family members will help get the message across to people of other ethnic groups. It is important to figure out whether some other factors may be influencing your style toward a particular patient and if that is appropriate. How might the other person's age, race, socioeconomic status, or gender affect his or her responses to you? We must continually work to update our communication competencies. Internal organizational communication is rapidly becoming electronic. Some hospital agencies are increasingly relying on digital communication, eliminating many of the nuances communicated nonverbally.

INTERPERSONAL COMPETENCE

Nurse-patient communication processes are based on the nurse's interpersonal competence and the situations that nurses find themselves in. Higher levels of anxiety affect your communication (Fletcher, McCallum, & Peters, 2016). **Interpersonal competence** develops as you come to understand the complex cognitive, behavioral, and cultural factors that influence communication. This understanding, together with the use of a broad range of communication skills, can help you to interact positively with your patients as they attempt to cope with multiple demands. Developing good communication skills will increase your competent communication. Such skills are identified as among the attributes of expert nurses with the most clinical credibility. In dealing with a patient in the sociocultural context of the health care system, two kinds of abilities are required: social cognitive competency and message competency.

Social cognitive competency is the ability to interpret message content within interactions from the point of view of each of the participants. By embracing your patients' perspectives, you begin to understand how they organize information and formulate goals. This is especially important when your patients' ability to communicate is impaired by a mechanical barrier such as a ventilator. Patients who have recovered from critical illnesses requiring ventilator support report that they felt fear and distress during this experience.

EXERCISE 6.1   Simulation Exercise My Communication Style: Quick Profile

Purpose: To Develop Self-Reflection

Procedure: Answer the following:

1. I prefer to
   - Get my way.
   - Follow the rules.
   - Avoid confrontation.
2. My verbal tone is most often
   - Warm.
   - Enthusiastic.
   - Determined.
3. If we have a difference of opinion, I usually want to
   - Dominate.
   - Compromise.
   - Give in.
4. In a social group situation, I sometimes
   - Fail to give my opinion.
   - Am very, very polite.
   - Digress from the topic.
   - Become irritated with those who disagree with me.
5. My friends have told me that
   - I talk using my hands.
   - I smile a lot.
   - I can't sit still.

Analytical Reflection

Compare your answers with book content on style. Analyze how these factors might affect your nurse-patient relationships.

Message competency refers to the ability to use language and nonverbal behaviors strategically in the intervention phase of the nursing process to achieve the goals of the interaction. Communication skills are used as a tool to influence patients to maximize their adaptation. Think how it feels when your patient sees you smile and hears you say, "That's impressive; you have successfully self-injected your insulin!"

STYLE FACTORS THAT INFLUENCE RELATIONSHIPS

The establishment of trust and respect in an interpersonal relationship with a patient and family is dependent on an effective, ongoing communication style. Having knowledge is not sufficient to guarantee its successful application. For example, providers who sit at eye level, at an optimal distance (**proxemics**), without furniture in between (special configuration) will likely have more eye contact and use more

SIMULATION EXERCISE 6.2 **Gender Bias**

Purpose
To create discussion about gender bias.

Procedure
In small groups, read and discuss the following comments that are made about care delivery on a geriatric psychiatric unit by staff and students: "Male staff tend to be slightly more confident and to make quicker decisions. Women staff are better at the feeling things, like conveying warmth."

Analytical Reflection
1. Reflect as to the effect of gender on perceptions of comments. Determine whether these comments are made by male or female staff.
2. Analyze their accuracy. Be sure to support with evidence from the text.
3. Can you truly generalize attributes to any male and female individuals?

SIMULATION EXERCISE 6.3 **Self-Analysis of Video Recording**

Purpose
To increase awareness of students' own style.

Procedure
With a partner, role-play an interaction between nurse and patient. Use the video capacity of your cell phone to record a 1- to 2-minute interview with the camera focused on you. The topic of the interview could be "identifying health promotion behaviors" or something similar.

Reflective Analysis
Analyze playbacks in a group. What postures were used? What nonverbal messages were communicated? How? Were verbal and nonverbal messages congruent?

BOX 6.1 **Suggestions to Improve Your Communication Style**

- Adapt yourself to your patient's cultural values.
- Use nonverbal communication strategies, such as
  - Maintaining eye contact
  - Displaying pleasant, animated facial expressions
  - Smiling often
  - Nodding your head to encourage talking
  - Maintaining an attentive, upright posture and sitting at the patient's level, leaning forward slightly
  - Attending to proper proximity and increasing space if the patient shows signs of discomfort, such as averting his or her gaze, or swinging his or her legs.
- Using touch if appropriate to the situation
- Using active listening and responding to patient's cues
- Using verbal strategies to engage your patient
  - Using humor, but avoiding gender jokes
  - Attending to proper tone and pitch, avoiding an overly loud voice
  - Avoiding jargon
  - Using nonjudgmental language and open-ended questions
  - Listening and avoiding jumping in too soon with problem solving
  - Verbalizing respect
  - Asking permission before addressing a client by his or her first name
  - Conveying caring comments
  - Using confirming, positive comments

an adult who says, "That's cool," might be referring to the temperature, whereas another might be conveying satisfaction. In health care, the "food pyramid" is understood by nurses to represent the basic nutritional food groups needed for health; however, the term may have limited meaning for others.

Medical Jargon

Beginning nursing students often report confusion while learning all the medical terminology required for their new role. Remembering our own experiences, we can empathize with patients who are attempting to understand the **medical jargon** involved in health care. Careful explanations help overcome this communication barrier. For successful communication, the words we use should have a similar meaning to both individuals in an interaction. An important part of the communication process is the search for a common vocabulary so that the message sent is the same as the one received. Consider the oncology nurse who

therapeutic touching. Adapting your style to fit your patient's needs encourages them to accept your message and to understand it better (Hawthorn, 2015). Box 6.1 contains suggestions to improve your own professional style of communicating.

Slang and Jargon

Different age groups even in the same culture may attribute different meanings to the same word. For example, develops a computer databank of cancer treatment terms. While she is admitting Mr. Michaels as a new patient, the nurse uses an existing template model on her computer to create an individualized terminology sheet with just the words that would be encountered by him during his course of chemotherapy.

Responsiveness of Participants

How responsive the participants are affects the depth and breadth of communication. Reciprocity affects not only the relationship process but also patient health outcomes. Some people are naturally more verbal than others. It is easier to have a therapeutic conversation with extroverted patients who want to communicate. You will want to increase the responsiveness of those who are less verbal and enhance their responsiveness. Verbal and nonverbal approval encourages patients to express themselves. Elsewhere, we discuss skills that promote responsiveness, such as active listening, demonstrations of empathy, and acknowledgment of the content and feelings of messages. Sometimes acknowledging the difficulty your patients are having in expressing their feelings, praising your patients' efforts, and encouraging them to use more than one route of communication will help. Such strategies demonstrate interpersonal sensitivity. Listening to the care experience of a patient, responding to verbal or nonverbal cues, and avoiding "talking down" encourages communication and may improve compliance with the treatment regimen. Simulation Exercise 6.4 will help you practice the use of confirming responses.

Roles of Participants

Paying attention to the **roles relationship** among the communicators may be just as important as deciphering the content and meaning of the message. The relationships between the roles of the sender and those of the receiver influence how the communication is likely to be received and interpreted. The same constructive criticism made by a good friend and by one's immediate supervisor is likely to be interpreted differently, even though the content and style are similar. Communication between subordinates and supervisors is far more likely to be influenced by power and style than by gender. When roles are unequal in terms of power, the more powerful individual tends to speak in a more dominant style. This is discussed in Chapters 22 and 23.

Context of the Message

Communication is always influenced by the environment in which it takes place. It does not occur in a vacuum but is shaped by the situation in which the interaction occurs.

SIMULATION EXERCISE 6.4 Confirming Responses

Purpose
To increase students' skills in using confirming communication.

Procedure
Formulate a better way to rephrase the same message. Evaluate whether it is easier for you to send a positive, confirming message or a disconfirming, negative message:
1. "Three of your 14 blood sugars this week were too high. What did you do wrong?"
2. "Your blood pressure is dangerously high. Are you eating salty foods again?"
3. "You gained 5 pounds this week. Can't you stick to a simple diet?"

Reflective Analysis
Suggest better rephrasing to communicate the same message. Was it relatively easy to send a positive, confirming message?

Taking time to evaluate the physical setting and the time and space in which the contact takes place—as well as the psychological, social, and cultural characteristics of each individual involved—gives you flexibility in choosing the most appropriate context.

Involvement in the Relationship

Relationships generally need to develop over time because communication changes during different phases of the relationship. Studies show that physicians, nurses, and other health care workers respond to patients' concerns less than half the time. Responses tend to focus on physical care and often do not address social emotional care. These days, nurses working with hospitalized patients have less time to develop relationships, whereas community-based nurses may have greater opportunities. To begin to explore ethical problems in your nursing relationships, consider the ethical dilemma provided.

Use of Humor

As discussed elsewhere, research has associated the use of humor with stress relief, diffusion of conflict, enhancement of learning, and improved communication in nurse-patient relationships (Canha, 2016). Can you incorporate humor into your relationships without using disparagement?

ADVOCATE FOR CONTINUITY OF CARE

We have learned that patients, evaluation of positive health care communication is higher when they consistently relate to the same individuals providing their care. These providers are more likely to listen to them, to explain things clearly, to spend enough time with them, and to show them respect. Because physicians, nurses and other team members communicate differently with patients, it is crucial for them to pool information.

SUMMARY

Communication involves more than an exchange of verbal and nonverbal information. As our population becomes more diverse, we are challenged to provide patient-centered care that is sensitive to culture, race, ethnicity, gender, and sexual orientation. The recurring theme in this chapter is that you can adapt your communication style to better suit individual patients. Modifying your style to provide more effective communication promotes safer care and better health outcomes. This chapter offers suggestions for styles of verbal and nonverbal communication as well as a discussion of cultural and gender differences. Style factors that affect the communication process include the responsiveness and role relationships of the participants, the types of responses and context of the relationships, and the level of involvement in the relationship. Skills are suggested, such as using confirming responses to acknowledge the value of a person's communication. More nonverbal strategies to facilitate nurse-patient communication are discussed in later chapters.

> **ETHICAL DILEMMA: What Would You Do?**
> Katy Collins, RN, is a new grad who learns that a serious error that harmed a patient has occurred on her unit. She realizes that if staff continues to follow the existing protocol, this error could occur again. In a team meeting led by an administrator, Katy raises this issue in a tentative manner. The leader speaks in a loud, decisive voice and states that he wants input from the staff nurses. However, he glances at the clock, gazes over Katy's head, and maintains a bored expression. Katy gets the message that the administration wants to smooth over the error, bury it, and go on as usual rather than using resources and time to correct the underlying problem.
> 1. What ethical principle is being violated in this situation?
> 2. What message does the administrator's behavior convey?
> 3. Explain the congruence. Draw conclusions about how you would change the nonverbal message to make it congruent.

DISCUSSION QUESTIONS

1. Use Simulation Exercise 6.2 to apply your knowledge about the influence of gender on communication.
2. In a loud, commanding voice, a nurse tells an immediate postoperative patient to take deep breaths every 20 minutes despite the pain it causes. Describe three possible reactions that might occur. Formulate ways to make this intervention more effective.

REFERENCES

Ahmadian, S., Azarshahi, S., & Paulhus, D. L. (2017). Explaining Donald Trump via communication style. *Personality & Individual Differences, 107*, 49–53.

Asan, O., Young, H. N., Chewing, B., & Montague, E. (2015). How physician HER screen sharing affects patient and doctor nonverbal communication in primary care. *Patient Education Counseling, 98*(3), 1–11.

Atenstaedt, R. (2012). Touch in the consultation. *British Journal of General Practice. 62*(596), 147–148.

Canha, B. (2016). Using humor in treatment of substance use disorders: worthy of further investigation. *Open Nursing Journal, 10*, 37–44.

Claramita, M., Tuah, R., Riskione, P., Prabandari, Y. S., & Effendy, C. (2016). Comparison of communication skills between trained and untrained students using a culturally sensitive nurse-client communication guide in Indonesia. *Nurse Education Today, 36*, 236–241.

Crawford, T., Candlin, S., & Roger, P. (2017). New perspectives on understanding cultural diversity in nurse-patient communication. *Collegian, 24*, 63–69.

Cuddy A. Your body language may shape what you are. n.d. on TED Talks, www.ted.com/search?q=amy+cuddy.

Fletcher, I., McCallum, R., & Peters, S. (2016). Attachment styles and clinical communication performance in trainee doctors. *Patient Education & Counseling, 99*, 1852–1857.

Giles, H. (n.d.). Communication accommodation theory. Retrieved from www.public.iastate.edu/~mredmond/SpAccT.htm.

Hargestam, M., Hultin, M., Brulin, C., & Jacobsson, M. (2016). Trauma team leaders nonverbal communication: video registration during trauma team training. *Scandinavian Journal of Trauma, Resuscitation and Emergency Medicine, 24*, 1–2.

Hawthorn, M. (2015). The importance of communication in sustaining hope at the end of life. *British Journal of Nursing, 24*(13), 702–705.

Kee, J. W. Y., Khoo, H. S., Lim, I., & Koh, M. Y. H. (2017). Communication skills in patient-doctor interactions. *Health Professions Education, ScienceDirect, in press*, available on-line April, 2017.

Kozlowska, L., & Doboszynska, A. (2012). Nurses' nonverbal methods of communicating with patients in the terminal phase. *International Journal of Palliative Nursing, 18*(1), 40–46.

Lang, C. (2016). Nursing and importance of body language. *Nursing, 46*(4), 48–49.

Moss, J. L., Reiter, P. L., Rimer, B. K., & Brewer, N. T. (2016). Collaborative patient-provider communication and uptake of adolescent vaccines. *Social Science & Medicine, 159*, 100–107.

Philip, S., Manias, E., & Woodward-Kron, R. (2015). Nurse educator perspectives of overseas qualified nurses' intercultural clinical communication: Barriers, enablers, and engagement strategies. *Journal of Clinical Nursing, 24*, 2628–2637.

Quality and Safety Education for Nurses (QSEN). (n.d.). Teamwork & collaboration (QSEN competencies: Online teaching modules). www.QSEN.org/.

Sharpe, B., & Hemsley, B. (2016). Improving nurse-patient communication with patients with communication impairments: Hospital nurses' views on the feasibility of using mobile communication technologies. *Applied Nursing Research, 30*, 228–236.

Sicoli, M. A., Stivers, T., Enfield, N. J., & Levinson, S. C. (2015). Marked initial pitch in questions signals marked communication function. *Language & Speech, 58*(2), 204–223.

Warren, E. (2015). Communication with patients. *Practice Nurse, 45*(9), 1–6.

Watts, K. J., Meiser, B., Zilliacus, E., Kaur, R., Taouk, M., Girgis, A., et al. (2017). Communication with patients from minority backgrounds: Individual challenges experienced by oncology health professionals. *European Journal of Oncology Nursing, 26*, 83–90.

White, R. O., Chakkalakal, R. J., Presley, C. A., Bian, A., Schildcrout, J. S., Wallstonet, et al. (2016). Perceptions of provider communication among vulnerable patients with diabetes: influences of medical mistrust and health literacy. *Journal of Health Communication, 21*(suppl), 127–134.

7

Intercultural Communication

Elizabeth C. Arnold

OBJECTIVES

At the end of the chapter, the reader will be able to:

1. Define *culture* and related terms.
2. Discuss key dimensions of intercultural communication.
3. Describe the concept of cultural competence.
4. Discuss the role of the National CLAS Standards.
5. Discuss characteristics of selected cultures as they relate to.

INTRODUCTION

Health care professionals and their patients each bring a personalized cultural background and perspective, with associated values and beliefs, to health care discussions. A person's culture will influence the way relevant information is interpreted and acted upon by an individual patient and his or her family. Each patient's social class, religious beliefs and spirituality, education, and family norms also influence patient preferences and values (Douglas et al., 2014). National Standards for Culturally and Linguistically Appropriate Services (CLAS) in Health and Health Care mandate close attention to honoring diversity in all aspects of health communication.

Understanding cultural variations in communication is a critical nursing competency in contemporary health care. The purpose of this chapter is to introduce students to common cultural patterns that nurses may encounter in health care settings. Included in the chapter are applications associated with the nation's four major cultural groups. This background can serve to improve the safety and quality of health care delivery for patients from different cultures.

BASIC CONCEPTS

The racial and ethnic distribution of the US population today reports a 62.6% non-Latino Caucasian majority population, 17% Hispanic or Latino ethnicity, 13.2% African American, and 5% Asian (US Census Bureau, 2015). Each minority population adds a personalized cultural context to how they understand and interpret accepted health habits and explanatory models of health and illness. By 2050, minority groups are projected to make up 54% of the population in the United States (Florczak, 2013).

Each cultural group develops shared stories, values, beliefs, and practices, which are shaped by both their history and geography (Fang, Sixsmith, Sinclair, & Horst, 2015). Cultural values about treatment options, ethnic and religious beliefs about key issues, and dietary habits influence health behaviors and clinical outcomes (Flores, 2006). Significant health disparities exist among the culturally and linguistically diverse people living in the United States, when comparing the non-Latino Caucasian population with other culturally and linguistically diverse people (US Department of Health and Human Services [DHHS], 2015).

The Institute of Medicine (IOM, 2002a) report on *Speaking of Health* established guidelines to promote more effective communication practices in diverse communities. Nurses need to view cultural diversity as a solid dimension of effective health care.

BASIC CONCEPTS

Definitions

Culture is a complex social concept, consisting of family customs, beliefs and values, political systems, and ethnic identities held by a particular group of people. Cultural competence is considered as both an ethical standard and a legal standard (Office of Minority Health, 2014).

Alexander (2008) suggests that, "Each individual, family, and community represents a unique blend of overlapping and intersecting cultural elements in which the whole is greater than the sum of the parts" (p. 416). To further complicate matters, when more than one culture helps to explain a person's health behavior, they do not necessarily support each other. It is important to avoid making assumptions about the degree to which patients embrace particular cultural beliefs because of issues like acculturation, and significant life experiences.

Culture in Health Care

In health care, culture provides a relevant context for understanding how patients and families experience health and illness. Cultural beliefs and values help explain how people approach shared decision making and participate in patient-centered self-management care (Fig. 7.1). In high-context cultures, such as Asian and Latino cultures, family involvement in decision making is desirable, and family-centered decision making tends to prevail over self-determination (Berkman & Ko, 2010).

Culture plays a particularly significant role in health-related life transitions, such as birth, death, old age, and terminal illness. Understanding embedded cultural considerations in health care delivery enhances compliance with treatment. Culture acts as a crucial filter through which people "learn how to be in the world, how to behave, what

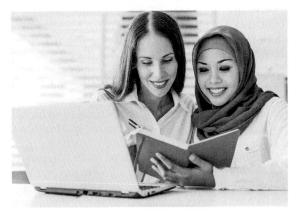

Fig. 7.1 Cultural differences influence how people interpret illnesses and manage treatment options.

to value, and what gives meaning to existence" (Schim & Doorenbos, 2010, p. 256).

The concept of culture extends beyond a specific ethnic background or country of origin (Betancourt, 2004). *Culture* is a term applied to professional and organizational systems. Ellison (2015) states that "the culture of an organization is the sum of the organization's beliefs, norms, values, mission, philosophies, traditions, and sacred cows" (p. 48) and "to subgroups within a dominant culture, including religious denominations, sports and educational groups, and lifestyle orientations."

HOW CULTURE IS LEARNED

We are born into a culture; however, culture is not an inborn characteristic. Initially, culture is learned through family and then through other social institutions, such as school, church affiliations, and community contacts (Giger, 2013). As children learn language from their primary caregivers, and later refine their language skills in school, they simultaneously integrate the cultural attitudes, meanings, values, and thought patterns that inform their words. Immigrants acquire a cultural identity through a two-step interpersonal process in which the person transitions from adhering to traditional cultural beliefs and values in a country of origin toward full adoption of the values and beliefs of culture. Efforts to understand and influence health behaviors of culturally diverse patients are best achieved at the community level (Kline & Huff, 2008).

Acculturation

Acculturation describes how immigrants from a different culture learn and choose to adapt to the behavior and norms of a different, new culture, which holds different expectations. This can be a complicated process because it includes embracing new social, hierarchal, and kinship relationships, consistent with an unfamiliar cultural context (Page, 2005). Becoming acculturated creates stress due to the competing pressures of reconciling a familiar cultural identity with the need to adopt new customs essential to functioning effectively in the adopted culture (Marsiglia & Booth, 2015). Exploring your patient's level of acculturation as it relates to culturally based explanatory models of illness, traditional health behaviors, and their potential impact on health care matters (Hardin, 2014).

Assimilation occurs when an individual from a different culture fully adopts the behaviors, customs, and values of the mainstream culture as part of his or her social identity. To become fully assimilated, immigrants must conform and adapt to the norms of the new culture. This is a gradual process. By the third generation, many immigrants may have little knowledge of their traditional culture and language or allegiance to their original heritage (Bacallao & Smokowski, 2005; Schwartz, Montgomery, & Briones, 2006). Box 7.1 summarizes points of cultural diversity in health care.

Cultural Patterns

Cultural patterns describe the social customs, expected behaviors, cultural beliefs, values, and language passed down from generation to generation by a group of people (Giger et al., 2007). These patterns are informally transmitted through the family, and formally through other affiliations such as school, work, and church.

Cultural patterns become an essential part of personal identity. This is because we learn them from the people who are important to us and/or through events that touch us deeply. Some cultural patterns are further indoctrinated through religious ceremonies, such as baptisms, bar mitzvahs, confirmations, and end of life rituals.

Cultural patterns and beliefs dictate personal preferences and influence how people process and interpret incoming information. Social factors, such as class and literacy level, further distinguish individual response patterns within a culture (Weiner, McConnell, Latella, & Ludi, 2013). Although cultural traditions evolve over time, remainders from the past still influence the behavior of many people either directly or indirectly.

Simulation Exercise 7.1, examining personal cultural patterns, offers you an opportunity to reflect on your own cultural heritage and examine what is fundamental about its influence on you.

BOX 7.1   Points of Cultural Diversity in Health Care

People's feelings, attitudes, and behavioral standards
Ways of living, language, and habits
How people relate to others, including attitudes about health professionals
Nutrition and diet
Personal views of what is right and wrong
Perspectives on health, illness, and death, including appropriate rituals
Hearing about and discussing negative health information
Decisional authority, role relationships, and truth-telling practices
Child-rearing practices
Use of advance directives, informed consent, and patient autonomy (Calloway, 2009; Carrese & Rhodes, 2000; Karim, 2003; Searight & Gafford, 2005)

Cultural Diversity

Cultural diversity is a term used to describe social variations between cultural groups. Unrecognized and/or unaccepted differences among different cultural groups can present significant difficulties in communication and relationships. Lack of exposure to and/or understanding of the normal patterns of people from other cultures decreases acceptance, reinforces stereotypes, and creates prejudice. People tend to notice differences related to language, manners, mannerisms, and behaviors in people of different cultures in ways that do not happen with people from their own culture (Spence, 2001).

Physiological risk factors and vulnerabilities are more apparent in certain ethnic cultures than others. For example, American Indians have a higher incidence of alcoholism. Chinese Americans demonstrate a higher incidence of hypertension (Chen & Hu, 2014). Tay Sachs disease is found almost exclusively in the Jewish population. Likewise, the incidence of sickle cell anemia is similarly found in African Americans.

SIMULATION EXERCISE 7.1   Cultural Authenticity

Purpose
To help students appreciate the importance of understanding your own culture as a basis for understanding culture relationships in health care.

Procedure
1. Write a one-page story about your own culture and/or ethnic background as you understand it.
2. Describe in what ways family and social customs or culture-bound traditions have influenced your sense of personal development, career and leisure choices, opportunities, values, and so forth.
3. Discuss how personal understanding of your cultural background has changed over time.
4. Identify how knowing about one's own culture informs cultural sensitivity to others in health care situations.
5. Briefly answer the question, "Does my story represent my cultural authenticity?"

Discussion
1. Share your culture story in small groups of three to four students.
2. As a class, discuss how personal culture can influence health behaviors.
3. Identify common themes.
4. Discuss how culturally authentic knowledge prevents unconscious projection of a personal cultural context on a patient from a different culture.

TABLE 7.1   Definitions Associated With Culture

Concept	Definition
Subculture	A smaller group of people living within the dominant culture with a distinct lifestyle, shared beliefs, and expectations that set them apart from the mainstream (Drench et al., 2009). Example: Amish, Mormons.
Ethnicity	Group of people who share a common social identity based on ancestral, national, or cultural experiences (Day-Vines et al., 2007).
Ethnocentrism	Belief that one's own culture is superior to all others, and should be the norm (Lewis, 2000).
Cultural relativism	Concept that each culture is unique and should be judged only on the basis of its own values and standards (Aroian & Faville, 2005).

Adapted from Aroian, K., & Faville, K. (2005). Reconciling cultural relativism for a clinical paradigm: What's a nurse to do? *Journal of Professional Nursing, 21*(6):330, 2005; Day-Vines, N., Wood, S., Grothaus, T., Craigen, L., Holman, A., Dotson-Blake, K., Douglass, M. J. (2007). Broaching the subjects of race, ethnicity and culture during the counseling process. *Journal of Counseling & Development* 85:401–409; and Drench, M., Noonan, A., Sharby, N., & Ventura S. H. (2009). *Psychosocial aspects of health care* (2nd ed.). Upper Saddle River, NJ: Pearson Prentice Hall.

Diversity can exist *within* a culture. In fact, more differences occur among individuals within a culture than between cultural groups, related to differences in educational and socioeconomic status (SES), age, gender, and life experiences (Drench, Noonan, Sharby, & Ventura, 2009). Within the same culture, individuals with radically different philosophies, social patterns, and sanctioned behaviors coexist, sometimes peacefully, and other times in conflict with each other. Consider, for example, the divisive political differences between liberal and conservatives voters, the disagreements between faith beliefs, and different social expectations of the very poor versus the very rich.

Despite historic legislation designed to make quality health care opportunities available to everyone, progress has been slow, and prejudicial attitudes continue to play a role in not ending unequal treatment for minority populations. Box 7.1 identifies points of cultural diversity in health care.

Culture diversity is an issue within the health care profession (Table 7.1). Minority nurses account for only 16.8% of the professional nursing workforce (Isaacson, 2014). Minorities comprise only about 3% of medical school faculty and about 17% of public health officers (Betancourt, Green, & Carrillo, 2003). Increasing the number of culturally diverse health professionals in the workforce must be an area of emphasis to help ensure equity and understanding in health care. Simulation Exercise 7.2 provides an opportunity to study components of cultural diversity within the profession.

WORLDVIEW

Worldview is defined as, "the way people tend to look out upon their world or their universe to form a picture or value stance about life or the world around them"

SIMULATION EXERCISE 7.2   Diversity in the Nursing Profession

Purpose

To help students learn about the experience of nurses from a different ethnic group.

Procedure

1. Each student will interview a registered nurse from an ethnic minority group different from their own ethnic origin.
2. The following questions serve as an interview guide:
   a. In what ways was your educational experience more difficult or easier as a minority student?
   b. What do you see as the barriers for minority nurses in our profession?
   c. What do you see as the opportunities for minority nurses in our profession?
   d. What do you view as the value of increasing diversity in the nursing profession for health care?
   e. What do you think we can do as a profession and personally to increase diversity in nursing?
3. Write a one- to two-page narrative report about your findings to be presented in a follow-up class.

Discussion

1. What were the common themes that seemed to be present across narratives?
2. In what ways, if any, did doing this exercise influence your thinking about diversity?
3. Did you find any of the answers to the interview questions disturbing or surprising?
4. How could you use this exercise to become culturally competent?

TABLE 7.2   Purnell's Domains of Cultural Assessment

Domains of Cultural Assessment	Sample Areas for Inquiry
Personal heritage	Country of origin, reasons for migration, politics, class distinctions, education, social and economic status
Communication	Dominant language and dialects, personal space, body language and touch, time relationships, greetings, eye contact
Family roles and organization	Gender roles; roles of extended family, elders, head of household; family goals, priorities, and expectations; lifestyle differences
Workforce issues	Acculturation and assimilation, gender roles, temporality, current and previous jobs, variance in salary and status associated with job changes
Bioecology	Genetics, hereditary factors, ethnic physical characteristics, drug metabolism
High-risk health behaviors	Drugs, nicotine and alcohol use, sexual behaviors
Nutrition	Meaning of food, availability and food preferences, taboos associated with food, use of food in illness
Pregnancy and childbearing	Rituals and constraints during pregnancy, labor and delivery practices, newborn and postpartum care
Death rituals	How death is viewed, death rituals, preparation of the body, care after death, use of advance directives, bereavement practices
Spirituality	Religious practices, spiritual meanings, use of prayer
Health care practices	Traditional practices, religious health care beliefs, individual versus collective responsibility for health, how pain is expressed, transplantation, mental health barriers
Health care practitioners	Use of traditional and/or folk practitioners, gender role preferences in health care

Adapted from Purnell, J. D., & Paulanka, B. J. (2013). *Transcultural health care: A culturally competent approach* (4th ed.). Philadelphia: F.A. Davis.

(Leininger & McFarland, 2006, p. 15). A person's worldview describes each *individual's* point of view or perspective about the larger social culture. Each person's worldview acts as a working model of a *personalized* interpretation of the patient's cultural values and customs. It acts as a perceptual lens through which an individual or cultural group interprets and interacts with a created universe. For example, teenagers and older adults can have similar overall beliefs about their culture. But, their worldviews can be polar opposites because of their experiential life events and age differences. This difference in concept is important in intercultural communication. Table 7.2 provides sample assessment questions nurses can use when the patient comes from a different culture.

Health Disparities

The nation's health agenda, *Healthy People 2020*, defines **health disparity** as "a particular type of health difference that is closely linked with a person's social, economic, and/or environmental disadvantage." The inequity present in health disparities influences a person's capacity to achieve positive health outcomes, experience satisfaction with treatment, and achieve healthy well-being through normal channels.

Health disparities adversely affect certain populations and groups of people who have systematically experienced greater obstacles to health care. Disparities can reflect an ethnic group; a religion; SES; education, gender, and age; mental health; and cognitive, sensory, or physical disability. Sexual orientation or gender identity, geographic locale, and physical or mental disability create informal disparities, historically linked to discrimination, but not always recognized as a challenge to equity in health care.

ETHNICITY AND RELATED CONCEPTS

Ethnicity describes a person's awareness of a shared cultural heritage with others based on common racial, geographic, ancestral, religious, or historical bonds. People develop a sense of identity associated with a particular heritage that passes from generation to generation. Ethnicity creates a sense of belonging and inspires a strong commitment to associated values and practices.

The term *ethnicity* represents a sociopolitical construct. It is *not* a descriptor of race or physical features (Ford & Kelly, 2005). People with similar skin color and features can have a vastly different ethnic heritage. For example, consider the difference between a person of Jamaican heritage versus African American descent. Ethnicity can also reflect spiritually based values and membership, for example, the Amish represent a religious sect within the larger social culture with an unique of behavioral differences (Donnermeyer & Friedrich, 2006). A relevant question is to ponder, what does it mean for you to be a member of a particular subculture (e.g., Latino American, Asian American, Jewish, Muslim, or Catholic)?

Ethnocentrism

Ethnocentrism is defined as a belief that one's own culture is superior to others. The concept of ethnocentrism can foster the belief that one's culture has the right to impose its standards of "correct" behavior and values on another culture.

Neuliep (2015) proposes that "ethnocentrism is essentially descriptive, not necessarily pejorative" (p. 206). Taking pride in one's culture is appropriate, but when a person fails to respect the value of other cultures or assumes that one culture is superior to another, can often result in stereotypes and prejudice. Prejudice can be directed toward an ethnic group as a whole or toward an individual associated with the group. The deadly consequences of unchecked prejudice were evidenced in the persecution of innocent people during Hitler's regime, and currently in Syria. Strong prejudice continues today with terrorist attacks and targeted violence against perceived "outsider" groups, such as Muslims, which are embedded in ethnocentric values and extreme sectarian differences between certain cultural groups.

The IOM (2003) identifies economic status and social class as components of diversity related to health risk and treatment outcomes. Other examples include physical or mental disability, sexual orientation, ageism, morbid obesity, and unusual physical or personal characteristics.

Case Example

"I knew a man who had lost the use of both eyes. He was called a blind man. He could also be called an expert typist, a conscientious worker, a good student, a careful listener, and a man who wanted a job. But he couldn't get a job in the department store order room where employees sat and typed orders, which came over the phone. The personnel man was impatient to get the interview over. 'But you are a blind man,' he kept saying, and one could almost feel his silent assumption that somehow the incapability in one aspect made the man incapable in every other. So blinded by the label was the interviewer that he could not be persuaded to look beyond it" (Allport, 1979, p. 178).

Cultural Relativism

Cultural relativism holds that each culture is unique, and its merits should be judged only on the basis of its own values and standards. Behaviors viewed as unusual from outside a culture can make perfect sense when they are evaluated within a cultural context (Aroian & Faville, 2005).

Case Example: Benjamin Franklin's Comments on Native Americans

"Savages we call them, because their Manners differ from ours, which we think the Perfection of Civility; they think the same of theirs. Perhaps if we could examine the Manners of Different Nations with Impartiality, we should find no people so rude, as to be without any Rules of Politeness; nor any so polite, as not to have some Remains of Rudeness" (Benjamin Franklin, quoted in Jandt, 2017, p. 76).

Intercultural Communication

Intercultural communication refers to conversations taking place between people from different cultures. The concept embraces differences in perceptions, language, and nonverbal behaviors and results in a recognition of different interpretive contexts (Samovar, Porter, McDaniel, & Roy, 2008). It is a primary means of sharing meaning and developing relationships between people of different cultures. Effective intercultural interactions take place within "transcultural caring relationships" (Pergert, Ekblad, Enskar, & Björk, 2007, p. 318). This means that the patient's *perception* of his or her relationship with the nurse can be just as important as the words used in the communication.

Case Example

A Chinese first-time mother, tense and afraid as she entered the transition phase of labor, spoke no English. Her husband spoke very little and saw birthing as women's work. Callister (2001) relates, "The nurse could feel palpable tension that filled the room. The nurse could not speak Chinese either, but she tried to convey a sense of caring, touching the woman, speaking softly, modeling supportive behavior for her husband and helping her to relax as much as possible. The atmosphere in the room changed considerably with the calm competence and quiet demeanor of the nurse. Following the birth, the father conveyed to her how grateful he was that she spoke Chinese. She tactfully said, 'Thank you, but I don't speak Chinese.' He looked at her in amazement and said with conviction, 'You spoke Chinese.' The language of the heart transcends verbal communication" (p. 212).

Language

Developing a common understanding of the issues inDifferent languages create and express different personal realities (Purnell, Purnell, & Paulanka, 2008). Understanding vocabulary and grammar is not enough. Cultural language competence requires "knowing what to say, and how, when, where, and why to say it" (Hofstede, Pedersen, & Hofsted, 2002, p. 18).

Within the same language, words can have more than one meaning. For example, the words *hot, warm,* and *cold* can refer to temperature, to impressions of strong personal characteristics, or to responses to new ideas (Sokol & Strout, 2006). Idioms are particularly problematic because they represent a nonliteral expression of an idea. Neuliep (2015) describes a common use of the word *bomb* to indicate a strong performance on an exam. In the United States, the word *bomb* is used to express doing poorly on an examination. Nonverbal behaviors, particularly gestures and eye contact, can have very different meanings in various cultures. What is appropriate in one culture can be thought of as discourteous or insulting in another culture (Anderson & Wang, 2008).

Even when a patient speaks good English, it is best to use clear simple language rather than complex words and to speak slowly. Despite having relatively strong verbal skills in an adopted language, many people with English as a second language lack the complex vocabulary in English needed to quickly grasp what is being said. Think about your own experiences learning a foreign language in school. You probably were more comfortable expressing yourself in simple terms, basically because you did not have the more complex vocabulary needed to understand language nuances and multiple meanings. You could attend to the conversation better when the words were spoken slowly with spacing between words. Frequent checks for understanding facilitate communication with culturally diverse patients.

High-Context Versus Low-Context Communication Style

Understanding the implications of differences between high- and low-context culturally based communication styles is an important dimension of intercultural communication. Drawn from Hall's (1976) seminal work, high-context cultures prefer an indirect communication style in which much of the shared information is implicit. High-context communication styles are associated with collectivistic cultures; they are characterized by a "we" consciousness and a strong emphasis on group loyalty and harmony. The relationship is more important than the task in communication (Hofstede, 2011). Trust is a critical dimension in communication, and the words are not as important as the tone of voice and perception of interpersonal relations. Asia, Africa, South America, and parts of the Middle East are considered high-context collective cultures.

In low-context individualistic cultures, Hofstede (2011) suggests that the "task prevails over relationship" (p. 11). Information is reality based and explicitly conveyed. Precise words are taken literally and lead to mutually determined actions. North American and Western European cultures are considered low-context cultures.

APPLICATIONS

Importance of Culture in Health Care Communication

We currently live in a global society, created by dramatic changes in immigration patterns and instant technological connectivity. Samovar, Porter, McDaniel, and Roy (2014) noted, "The forces of globalization have created an environment where cross-cultural awareness and intercultural communication competence are daily necessities" (p. 3).

Most industrialized nations are becoming multiethnic, with majority population percentages becoming significantly smaller. Minority populations represent a critical and expanding component of health care consumers in our nation.

The Institute of Medicine (2002b, 2003) identifies ineffective communication as a significant source of health disparities, that is, unequal care and health outcomes among minority populations in the United States. This makes the nurse's ability to communicate and function effectively with culturally diverse patients even more important as nurses frequently have the most consistent and continuous contact with people seeking medical treatment and health

DEVELOPING AN EVIDENCE-BASED PRACTICE

Purpose: The purpose of this study was to describe the key findings of global nursing found in empirical nursing studies, through descriptive data synthesis of peer-reviewed articles in the field of nursing education and practice.

Method: Commonly used sources (Cinahl Complete, PubMed, PsycINFO and Scopus) were examined using "Global Nursing" as the search descriptor.

Only nursing articles published in peer-reviewed scientific journals were used for analysis. Nonnursing articles, review articles, and those published in nonscientific journals were not accepted. After careful culling and a final selection of relevant articles, a total of 54 articles were included for full-text reading.

Findings: The articles provided findings that could be described across five categories: global nursing arena, global nursing working environments, global nursing workforce management, global nursing competencies, and global nursing networking. These categories encompassed the major professional aspects of global nursing.

Implications for Nursing Practice: Findings from careful review analysis of serious published research studies can provide policy makers, other researchers, educators, and students with a better understanding of the dimensions of global nursing. Contemporary nurses need to have a strong understanding of the nuances and professional aspects of global nursing to ensure cultural competence in the nursing profession.

From Kraft, M., Kastel, A., Eriksson, H., & Hedman, A. M. (2017). Global nursing—a literature review in the field of education and practice. *Nursing Open, 4*(3), 122–123.

information. Self-awareness and careful reflection can help you appreciate how your own cultural beliefs and values can influence communication with patients from different cultures.

Another component of effective intercultural communication relates to developing knowledge of common behavioral response patterns associated with different cultures, and worldviews. Understanding cultural patterns helps normalize behaviors, attitudes, and values as being different, rather than as being wrong or inferior.

Health Disparities

Healthy People 2020 defines a health disparity as "a particular type of health difference that is closely linked with social, economic, and/or environmental disadvantage."

Health disparities create an increased health burden on certain segments of the population, particularly those with the least ability to correct their health situation (Wheeler & Bryant, 2017). In 2002, the Institute of Medicine reported that people of color and ethnic minorities received a lower quality of care even when insurance and income were considered. Since then, other research studies have validated this finding (Giger, 2013).

The *National Healthcare Quality and Disparities Report* (DHHS, 2007) confirms that minority status accounts for major differences and inequality in the quality of health care related to access, screenings, and level of care. The National Center for Health Statistics (2018) indicates that ethnic and racial minorities, which make up 30% of the adult population and almost 40% of the US population younger than 18, have greater mortality and morbidity rates (Edwards, 2009). The National Center for Health Statistics is the nation's principal health statistics agency. This agency offers health statistics, used to describe population characteristics, race and ethnicity and relevant disparities in health status among Americans. Increasing the number of culturally diverse nurses within the profession has been identified as key to increasing cultural responsiveness in health care (Lowe & Archibald, 2009). By 2050, ethnic minorities are expected to become a numerical majority (Giger, 2013; Sue & Sue, 2003).

National Culturally and Linguistically Appropriate Services Standards

In April 2017, the Office of Minority Health of the DHHS published a revised culturally and linguistically appropriate services (CLAS) policies and practices document. Known as the National Standards for Culturally and Linguistically Appropriate Services in Health and Health Care, the CLAS document provides a national blueprint for advancing health equity by reducing health disparities (DHHS, 2017).

The overarching CLAS standard is to provide effective, equitable, understandable, and respectful quality care and services that are responsive to diverse cultural health beliefs and practices, preferred languages, health literacy, and other communication needs. Five population groups were identified, including people with: disabilities, low health literacy, limited English proficiency, racial/ ethnic minorities, and sexual and gender minorities.

Specific objectives designed to improve the accessibility and quality of service for diverse populations. A related goal is to provide services in a manner that respects the personalized cultural perspectives of diverse populations. Simulation Exercise 7.3 examines values and perceptions associated with different cultures.

SIMULATION EXERCISE 7.3 Values and Perceptions Associated With Different Cultures

Purpose

To help students appreciate values and generalized perceptions associated with different cultures.

Procedure

1. Select a specific ethnic culture.
2. Interview someone from that culture, and ask them to tell you about their culture as related to family values, religion, what is important in social interaction, health care beliefs, and end-of-life rituals.
3. Write a short report on your findings.
4. Share your written report with your classmates.

Discussion

1. What important values did you uncover?
2. In what ways did the person's answers agree or disagree with the generalized cultural characteristics of the culture?
3. What did you learn from doing this exercise that you could use in your clinical practice with culturally diverse patients?

Cultural Competence

Cultural competence is defined as "a set of cultural behaviors and attitudes integrated into the practice methods of a system, agency, or its professionals that enables them to work effectively in cross-cultural situations" (Sutton, 2000, p. 58). The concept represents a process, not an event. The IOM (2003) and the American Association of Colleges of Nursing (AACN, 2008) identify cultural competence as an essential skill set required for professional nurses and other health care providers.

Developing competence begins with *cultural humility,* defined as a process of openness, self-awareness, being egoless, and incorporating self-reflection and critique after willingly interacting with diverse individuals. The results of achieving cultural humility are mutual empowerment, respect, partnerships, optimal care, and lifelong learning (Foronda et al., 2018, p. 213).

This involves self-awareness of your own cultural values, attitudes, and perspectives, followed by developing knowledge and acceptance of cultural differences in others (Gravely, 2001; Leonard & Plotnikoff, 2000). Value judgments are hard to eliminate, particularly those outside of awareness. Self-awareness allows you to own your own biases and not project them onto patients.

Cultural sensitivity is an integral part of competence. The Office of Minority Health (DHHS, 2018) defines *cultural sensitivity* as "the ability to be appropriately responsive to the attitudes, feelings, or circumstances of groups of people that share a common and distinctive racial, national, religious, linguistic, or cultural heritage" (p. 131). Cultural sensitivity emphasizes an openness to different cultural beliefs and values, with a corresponding willingness to incorporate the patient's cultural values in care whenever possible. Cultural sensitivity facilitates care and self-management of health conditions. It is hard for patients to overlook a significant tradition. When health recommendations conflict with their worldview, patients are less likely to follow them. Cultural sensitivity is key to safe care (Knoerl, 2011).

Nurses demonstrate cultural sensitivity by using neutral words and behaviors, which are respectful of the patient's culture, and avoiding could be interpreted as offensive (AACN, 2008). A valuable way to learn about another person's culture is to spend time with them and to ask frequent questions about what is important to them about their culture. Smaller ethnic groups within the larger population group are sometimes referred to as "minority" (Jandt, 2017, p. 13).

Minority populations, especially new immigrants, have special problems with access and continuity of health care. They often are marginalized economically, occupationally, and socially in ways that adversely affect their access to mainstream health care. Accessing health care can be so frustrating that they give up when they meet even small obstacles. A secondary issue is a lack of knowledge and experience with how to obtain services. Undocumented immigrants have an added burden of fearing deportation if their legal status is revealed (Chung, Bernak, Otiz, & Sandoval-Perez, 2008). Nurses can help patients successfully navigate the health care system. Patients also appreciate providers who orient them to the clinical setting and set the stage for a comfortable encounter.

CARE OF THE CULTURALLY DIVERSE PATIENT

This section describes the integration of cultural sensitivity into the assessment, diagnosis and treatment planning, implementation, and evaluation of patient-centered professional nursing care. Having knowledge and an accepting attitude about health traditions associated with different cultures increases patient comfort and engagement with caregivers. Hulme (2010) distinguishes between the folk domain and alternative health care remedies. She emphasizes the need to understand the patient's health care traditions, which are "specific to—and fundamentally a part of—an individual's culture" (p. 276).

Building Rapport

When meeting a patient for the first time, you should introduce yourself and identify your role.

- Calling the patient by title and last name shows respect. Strive to pronounce the name correctly. Always ask if you are not sure.
- Speak clearly, and spend time with the patient before asking assessment questions to make the patient and/or family comfortable.
- Avoid assumptions or interpretations about what you are hearing without validating the information.
- Allot more time to conduct a health assessment to accommodate language needs and cultural interpretations.
- Take the position of an interested learner when inquiring about cultural values and standards of behavior.
- Inquire about individual perceptions, along with cultural explanatory models associated with the illness and preferences for treatment.
- Explain treatment procedures at every opportunity, and alert patients ahead of time of potential discomfort.
- Ask permission and explain the necessity for any physical examination or use of assessment tools.

Theoretical Frameworks

Madeleine Leininger's Theory of Culture Care (Leininger & McFarland, 2006) is recognized as the first major theory-based approach to describe the nature of culture in health care from a nursing perspective. Leininger believes that nurses must have knowledge about diverse cultures to provide care that fits the patient; in today's world, this would be viewed as an essential component of patient-centered care.

Purnell's Model

Larry Purnell (2008) considers cultural competence from a macro level (global society, community, family, down to the micro level of the person).

Using Purnell's domains as a framework for understanding individual differences allows for a comprehensive cultural assessment leading to a culturally congruent, individualized, patient-centered approach to patient care. Understanding the patient's cultural explanation for the health problem is essential, as different cultures frame illness and its causes in various ways. For example, in Asian cultures, depression is characterized as "sadness," rather than a mental disorder. It is not uncommon for Asian and Arab Israeli women to believe that breast cancer is God's will or fate (Baron-Epel, Friedman, & Lernau, 2009; Kim & Flaskerud, 2008). Table 7.3 provides sample questions to assess patient preferences when the patient is from a different culture.

Cultural Implications in Patient-Centered Decision Making

National health-reform expectations for patient-centered care call for a shared patient-centered understanding of illness, diagnosis, and prognosis. This expectation may require adaptation with diverse cultural groups. For example, certain cultures have strong beliefs about providing direct disclosure of diagnosis and prognosis to patients. Asian and Hispanic cultures traditionally prefer family-centered decision making about care for a family member with a terminal diagnosis (Kwak & Haley, 2005). The family then decides when and if the disclosure should be made to the patient. This contingency comes up often enough to warrant your full attention to its implications for care.

Careful, unhurried discussion and inclusion of family members in the decision-making processes can be helpful. This can although informed consent forms require full disclosure, the cultural acceptability of autonomous informed consent can be an ethical issue when interacting with patients who hold different cultural values (Calloway, 2009). When a patient authorizes the family to discuss diagnosis and make treatment decisions, this patient's preference should be honored. Exploration of each patient's preferences about disclosure should take place early in the clinical relationship.

WORKING WITH LANGUAGE BARRIERS

Patients from different cultures often identify language barriers as the most frustrating aspect of communication in health care situations. Limited language proficiency is a fundamental barrier to a patient's full participation in learning self-management strategies and a factor influencing patient safety. For example, in addition to obtaining knowledge about cultural differences, health providers must learn from their patients how these differences influence treatment decisions (Vaughn, Jacquez, & Baker, 2009).

Even if the patient speaks English, always allow additional time for communication processing. People with English as a second language tend to think and process information in their native language, translating back and forth from English. Language also involves subtleties of meaning (IOM, 2002b, p. 232). Internal interpretation of a message is often accompanied by visual imagery reflecting the person's cultural beliefs and experiences. (This can change the meaning of the original message, with neither party having an awareness of the differences in interpretation.) Examples of sample questions you might want to ask are presented in Table 7.3 seems to be taking more time than usual or seems more

TABLE 7.3 Assessing Patient Preferences When the Patient Is From a Different Culture

Areas to Assess	Sample Assessment Questions
Explanatory models of illness	"What do you think caused your health problem? Can you tell me a little about how your illness developed?"
Traditional healing processes	"Can you tell me something about how this problem is handled in your country? Are there any special cultural beliefs about your illness that might help me give you better care? Are you currently using any medications or herbs to treat your illness?"
Lifestyle	"What are some of the foods you like? How are they prepared? What do people do in your culture to stay healthy?"
Type of family support	"Can you tell me who in your family should be involved with your care? Who is the decision maker for health care decisions?"
Spiritual healing practices and rituals	"I am not really familiar with your spiritual practices, but I wonder if you could tell me what would be important to you so we can try to incorporate it into your care plan."
Cultural norms about personal care	"A number of our patients have special needs around personal care, of which we are not always aware. I am wondering if this is true for you and if you could help me understand what you need to be comfortable."
Truth-telling and level of disclosure	Ask the family about cultural ways of talking about serious illness. In some cultures, the family knows the diagnosis/prognosis, which is not told to the ill person (e.g., Hispanic, Asian).
Ritual and religious ceremonies at time of death	Ask the family about special rituals and religious ceremonies at time of death.

anxious. It is important to speak slowly and clearly; use simple words; and avoid slang, technical jargon, and complex sentences.

Validation

Validation is an important communication strategy with culturally diverse patients, as word meanings are not the same even within a culture (Giger, 2013). In many cultures, there is a tendency to view health professionals as authority figures, treating them with deference and respect. This value can be so strong that a patient will not question the nurse or in any way indicate mistrust of professional recommendations. They just do not follow the professional advice. Using teach-back and having patients repeat process instructions improves compliance.

Use of Interpreters

Federal law (Title VI of the Civil Rights Act) mandates the use of a trained interpreter for any patient experiencing communication difficulties in health care settings due to language. Interpreters should have a thorough knowledge of the culture and the language. Interpreters should be carefully chosen, keeping in mind variations in dialects and

differences in the gender and social status of the interpreter and the patient if these factors are likely to be an issue. There are quality assurance and ethical issues associated with the use of untrained interpreters, such as family, friends, or ancillary staff. They may not be familiar with medical terminology and unintentionally may misrepresent the meaning of a message. The patient may or may not want a relative, friend, or nonprofessional staff to "know their business" or have access to subjective information (Messias, McDowell, & Estrada, 2009). Box 7.2 provides guidelines for the use of interpreters in health care interviews.

Time Orientation

Culturally, clock time versus activity time can reflect cultural standards (Galanti, 2015). This can be a major issue when appointments or medications are involved. Precise time frames are important in low-context cultures (North America and Western Europe). People in these cultures are accustomed to setting and meeting exact time commitments for appointments and taking medications. In high-context cultures, individuals do not consider commitment to a future appointment as important as attending to what is happening in the moment. Contrast the

BOX 7.2   Guidelines for Using Interpreters in Health Care

Whenever possible, the translator should not be a family member.

Orient the translator to the goals of the clinical interview and expected confidentiality.

Look directly at the patient when either you or the patient is speaking.

Ask the translator to clarify anything that is not understood by either you or the patient.

After each completed statement, pause for translation.

difference in time orientation of a clock-conscious German person with that of his Italian counterpart in the following case example.

Case Example

The Germans and Swiss love clock-regulated time, for it appears to them as a remarkably efficient, impartial, and very precise way of organizing life—especially in business. For Italians, on the other hand, time considerations will usually be subjected to human feelings. "Why are you so angry because I came at 9:30?" an Italian asks his German colleague. "Because it says 9 a.m. in my diary," says the German. "Then why don't you write 9:30 and then we'll both be happy?" is a logical Italian response. The business we have to do and our close relations are so important that it is irrelevant at what time we meet. The meeting is what counts (Lewis, 2000, p. 55).

Communication Principles

Culturally diverse patients respond better to health care providers who ask about and incorporate cultural and social knowledge of patient values into care Knoerl (2011). Framing interventions that the patient recognizes as familiar and valid and openly discussing differences in backgrounds, norms, and health practices builds trust. Simulation Exercise 7.4 provides experience with culture assessment interviews.

FRAMING PATIENT TEACHING WITH CULTURALLY DIVERSE PATIENTS

The **LEARN** model is used to frame clinical teaching and coaching encounters with culturally diverse patients.

- Listen carefully to patient perceptions and the words the patient uses. Ask the patient to describe the illness

SIMULATION EXERCISE 7.4   Key Informant Cultural Assessment Exercise

Purpose
To provide practice with assessment related to cultural information.

Procedure
Each person is a key informant about your own culture. Pair off with another student. Interview your student partner about his or her cultural background as related to the questions below. Guide the interview process so that you address all questions.

1. From where did your family originate?
2. What cultural values are held in your family?
3. What do you believe about the gender roles of men and women? Are your beliefs different or consistent with those of your parents?
4. How much physical distance do you need for comfort in social interactions?
5. Who are the decision makers in your family, and to whom do you look for guidance in important matters?
6. What are your definitions of health and well-being?
7. If you needed health care, how would you respond to this need, and what would be your expectations?
8. In a health care situation, what would be the role of your family?
9. In a health care situation, how important would religion be, and what would you need for spiritual comfort?
10. What do you like and dislike about your cultural background?

Discussion
1. What was it like to be the interviewer? The interviewee?
2. How difficult was it for you to really identify some of the behaviors and expectations that are a part of your cultural self?
3. Were you surprised with any of your answers? If so, in what ways?
4. How can you use this exercise in communicating with patients from culturally diverse backgrounds?

or injury, how it occurred, and what the patient believes caused it.

- Explain what the patient needs to understand about his or her condition or treatment, incorporating patient's words and explanatory models.
- Acknowledge cultural differences between nurse and patient viewpoints, without devaluing the patient's viewpoint. Respect cultural sources of health care,

and incorporate culturally acceptable treatments and interventions when possible. Ask about cultural and family treatment considerations. Use frequent validation to ensure the cultural appropriateness of provider assumptions.

- **Recommend what the patient should do.** Frame treatment suggestions using a culturally acceptable care process. Invite patient participation in developing a plan that is culturally authentic and therapeutic.
- **Negotiate with the patient** to culturally adapt constructive self-management strategies based on patient input. Negotiation of cultural acceptability is fundamental to patient compliance. Familiarity with formal and informal sources of health care, such as churches, shamans, medicine men and women, curanderos, and other faith healers, provides additional patient support.

Informed Consent and Advance Directives in a Cultural Context

Issues of informed consent and other legal documents need to be reframed within a cultural context (Calloway, 2009). Without full disclosure, consent forms are not valid.

Philosophical differences about end-of-life care exist between Western values and those of the four major minority groups. Many minority patients believe in prolonging life and are reluctant to use advance directives (Thomas, 2001). Simulation Exercise 7.5 provides an opportunity to explore the role of cultural assessment questions in care planning.

Key Cultural Groups

Wilson (2011) notes that "domains such as family roles, health care practices, religion, and communication are essential attributes that define an individual's culture" (p. 222). These attributes provide a framework for identifying common cultural features of the four major minority cultures in the United States as discussed in the following sections.

Culture plays a significant role in shaping people's health-related beliefs, values, and behaviors (Betancourt, 2004). As you review each culture overview, keep in mind that cultural descriptors should be treated as generalized impressions. Galanti (2015) distinguishes between generalizations, which can be helpful, and stereotypes, which overlook individual variants in culture values leading to an inaccurate descriptor.

Case Example

"An example is the assumption that Mexicans have large families. If I meet Rosa, a Mexican woman, and I say to myself, 'Rosa is Mexican; she must have a large family,' I am stereotyping her. But if I think Mexicans often have large families and wonder whether Rosa does, I am making a generalization" (Galanti, 2015, p. 7).

SIMULATION EXERCISE 7.5 Applying Cultural Sensitivity to Care Planning

Purpose
To practice cultural sensitivity in care planning.

Procedure
This can be done in small even-numbered groups rather than as an individual exercise.
1. Out of class, create a written clinical scenario based on a culturally diverse patient you have cared for recently. Identify ethnic or cultural factors present in the patient's nursing needs.
2. Trade scenarios with another student.
3. Write what should be included in a culturally sensitive care plan.
4. Discuss each of the care plans, and make any revisions.

Discussion
1. What were the areas of agreement and disagreement about the care plan?
2. What questions would you need to ask to clarify needs?
3. In developing the plan, did you find any additional needs?
4. How could you use this exercise to improve your clinical practice?

HISPANIC/LATINO CULTURE

Hispanic Americans account for 16.7% of the population of the United States (Office of Minority Health and Health and Health Equity [OMHHE], n.d.), making them the largest minority group in the United States. This figure is projected to increase to 29% by 2050. Identifying themselves as Hispanics, or Latinos, this population is more racially diverse and represents a wider range of cultures than other minority groups. Within the Hispanic/Latino populations are Mexican Americans (Chicanos), Puerto Ricans, Cubans, individuals from the Dominican Republic, and South or Central America (Hardin, 2014).

Current growth of the Hispanic population in the United States consists mainly of first-generation and younger immigrants with lower SES and undocumented legal status. Many do not speak English, or do not speak it well enough to negotiate the US health care system. Implementation of bilingual and ESOL education programs in schools acknowledges the significance of the growth of the Hispanic population and social repositioning of diversity as a fact of life in the United States. More and more US communities with larger Hispanic populations use both English and Spanish signage and directions.

Family and Gender Roles

The family (familismo) is the center of Hispanic life and serves as a primary source of emotional support. Hispanic patients are considered "family members first, and individuals second" (Pagani-Tousignant, 1992, p. 10).

Ayon, Marsiglia, and Bermudez-Parsai (2010) describe *familismo* as representing a strong family loyalty with corresponding responsibilities for ensuring the family's stability. The "family" includes immediate and extended family members; it is considered a protective factor in promoting the mental health and individual well-being of family members. Familismo can extend to helping immigrant family members adjust and navigate the health care system. Family units tend to live in close proximity with one another. Close friends are considered a part of the family unit. Family support and practices can be easily integrated into patient care, sometimes with a little assist from the nurse. It is important to explore the meaning of family to the patient, especially in times of stress. When asking "who" the "family" is for the patient, especially in clinical situations involving life transitions, is important assessment data.

Family opinions are sought in decision-making processes. Family members show their love and concern in health care situations by pampering the patient. Gender roles are rigid, with the father viewed as the head of the household and primary decision maker. Latino women are socialized to serve their husbands and children without question (*la sufrida*, or the long-suffering woman; Pagani-Tousignant, 1992). The nurse needs to be sensitive to gender-specific cultural values in treatment situations.

Religion

Hispanic patients are predominantly Roman Catholic. Latino families have strong cultural values and beliefs about the sanctity of life. Receiving the sacraments is important and calls for family celebration. The final sacrament in the Roman Catholic Church, anointing of the sick, offers comfort to patients and families. Faith in God is closely linked with the Hispanic population's understanding of health care problems. Their relationship with God is an intimate one, which may include personal visions of God or saints. This should not be interpreted as a hallucination. Hispanic patients view health as a gift from God, related to physical, emotional, and social balance (Kemp, 2004). Many believe that illness is the result of a great fright (*susto*), or falling out of favor with God. Santeros are folk healers whose healing powers derive from the power of the saints. Santeros may prescribe the lighting of candles or incense and the use of herbs and ointments, which are purchased from a spiritual pharmacy.

Health Beliefs and Practices

Latinos have a lower prevalence of chronic disorders in general compared to the nation's overall population, with the exception of diabetes (Livingston, Minushkin, & Cohn, 2008). They are less likely to have a regular health provider and more likely to use the formal health care system episodically, as a short-term problem-solving strategy for health problems.

Many Hispanic patients are illegal immigrants, making them ineligible for health insurance. A source of health care outside the family is the use of *curanderos* (local folk healers and herb doctors) for initial care. The *curandera* uses a combination of prayers, healing practices, medicines, and herbs to cure illness (Amerson, 2008).

Latino patients may identify a *"hot-cold balance,"* referring to a cultural classification of illness resulting from an imbalance of body humors, as essential for health. When a person loses balance, illness follows (Juckett, 2013). So-called cold health conditions are treated with hot remedies, and vice versa. Mental illness is not addressed as such. Instead, a Hispanic patient will talk of being sad *(triste)*. Modesty is important to Hispanic women. Women may be reluctant to express their private concerns in front of their children, even adult children.

It is not uncommon for patients to share medications with other family members. Aponte (2009) suggests that nurses should ask Hispanic patients about the use of folk medicine and explain, if needed, the reason and importance of sharing this information with the nurse. A proactive prevention approach tailored to the health care needs of this minority population is essential.

Communication and Social Interaction Patterns

Spanish is the primary language spoken in all Latin American countries except Brazil (Portuguese) and Haiti (French). Hispanics are an extroverted people who value interpersonal relationships. They tend to trust feelings more than facts.

Strict rules govern social relationships *(respecto)*, which is characterized by a respect for hierarchical family roles, with higher status being given to older individuals and to male over female individuals. Nurses are viewed as authority figures to be treated with respect. Patients hesitate to ask questions, so it is important to ask enough questions to ensure that your patients understand their diagnosis and treatment plan (Aponte, 2009).

Hispanic patients look for warmth, respect, and friendliness *(personalismo)* from their health care providers. It is important to ask about their well-being and to take extra time finding out what they need. They value smooth social relations and avoid confrontation and criticism. Hispanic people are sensitive and easily hurt.

The Latino culture is a high-context culture from a communication perspective. Hispanic patients need to develop trust *(confianza)* in the health care provider. They do this by making small talk before getting down to the business of discussing their health problems. Knowing the importance of *confianza* to the Hispanic patient allows nurses to spend initial time engaging in general topics before moving into assessment or care (Knoerl, 2007).

AFRICAN AMERICAN CULTURE

African Americans account for approximately 14.2% of the US population (OMHHE, n.d.), making them the second largest minority group in the nation. Purnell et al. (2008) note, "Black or African American refers to people having origins in any of the black racial groups of Africa, and includes Nigerians and Haitians or any person who self-designates this category regardless of origin" (p. 2). Although African Americans are represented in every socioeconomic group, approximately one-third of them live in poverty (Spector, 2004).

For too many African American patients, their cultural heritage traces back to cultural oppression (Eiser & Ellis, 2007). This unfortunate legacy colors their expectations around health care issues and explains the mistrust many African Americans have about the US health care system (Wilson, 2011). African Americans need to experience feeling respected by their caregivers to counteract a sense of powerlessness and lack of confidence they sometimes feel in health care settings.

The African American worldview consists of four fundamental characteristics:
* *Interdependence:* feeling interconnected and as concerned about the welfare of others as of themselves
* *Emotional vitality:* expressed with intensity and animation in lifestyle, dance, language, and music
* *Harmonious blending:* "going with the flow" or natural rhythm of life
* *Collective survival:* sharing and cooperation is essential to everyone surviving and succeeding (Parham, White, & Ajamu, 2000)

Family and Gender Roles
The family is considered the "primary and most important tradition in the African American community" (Hecht, Ronald, & Jackson, 2003, p. 2). Women are often considered the head of the family, consistent with vestiges of a matriarchal tradition in many earlier African villages. Many low-income African American children grow up in extended families.

Older African American women are referred to as "the backbone" of the African American family and community (Carthron, Bailey, & Anderson, 2014). Women take on multiple roles in their church and community and often assume caregiving responsibilities for working parents. When assessing family, be sure to ask about grandparents, particularly grandmothers, as being primary or supportive caregivers for children and adolescents.

Loyalty to the extended family is a dominant value in the African American culture, and family members rely on one another for emotional and financial support (Purnell et al., 2008). The combination of strong kinship bonds and the value of "caring for one's own" are important principles in the African American culture (Sterritt & Pokorny, 1998). When planning interventions, take advantage of kinship bonds, and incorporate family members as a supportive network. Family members want to be involved when one of their members is ill. It is not unusual to have five or six people descend on a patient's hospital room.

RELIGION AND SPIRITUAL PRACTICES

Spirituality is an important dimension of life for people of African American ancestry. Faith represents a personal connected relationship with God, or a higher being, experienced as an essential life support. Honoring God, self, and others is important for personal health (Lewis, Hankin, Reynolds, & Ogedegbe, 2007). Religions participation has a positive infuence on improved health status and qualitoy of life for African Americans (Asron et al., 2003).

The church serves the dual purpose of providing a structure for meeting spiritual needs and functioning as a primary social, economic, and community life center. Chambers and Higgins (1997) explain, "Since its inception, the black church has been more than a place of worship for African Americans. It is where the community has gathered to lobby for freedom and equal rights" (p. 42).

African American political leaders (e.g., Jesse Jackson and Dr. Martin Luther King, Jr.) are revered as influential church leaders. Major religions include Christianity (predominantly Protestant and Pentecostal) and Islam.

Prayer and the "laying on of hands" are important to many African American patients (Purnell et al., 2008). Readings from the Bible and gospel hymns are sources of support during hospitalization. Because of the central meaning of the church in African American life, incorporating appropriate clergy as a resource in treatment, and especially at the end of life, is a useful strategy. Barton-Burke, Smith, Frain, and Loggins (2010) suggest that care interventions should address the patient's spiritual needs.

African Americans account for approximately 30% of the US Muslim population. Islam influences all aspects of life. Muslim patients are expected to follow the Halal (lawful) diet, which calls for dietary restrictions on eating pork or pork products and drinking alcohol (Rashidi & Rajaram, 2001).

Health Beliefs and Practices

African Americans suffer more health disparities than any other minority population (Hopp & Herring, 2014). They have higher rates of hypertension, adolescent pregnancy, diabetes, heart disease, and stroke, and male African Americans have a significantly greater chance of developing cancer and of dying of it (Spector, 2004). Lower-income African American patients statistically are less likely to use regular preventive health services. Many African Americans use emergency departments as a major health care resource, in part because of cost (Lynch & Hanson, 2004).

African Americans tend to rely on informal helping networks in the community, particularly those associated with their churches, until a health problem becomes a crisis. Purnell et al. (2008) advise engagement of the extended family system, particularly grandmothers, in providing support and health teaching when working with African Americans in the community.

Communication and Social Interaction

Establishing trust is essential for successful communication with African American patients. Allowing these patients to have as much control over their health care as possible reinforces self-efficacy and promotes self-esteem. Recognizing and respecting African American values of interdependence, emotional vitality, and collective survival helps facilitate confidence in health care. Awareness of community resources in the African American community and incorporation of informal care networks, such as the church, neighbors, and extended family, can help provide culturally congruent continuity of care.

ASIAN AMERICAN

As of 2010, Asian Americans were estimated to make up 4.8% of the US population and represented the fastest-growing minority group (Hoeffel, Rastogi, Kim, & Shahid, 2012; OMHHE, n.d.) of all major ethnic groups. Asians and Pacific Islanders comprise more than 32 ethnic groups, among them people from China, the Philippines, Japan, Vietnam, Laos, Cambodia, and India (Hardin, 2014). Even within the same geographic grouping, significant cultural differences exist. For example, in India, there are more than 350 "major languages," with 18 being acknowledged as "official languages," and a complex caste system defines distinctive behavioral expectations for gender roles within the broader culture (Chaudhary, 2004).

Asian cultures value hard work, education, and going with the flow of events. There is an emphasis on politeness and correct behavior. The appropriate cultural behavior is to put others first and to avoid conflict. This standard creates an indirect style in communication that is not always understandable to cultures that use a more direct communication style.

Traditionally, Asian patients exercise emotional restraint in communication and exhibit stoicism with pain. They control their facial expressions. Interpersonal conflicts are not directly addressed, and challenging an expert is not favored. Jokes and humor are usually not appreciated because "the Confucian and Buddhist preoccupation with truth, sincerity, kindliness and politeness automatically eliminates humour techniques such as sarcasm, satire, exaggeration and parody" (Lewis, 2000, pp. 20–21).

Family and Gender Roles

Asian culture is contextual and collectivistic. Families traditionally live in multigenerational households, with extended family members providing important social support. Individual privacy is uncommon. The Asian culture places family before individual welfare. Family members will sacrifice their individuality, if needed, for the good of the family.

There is a need to avoid "loss of face" because loss of face brings shame to the whole family, including ancestors. Chinese parenting stresses parental control and emotional restraint (Ho, 2014).

The family can consist of the nuclear family, grandparents, and other relatives all living together or a split family, in which some family members are in the United States and other nuclear family members live in their country of origin. There is family pressure on younger members to do well academically, and the behavior of individual members is considered within the context of its impact on the family as a whole. Family members are obligated to assume a great deal of responsibility for one another, including ongoing financial assistance. Older children are responsible for the well-being of younger children.

The family is a powerful force in maintaining the religious and social values in Asian cultures. "Good health" is described as having harmonious family relationships and a balanced life (Harrison et al., 2005). Family communication takes place through prescribed roles and obligations, taking into account family roles, age, and position in the family. The husband (father) is the primary authority and decision maker. He acts as the family spokesperson in crisis situations, and his decisions are considered absolute. Authority is passed down from the father to the oldest son.

Elders in the Asian community are highly respected and well taken care of by younger members of the family

(Pagani-Tousignant, 1992). The wisdom of the elders helps guide younger family members on many life issues, including major health decisions (Davis, 2000).

Tradition strongly regulates individual behavior. Traditional Chinese culture does not allow patients to discuss the full severity of an illness; this creates challenges for mutual decision making based on full disclosure, which is characteristic of Western health care. Family members take an active role in deciding whether a diagnosis should be disclosed to a patient. They are frequently the recipients of this information before the patient is told of the diagnosis, prognosis, and treatment options.

Religion and Spiritual Practices

Religion plays an important role in Asian society, with religious beliefs tightly interwoven into virtually every aspect of daily life. Referred to as "Eastern religions," major groups include Hindus, Buddhists, and Muslims.

Hinduism is not a homogeneous religion. It represents a living faith and a philosophical way of life with diverse doctrines, religious symbols, and moral and social norms (Michaels, 2003). Hinduism represents a pragmatic philosophy of life that articulates harmony with the natural rhythms of life, and "right" or "correct" principles of social interaction and behavior. The *veda* refers to knowledge passed through many generations from ancient sages, which combined with Sanskrit literature provides the "codes of ritual, social and ethical behavior, called dharma, which that literature reveals" (Flood, 1996, p. 11). Hindus are vegetarians: It is against their religion to kill living creatures. Sikhism is a reformed variation of Hinduism in which women have more rights in domestic and community life.

Buddhism represents a philosophical approach to life that identifies fate, which is referred to as the four noble truths. Buddhists believe:

1. All life is suffering.
2. Suffering is caused by desire or attachment to the world.
3. Suffering can be extinguished by eliminating desire.
4. The way to eliminate desire is to live a virtuous life (Lynch & Hanson, 2004).

Buddhists follow the path to enlightenment by leading a moral life, being mindful of personal thoughts and actions, and by developing wisdom and understanding. Buddhists pray and meditate frequently. They eat a vegetarian diet, and alcohol, cigarettes, and drugs are not permitted.

The Muslim religion (Islam) describes a way of life. Muslims adhere to the Quran/Koran, the holy teachings of Muhammad. Faith, prayer, giving alms, and making a yearly pilgrimage to Mecca are requirements of the religion. Identified as an Eastern monotheistic religion, Islam is practiced throughout the world. Followers are called Muslims. Allah is identified as a higher power or God. Muhammad is his prophet. Muslims submit to Allah and follow Allah's basic rules about everything from personal relationships to business matters, including personal matters, such as dress and hygiene. Islam has strong tenets that affect health care, an important one being that God is the ultimate healer.

Dietary Restrictions Center on consuming halal (Lawful) Food

Excluded from the diet are pork, pork products, and alcohol. In the hospital, Muslims can order kosher food because it meets the requirements for halal (Davidson, Boyer, Casey, Matzel, & Walden, 2008). The Muslim patient values physical modesty. The family may request that only female staff care for female family members. Physical contact, eye contact, touch, and hugs between members of the opposite sex who are not family are avoided (McKennis, 1999).

Muslims believe death is a part of Allah's plan, so to fight the dying process with treatment is wrong. They believe that the dying person should not die alone. A close relative should be present, praying for God's blessing or reading the Quran/Koran. Once a person actually dies, it is important to perform the following: turn the body toward Mecca; close the person's mouth and eyes and cover the face; straighten the legs and arms; announce the death to relatives and friends; bathe the body (with men bathing men and women bathing women); and cover the body with white cotton (Servodido & Morse, 2001).

Health Care Beliefs and Practices

Health is based on the Ayurveda principle, which requires harmony and balance between yin and yang, as the two energy forces required for health (Louie, 2001). A blockage of *qi*, defined as the energy circulating in a person's body, creates an imbalance between yin (negative energy force) and yang (positive energy force), resulting in illness (Chen, 2001). Yin represents the female force, containing all the elements that represent darkness, cold, and weakness. Yang symbolizes the male elements of strength, brightness, and warmth. Ayurveda emphasizes health promotion and disease prevention.

The influence of Eastern health practices and alternative medicine is increasingly incorporated into the health care of all Americans. Many complementary and alternative medical practices in the United States (acupuncture, botanicals, and massage and therapeutic touch) trace their roots to Eastern holistic health practices. Acupressure and herbal medicines are among the traditional medical practices used by Asian patients to reestablish the balance between yin and yang. In some Asian countries, healers use a process of "coining," in which a coin is heated and vigorously rubbed on the body to draw illness out of the body. The resulting welts can mistakenly be attributed to child abuse if this practice is not understood. Traditional healers, such as Buddhist monks, acupuncturists, and herbalists, also may be consulted when someone is ill.

Asian patients typically respond better to a formal relationship and an indirect communication style characterized by polite phrases and marked deference. They work better with well-defined boundaries and clear expectations (Galanti, 2015). The patient waits for the information to be offered by the nurse as the authority figure. Sometimes this gets interpreted as timidity. A better interpretation is that the patient is deferring to the health professional's expertise.

Sometimes it is difficult to tell what Asian patients are experiencing. Facial expressions are not as flexible, and words are not as revealing as those of people in other cultures. Asian patients may not request pain medication until their pain is quite severe (Im, 2008). Asking the patient about pain and offering medication as normal clinical management is usually necessary.

Health care concerns include a higher-than-usual incidence of tuberculosis, hepatitis B, and liver cancer (OMHHE, n.d.). Asian men may have a difficult time disclosing personal information to a female nurse unless the nurse explains why the data are necessary for care. This is because, in serious matters, women are not considered as knowledgeable as men. Asian patients may be reluctant to be examined by a person of the opposite sex, particularly if the examination or treatment involves intimate areas.

SOCIAL INTERACTION PATTERNS

Communication behaviors in the Asian culture are characterized by mutuality, respect, and honesty (Chen, 2007). Health care providers are considered health experts, and there is a significant social hierarchal gap between providers and patients related to decision making. Another variable in decision making is the opinion of senior family members. (They are expected to provide specific advice and recommendations.) Asian patients prefer a polite, friendly, but formal approach in communication. They appreciate clinicians willing to provide advice in a matter-of-fact, concise manner (Lynch & Hanson, 2004). Always ask what a behavior means to a patient, as misinterpretations can easily occur.

Asian patients favor harmonious relationships. Confrontation is avoided; patients will nod and smile in agreement, even when they strongly disagree (Cross & Bloomer, 2010). Nurses need to ask open-ended questions and clarify issues throughout an interaction. If you use questions that require a yes or no answer, the answer may reflect the patient's polite deference rather than an honest response. Explain treatment as problem solving, ask the patient how things are done in his or her culture, and work with your Asian patient to develop culturally congruent solutions.

NATIVE AMERICAN PATIENTS

Native Americans represent the smallest racial minority in the United States (Cesario, 2001). They account for 1.7% of the US population (OMHHE, n.d.). American Indians and Alaska natives trace their origins to the original populations of North, Central, and South America. There are more than 500 federally recognized tribes and another 100 tribes or bands that are state-recognized but are not recognized by the federal government. Native Americans include First or Original Americans, American Indians, Alaskan Natives, Aleuts, Eskimos, Metis (mixed blood), or Amerindians. Most will identify themselves as members of a specific tribe (Garrett & Herring, 2001). Tribal identity is maintained through regular powwows and other ceremonial events. Like other minority groups with an oppressed heritage, the majority of Native Americans are poor and undereducated, with associated higher rates of social and health problems (Hodge, & Rodriguez'g Hodge, 2014).

Family and Gender Roles

The family is highly valued by Native Americans. Multigenerational families live together in close proximity. When two individuals marry, the marriage contract implicitly includes attachment and obligation to a larger kinship system (Red Horse, 1997). Both men and women feel a responsibility to promote tribal values and traditions through their crafts and traditional ceremonies. However, women are identified as their culture's standard bearers. A Cheyenne proverb graphically states, "A nation is not conquered until the hearts of its women are on the ground. Then it is done, no matter how brave its warriors nor how strong its weapons" (Crow Dog & Erdoes, 1990, p. 3). Cheshire (2001) also notes, "It is the women—the mothers, grandmothers and aunties—that keep Indian nations alive" (p. 1534).

Gender roles are egalitarian, and women are valued. Being a mother and auntie gives a social standing as a life giver, which is related to the survival of the tribe (Barrios & Egan, 2002). Because the family matriarch is a primary decision maker, her approval and support may be required for compliance with a treatment plan (Cesario, 2001).

Native American culture is highly contextual. Identifying and including from the outset all those who will be taking an active part in the care of the patient recognizes the communal nature of family involvement in health care. For the Native American patient, family may also include members of an immediate tribe or its spokesperson.

Spiritual and Religious Practices

The religious beliefs of Native Americans are embedded in nature and the earth. There is a sense of sacredness in everyday living between "grandmother earth" and "grandfather sky" that tends to render the outside world extraneous (Kavanagh, Absalom, Beil, & Schliessmann, 1999, p. 25).

Health Beliefs and Practices

Native Americans suffer from greater rates of mortality from chronic diseases such as tuberculosis, alcoholism, diabetes, and pneumonia. Domestic violence, often associated with alcoholism, is a significant health concern. Pain assessment is important because Native American patients tend to display a stoic response to pain (Cesario, 2001). Health concerns of particular relevance to the Native American population are unintentional injuries (of which 75% are alcohol related), cirrhosis, alcoholism, and obesity. Homicide and suicide rates are significantly greater for Native Americans (Meisenhelder & Chandler, 2000).

Illness is viewed as a punishment from God for some real or imagined imbalance with nature. Native Americans believe illness to be divine intervention to help the individual correct evil ways, and spiritual beliefs play a significant role in the maintenance and restoration of health (Cesario, 2001; Meisenhelder & Chandler, 2000). Spiritual ceremonies and prayers form an important part of traditional healing activities, and healing practices are strongly embedded in religious beliefs. Recovery occurs after the person is cleansed of "evil spirits."

Medical help is sought from tribal elders and shamans (highly respected spiritual medicine men and women) who use spiritual healing practices and herbs to cure the ill member of the tribe (Pagani-Tousignant, 1992). For example, spiritual and herbal tokens, or medicine bags, placed at the bedside or in an infant's crib are essential to the healing process and should not be disturbed (Cesario, 2001). Native Americans view death as a natural process, but they fear the power of dead spirits and use numerous tribal rituals to ward them off.

Social Interaction Patterns

Respect is a core value in American Indian and Alaskan Native cultures (Hodge & Rodriguez'g Hodge, 2014). Building a trusting relationship with the health care provider is important to the Native American patient. They respond best to health professionals who stick to the point and do not engage in small talk. Conversely, they love storytelling and appreciate humor.

Nurses need to understand the value of nonverbal communication and taking time in conversations with Native American patients. Direct eye contact is considered disrespectful. Listening is considered a sign of respect and essential to learning about the other (Kalbfleisch, 2009). The patient is likely to speak in a low tone. Native Americans are private people who respect the privacy of others and prefer to talk about the facts rather than the emotions surrounding them.

Native Americans live in present time. They have little appreciation of scheduled time commitments, which in their mind do not necessarily relate to what needs to be achieved. For Native Americans, being on time or taking medications with meals (when three meals are taken on one day and two meals are eaten on another day) has little relevance (Kavanagh, Absalom, Beil & Schliessmann, 1999). Understanding time from a Native American perspective decreases frustration. Calling the patient before making a home visit or to remind the patient of an appointment is a useful strategy.

Verbal instructions delivered in a storytelling format are more familiar to Native Americans (Hodge, Pasqua, Marquez, & Geishirt-Cantrell, 2002). The preferred learning style is observational and oral. Written instructions and pamphlets are not well received. Native Americans are experiential learners.

Case Example

When the nurse is performing a newborn bath demonstration, the Native American mother is likely to watch from a distance, avoid eye contact with the demonstrator, ask few or no questions, and decline a return demonstration. This learning style should not be seen as indifference or lack of understanding. Being an experiential learner, the Native American woman is likely to assimilate the information provided and simply give the newborn a bath when it is needed (Cesario, 2001, p. 17).

POVERTY: HIDDEN PSYCHOSOCIAL CULTURE

Poverty is a difficult, but important, sociocultural concept, particularly in today's uncertain economy. Commitment to the health of vulnerable populations and the elimination of health disparities is identified as one of the five competencies required to provide culturally competent care; it is an overarching goal for Healthy People 2020.

Recent research suggests that SES "drives health disparities more than minority status" (Barton-Burke et al., 2010, p. 158). The plight of those who fall below the poverty line is significant enough to warrant special consideration of their needs in health care settings. Raphael (2009) notes, "Poverty is not only the primary determinant of children's intellectual, emotional, and social development but also an excellent predictor of virtually every adult disease known to medicine" (p. 10).

People living in poverty have to think carefully about seeking medical attention for anything other than an emergency. The emergency department becomes a primary health care resource for the very poor, and health-seeking behaviors tend to be crisis oriented. Things that most of us take for granted, such as food, housing, clothing, the chance for a decent job, and the opportunity for education, are not available or are insufficient to realistically meet human needs. People at the poverty level have to worry on a daily basis about how to provide for basic human needs. Usually they are less educated and have more limited knowledge of healthy lifestyle-promoting activities.

Lack of essential resources is associated with political and personal powerlessness (Reutter et al., 2009). The idea that the poor can exercise choice, or make a difference in their lives, is not necessarily part of their worldview. People living in poverty overlook opportunities simply because their life experience tells them that they cannot trust their own efforts to produce change. They want, but do not really expect, their health providers to help. This mindset prompts people living in poverty to avoid and distrust the health care system for anything other than emergencies. If they *are* treated less favorably than people with money or good insurance, this further exacerbates their sense of helplessness in the health care system. Care strategies require a proactive, persistent, patient-oriented approach to helping patients and families self-manage health problems.

Respect for the human dignity of the poor patient is a major component of proactive culturally competent care. This means that the nurse pays strict attention to personal biases and stereotypes so as not to distort assessment data or impede caring implementation of nursing interventions. It means treating each patient as "culturally unique" with a set of assumptions and values regarding the disease process and its treatment and acting in a nonjudgmental manner that respects the patient's cultural integrity (Haddad, 2001). Ethics become particularly important in patient situations requiring informed consent, health care decision-making, and involvement of family and significant others, treatment access and care choices, and decisions about end-of-life care.

SUMMARY

This chapter explores the intercultural communication that takes place when the nurse and patient are from different cultures. Culture is defined as a common collectivity of beliefs, values, shared understandings, and patterns of behavior of a designated group of people. Culture needs to be viewed as a human structure with many variations in meaning.

Related terms include *cultural diversity*, *cultural relativism*, *subculture*, *ethnicity*, *ethnocentrism*, and *ethnography*. Each of these concepts broadens the definition of culture. *Intercultural communication* is defined as a communication in which the sender of a message is a member of one culture and the receiver of the message is from a different culture. Different cultures create and express different personal realities.

A *cultural assessment* is defined as a systematic appraisal of beliefs, values, and practices conducted to determine the context of patient needs and to tailor nursing interventions. It is composed of three progressive, interconnecting elements: a general assessment, a problem-specific assessment, and the cultural details needed for successful implementation.

Knowledge and acceptance of the patient's right to seek and support alternative health care practices dictated by culture is important. They can make a major difference in compliance and successful outcome. Health care professionals sometimes mistakenly assume that illness is a single concept, but illness is a personal experience strongly colored by cultural norms, values, social roles, and religious beliefs. Interventions that take into consideration the specialized needs of the patient from a culturally diverse background follow the mnemonic LEARN: Listen, Explain, Acknowledge, Recommend, and Negotiate.

Some basic thoughts about the traditional characteristics of the largest minority groups (African Americans, Hispanics, Asians, Native Americans) living in the United States, relating to communication preferences, perceptions about illness, and family, health, and religious values, are included in the chapter. The culture of poverty is also discussed.

ETHICAL DILEMMA: What Would You Do?

Antonia Martinez is admitted to the hospital and needs immediate surgery. She speaks limited English, and her family is not with her. She is frightened by the prospect of surgery and wants to wait until her family can be with her to help her make the decision about surgery. As a nurse, you feel there is no decision to be made: She must have the surgery, and you need to get her consent form signed now. What would you do?

DISCUSSION QUESTIONS

1. In what ways does your cultural identity influence the way you think, feel, and act toward someone of another culture?
2. Think of a person or a patient from another culture, and describe how you think that this person perceives or responds to you as someone from a different culture.
3. In what ways is your patient's culture similar or different from yours?

REFERENCES

Alexander, G. (2008). Cultural competence models in nursing. *Critical Care Nursing Clinics of North America, 20,* 415–421.

Allport, G. (1979). *The Nature of Prejudice.* Reading, MA: Addison-Wesley.

American Association of Colleges of Nursing (AACN). (2008). The essentials of baccalaureate education for professional nursing practice. Retrieved from: http://www.aacn.nche.edu/educationresources/BaccEssentials08.pdf.

Amerson, R. (2008). Reflections on a conversation with a curandera. *Journal of Transcultural Nursing, 19*(4), 384–387.

Anderson, P., & Wang, H. (2008). Beyond language: Nonverbal communication across cultures. In L. Samovar, R. Porter, & E. McDaniel (Eds.), *Intercultural Communication: A reader* (12th ed.). Belmont, CA: Wadsworth.

Aponte, J. (2009). Addressing cultural heterogeneity among Hispanic subgroups by using campinha-bacote's model of cultural competency. *Holistic Nursing Practice, 23*(1), 3–12; quiz 13–14.

Aroian, K., & Faville, K. (2005). Reconciling cultural relativism for a clinical paradigm: What's a nurse to do? *Journal of Professional Nursing, 21*(6), 330.

Asron, K., Levine, D., & Burstin, H. (2003). African American church participation and health care practices. *Journal of General Internal Medicine, 18,* 908–913.

Ayon, C., Marsiglia, F., & Bermudez-Parsai, M. (2010). Latino family mental health: Exploring the role of discrimination and familismo. *Journal of Community Psychology, 38*(6), 742–756.

Bacallao, M., & Smokowski, P. (2005). "Entre dos mundos" (between two worlds): Bicultural skills with Latino immigrant families. *Journal of Primary Prevention, 26*(6), 485–509.

Baron-Epel, O., Friedman, N., & Lernau, O. O. (2009). Fatalism and mammography in a multicultural population. *Oncology Nursing Forum, 36*(3), 353–361.

Barrios, P. G., & Egan, M. (2002). Living in a bicultural world and finding the way home: Native women's stories. *Affilia, 17,* 206–228.

Barton-Burke, M., Smith, E., Frain, J., & Loggins, C. (2010). Advanced cancer in underserved populations. *Seminars in Oncology Nursing, 26*(3), 157–167.

Berkman, C., & Ko, E. (2010). What and when Korean American older adults want to know about serious illness, *Journal of Psychosocial Oncology, 28*:244–259.

Berlin, E., Fowkes, W. (1982). A teaching framework for cross cultural health care. *The Western Journal of Medicine, 139*(6), 934–938.

Betancourt, J. (2004). Cultural competence—marginal or mainstream movement. *New England Journal of Medicine, 35*(10), 953–955.

Betancourt, J., Green, A., & Carrillo, J. (2003). Defining cultural competence: A practical framework for addressing racial/ethnic disparities in health and health care. *Public Health Report, 118,* 293–302.

Black, P. (2008). A guide to providing culturally appropriate care. *Gastrointestinal Nursing, 6*(6), 10–17.

Callister, L. (2001). Culturally competent care of women and newborns: Knowledge, attitude, and skills. *Journal of Obstetric, Gynecologic, & Neonatal Nursing, 30*(2), 209–215.

Calloway, S. (2009). The effect of culture on beliefs related to autonomy and informed consent. *Journal of Cultural Diversity, 16*(2), 68–70.

Campinha-Bacote, J. (2011). Delivering patient-centered care in the midst of a cultural conflict: The role of cultural competence. *Online Journal of Issues in Nursing, 16*(2), 5.

Canales, M., & Howers, H. (2001). Expanding conceptualizations of culturally competent care. *Journal of Advanced Nursing, 36*(1), 102–111.

Carthron, D., Bailey, D., & Anderson, R. (2014). The "invisible caregiver": Multicaregiving among diabetic African American grandmothers. *Geriatric Nursing, 35,* S32–S36.

CDC. (Page last updated March 14, 2014). *Healthy People 2020 social determinants of health.* Retrieved from: http://www.cdc.gov/socialdeterminants/Definitions.html.

Centers for Disease Control and Prevention. (2014). CDC health disparities and inequalities report—United States. Retrieved from: http://www.cdc.gov/mmwr/pdf/other/su6001.pdf.

Cesario, S. (2001). Care of the native american woman: Strategies for practice, education and research. *Journal of Obstetric, Gynecologic, & Neonatal Nursing, 30*(1), 13–19.

Chambers, V., & Higgins, C. (1997). Say amen, indeed. *American Way, 30*(4), 38–102.

Chao, G., & Moon, H. (2005). The cultural mosaic: a metatheory for understanding the complexity of culture. *Journal of Applied Psychology, 90,* 1120–1140.

Chaudhary, N. (2004). *Listening to culture: constructing reality from every day talk.* Thousand Oaks, CA: Sage Publications, Inc.

Chen, M., & Hu, J. (2014). Health disparities in Chinese Americans with hypertension: a review, International. *Journal of Nursing Sciences*, 1(3), 318–322.

Cheshire, T. (2001). Cultural transmission in urban American Indian families. *American Behavioral Scientist*, 44(9), 1528–1535.

Cross, W., & Bloomer, M. (2010). Extending boundaries: Clinical communication with culturally and linguistically diverse mental health patients and carers. *International Journal of Mental Health Nursing*, 19, 268–277.

Crow Dog, M., & Erdoes, R. R. (1990). *Lakota Woman*. New York: Grove Weidenfeld.

Davidson, J., Boyer, M., Casey, D., Matzel, S. C., & Walden, C. D. (2008). Gap analysis of cultural and religious needs of hospitalized patients. *Critical Care Nursing Quarterly*, 31(2), 119–126.

Davis, R. (2000). The convergence of health and family in the Vietnamese culture. *Journal of Family Nursing*, 6(2), 136–156.

Day-Vines, N., Wood, S., Grothaus, T., Craigen, L., Holman, A., Dotson-Blake, K., et al. (2007). Broaching the subjects of race, ethnicity and culture during the counseling process. *Journal of Counseling & Development*, 85, 401–409.

Donnermeyer, J., & Friedrich, L. (2006). Amish Society: An overview reconsidered. *Journal of Multicultural Nursing*, 12(3), 36–43.

Douglas, M., Rosenkoetter, M., Pacquiao, D., Callister, L., et al. (2014). Guidelines for implementing culturally competent nursing. *Journal of Transcultural Nursing*, 1:25(2), 109–121.

Drench, M., Noonan, A., Sharby, N., & Ventura, S. H. (2009). *Psychosocial Aspects of Health Care* (2nd ed.). Upper Saddle River, NJ: Pearson Prentice Hall.

Edwards, K. (2009). Disease prevention strategies to decrease health disparities. *Journal of Cultural Diversity*, 16(1), 3–4.

Eiser, A., & Ellis, G. (2007). Cultural competence and the African American experience with health care: The case for specific content in cross-cultural education. *Academic Medicine*, 82, 176–183.

Ellison, D. (2015). Communication skills. *Nursing Clinics of North America*, 50(1), 45–57.

Escallier, L. A., Fullerton, J. T., & Messina, B. A. (2011). Cultural competence outcomes assessment: A strategy and model. *International Journal of Nursing & Midwifery*, 3(3), 35–42.

Fang, M., Sixsmith, J., Sinclair, S., & Horst, G. (2015). A knowledge synthesis of culturally- and spiritually-sensitive end-of-life care: Findings from a scoping review. *Journal of Palliative Care*, 31(3) 201–201.

Flood, G. (1996). *An Introduction to Hinduism*. Cambridge: Cambridge University Press.

Florczak, K. (2013). Culture: Fluid and complex. *Nursing Science Quarterly*, 26(1), 12–13.

Flores, G. (2006). Language barriers to health care in the United States. *New England Journal of Medicine*, 229–231.

Ford, M., & Kelly, P. (2005). Conceptualizing and categorizing race and ethnicity in health services research. *Health Services Research*, 40(5 pt 2), 1658–1675.

Foronda, C. L., Baptiste, D. L., Pfaff, T., Velez, R., Reinholdt, M., Sanchez, M., et al. (2018). Cultural competency and cultural humility in simulation-based education: An integrative review. *Clinical Simulation in Nursing*, 15, 42–60.

Galanti, G. (2015). *Caring for Patients from Different Cultures* (5th ed.). Philadelphia: University of Pennsylvania Press.

Garrett, M., & Herring, R. (2001). Honoring the power of relations: Counseling Native adults. *Journal of Humanistic Counseling Education and Development*, 40(20), 139–140.

Giger, J. N. (2013). *Transcultural nursing: Assessment and intervention* (6th ed.). Philadelphia: Mosby.

Giger, J. N. (2017). *Transcultural nursing: Assessment and intervention* (7th ed.). MO: St. Louis.

Giger, J., Davidhizar, R., Purnell, L., Harden, J. T., Phillips, J., & Strickland, O. (2007). American academy of nursing expert panel report: Developing competence to eliminate health disparities in ethnic minorities and other vulnerable populations. *Journal of Transcultural Nursing*, 18(2), 95–102.

Grady, A. M. (2014). Enhancing cultural competency in home care nurses caring for Hispanic/Latino patients. *Home Healthcare Nurse*, 32(1), 24–30.

Gravely, S. (2001). When your patient speaks Spanish—and you don't. *Registered Nurse Journal*, 64(5), 64–67.

Haddad, A. (2001). Ethics in action. *Registered Nurse Journal*, 64(5), 25–26, 30.

Hall, E. (1976). *Beyond Culture*. Garden City, NY: Doubleday.

Hardin, S. (2014). Ethnogeriatrics in critical care. *Critical Care Nursing Clinics of North America*, 26, 21–30.

Harrison, G., Kagawa-Singer, M., Foerster, S., Lee, H., Pham Kim, L., Nguyen, T. N., et al. (2005). Seizing the moment. *Cancer*, 15(104–112), 2962–2968.

Hawley, S., & Morris, A. (2017). Cultural challenges to engaging patients in shared decision making. *Patient Education and Counseling*, 100, 24–81.

Hecht, G., Ronald, L., & Jackson, L. (2003). *African American Communication: Identity and Cultural Interpretation*. Mahwah, NJ: Erlbaum.

Ho, G. (2014). Acculturation and its implications on parenting for Chinese immigrants. *Journal of Transcultural Nursing*, 25(2), 145–158.

Hodge, F., & Rodriguez'g Hodge, C. (2014). Health and disease of American Indian and Alaska Native populations: An overview. In R. Huff, & M. Kline (Eds.), *Promoting Health in Multicultural Populations* (2nd ed.) (pp. 270–291). Thousand Oaks, CA: Sage Publications.

Hodge, F. S., Pasqua, A., Marquez, C. A., & Geishirt-Cantrell, B. (2002). Utilizing traditional storytelling to promote wellness in American Indian communities. *Journal of Transcultural Nursing*, 13(1), 6–11.

Hoeffel, E., Rastogi, S., Kim, M., & Shahid, H. (2012). The Asian population: 2010 census briefs. Retrieved from: www.census.gov/rpod/cen2010/briefs/c2010br-11pdf. Issued, March 2012.

G. Hofstede, Dimensionalizing cultures: The Hofstede model in context, *online readings in psychology and culture*. Retrieved from: https://doi.org/10.9707/2307.0919.1014. 2011. 2. 1

Hofstede, G., Pedersen, P., & Hofsted, G. H. (2002). *Exploring Culture: Exercises, Stories, and Synthetic Cultures.* Yarmouth, ME: Intercultural Press, Inc.

Hopp, J., & Herring, R. P. (2014). Promoting health among Black Americans: An overview. In R. Huff, & M. Kline (Eds.), *Promoting Health in Multicultural Populations* (2nd ed.) (pp. 238–269). Thousand Oaks, CA: Sage Publications.

Hulme, P. (2010). Cultural considerations in evidence-based practice. *Journal of Transcultural Nursing, 21*(3), 271–280.

Im, E. (2008). The situation specific theory of pain experience for Asian American cancer patients. *Advances in Nursing Science, 31*(4), 319–331.

Institute of Medicine (IOM). (2002a). *Speaking of Health: Assessing Health Communication Strategies for Diverse Populations.* Washington, DC: National Academy Press.

Institute of Medicine (IOM). (2002b). *Unequal Treatment. What Healthcare Providers Need to Know About Racial and Ethnic Disparities in Healthcare.* Washington, DC: National Academy Press.

Institute of Medicine (IOM). (2011). *The Future of Nursing: Leading Change, Advancing Health.* Washington, DC: National Academy Press.

Institute of Medicine (IOM). (2003). *Unequal treatment: Confronting racial and ethnic disparities in health care.* Washington, DC: National Academy Press.

Isaacson, M. (2014). Clarifying concepts: Cultural humility or competence. *Journal of Professional Nursing, 30,* 251–258.

Jacob, J., Gray, B., & Johnson, A. (2013). The Asian American family and mental health: Implications for child health professionals. *Journal of Pediatrics Care, 27*(3), 180–188.

Jandt, F. (2003). *An Introduction to Intercultural Communication: Identities in a Global Community.* Thousand Oaks, CA: Sage Publications.

Jirwe, M., Gerrish, K., Keeney, S., & Emami, A. (2009). Identifying the core components of cultural competence: Findings from a Delphi study. *Journal of Clinical Nursing, 18,* 2622–2634.

Juckett, G. (2013). Caring for Latino patients. *American Family Physician, 87*(1), 48–54.

Kalbfleisch, P. (2009). Effective health communication in native populations in North America. *Journal of Language and Social Psychology, 28*(2), 158–173.

Karim, K. (2003). Informing cancer patients: Truth telling and culture. *Cancer Nursing Practice, 2,* 23–31.

Kavanagh, K., Absalom, K., Beil, W., & Schliessmann, L. (1999). Connecting and becoming culturally competent: A Lakota example. *Advances in Nursing Science, 21*(3), 9–31.

Kemp, C. (2004). *Mexican & Mexican-Americans: Health Beliefs & Practices.* Cambridge: Cambridge University Press.

Kim, S., & Flaskerud, J. (2008). Does culture frame adjustment to the sick role? *Issues in Mental Health Nursing, 29,* 315–318.

Kleinman, A., & Benson, P. (2006). Anthropology in the clinic: the problem of cultural competency and how to fix it. *PLOS Medicine, 3,* 1672–1675.

Kline, M., & Huff, R. (2008). Health promotion in multicultural populations. In Kline M, Huff R, editors, ed 2, Thousand Oaks, CA: Sage Publications.

Knoerl, A. M. (2007). Cultural considerations and the Hispanic cardiac patient. *Home Health Care Nurse, 25*(2), 82–86.

Knoerl, A. M., Esper, K., & Hasenau, S. (2011). Cultural sensitivity in patient health education. *Nursing Clinics of North America, 46*(3), 335–340.

Kozub, M. L. (2013). Through the eyes of the other: Using event analysis to build cultural competence. *Journal of Transcultural Nursing, 24*(3), 313–318.

Kraft, M., Kastel, A., Eriksson, H., & Hedman, A. M. (2017). Global nursing—a literature review in the field of education and practice. *Nursing Open, 4*(3), 122–123.

Kwak, J., & Haley, W. (2005). Current research findings on end-of-life decision making among racially or ethnically diverse groups. *Gerontologist, 45*(5), 634–641.

Lai, D., & Surood, S. (2008). Predictors of depression in aging South Asian Canadians. *Journal of Cross-Cultural Gerontology, 23*(1), 57–75.

Leininger, M., & McFarland, R. (Eds.). (2006). *Culture Care Diversity and Universality: A Worldwide Nursing Theory.* Sudbury, MA: Jones and Bartlett.

Leonard, B., & Plotnikoff, G. (2000). Awareness: the heart of cultural competence. *AACN Clinical Issues, 11*(1), 51–59.

Lewis, R. (2000). *When cultures collide: managing successfully across cultures.* London: Nicholas Brealey Publishing.

Lewis, L., Hankin, S., Reynolds, D., & Ogedegbe, G. (2007). African American spirituality: a process of honoring God, others and self. *Journal of Holistic Nursing, 25*(1), 16–23.

Littlejohn-Blake, S., & Darling, C. A. (1993). Understanding the strengths of African American families. *Journal of Black Studies, 23*(4), 460–471.

Livingston, G., Minushkin, S., & Cohn, D. (2008). Hispanics and health care in the United States: access, information and knowledge, Pew Hispanic Center and Robert Wood Johnson foundation. www.pewhispanic.org/files/reports/91.pdf.

Louie, K. (2001). White paper on the health status of Asian-Americans and Pacific Islanders and recommendations for research. *Nursing Outlook, 49,* 173–178.

Lowe, J., & Archibald, C. (2009). Cultural diversity: The intention of nursing,. *Nursing Forum, 44*(1), 11–18.

Lynch, E., & Hanson, M. (2004). *Developing cross-cultural competence: A guide for working with children and families* (3rd ed.). Baltimore, MD: Paul H. Brookes Publishing Co.

Marsiglia, F., & Booth, J. (2015). Cultural adaptation of interventions in real practice settings. *Research on Social Work Practice, 25*(4), 423–432.

McClimens, A., Brewster, J., & Lewis, R. (2014). Recognizing and respecting patients cultural diversity. *Nursing standard, 12*(28), 45–52.

McFarland, M. R., & Wehbe-Alamah, H. B. (Eds.). (2015). *Leininger's Culture Care Diversity and Universality: A World Wide Nursing Theory.* Burlington, MA: Jones and Bartlet Learning.

McKennis, A. (1999). Caring for the Islamic patient. *AORN Journal, 69*(6), 1185–1206.

Meisenhelder, J. B., & Chandler, E. N. (2000). Faith, prayer, and health outcomes in elderly Native Americans. *Clinical Nursing Research, 9*(2), 191–204.

Messias, D., McDowell, L., & Estrada, R. (2009). Language interpreting as social justice work: Perspectives of formal and informal healthcare interpreters. *Advances in Nursing Science, 32*(2), 128–143.

Michaels, A. (2003). *Hinduism: Past and Present.* Princeton, NJ: Princeton University Press.

Migration Policy Institute. (2011). U.S. in focus: Chinese immigrants in the United States. Retrieved from: http://www.migrationinformation.org/usfocus/display.cfm?id=685 Google Scholar.

National Center for Cultural Competence. (2014). The compelling need for cultural competence. [Georgetown University.] Retrieved from: http://nccc.georgetown.edu/foundations/need.html.

Neuliep, J. (2015). *Intercultural Communication: A Contextual Approach.* (6th ed.).Thousand Oaks, CA: Sage Publications.

Office of Minority Health. (2014). Culturally competent nursing care. Retrieved from: https://ccnm.thinkculturalhealth.hhs.gov/.

Office of Minority Health and Health Equity (OMHHE). (n.d.) Available at: http://www.cdc.gov/minorityhealth.

Pagani-Tousignant, C. (1992). *Breaking the Rules: Counseling Ethnic Minorities.* Minneapolis, MN: The Johnson Institute.

Page, J. B. (2005). The concept of culture: A core issue in health disparities. *Journal of Urban Health, 82*(2 Suppl. 3), iii35–iii43.

Parham, T. A., White, J. L., & Ajamu, A. (2000). *The Psychology of Blacks: An African Centered Perspective.* Upper Saddle River, NJ: Prentice Hall.

Pergert, P., Ekblad, S., Enskar, K., & Björk, O. (2007). Obstacles to transcultural caring relationships: experiences of health care staff in pediatric oncology. *Journal of Pediatric Oncology Nursing, 24*(6), 314–328.

Purnell, J. D. (2008). *Guide to Culturally Competent Health Care* (2nd ed.). Philadelphia, PA: F.A. Davis.

Purnell, L., Purnell, J. D., & Paulanka, B. J. (2008). *Transcultural Health Care: A Culturally Competent Approach* (3rd ed.). Philadelphia, PA: F.A. Davis.

Raphael, D., & Poverty (2009). Human development, and health in Canada: Research, practice, and advocacy dilemmas. *Canadian Journal of Nursing Research, 41*(2), 7–18.

Red Horse J. (1997). Traditional American Indian family systems, families, systems and health. *15*(3), 243–250.

Reutter, L., Stewart, M., Veenstra, G., Love, R., Raphael, D., & Makwarimba, E. (2009). Who do they think we are anyway? perceptions and responses to poverty stigma. *Qualitative Health Research, 19*(3), 297–311.

Salas-Lopez, D., Soto-Greene, M., Bolder, C., & Like, R. C. (2014). *Infusing Cultural Competency into Health Professions Education: Best and Promising Practices.* University of Medicine and Dentistry of New Jersey–Robert Wood Johnson Medical School. Retrieved from: http://njms.rutgers.edu/culweb/.

Samovar, L. L., Porter, R. R., McDaniel, E. E., & Roy, C. S. (2008). *Intercultural Communication: A reader* (12th ed.). Belmont, CA: Wadsworth.

Samovar, L., Porter, R., McDaniel, E., & Roy, C. (2014). *Intercultural Communication: A reader.* Boston, MA: Cengage Learning.

Schim, S., & Doorenbos, A. (2010). A three-dimensional model of cultural congruence: framework for intervention. *Journal of Social Work in End-of-Life & Palliative Care, 6*(3–4), 256–270.

Schwartz, S., Montgomery, M., & Briones, E. (2006). The role if identity in acculturation among immigrant people: Theoretical propositions, empirical questions, and applied recommendations. *Human Development, 49*, 1–30.

Searight, H., & Gafford, J. (2005). Cultural diversity at the end of life: issues and guidelines for family physicians. *American Family Physician, 71*, 3.

Servodido, C., & Morse, E. (2001). End of life issues. *Nursing Spectrum, 11*(8DC), 20–23.

Shen, Z. (2014). Cultural competence models and cultural competence assessment instruments in nursing: A literature review. *Journal of Transcultural Nursing*, 1–14.

Sokol, R., & Strout, S. (2006). A complete theory of human emotion: The synthesis of language, body, culture and evolution in human feeling. *Culture & Psychology, 12*(10), 115–123.

Spector, R. (2004). *Cultural Diversity in Health and Illness* (8th ed.). Upper Saddle River, NJ: Pearson Prentice Hall.

Spence, D. (2001). Prejudice, paradox, and possibility: Nursing people from cultures other than one's own. *Journal of Transcultural Nursing, 12*(2), 100–106.

Sterritt, P., & Pokorny, M. (1998). African American caregiving for a relative with Alzheimer's disease. *Geriatric Nursing, 19*(3), 127–128 133–134.

Sue, D. W., & Sue, S. (2003). *Counseling the Culturally Diverse: Theory and Practice* (4th ed.). New York: Wiley.

Susilo, A. P., van Dalen, J., Scherpbier, A., Tanto, S., Yuhanti, P., & Ekawati, N. (2013). Nurses' roles in informed consent in a hierarchical and communal context. *Nursing Ethics, 20*, 413–425.

Sutton, M. (2000). Cultural competence. *Family Practice Management, 7*(9), 58–62.

The Office of Minority Health of the DHHS. (2018). The national standards for culturally and linguistically appropriate services in health and health care.

Thomas, N. (2001). The importance of culture throughout all of life and beyond. *Holistic Nursing Practice, 15*(2), 40–46.

Underwood, S., Buseh, A., Kelber, S., Stevens, P. E., & Townsend, L. (2013). Enhancing the participation of African Americans in health-related genetic research: Finding of a collaborative academic and community based research study. *Nursing Research and Practice, 2013*, 749563, 2013. https://doi.org/10.1155/2013/749563. Epub 2013 Dec 4.

US Census Bureau. (2015). US Census Bureau An Aging World, Report Number P95-16-1.

US Department of Health and Human Services (DHHS). (2001). *National Standards for Cultural and Linguistically Appropriate Services in Health Care*, Washington, DC, final report Author.

US Department of Health and Human Services (DHHS). (2006a). *National Healthcare Disparities Report.* Rockville, MD: Author.

US Department of Health and Human Services (DHHS). (2006b). National health care disparities. Retrieved from:

Monorityhealth.hhs.gov/npa/files/toolkit/NPA_Toolkit.pdf Google Scholar.

US Department of Health and Human Services (DHHS). (2010). *Healthy People 2020: Disparities*. Retrieved from: http://healthypeople.gov/2020/about/Disparities. About.aspx.

US Department of Health and Human Services (DHHS). (2014). *National Standards for Culturally and Linguistically Appropriate Services in Health Care*. Washington, DC: Author. www.omhrc.gov/assets/pdf/checked/finalreport.pdf.

US Department of Health and Human Services (DHHS), *Healthy People*. 2014b, 2020, Retrieved from: http://www.healthypeople.gov/2020/.

US Department of Health and Human Services (DHHS). (2015). Office of Minority Health. National CLAS standards. Retrieved from: https://www.thinkculturalhealth.hhs.gov/content/clas.asp.

US Department of Health and Human Services: *Office of Minority Health. (n.d.-a). Closing the health gap*, Retrieved from: http://minorityhealth.hhs.gov/templates/content.aspx?ID=2840 Google Scholar.

US Department of Health and Human Services: *Office of Minority Affairs. (n.d.-b). National standards on culturally and linguistically appropriate services (CLAS)*, Retrieved from: http://minorityhealth.hhs.gov/templates/browse.aspx?lvl=2&lvlID=15 Google Scholar.

Vaughn, L., Jacquez, F., & Baker, R. (2009). Cultural health attributions, beliefs, and practices: Effects on health care and medical education, *Open Medical Education J, 2*, 64–74.

Weiner, L., McConnell, D., Latella, L., & Ludi, E. (2013). Cultural and religious considerations in pediatric palliative care. *Palliat Support Care, 11*(1), 47–67.

Wheeler, S., & Bryant, A. (2017). Racial and ethnic disparities in health care. *Obstetrics and Gynecology Clinics of North America, 44*, 1–11.

Wilson, A. E. (2009). Fundamental causes of health disparities: a comparative analysis of canada and the united states. *International Sociology, 24*(1), 93–113.

Wilson, L. (2011). Cultural competency: beyond the vital signs. delivering holistic care to African Americans. *Nursing clinics of North America, 46*, 219–232.

World Health Organization. (n.d). *What are the social determinants of health?* Retrieved from: http://www.int/social determinants/en

Wu, E., & Martinez, M. (2006). Taking cultural competency from theory to action. Retrieved from: www.commonwealthfund.org/publications_show.htm?doc_id=ic=414097 Google Scholar.

Web Resources

http://www.diversityrx.org.
http://www.minorityhealth.hhs.gov.
http://www.ceh.org.au.
http://www.hispanichealth.org.

US Department of Health and Human Services: *The Secretary's Advisory Committee on National Health Promotion and Disease Prevention Objectives for 2020. Phase I report: Recommendations for the framework and format of Healthy People 2020 [Internet]. Section IV: Advisory Committee findings and recommendations [cited 2010 January 6]*, Retrieved from: http://www.healthypeople.gov/sites/default/files/PhaseI_0.pdf.

Communicating in Groups

Elizabeth C. Arnold

OBJECTIVES

At the end of the chapter, the reader will be able to:
1. Define group communication in health care.
2. Identify the characteristics of small group communication in contemporary health care.
3. Describe the stages of small group development.
4. Discuss theory-based concepts of group dynamics.
5. Apply group concepts in therapeutic groups.
6. Compare and contrast different types of therapeutic groups.
7. Apply concepts of group dynamics to work groups.
8. Discuss differences in small group communication and team communication.

INTRODUCTION

In clinical practice, group communication formats are used extensively as a major means of communication for clinical knowledge sharing and decision making. The diversity of opinions is not available in individual formats. Group communication provides unique opportunities for students to learn how to express, and defend, their ideas in task, project, and discussion groups. In group settings, each participant brings his or her own personal perspective and draws from distinctive experiences of other members. Knowledge sharing is not the only advantage of group interaction. Group membership can create productive relationships with other group members that might not occur otherwise.

Chapter 8 focuses on small group communication in contemporary health care. The chapter identifies theory-based concepts related to small group dynamics and processes and describes group role functions as a foundation for interactive applications in clinical and work groups. The chapter concludes with a discussion of applications for clinical and work groups.

BASIC CONCEPTS

Rothwell (2013) defines a **group** as "a human communication system composed of three or more individuals, interacting for the achievement of some common goal(s) who influence and are influenced by each other" (p. 36). Unlike communication in individual relationships, there are multiple inputs, and responses to each conversational segment in a group format.

Group relationships are interdependent. Each group member's contribution has an influence on the behavior and responses of other group members. In this way, group communication shares a key characteristic with system and team concepts (see Chapters 1 and 23). However, while a team is a group, a group is not a team. Over time, a group culture emerges, supported by stories, myths, and metaphors about the group and how it functions.

Primary and Secondary Groups

"Membership in groups is inevitable and universal" (Johnson & Johnson, 2014, p. 2). Groups are categorized as primary or secondary. **Primary groups** are characterized by an informal structure and close personal relationships. Group membership in primary groups is automatic (e.g., in a family) or voluntarily chosen because of a strong common interest (e.g., long-term friendship). There are no previously determined end dates. Primary groups have an important influence on self-identity and the development of socialization skills.

Secondary groups represent time-limited group relationships with an established beginning and end. Group size is determined by its goals and functions. In contrast with primary groups, secondary groups have a prescribed formal structure, a designated leader, and specific goals

(Forsyth, 2010). When the group completes its task, or achieves its goals, the group ends.

People join secondary groups to meet short-term established goals, to develop knowledge and skills, or because it is required by the larger community system to which the individuals belong. Formal work groups, which are critical to the accomplishment of predetermined organizational goals, are also classified as secondary groups as are therapy and support groups. Other group formats with a work-related rather than friendship basis include social action, specific task, clinical teams, and education groups.

Beebe and Masterson (2014) suggest that systems theory explains how a group as a system relates to smaller individual systems within it and to the larger organizational systems of which the group is a part. Exercise 8.1 presents the role that group communication plays in a person's life.

Group Communication in Health Care

Counseling and therapy groups, psychoeducation, work groups, and interprofessional clinical teams functioning within a larger health care system setting rely on aspects of group communication to achieve designated goals in health care settings. Multiple informational inputs available in small groups are an invaluable input resource in professional clinical education.

Nurses are increasingly involved in task forces and committees to help strengthen health systems and improve clinical outcomes within the profession, on interprofessional health care teams, and within the larger community (Yang, Woomer, & Matthews, 2012). In the community, nurses come together with other health professionals and concerned citizens to advocate for clinical approaches that address specific and global health needs in the community. Examples include citizen advisory groups to advocate for the needs of the elderly, mental health, drug abuse, and disabled or mentally retarded citizens.

In your nursing program, group communication provides a central means of communicating with other students and health professionals within and between clinical settings. As you work with other students in small group formats to complete educational projects or engage in related reflective analysis discussions of simulated and experiential clinical scenarios, you are using group communication skills. Interprofessional education and practice collaboration, now a global initiative in health care, use small group communication as a fundamental form of interaction (see Chapter 23).

In 2002, the National Institute of Medicine made specific recommendations for nursing and other clinically based programs to offer collaborative training opportunities with different professionals working together as a unit in hospitals and other clinical sites.

Group learning formats use group communication concepts and simulated group experiences to help students to develop critical thinking about coordinated interprofessional clinical approaches in clinical settings. Clinical simulations prepare students experientially to work together in prototype situations similar to those they will encounter in actual practice. Students share information, question and negotiate with one another, and communicate with standardized patients in simulated clinical scenarios. They begin to experientially understand the practices, processes, and concerns of their own and other disciplines in a system-based therapeutic approach to patient-centered care. Reflective analysis group discussions and negotiating roles are critical components of interdisciplinary team learning processes (Michaelsen & Sweet, 2008).

CHARACTERISTICS OF SMALL GROUP COMMUNICATION THERAPY

Group Purpose

The group purpose provides the rationale for a group's existence (Powles, 2007). Purpose provides direction for

---

EXERCISE 8.1   Groups in Everyday Life

Purpose
To help students gain an appreciation of the role group communication plays in their lives.

Procedure
1. Write down all the groups in which you have been a participant (e.g., family, scouts, sports teams, and community, religious, work, and social groups).
2. Describe the influence membership in each of these groups had on the person you are today.
3. Identify the ways in which membership in different groups were of value in your life.

Discussion
1. How similar or dissimilar were your answers from those of your classmates?
2. What factors account for differences in the quantity and quality of your group memberships?
3. How similar were the ways in which membership enhanced your self-esteem?
4. If your answers were dissimilar, what makes membership in groups such a complex experience?
5. Could different people get different things out of very similar group experiences?
6. What implications does this exercise have for your nursing practice?

group decisions and influences the type of communication and activities required to meet group goals. For example, the purpose of group therapy would be to improve the interpersonal functioning of individual members. In a work group, the purpose would support a better solution to implementation of a specific work-related issue, such as wait times, transfer processes, or introduction of a new program or process. The purpose of a health team would be to deliver quality health care to assigned patients. The purposes of different group types are presented in Table 8.1.

Group Goals

Group goals define expected therapeutic outcomes in a process group or describe a defined work outcome in a task group, indicating goal achievement. Goals serve as benchmarks for successful achievement. Matching group goals with member needs and characteristics is essential in counseling and therapeutic groups. In work groups, the match should be between group members' expertise/skills, interests, and goal requirements.

General group goals should be of interest to the group members. Group members need to understand and commit to achieving group goals. Goals need to be achievable, measurable, and within the capabilities of group membership. A good match energizes a group; members develop commitment and interest because they perceive the group as having value.

Group Size

Group purpose dictates group size. Patient-centered therapeutic groups consist of six to eight members. With fewer than five members, deep sharing tends to be limited. If one or more members are absent, group interaction can become intense and uncomfortable for the remaining members. Powles (2007) argues that "the threesome rarely leads to solid group formation or a productive group work" (p. 107). Education-focused groups, such as medication, psychoeducation, diagnosis, skill training, and treatment groups can have 10 or more members. Membership on interdisciplinary teams varies, depending in part on patient needs. They typically reflect the essential number of health care professionals needed to coordinate and share care responsibility for a common patient population.

Group Member Composition

Careful selection of group members should be based on functional similarity, commitment to identified group goals, and basic knowledge of how group communication processes enable goal achievement. A person's capacity to derive benefit from the group and to contribute to group goals is a critical requirement for patient therapy groups (Yalom & Leszcz, 2005).

Functional similarity is defined as choosing the group members who are similar enough—intellectually, emotionally, and experientially—to interact with one another in a meaningful way. A one-of-a-kind group member is at a disadvantage from an acceptance perspective. For example, an older highly educated adult placed in a therapy group of young adults with limited verbal and educational skills or a single adolescent girl placed in a group of similar-aged boys can be a group casualty or scapegoat, simply because of personal characteristics beyond that individual member's control. In a different group, with members having similar intellectual, emotional, and life experiences, the treatment outcomes might be quite different.

Participation can be compromised by a "one-of-a-kind" significant emotional difference, for example, acute psychosis that would interfere with meaningful communication. Group therapy is contraindicated for an acutely psychotic, actively suicidal, paranoid, excessively hostile, or impulsive patient until symptoms are brought under control.

TABLE 8.1 Therapeutic Group Type and Purpose	
Group	**Purpose**
Therapy	Reality testing, encouraging personal growth, inspiring hope, strengthening personal resources, developing interpersonal skills
Support	Giving and receiving practical information and advice, supporting coping skills, promoting self-esteem, enhancing problem-solving skills, encouraging patient autonomy, strengthening hope and resiliency
Activity	Getting people in touch with their bodies, releasing energy, enhancing self-esteem, encouraging cooperation, stimulating spontaneous interaction, supporting creativity
Health education	Learning new knowledge, promoting skill development, providing support and feedback, supporting development of competency, promoting discussion of important health-related issues

In work (task) groups, functional similarity consists of choosing members with complementary experiential knowledge or skill sets, plus the interest, commitment, and essential skills to contribute to group goals. This type of functional match produces a higher level of group performance and member satisfaction.

Interpersonal compatibility among group members is desirable, as this can enhance task interdependence and the desire to work together as a group. On the other hand, differences in outlook and opinion can enrich group conversation, if not extreme. Group members from different backgrounds have diverse life experiences, which can help group members consider alternative viewpoints. Working through differences to achieve consensus makes the group process a richer experience, and the outcome will reflect a broader consensus. Exercise 8.2 provides an opportunity to explore the concept of functional similarity.

Group Norms

Group norms refer to the unwritten behavioral rules of conduct expected of group members. Norms provide needed predictability for effective group functioning and make the group safe for its members. There are two types of norms: universal and group specific.

Universal norms are explicit behavioral standards, which must be present in all groups to achieve effective outcomes. Examples include confidentiality, regular attendance, and using the group as the forum for discussion rather than individual discussion with members outside of the group (Burlingame et al., 2006). Unless group members in process groups believe that personal information will not be shared outside the group setting (confidentiality), trust will not develop. Regular attendance at group meetings is critical to group stability and goal achievement. Even if the member is a perfect fit with group goals, he or she must fully commit to regular attendance and full participation. Personal relationships between group members outside of the group also threaten the integrity of the group.

Group-specific norms are constructed by group members. They represent the shared beliefs, values and unspoken operational rules governing group functions (Rothwell, 2013). Norms help define member interactions. They are often implicit. Examples include the group's tolerance for lateness, use of humor, or confrontation, and talking directly to other group members rather than about them. Exercise 8.3 can help you develop a deeper understanding of group norms.

EXERCISE 8.2 Exploring Functional Similarity

Purpose
To provide an experiential understanding of functional similarity.

Procedure
1. Break class into groups of four to six people.
2. One person should act as a scribe.
3. Identify two characteristics or experiences that all members of your group have in common other than that you are in the same class.
4. Identify two things that are unique to each person in your group (e.g., only child, never moved from the area, born in another country, unique skill or life experience).
5. Each person should elaborate on both the common and different experiences.

Discussion
1. What was the effect of finding common ground with other group members?
2. In what ways did finding out about the uniqueness of each person's experience add to the discussion?
3. Did anything in either the discussion of commonalities or differences in experience stimulate further group discussion?
4. How could you use what you have learned in this exercise in your clinical practice?

EXERCISE 8.3 Identifying Norms

Purpose
To help identify norms operating in groups.

Procedure
1. Divide a piece of paper into three columns.
2. In the first column, write the norms you think exist in your class or work group. In the second column, write the norms you think exist in your family. Examples of norms might be as follows: no one gets angry, decisions are made by consensus, assertive behaviors are valued, missed sessions and lateness are not tolerated.
3. Share your norms with the group, first related to the school or work group and then to the family. Place this information in the third column.

Discussion
1. What were some of the differences in existing norms for school and work and family?
2. Were there any universal norms on either of your lists?
3. Was there more or less consistency in overall student responses about class and work group norms and family norms? If so, what would account for it?

Group Role Positions

A person's role position in the group corresponds with the status, power, and internal image that other members in the group hold of the member. Group members assume, or are ascribed, roles that influence their communication and the responses of others in the group. They usually have trouble breaking away from roles they have been cast in despite their best efforts. For example, people will look to the "helper" group member for advice, even when that person lacks expertise or personally needs the group's help. That identified "helper" member may suffer because he or she does not always receive the help he or she needs. Other times, group members project a role position onto a particular group member that represents a hidden agenda or an unresolved issue for the group as a whole. Projection is largely unconscious, but it can be destructive to group functioning (Moreno, 2007). For example, if the group as a whole seems to scapegoat, ignore, defer to, or consistently idealize one of its members, this group projection can compromise the group's effectiveness because of an unrealistic focus on one group member. Exercise 8.4 considers group role-position expectations.

Group Dynamics

Group dynamics is a term used to describe the communication processes and behaviors that occur during the life of the group (Forsyth, 2010). These underlying forces represent a complex blend of individual and group characteristics that interact with each other to achieve the group purpose. Bernard et al. (2008) categorized the primary forces operating in groups as individual dynamics (member variables), interpersonal dynamics (group communication variables), and group as a whole dynamics related to purpose, norms, etc. Factors influencing group dynamics are displayed in Fig. 8.1. The group leader is charged with integrating these multiple variables into a workable group process. Group work can enhance member confidence, interpersonal skills, and cultural awareness (Forehand, et. al., 2016).

Group Process

Group process refers to the structural development of small group relationships. (Tuckman & Jensen, 1977) *Tuckman's (1965) five-stage model of small group development* (forming, storming, norming, performing, and

---

EXERCISE 8.4   Headbands: Group Role Expectations

Purpose

To experience the pressures of role expectations on group performance.

Procedure

1. Break the group up into a smaller unit of six to eight members. In a large group, a small group performs while the remaining members observe.
2. Make up mailing labels or headbands that can be attached to or tied around the heads of the participants. Each headband is lettered with directions on how the other members should respond to the role. Examples:
   - Comedian: laugh at me
   - Expert: ask my advice
   - Important person: defer to me
   - Stupid: sneer at me
   - Insignificant: ignore me
   - Loser: pity me
   - Boss: obey me
   - Helpless: support me
3. Place a headband on each member in such a way that the member cannot read his or her own label, but the other members can see it easily.
4. Provide a topic for discussion (e.g., why the members chose nursing, the women's movement), and instruct

each member to interact with the others in a way that is natural for him or her. Do not role-play; be yourself. React to each member who speaks by following the instructions on the speaker's headband. You are not to tell one another what the headbands say, but simply to react to them.

5. After about 20 min, the facilitator halts the activity and directs each member to guess what his or her headband says and then to take it off and read it.

Discussion

Initiate a discussion, including any members who observed the activity. Possible questions include the following:

1. What were some of the problems of trying to be yourself under conditions of group role pressure?
2. How did it feel to be consistently misinterpreted by the group—to have them laugh when you were trying to be serious or ignore you when you were trying to make a point?
3. Did you find yourself changing your behavior in reaction to the group treatment of you—withdrawing when they ignored you, acting confident when they treated you with respect, giving orders when they deferred to you?

Modified from Pfeiffer, J., & Jones, J. (1977). *A handbook of structured experiences for human relations training* (Vol VI). La Jolla, CA: University Associate Publishers.

adjourning) describes the most commonly used framework for the structural development and relationship process of small groups. Stages of group development are applicable to work groups and therapeutic groups. Each sequential phase of group development has its own set of tasks, which build and expand on the work of previous phases.

Forming

The forming phase begins when members come together as a group. Members enter group relationships as strangers to one another. The leader orients the group to the group's purpose, and asks members to introduce themselves. The information each person shares about himself or herself should be brief and relate to personal data relevant to achieving the group's purpose.

During the forming phase, the leader introduces universal norms (group ground rules) for attendance, participation, and confidentiality. Getting to know one another, finding common threads in personal or professional experience, and acceptance of group goals and tasks are initial group tasks. Members have a basic need for acceptance, so communication is more tentative than it will be later when members know and trust one another.

Storming

The storming phase focuses on power and control issues. Members use testing behaviors around boundaries, communication styles, and personal reactions with other members and the leader. Characteristic behaviors may include disagreement with the group format, topics for discussion, the best ways to achieve group goals, and comparisons of member contributions. Setting group goals evolves from a brainstorming discussion of alternative concerns generated by its members that the group might pursue. The next step is to choose the most promising issues to focus on as top priority concerns the group feels it can address. Although the storming phase is uncomfortable, successful resolution leads to the development of group-specific norms.

Norming

In the norming phase, individual goals become aligned with group goals. Group-specific norms help create a supportive group climate characterized by dependable fellowship and purpose. These norms make the group "safe," and members begin to experience the cohesiveness of the group as "their group." The group holds its members accountable and challenges individual members who fail to adhere to expected norms.

Brainstorming consists of the group members thinking of as many ideas as possible related to resolving an identified issue. Criticism of any ideas and/or statements of judgment are not permitted in the early stages of brainstorming. Later, the group members will begin to prioritize which potential solutions are the most workable.

Cohesiveness is defined as the relational bonds that link members of a group to one another and to the group as a whole. A sense of interconnection is the basis for group identity. It is an essential characteristic of optimum group productivity. It develops when all group members accept group-specific behavioral standards as operational norms for the group and view the group as a united whole. Sources of cohesiveness include shared goals, working through and solving problems, and the nature of group interaction.

Performing

Most of a group's work gets accomplished in the performing phase. This phase of group development is characterized by interdependence, acceptance of each member as a person of value, and the development of group cohesion. Members feel loyal to the group and engaged in its work. They are comfortable taking risks and are invested enough in one another and the group process to offer constructive comments without fearing censure from other members.

Adjourning

Tuckman introduced the adjourning phase as a final phase of group development at a later date (Tuckman & Jensen, 1977). This phase is characterized by reviewing what has been accomplished, reflecting on the meaning of the group's work together, creating deliverables, and making plans to move on in different directions.

Group Role Functions

Functional roles differ from the positional roles that group members assume. Group roles relate to the type

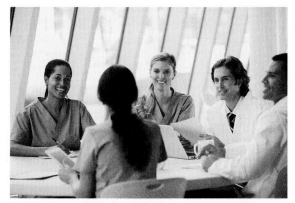

Fig. 8.1 Group dynamics describe the communication processes and behaviors' that occur during the life of a group. Copyright © monkeybusinessimages/iStock/Thinkstock.

BOX 8.1 Task and Maintenance Functions in Group Dynamics

Task Functions: Behaviors Relevant to the Attainment of Group Goals

- **Initiating:** Identifies tasks or goals; defines group problem; suggests relevant strategies for solving problem
- **Seeking information or opinion:** Requests facts from other members; asks other members for opinions; seeks suggestions or ideas for task accomplishment
- **Giving information or opinion:** Offers facts to other members; provides useful information about group concerns
- **Clarifying, elaborating:** Interprets ideas or suggestions placed before group; paraphrases key ideas; defines terms; adds information
- **Summarizing:** Pulls related ideas together; restates key ideas; offers a group solution or suggestion for other members to accept or reject
- **Consensus taking:** Checks to see whether group has reached a conclusion; asks group to test a possible decision.

Maintenance Functions: Behaviors That Help the Group Maintain Harmonious Working Relationships

- **Harmonizing:** Attempts to reconcile disagreements; helps members reduce conflict and explore differences in a constructive manner
- **Gatekeeping:** Helps keep communication channels open; points out commonalties in remarks; suggests approaches that permit greater sharing
- **Encouraging:** Indicates by words and body language unconditional acceptance of others; agrees with contributions of other group members; is warm, friendly, and responsive to other group members
- **Compromising:** Admits mistakes; offers a concession when appropriate; modifies position in the interest of group cohesion
- **Setting standards:** Calls for the group to reassess or confirm implicit and explicit group norms when appropriate

Note: Every group needs both types of functions and needs to work out a satisfactory balance of task and maintenance activity.

Modified from Rogers, C. (1972). The process of the basic encounter group. In R. Diedrich, & H. A. Dye (Eds.), *Group procedures: Purposes, processes and outcomes*. Boston: Houghton Mifflin.

---

of member contributions needed to achieve group goals. Benne and Sheats (1948) described constructive role functions as the behaviors members use to move toward goal achievement (task functions) and behaviors designed to ensure personal satisfaction (maintenance functions).

Balance between task and maintenance functions increases group productivity. When task functions predominate, member satisfaction decreases, and a collaborative atmosphere is diminished. When **maintenance** functions override task functions, members have trouble reaching goals. Members do not confront controversial issues, so the creative tension needed for successful group accomplishment is compromised. Task and maintenance role functions found in successful small groups are listed in Box 8.1.

Benne and Sheats (1948) also identified nonfunctional role functions. *Self-roles* are roles a person unconsciously uses to meet self-needs at the expense of other members' needs, group values, and goal achievement. Self-roles, identified in Table 8.2, detract from the group's work and compromise goal achievement by taking time away from group issues and creating discomfort among group members.

TABLE 8.2 Nonfunctional Self-Roles

Role	Characteristics
Aggressor	Criticizes or blames others, personally attacks other members, uses sarcasm and hostility in interactions
Blocker	Instantly rejects ideas or argues an idea to death, cites tangential ideas and opinions, obstructs decision making
Joker	Disrupts work of the group by constantly joking and refusing to take group task seriously
Avoider	Whispers to others, daydreams, doodles, acts indifferent and passive
Self-confessor	Uses the group to express personal views and feelings unrelated to group task
Recognition seeker	Seeks attention by excessive talking, trying to gain leader's favor, expressing extreme ideas or demonstrating peculiar behavior

Modified from Benne, K. D., & Sheats, P. (1948). Functional roles of group members. *Journal of Social Issues, 4*(2), 41–49.

APPLICATIONS TO HEALTH-RELATED GROUPS

In clinical settings, a health-related group purpose and goals dictate group structure, membership, and format. For example, a medication group would have an educational purpose. A group for parents with critically ill children would have a family support design, while a therapy group would have restorative healing functions. Activity groups are used therapeutically with children and with chronically mentally ill patients who have difficulty fully expressing themselves verbally. Exploration of personal feelings would be limited and related to the topic under discussion in an education group. In a therapy group, such probing would be encouraged.

Group Membership

Therapeutic and support groups are categorized as closed or open groups, and as having homogeneous or heterogeneous membership (Corey & Corey, 2013). *Closed therapeutic* groups have a selected membership with an expectation of regular attendance for an extended time period. Group members may be added, but their inclusion depends on a match with group-defined criteria. Most psychotherapy groups fall into this category. *Open groups* do not have a defined membership. Most community support groups are open groups. Individuals come and go depending on their needs. One week the group might consist of two or three members and the next week 15 members. Some groups, such as Alcoholics Anonymous, have open meetings that anyone can attend and "closed" meetings that only alcoholic members can attend.

Having a homogeneous or heterogeneous membership identifies member characteristics. *Homogeneous* groups share common characteristics, for example, diagnosis (e.g., breast cancer support group) or a personal attribute (e.g., gender, or age). Twelve-step programs for alcohol or drug addiction, eating disorders, and gender-specific consciousness-raising groups are familiar examples of homogeneous groups. Psychoeducation (e.g., medication groups) groups often have a homogeneous membership related to particular medications or a diagnosis.

Heterogeneous groups represent a wider diversity of member characteristics and personal issues. Members vary in age, gender, and psychodynamics. Most psychotherapy and insight-oriented personal growth groups have a heterogeneous membership.

Creating the Group Environment

Privacy and freedom from interruptions are key considerations in selecting an appropriate location. A sign on the door indicating that the group is in session is essential for privacy. Seating should be comfortable and arranged in a circle so that each member has face-to-face contact with all other members. Being able to see facial expressions and to respond to several individuals at one time is essential to effective group communication. Often group members choose the same seats in therapy groups. When a member is absent, that seat is left vacant.

Therapy groups usually meet weekly at a set time. Support groups meet at regular intervals, more often monthly. Educational groups meet for a predetermined number of sessions and then disband. Unlike individual sessions, which can be convened spontaneously in emergency situations, therapeutic groups meet only at designated times. Most therapeutic and support groups meet for 60 to 90 minutes on a regular basis with established, agreed-on meeting times. Groups that begin and end on time foster trust and predictability.

GROUP LEADERSHIP

Group leadership is based on two assumptions: (1) group leaders have a significant influence on group process; and (2) most problems in groups can be avoided or reworked productively if the leader is aware of and responsive to the needs of individual group members, including the needs of the leader (Corey & Corey, 2013).

Effective leadership requires adequate knowledge of the topic, preparation, professional attitudes and behavior, responsible selection of members, and an evidence-based approach. Personal characteristics demonstrated by effective group leaders include commitment to the group purpose; self-awareness of personal biases and interpersonal limitations, careful preparation of the group, and an accepting attitude toward group members. Knowledge of group dynamics, training, and supervision are additional requirements for leaders of psychotherapy groups. Health education group leaders need to have expertise about the topic to be discussed.

Throughout the group's life, the group leader models an attitude of caring, objectivity, and integrity. Effective leaders are good listeners; they can adapt their leadership style to fit the changing needs of the group. They respectfully support the reliability of group members as equal partners in meeting group goals. Successful leaders trust the group process enough to know that group members can work through conflict and difficult situations. The bonds that build between group members are real. Leaders know that even mistakes can be temporary setbacks and can be used for discussion to promote group member growth (Rubel & Kline, 2008).

INFORMAL GROUP LEADERS

Informal power is given to members who best clarify the needs of the other group members or who move the group toward goal achievement. Informal leaders develop within the group because they have a good grasp of the situational demands of the task at hand. They are not always the group members making the most statements. Some individuals, due to the force of their personalities, knowledge, or experience, will emerge as informal leaders within the group.

Ideally, group leadership is a shared function of all group members, with many opportunities for different informal leaders to divide up responsibility for achieving group goals.

Emergent informal leaders become the voice of the group. Their comments are equated with those of the designated leader. Emergent leaders are more willing to take an active role in making a recommendation and generally move the group task forward.

Case Example

Al is a powerful informal leader in a job search support group. Although he makes few comments, he has an excellent understanding of and sensitivity to the needs of individual members. When these are violated, Al speaks up, and the group listens.

Co-Leadership

Co-leadership represents a form of shared leadership found primarily in therapy and support groups. It is desirable for several reasons. The co-leader adds another perspective related to processing group dynamics. Co-leaders can provide a wider variety of responses and viewpoints that can be helpful to group members. When one leader is under fire, it can increase the other leader's confidence, knowing that an opportunity to process the session afterward is available.

Respecting and valuing each other, with sensitivity to a co-leader's style of communication, is characteristic of effective co-leadership (Corey & Corey, 2013). Problems can arise when co-leaders have different theoretical orientations or are competitive with each other. Needing to pursue solo interpretations rather than explore or support the meaning of a co-leader's interventions is distracting to the group. Yalom and Leszcz (2005) state: "You are far better off leading a solo group with good supervision than being locked into an incompatible co-therapy relationship" (p. 447).

Co-leaders should spend sufficient prep time together prior to meeting with a therapy group to ensure personal compatibility and to come to consensus regarding an understanding of the group purpose. Co-leaders need to process group dynamics together, preferably after each meeting. Processing group dynamics allows leaders to consider different meanings and to evaluate what happened in the group session and what might need to be addressed to productively move the group ahead.

DEVELOPING AN EVIDENCE-BASED PRACTICE

Purpose

The purpose of this study was to explore the impact of interprofessional team composition on team dynamics, related to conflict and open-mindedness. Using a cross-sectional correlational design, survey data from 218 team members of 47 interprofessional teams in an acute care setting were analyzed to investigate two moderated mediation pathways.

Results

Study results demonstrated a significant relationship between interprofessional composition and affective conflict for teams rated highly for individualized professional identification.

Practice Implications

Study results indicate the need to develop a shared group identity with reinforcement of shared values related to patient care as a means of improving interprofessional team communication dynamics.

Mitchell, R., Parker, V., Giles, M., & Boyle, B. (2014). The ABC of health care team dynamics: Understanding complex affective, behavioral, and cognitive dynamics in interprofessional teams. *Health Care Management Review, 39*(1), 1–9.

APPLICATIONS

Therapeutic Groups

Group communication is more complex than individual conversations because each member brings a different set of perspectives, perception of reality, communication style, and personal agenda to the group. It can also be a more powerful communication modality. Counselman (2008) refers to the power of a group as being able to resonate with a member's experience, change behaviors, and strengthen emotions as being unparalleled. "Group demonstrates that there truly are multiple realities" (p. 270).

A major difference between group and individual communication is that the leader relates to the group as a whole, instead of with only one person. The leader joins member responses and themes together and/or points to

TABLE 8.3   Therapeutic Factors in Groups

Installation of hope	Occurs when members see others who have overcome problems and are successfully managing their lives
Universality	Sharing common situations validates member experience, decreases sense of isolation: "Maybe I am not the only one with this issue."
Imparting information	New shared information is a resource for individual members and stimulates further discussion and the learning of new skills.
Imitative behavior	Members learn new behaviors through observation and the modeling of desired actions and gain confidence in trying them, e.g., managing conflict, receiving constructive criticism.
Socialization	Group provides a safe learning environment in which to take interpersonal risks and try new behaviors.
Interpersonal learning	Group acts as a social microcosm; focus is on members learning about how they interact and getting constructive feedback and support from others.
Cohesiveness	Sense of we-ness. Emphasizes personal bonds and commitment to the group. Members feel acceptance and trust from others. Cohesiveness serves as the foundation for all curative factors.
Catharsis	Expression of emotion that leads to receiving support and acceptance from other group members.
Corrective recapitulation of primary family	Allows for recognition and handling of transference issues in therapy groups. This helps group members to avoid repeating destructive interaction patterns in the "here and now."
Altruism	Providing help and support to other group members enhances personal self-esteem.
Existential factors	Highlights primary responsibility for taking charge of one's life and the consequences of their actions, creating a meaningful existence.

Adapted from Yalom, I., & Leszcz, M. (2005). *The theory and practice of group psychotherapy* (5th ed.). New York: Basic Books.

conversational differences as providing broader information. Instead of immediately responding to individual members, group leaders highlight different options by engaging additional group responses.

Making important connections among multiple realities offers different possibilities to individual patients to learn about and test out new interpersonal communication skills. Table 8.3 displays therapeutic factors found in therapeutic group formats.

Pregroup Interview

Adequate preparation of group members in pregroup interviews enhances the effectiveness of therapeutic groups (Yalom & Leszcz, 2005). A pregroup interview makes the transition into the group easier as group members have an initial connection with the leader and an opportunity to ask questions before committing to the group. Reservations held by either the leader or potential group member are handled beforehand. The description of the group and its members should be short and simple, as this information will be repeated in initial meetings.

Forming Phase

How well leaders initially prepare themselves and group members has a direct impact on building the trust needed within the group (Corey & Corey, 2013). The forming phase in therapeutic groups focuses on helping patients establish trust in the group and with one another. Communication is tentative. Members are asked to introduce themselves and share a little of their background or reason for coming to the group. An introductory prompt such as, "What would you most like to get out of this group?" helps the patients link personal goals to group goals.

In the first session, the leader introduces group goals. Clear group goals are particularly important to provide a frame for the group in its initial session. Even if the members know one another, it is helpful to ask each group member to introduce himself or herself and tell what they would like to get out of the experience. The leader clarifies how the group will be conducted and what the group can expect from the leader, and from each other, regarding group goals. Orienting statements may need to be restated in subsequent early sessions, especially if there is a lot of anxiety in the group.

The leader will also introduce universal behavioral norms such as confidentiality, regular attendance, and mutual respect (Corey & Corey, 2013). Confidentiality is harder to implement with group formats because members are not held to the same professional ethical standards as the group leader. However, for the integrity of the group, all members need to commit to confidentiality as a universal group norm (Lasky & Riva, 2006).

Storming Phase

The storming phase focuses on the differences among group members rather than the commonalities. It is usually characterized by some disagreements among group members. This is normal behavior as group members feel more comfortable with expressing authentic opinions. The leader plays an important facilitative role in the storming phase by accepting differences in member perceptions as being expected and growth producing. By affirming genuine but different strengths in individual members, leaders model handling conflict with productive outcomes. Linking constructive themes while identifying the nature of the disagreement is an effective modeling strategy. These discussions are important. However, if members test boundaries through sexually provocative statements, flattery, or insulting remarks, the leader should step in and promptly set limits. Refer to the work of the group as being of the highest priority, and tactfully ask the person to align remarks with the group purpose. Working through conflicts allows members to take stands on their personal preferences without being defensive and to compromise when needed. Conflict issues in groups are informants of what is important to group members and how individual members handle difficult emotions. Resolution leads to the development of cohesion.

Norming Phase

Once initial conflict is resolved in the storming phase, the group moves into the norming phase. Tasks in the norming phase center on the development of the implicit group developed rules governing their group behaviors. Group-specific norms develop spontaneously through group-member interactions. They represent the group's shared expectations of its members. For example, lateness may not be tolerated. The group leader encourages member contributions and emphasizes cooperation in recognizing each person's talents and contributions related to group goals. Successful short-term groups focus on here-and-now interactions, giving practical feedback, sharing personal thoughts and feelings, and listening to one another (Corey & Corey, 2013).

> **BOX 8.2   Communication Principles to Facilitate Cohesiveness**
>
> - Group tasks should be within the membership's range of ability and expertise.
> - Comments and responses should be nonevaluative, focused on behaviors rather than on personal characteristics.
> - The leader should point out group accomplishments and acknowledge member contributions.
> - The leader should be empathetic and teach members how to give effective feedback.
> - The leader should help group members view and work through creative tension as being a valuable part of goal achievement.

Cohesion begins to develop as a sharing of feelings deepens the trust in the group as a safe place. *Cohesion* describes the emotional bonds members have for one another and underscores the level of member commitment to the group (Yalom & Leszcz, 2005). Research suggests that cohesive groups experience more personal satisfaction with goal achievement and that members of such groups are more likely to join other group relationships. In a cohesive group, members demonstrate a sense of common purpose, a caring commitment to one another, collaborative problem solving, a sense of feeling personally valued, and a team spirit (Powles, 2007). See Box 8.2 for communication principles that facilitate cohesiveness.

Performing Phase

The performing phase is similar to the working phase in individual relationships; members focus on problem solving and developing new behaviors. This phase is where the group's serious work takes center stage. The group leader is responsible for keeping the group on task to accomplish group goals. Group members are responsible for working with the group leader(s) to maintain a supportive group-work environment. If group members seem to be moving off track, asking open-ended questions or verbally observing group processes can restore forward movement. Modeling respect, empathy, appropriate self-disclosure, and ethical standards helps ensure a supportive group climate. Working together and participating in another person's personal growth allows members to experience one another's personal strengths and the collective caring of the group. Of all the possibilities that can happen in a group, individual members report feeling affirmed and respected by other group members as being most valuable.

Because members function interdependently, they are able to work through disagreements and difficult issues in ways that are acceptable to each individual and the group. Effective group leaders trust group members to develop their own solutions, but they call attention to important group dynamics when needed. This can be introduced with a simple statement, such as, "I wonder what is going on here right now" (Rubel & Kline, 2008). Feedback should be descriptive and specific to the immediate discussion. As with other types of constructive feedback, the feedback should focus only on modifiable behaviors. Think about how you can word your message so that it helps a member better understand the impact of a behavior, to make sense of an experience, and to grow from the experience.

Monopolizing

Monopolizing is a negative form of power communication used to advance a personal agenda without considering the needs of others. It may not be intentional, but rather a member's way of handling anxiety. When one member monopolizes the conversation, there are several ways the leader can respond. Acknowledging this person's contribution and broadening the input with a short open-ended question, such as, "Has anyone else had a similar experience?" can redirect the attention to the larger group. Looking in the direction of other group members as the statements are made encourages alternative member responses. If a member continues to monopolize the conversation, the leader can respectfully acknowledge the person's comment and refocus the issue within the group directly, "I appreciate your thoughts, but I think it would be important to hear from other people as well. What do you think about this, Jane?" or "We don't have much time left, I wonder if anyone else has a comment or something they need to talk about."

Adjourning Phase

The final phase of group development, termination or adjournment, ideally occurs when the group members have achieved desired outcomes. The termination phase is about task completion and disengagement. The leader encourages the group members to express their feelings about one another with the stipulation that any concerns the group may have about an individual member or suggestions for future growth be stated in a constructive way. The leader should present his or her comments last and then close the group with a summary of goal achievement. By waiting until the group ends to share closing comments, the leader has an opportunity to soften or clarify previous comments and to connect cognitive and feeling elements that need to be addressed. The leader needs to remind members that the norm of confidentiality continues after the group ends

---

EXERCISE 8.5 Group Closure Activities

Purpose
To develop closure skills in small-group communication.

Procedure
1. Focus your attention on the group member next to you and think about what you like about the person, how you see him or her in the group, and what you might wish for that person as a member of the group.
2. After five minutes, your instructor will ask you to tell the person next to you to use the three themes in making a statement about the person. For example, "The thing I most like about you in the group is …"; "To me, you represent the _____ in the group"; and so on.
3. When all of the group members have had a turn, discussion may start.

Discussion
1. How did you experience telling someone about your response to him or her in the group?
2. How did you feel being the group member receiving the message?
3. What did you learn about yourself from doing this exercise?
4. What implications does this exercise have for future interactions in group relationships?

(Mangione, Forti, & Iacuzzi, 2007). Referrals are handled on an individual as-needed basis. Exercise 8.5 considers group closure issues.

TYPES OF THERAPEUTIC GROUPS

The group provides a microcosm of social dynamics in the larger world. Individuals tend to act in groups as they do in real life. Through group participation, patients can learn how others respond to them in a safe learning environment. The group provides an opportunity for individual members to practice new and different interpersonal skills (interpersonal learning).

The term *therapeutic*, as it applies to group relationships, refers to more than treatment of emotional and behavioral disorders. In today's health care arena, short-term groups are designed for a wide range of different patient populations as a first-line therapeutic intervention to either remediate problems or prevent them (Corey & Corey, 2013). Therapeutic groups offer a structured format that encourages a person to experience his or her natural healing potential (instillation of hope) and achieve higher levels of functioning. Other group members provide ideas and reinforce individual group members' resolve.

Therapeutic groups provide reality testing. People under stress lose perspective. Other group members can gently challenge cognitive distortions carried over from previous damaging relationships (corrective recapitulation of primary family relationships). Because of the nature of a therapy group, group members can say things to the patient that friends and relatives are afraid to say—and they are able to do so in a compassionate, constructive way. It becomes difficult for a troubled member to deny or turn aside the constructive observations and suggestions of five to six caring people who know and care about the member.

Inpatient Therapy Groups

Therapy groups in inpatient settings are designed to stabilize the patient's behavior enough for them to functionally transition back into the community. Here-and-now group interaction is the primary vehicle of treatment (Beiling, McCabe, & Antony, 2009). Since hospitalizations are brief, patients attend focused therapy groups on a daily basis. When situations cannot be changed, psychotherapy groups help patients accept that reality and move on with their lives by empowering and supporting their efforts to make constructive behavioral changes. The value of a short-term process group is the immediate interaction.

Deering (2014) suggests allowing a theme to emerge and then using it to stimulate interaction about possible ways to handle difficult issues. A hidden benefit of group therapy is the opportunity to experience giving and receiving help from others. Helping others is important, especially for people with low self-esteem, who feel they have little to offer others.

Leading Groups for Psychotic Patients

Staff nurses are sometimes called upon to lead or co-lead unit-based group psychotherapy on inpatient units (Clarke, Adamoski, & Joyce, 1998). Other times, staff nurses participate in community group meetings comprised mostly of psychotic patients. Because the demands of leadership are so intense with psychotic patients, co-leadership is recommended.

Co-therapists can share the group-process interventions, model healthy behaviors, offset negative transference from group members, and provide useful feedback to each other. Every group session should be processed immediately after its completion.

A directive, but flexible, leadership approach works best with psychotic patients. Active encouragement of group comments related to relevant concrete topics of potential interest facilitates communication. This strategy is more effective than asking patients to share their feelings. For example, the leader could ask the group to discuss how to handle a simple behavior in a more productive way. This type of discussion allows patients to feel more successful with their contributions. Full attention on the speaker and offering commendations for member effort and contributions are useful. Other members can be encouraged to provide feedback, and the group can choose the best solution.

Before the group begins, the leader should remind individual members that the group is about to take place. Some patients may want to leave the group before it ends. Viewed as anxiety, the leader can gently encourage the patient to remain for the duration of the group.

A primary goal in working with psychotic patients is to respect each person as a unique human being with a potentially valuable contribution. Although their needs are disguised as symptoms, you can help patients "decode" a psychotic message by uncovering the underlying theme and translating it into understandable language. Or, the leader might ask, "I wonder if anyone in the group can help us understand better what John is trying to say." Keep in mind how difficult it is for the psychotic patient to tolerate close interaction and how necessary it is for the patient to interact with others if the patient is to succeed in the outside environment.

Therapeutic Groups in Long-Term Settings

Therapeutic groups in long-term settings offer opportunities for socially isolated individuals to engage with others. Common types of groups include reminiscence, reality orientation, resocialization, remotivation groups, and activity groups.

Reminiscence Groups

Reminiscence groups focus on life review and/or pleasurable memories (Stinson, 2009). They are not designed as insight groups, but rather to provide a supportive, ego-enhancing experience. Each group member is expected to share a few memories about a specific weekly group focus (holidays, first day of school, family photos, songs, favorite foods, pets, etc.). The leader encourages discussion. Depending on the cognitive abilities of the group members, the leader will need to be more or less directive. Sessions are held on a weekly basis and meet for an hour.

Reality Orientation Groups

Used with confused patients, *reality orientation groups* help patients maintain contact with the environment and reduce confusion about time, place, and person. Reality orientation groups are usually held each day for 30 minutes. Nurses can use everyday props, such as a calendar, a clock, and pictures of the seasons to stimulate interest.

The group should not be seen as an isolated activity; what occurs in the group should be reinforced throughout the 24-hour period. For example, on one unit, nurses placed pictures of the residents in earlier times on the doors to their bedrooms.

Resocialization Groups

Resocialization groups are used with confused elderly patients who may be too limited to benefit from a remotivation group but still need companionship and involvement with others. Resocialization groups focus on providing a simple social setting for patients to experience basic social skills again, for example, eating a small meal together. Although the senses and cognitive abilities may diminish in the elderly, basic needs for companionship, interpersonal relationships, and a place where one is accepted and understood remain the same throughout the life span. Improvement of social skills contributes to an improved sense of self-esteem.

Remotivation Groups

Remotivation groups are designed to stimulate thinking about activities required for everyday life. Originally developed by Dorothy Hoskins Smith for use with chronically mentally ill patients, remotivation groups represent an effort to reach the unwounded areas of the patient's personality (i.e., those areas and interests that have remained healthy). Remotivation groups focus on tapping into strengths through discussions of realistic scenarios that stimulate and build confidence. They are successfully used in long-term settings, substance use prevention, with the chronically mentally ill, and in combination with recreational therapy (Dyer & Stotts, 2005). Group members focus on a defined everyday topic, such as the way plants or trees grow, or they might consist of poetry reading or art appreciation. Visual props engage the participants and stimulate more responses.

Therapeutic Activity Groups

Activity groups offer patients a variety of self-expressive opportunities through creative activity rather than through words. They are particularly useful with children and early adolescents (Aronson, 2004). The nurse functions as the group leader, or as a support to other disciplines in encouraging patient participation. Activity groups include the following:

- *Occupational therapy* groups allow patients to work on individual projects or to participate with others in learning life skills. Examples are cooking, art work, making ceramics, or activities of daily living groups. Tasks are selected for their therapeutic value and in response to patient interest. Life skills groups use a problem-solving

approach to help patients successfully negotiate interpersonal situations.
- *Recreational therapy groups* offer opportunities for patients to engage in leisure activities that release energy and provide a social format for learning interpersonal skills. Some people never learned how to build needed leisure activities into their lives.
- *Exercise or movement therapy groups* allow patients to engage in structured exercise. The nurse models the exercise behaviors, either with or without accompanying music, and encourages patients to participate. This type of group works well with chronically mentally ill patients and the elderly.
- *Art therapy groups* encourage patients to reveal feelings through drawing or painting. It is used in different ways. Patients are able to reveal feelings through expression of color and abstract forms when they have trouble putting their feelings into words. The art can be the focus of discussion. Children and adolescents may engage in a combined group effort to make a mural.
- *Poetry and bibliotherapy groups* select readings of interest and invite patients to respond to literary works. Sluder (1990) describes an expressive therapy group for the elderly in which the nurse leader first read free verse poems and then invited the patients to compose group poems around feelings, such as love or hate. Patients wrote free verse poems and read them in the group. In the process of developing their poetry, patients got in touch with their personal creativity.

Self-Help and Support Groups

Self-help and support groups provide emotional and practical support to patients and/or families experiencing chronic illness, crises, or the ill health of a family member. Held mostly in the community, peer support groups are led informally by group members rather than professionals, although often a health professional acts as an adviser. Criteria for membership is having a particular medical condition (e.g., cancer, multiple sclerosis) or being a support person (family of an Alzheimer victim). Self-help groups are voluntary groups, led by consumers and designed to provide peer support for individuals and their families struggling with mental health issues. Support groups have an informational function in addition to social support (Percy, Gibbs, Potter, & Boardman, 2009). Nurses are encouraged to learn about support group networks in their community. Exercise 8.6 offers an opportunity to learn about them.

Self-help groups are often associated with hospitals, clinics, and national health organizations. They provide a place for people with serious health care problems to interact with others experiencing similar physical or emotional problems.

Educational Groups

Community health agencies sponsor educational groups to impart important knowledge about lifestyle changes needed to promote health and comfort and to prevent illness. Family education groups provide families of patients with the knowledge and skills they need to care for their loved ones.

Educational groups are time-limited group applications (e.g., the group might be held for four 1-hour sessions over a 2-week period or as an 8-week, 2-hour seminar). Examples of primary prevention groups are childbirth education, parenting, and stress reduction.

Medication groups offer patients and families effective ways to carry out a therapeutic medication regimen, while learning about a particular disorder. A typical sequence would be to provide patients with information about:
* the disorder and how the medication works to reduce symptoms;

* medications, including purpose, dosage, timing, side effects, and what to do when the patient does not take the medication as prescribed;
* what to avoid while on the medication (drug interactions, food restrictions, avoiding sun, etc.); and
* tests needed to monitor the medication.

Giving homework, written instructions, and materials to be read between sessions helps if the medication group is to last more than one session. Allowing sufficient time for questions and encouraging an open informal discussion of the topic mobilizes patient energy to share concerns and fears that might not otherwise come to light.

Discussion Groups

Functional elements found in effective discussion groups are found in Table 8.4.

Careful preparation, formulation of relevant questions, and use of feedback ensure that personal learning needs are met in discussion groups. Discussion group topics often include prepared data and group-generated material, which is then discussed in the group. Before the end

---

EXERCISE 8.6 Learning About Support Groups

Purpose
To provide direct information about support groups in the community.

Procedure
1. Directly contact a support group in your community. (Ideally, students will choose different support groups so a variety of groups are shared.)
2. Identify yourself as a nursing student, and indicate that you are looking at community support groups. Ask for information about the group (e.g., the time and frequency of meetings, purpose and focus of the group, how a patient joins the group, who sponsors the group, issues the group might discuss, and fee, if any).
3. Write a two-paragraph report including the information you have gathered, and describe your experience in asking for the support group information.

Discussion
1. How easy was it for you to obtain information?
2. Were you surprised by any of the informants' answers?
3. If you were a patient, would this information inform your decision to join the support group? If not, what else would be important to you?
4. What did you learn from doing this exercise that might be useful in your nursing practice?

TABLE 8.4 Elements of Successful Discussion Groups

Element	Rationale
Careful preparation	Thoughtful agenda and assignments establish a direction for the discussion and the expected contribution of each member.
Informed participants	Each member should come prepared so that all members are communicating with relatively the same level of information, and each is able to contribute equally.
Shared leadership	Each member is responsible for contributing to the discussion; evidence of social loafing is effectively addressed.
Good listening skills	Concentrates on the material, listens to content. Challenges, anticipates, and weighs the evidence; listens between the lines to emotions about the topic.
Relevant questions	Focused questions keep the discussion moving toward the meeting objectives.
Useful feedback	Thoughtful feedback maintains the momentum of the discussion by reflecting different perspectives of topics raised and confirming or questioning others' views.

of each meeting, the leader or a group member should summarize the major themes developed from the content material.

Equal group participation should be a group expectation. Although the level of participation is never quite equal, discussion groups in which only a few members actively participate are disheartening to group members and limited in learning potential. Referred to as *social loafing*, when individual group members fail to do their part of the work or skip or come late to group project meetings, it can be frustrating for other group members (Aggarwal & O'Brien, 2008). Because the primary purpose of a discussion group is to promote the learning of all group members, all members are charged with the responsibility of contributing their ideas and encouraging the participation of more silent members. As an individual group member, make it a practice to make at least one relevant contribution to the discussion in each group session. This practice will help you develop ease with group discussion, which is one of the most important skills you can develop as a representative of the nursing profession.

Cooperation, not competition, needs to be developed as a conscious group norm for all discussion groups. Strategies can include allowing more room for more reticent members by asking for their thoughts or opinions. Sometimes, when verbal participants keep quiet, a more reticent group member begins to speak. An invitation, for example, saying "I wonder what your experience of…has been" said tentatively and without pressure can invite the impressions of others. Exercise 8.7 provides an opportunity to explore potential group participation issues.

PROFESSIONAL TASK AND WORK GROUPS

Unlike therapeutic groups, task and work groups do not emphasize personal behavioral change as a primary focus (Gladding, 2011). Instead, organizations use work groups to identify problems, plan and implement changes to improve patient care, and engage in strategies to more effectively communicate with one another. Groups allow health professionals, staff, and involved stakeholders to more quickly develop and implement new evidence-based initiatives. Work groups (e.g., standing committees, ad hoc task forces, and quality circles) accomplish a wide range of tasks related to organizational goals. Involvement of affected stakeholders helps ensure the needed buy-in for recommendation acceptance.

Work groups are an embedded part of a larger organizational system, operating within a smaller work-related political culture. The small group operates as an adaptive open system (Beebe & Masterson, 2014; Tubbs, 2011). All aspects of group work should incorporate the values, norms, general mission, and philosophy of the larger work system. Group strategies, group activities, and methods of evaluation should be congruent with the philosophy and the goals of the larger organizational system to achieve maximum success (Mathieu, Maynard, Rapp, & Gilson, 2008).

Work groups are concerned with content and process. The content (task) is predetermined by organizational parameters or the charge given to the group. Effective group leaders need to have a strong working knowledge of task expectations and their relationship to existing content. Having sufficient available resources in terms of time,

---

EXERCISE 8.7   Addressing Participation Issues in Professional Discussion Groups

Purpose

To provide an opportunity to develop response strategies in difficult group participation issues.

Procedure

A class has been assigned a group project for which all participants will receive a common group grade. Develop a group understanding of the feelings experienced in each of the following situations and a way to respond to each. Consider the possible consequences of your intervention in each case.

1. Don tells the group that he is working full time and will be unable to make many group meetings. There are so many class requirements that he is not sure he can put much effort into the project, although he would like to help and the project interests him.

2. Martha is very outspoken in the group. She expresses her opinion about the choice of the group project and is willing to make the necessary contacts. No one challenges her or suggests another project. At the next meeting, she informs the group that the project is all set up and she has made all the arrangements.

3. Joan promises she will have her part of the project completed by a certain date. The date comes, and Joan does not have her part completed.

Discussion

1. What are some actions the participants can take to initiate a win-win solution and move the group forward?

2. How can you use this exercise as a way of understanding and responding effectively in group projects?

money, information, and member expertise is essential to achieving successful outcomes. Group membership should reflect stakeholders and key informants with the different skill sets needed to accomplish group goals. Essential member matching with task requirements includes matching with:

- group goals,
- identified expectations for group achievement,
- availability and meeting schedule, and
- capacity for ensuring deliverables.

Task groups usually take place within specified time frames and need consistent administrative support to flourish. Table 8.5 lists characteristics of effective versus ineffective task groups.

Leadership Styles

Effective leadership develops from leader characteristics, situational features, and member inputs working together with one another. The three types of leadership styles found in groups are authoritarian, democratic, and laissez-faire. Leaders demonstrating an **authoritarian leadership** style take full responsibility for group direction and control group interaction. Authoritarian leadership styles work best when the group needs a strong structure to function and there is limited time to reach a decision. **Democratic leadership** is a form of participatory leadership, which involves members in active discussion and shared decision making (Rothwell, 2013). Democratic leaders are goal-directed but flexible. They offer members a functional structure while preserving individual member autonomy. Group members

feel ownership of group solutions. **Laissez-faire leadership** is a disengaged form of leadership. The leader avoids making decisions and is minimally present emotionally or otherwise in the group even in crisis situations. Groups with laissez-faire leadership are likely to be less productive and satisfying to group members.

Another way to look at leadership styles in professional group life is by using a situational framework (Blanchard, Zigarmi, & Zigarmi, 2013). This format requires group leaders to match their leadership style to the situation and the maturity of the group members. A **situational leadership style** can be particularly adaptive in organizational group life when a new project is the object of group focus. The situational leader varies the amount of direction and support a group needs based on the complexity of the task and the follower's experience and confidence with achieving task or group goals.

Group maturity involves two forms of maturity: job maturity and psychological maturity related to the work. Job maturity refers to the level of group members' work abilities, skills, and knowledge, which is often consistent with job experience. Psychological job maturity refers to the group members' feelings of confidence, willingness, and motivation. The capacity and readiness of situational maturity play a role in the type of preferred leadership style necessary to accomplish goals. A basic assumption about leadership is that it should be flexible and adapted to group needs. Hershey and Blanchard describe four leadership styles, matched to employee's maturity levels in a particular work situation and dependent on their need for structure and direction.

TABLE 8.5   Characteristics of Effective and Ineffective Work Groups

Effective Groups	Ineffective Groups
Goals are clearly identified and collaboratively developed.	Goals are vague or imposed on the group without discussion.
Open, goal-directed communication of feelings and ideas is encouraged.	Communication is guarded; feelings are not always given attention.
Power is equally shared and rotates among members, depending on ability and group needs.	Power resides in the leader or is delegated with little regard to member needs. It is not shared.
Decision making is flexible and adapted to group needs.	Decision making occurs with little or no consultation. Consensus is expected rather than negotiated based on data.
Controversy is viewed as healthy because it builds member involvement and creates stronger solutions.	Controversy and open conflict are not tolerated.
There is a healthy balance between task and maintenance role functioning.	There is a one-sided focus on task or maintenance role functions to the exclusion of the complementary function.
Individual contributions are acknowledged and respected. Diversity is encouraged.	Individual resources are not used. Conformity and being a "company person," is rewarded. Diversity is not respected.
Interpersonal effectiveness, innovation, and problem-solving adequacy are evident.	Problem-solving abilities, morale, and interpersonal effectiveness are low and undervalued.

- Telling: high structure, low consideration
- Selling: high structure, high consideration
- Participating: high consideration, low structure
- Delegating: low consideration, low structure

Effective leaders adapt to the amount of structure required by changes in the group's maturity in working together. As the group matures, leaders turn more of the responsibility for the group productivity over to its members. Decision making is collaborative. The leader seeks member input, acts as a discussion facilitator, and seeks consensus.

Leader and Member Responsibilities

Leadership tasks in work groups include:
- forming the group structure and establishing the agenda for each meeting;
- clarifying the group's tasks and goals (providing background data and material if needed);
- notifying each member of meeting dates, times, and places;
- keeping group members focused on tasks;
- adhering to time limits; and
- concluding each meeting with a summarization of progress.

Group members should take responsibility for coming prepared to meetings, demonstrating respect for other members' ideas, and taking an active participatory role in the development of viable solutions. Affirming the contributions of team members helps build cohesion and investment in ensuring productive outcomes.

Task Groups

Pregroup Tasks

Successful work groups do not just happen. Before the group starts, participants should have a clear idea of what the group task commitment will entail in terms of time, effort, and knowledge—and be willing to commit to the task. Selected group members should have the experience, and enough in common, to engage in meaningful communication, relevant knowledge of the issues, and/or expertise needed for resolution, a willingness to make a contribution to the group solution, and the ability to complete the task.

Effective Group Planning

Effective planning should be considered a major focus of and raison d'être for participating in work groups. Successful outcomes reflect the responsible engagement of group members and careful planning. Berger (2014) defines planning as "a process that produces a plan or plans as its product" and suggests focusing on the *processes* in planning by:
- assessing the situation,
- deciding what goal or goals to pursue,
- creating or retrieving plans, and then
- executing them (p. 91).

Group communication is a thoughtful endeavor. The group leader should come to each meeting prepared with a clear agenda, an overview of key issues, and member concerns. Inviting members to submit agenda items and involving others in developing an agenda stimulates interest and commitment. The plan is more likely to become "our project" rather than a set of tasks. Nothing is more compelling than enthusiasm backed by facts and a willingness to work in tandem with others to make something important happen. The product is also usually better because it is the end result of many different inputs.

Structural Group Development

Forming

Even if members are known to one another, it is useful to have each person give a brief introduction that includes his or her reason for being part of the work group. The leader should explain the group's purpose and structural components (e.g., time, place, and commitment) and ask for buy-in. Member responsibilities should be outlined clearly with time for questions. A task group with vague or poorly understood goals or structure breeds boredom or frustration, leading to power struggles and inadequate task resolution.

Norming

To be successful, group norms should support accomplishment of stated goals. In general, all data developed within the group context should be kept confidential until officially ready for publication. Otherwise the grapevine can distort information and sabotage group efforts. Members should be accountable for regular attendance. If administrative staff is part of the group membership, they should attend all, or designated meetings. Few circumstances are more threatening to a work-related group than having a supervisor enter and exit the task group at will.

Performing

Most of the group's work gets accomplished in the performing phase, including development of recommendations and preparation of final reports. Leader interventions should be consistent, well defined, and supportive as the group works to fulfill its charge.

Brainstorming

Brainstorming is a commonly employed strategy used to generate solutions during the performing phase. Guidelines for brainstorming include:
- entertaining all ideas without censure;
- testing the more-promising ideas for relevance;
- exploring the consequences of each potential solution;
- identifying human and instrumental resources, including availability; and

- achieving agreement about the best-possible solutions. Exercise 8.8 provides an opportunity to experience brainstorming.

Group Think

Extreme cohesiveness can result in negative group phenomena, referred to as *group think*. Originally defined by Janis (1982), this interpersonal situation represents "a mode of thinking that people engage in when they are deeply involved in a cohesive in-group, when the members' striving for unanimity override their motivations to realistically appraise alternative courses of action" (p. 9).

Symptoms of group think occur when the approval of other group members becomes so important that it overrides a reasonable decision-making process or presents a group outcome that group members fundamentally do not agree with but agree with for the sake of harmony. Realistic evaluation of issues does not occur because group members minimize the conflict in an effort to reach consensus. Warning signs of group think are listed in Box 8.3. Group think can create dissatisfaction with goal achievement and produce unworkable solutions. Fig. 8.2 displays the characteristics of group think.

EXERCISE 8.8   Brainstorming: Selecting Alternative Strategies

Purpose

To help students use a brainstorming process for considering and prioritizing alternative options.

Procedure

You have two exams within the next 2 weeks. Your car needs servicing badly. Because of all the work you have been doing, you have not had time to call your mother, and she is not happy. Your laundry is overflowing the hamper. Several of your friends are going to the beach for the weekend and have invited you to go along. How can you handle it all?

1. Give yourself 5 min to write down all the ideas that come to mind for handling these multiple responsibilities. Use single words or phrases to express your ideas. Do not eliminate any possibilities, even if they seem farfetched.

2. In groups of three or four students, choose a scribe, and share the ideas you have written down. Discuss the relevant pros and cons of each idea.
3. Select the three most promising ideas.
4. Develop several small, concrete, achievable actions to implement these ideas.
5. Share the small group findings with the class group.

Discussion

1. In what ways were the solutions you chose similar or dissimilar to those of your peers?
2. Were any of your ideas or ways of achieving alternative solutions surprising to you or to others in your group?
3. What did you learn from doing this exercise that could help you and a patient generate possible solutions to seemingly impossible situations?

BOX 8.3   Warning Signs of Group Think

1. Illusion of invulnerability
2. Collective rationalization that disregards warnings
3. Belief in inherent morality of the decision
4. Stereotyped or negative views of people outside of the group
5. Direct pressure on dissenters to not express their concerns
6. Self-censorship—individual members with doubts do not express them
7. Illusion of unanimity in which majority view is held to be unanimous
8. Self-appointed "mindguards" within the group who withhold data that would be problematic or contradictory

Adapted from Janis, I. (1982). *Groupthink: Psychological studies of policy decisions and fiascoes* (2nd ed.). New York: Houghton Mifflin.

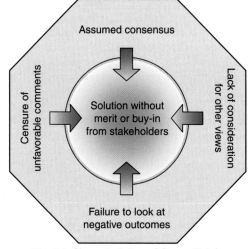

Fig. 8.2 Characteristics of Group Think.

Norms that diminish the potential impact of "group think" allow members to:
- hold different opinions from other group members,
- seek fresh information and outside opinions, and
- act as "devil's advocate" about important issues.

Adjourning Phase

Termination in work groups takes place when the group task is accomplished or at a designated ending time established earlier in the group's life. As the group moves toward its close, the leader should summarize the work of the group, allow time for processing the level of goal achievement, and identify any need for follow-up. Task groups typically disband once their initial charge is satisfied. They should not simply move on into a never-ending commitment without negotiation and the agreement of participants to continue with another assignment.

Groups Versus Teams

Teams and groups have certain characteristics in common, but there also are some clear differences. Team communication occurs as a continuous communication thread with multiple levels of formal and informal working arrangements (see Chapter 23). In 2003, the IOM report, *Health Professions Education: A Bridge to Quality*, identified the development and implementation of collaborative, multiskilled interdisciplinary teams as a key priority in providing safe, quality patient care.

Forsyth (2010) maintains that while teams are fundamentally groups having similar characteristics of interdependence, structure, and ways of interacting, there are notable differences. A health care team differs from a group in distinctive ways. First and foremost, it acts as a single coordinated unit of interprofessional providers. Team members have complementary skills or management responsibilities related to patient care as a deliverable project. They share accountability for goal achievement as an interdisciplinary team (Beebe & Masterson, 2014).

On an embedded team, members are expected to develop shared meanings related to defined health goals, achieve consensus and constructively manage conflict, coordinate their actions, and offer interpersonal support to one another. Implementation takes place through actions related to specified health goals. Communication takes place through electronic channels and communication face-to-face communication (see Chapter 23 for details of team communication).

The involved patient/family are considered part of the health team. Team roles, functions, and provider contributions are interconnected and reinforce each other in completing the work of the team, which is designed to achieve desired clinical outcomes. Discussion in team meetings focuses on collaborative problem solving and decision making, always with the goal of achieving effective coordination and implementation of quality patient-centered care for a particular set of patients.

Group member composition is different for interprofessional health care teams than for task or other types of work groups. The team brings together people with individual skills and abilities to function as a clinical unit with collaborative specialized tasks related to common patient-centered health goals. The number of members varies, and team composition needs to reflect specific health-related goals. Table 8.6 displays some of the differences between task groups and team communication.

TABLE 8.6 Differences Between Groups and Teams	
Working Group	**Team**
Strong, clearly focused leader	Shared leadership role
Individual accountability	Individual and mutual accountability
The group's purpose is the same as the broader organizational mission	Specific team purpose that the team itself delivers
Individual work products	Collective work products
Runs efficient meetings	Encourages open-ended discussion and active problem-solving meetings
Measures its effectiveness indirectly by its influence on others (e.g., financial performance of the business)	Measures performance directly by assessing collective work products
Discusses, decides, and delegates	Discusses, decides, and does real work together

Reprinted with permission from Katzenbach, J., & Smith, D. (1993). The discipline of teams. *Harvard Business Review, 71*(2):113. Reprint number 93201.

SUMMARY

Chapter 8 looks at the ways in which a group experience enhances patients' abilities to meet therapeutic self-care demands, provides meaning, and is personally affirming. The rationale for providing a group experience for patients is described. Group dynamics include individual member commitment, functional similarity, and leadership style. Group concepts related to group dynamics consist of purpose, norms, cohesiveness, roles, and role functions. Tuckman's phases of group development—forming, storming, performing, and adjourning—provide guidelines for group leaders.

In the forming phase of group relationships, the basic need is for acceptance. The storming phase focuses on issues of power and control in groups. Behavioral standards are formed in the norming phase that will guide the group toward goal accomplishment, and the group becomes a safe environment in which to work and express feelings. Most of the group's work is accomplished during the performing phase. Feelings of warmth, caring, and intimacy follow; members feel affirmed and valued. Finally, when the group task is completed to the satisfaction of the individual members, or of the group as a whole, the group enters an adjourning (termination) phase. Different types of groups found in health care include therapeutic, support, educational, and discussion focus groups.

ETHICAL DILEMMA: WHAT WOULD YOU DO?

Mrs. Murphy is 39 years old and has had multiple admissions to the psychiatric unit for bipolar disorder. She wants to participate in group therapy but is disruptive when she is in the group. The group gets angry with her monopolization of their time. She says she has just as much right as a group member to talk if she chooses. Mrs. Murphy's symptoms could be controlled with medication, but she refuses to take it when she is "high" because it makes her feel less energized. How do you balance Mrs. Murphy's rights with those of the group? Should she be required to take her medication? Or should she be excluded from the group if her behavior is not under her control? How would you handle this situation from an ethical perspective?

DISCUSSION QUESTIONS

1. How would you describe the differences between a work task group and a collaborative health care team?
2. How do active-listening strategies differ in group communication versus individual communication?
3. What do you see as potential ethical issues in group-communication formats?

REFERENCES

Aggarwal, P., & O'Brien, C. L. (2008). Social loafing on group projects: Structural antecedents and effects on student satisfaction. *Journal of Marketing Education, 30*(3), 255–264.

Aronson, S. (2004). Where the wild things are: The power and challenge of adolescent group work. *The Mount Sinai Journal of Medicine, New York, 71*(3), 174–180.

Beebe, S., & Masterson, J. (2014). *Communicating in small groups: principles and practices* (11 ed.). Boston: Pearson.

Beiling, P., McCabe, R., & Antony, M. (2009). *Cognitive-behavioral therapy in groups.* New York: Guilford Press.

Benne, K. D., & Sheats, P. (1948). Functional roles of group members. *Journal of Social Issues, 4*(2), 41–49.

Berger, C. (2014). Planning theory of communication: goal attainment through communicative action. In D. Braithwait, & P. Schrodt (Eds.), *Engaging theories in interpersonal communication: multiple perspectives* (2nd ed.). Thousand Oaks, CA: Sage Publications.

Bernard, H., Birlingame, G., Flores, P., Greene, L., Joyce, A., Kobos, J. C., et al. (2008). Clinical practice guidelines for group psychotherapy. *International Journal of Group Psychotherapy, 58*(4), 455–542.

Blanchard, K., Zigarmi, P., & Zigarmi, D. (2013). *Leadership and the one minute manager updated.* New York, NY: Harper Collins.

Burlingame, G., Strauss, B., Joyce, A., MacNair-Semands, R., Mackenzie, K., Ogrodniczuk, J., et al. (2006). *Core battery—revised.* New York: American Group Psychotherapy Association.

Clarke, D., Adamoski, E., & Joyce, B. (1998). In-patient group psychotherapy: The role of the staff nurse. *Journal of Psychosocial Nursing and Mental Health Services, 36*(5), 22–26.

Corey, M., & Corey, B. (2013). *Groups: Process and practice* (9th ed.). Pacific Grove, CA: Brooks/Cole.

Counselman, E. (2008). Reader's forum: Why study group therapy? *International Journal of Group Psychotherapy, 58*(2), 265–272.

Deering, C. G. (2014). Process oriented groups: Alive and well? *International Journal of Group Psychotherapy, 64*(2), 164–179.

Dyer, J., & Stotts, M. (2005). *Handbook of remotivation therapy.* Binghampton, NY: The Haworth clinical Practice Press.

Forehand, J., Leigh, K., Farrel, R., & Spurlock, A. (2016). Social dynamics in group work. *Teaching and Learning in Nursing, 11,* 62–66.

Forsyth, D. (2018). *Group dynamics* (6th ed.). Belmont, CA: Wadsworth Cengage Learning.

Gagnon, L., & Roberge, G. (2012). Dissecting the journey: Nursing student experiences with collaboration during the group work process. *Nurse Education Today, 32*(8), 945–950.

Gladding, S. (2011). *Groups: A counseling specialty* (6th ed.). Upper Saddle River: Merrill.

Institute of Medicine (IOM). (2003). *Report on health professions education: A bridge to quality.* Washington, DC: National Academies Press (IOM).

Janis, I. (1971). Groupthink 1982. *Psychology Today, 5,* 43–46.

Janis, I. L. (1982). *Victims of groupthink.* New York: Houghton Mifflin.

Janis, I. (1982). *Groupthink: Psychological studies of policy decisions and fiascoes* (2nd ed.). New York: Houghton Mifflin.

Johnson, D., & Johnson, F. (2014). *Joining together: Group theory and group skills* (11th ed). Edinburgh Gate: Pearson Education Limited.

Katzenbach, J., & Smith, J. (1993). The discipline of teams. *Harvard Business Review, 71*(2), 111–120.

Lasky, G., & Riva, M. (2006). Confidentiality and privileged communication in group psychotherapy. *International Journal of Group Psychotherapy, 56*(4), 455–476.

Mangione, L., Forti, R., & Iacuzzi, C. (2007). Ethics and endings in group psychotherapy: Saying good-bye and saying it well. *International Journal of Group Psychotherapy, 57*(1), 25–40.

Mathieu, J., Maynard, T., Rapp, T., & Gilson, L. (2008). Team effectiveness: A review of recent advancements and a glimpse into the future. *Journal of Management, 34,* 410–476.

Michaelsen, L. K., & Sweet, M. (2012). Team-based learning: Small group learning's next big step. *New Directions in Teaching and Learning.*

Moreno, K. J. (2007). Scapegoating in group psychotherapy. *International Journal of Group Psychotherapy, 57*(1), 93–104.

Percy, C., Gibbs, T., Potter, L., & Boardman, S. (2009). Nurse-led peer support group: Experiences of women with polycystic ovary syndrome. *Journal of Advanced Nursing, 65*(10), 2046–2055.

Powles, W. (2007). Reader's forum: Reflections on "what is a group?". *International Journal of Group Psychotherapy, 57*(1), 105–113.

Rothwell, D. (2013). *In mixed company.* Boston, MA: Wadsworth Cengage Learning.

Rubel, D., & Kline, W. (2008). An exploratory study of expert group leadership. *The Journal for Specialists in Group Work, 3*(2), 138–160.

Rutan, J. S., Stone, W., & Shay, J. (2007). *Psychodynamic group psychotherapy.* New York: The Guilford Press.

Sluder, H. (1990). The write way: Using poetry for self-disclosure. *Journal of Psychosocial Nursing and Mental Health Services, 28*(7), 26–28.

Stinson, C. (2009). Structured group reminiscence: An intervention for older adults. *Journal of Continuing Education in Nursing, 40*(11), 521–528.

Tubbs, S. (2011). *A systems approach to small group interaction* (11th ed.). Boston: McGraw Hill.

Tuckman, B. (1965). Developmental sequence in small groups. *Psychological Bulletin, 63*(6), 384–399.

Tuckman, B., & Jensen, M. (1977). Stages of small-group development revisited. *Group & Organization Management, 2*(4), 419–427.

Yalom, I., & Leszcz, M. (2005). *The Theory and practice of group psychotherapy* (5th ed.). New York: Basic Books.

Yang, K., Woomer, G., & Matthews, J. (2012). Collaborative learning among undergraduate students in community health nursing. *Nurse Education in Practice, 12*(2), 72–76.

WEB RESOURCES

- American Group Psychotherapy Association: www.groupsinc.org
- American Society of Group Psychotherapy and Psychodrama (ASGPP): www.asgpp.org

- Association for Specialists in Group Work Professional Training Standards: www.asgw.org/PDF/training_standards.pdf
- Best Practices Guidelines: www.asgw.org/PDF/best_Practices.pdf
- Principles for Diversity Competent Group Workers: www.asgw.org/PDF/Principles_for_Diversity.pdf

9

Self-Concept in Professional Interpersonal Relationships

Eileen O'Brien

OBJECTIVES

At the end of this chapter, the reader will be able to:

1. Define self-concept.
2. Describe the features and characteristics of self-concept.
3. Identify theoretical frameworks explaining self-concept.
4. Identify functional health patterns and nursing diagnoses related to disturbances in the pattern of self-concept.
5. Apply the nursing process in caring for patients with disturbances in the pattern of self-concept as related to body image, personal identity, and social role. *(role performance)*
6. Use therapeutic communication and interventions related to self-esteem issues.
7. Recognize and apply therapeutic communications that meet patient spiritual needs in health care.

INTRODUCTION

This chapter focuses on self-concept as a key dynamic in communication, therapeutic relationships, and self-management strategies. The chapter identifies basic concepts and frameworks related to the development of self-concept and describes its impact on individual development. The Application section discusses communication that strategies nurses can use with patients to empirically enhance self-concept in health care situations.

BASIC CONCEPTS

Definition

Self-concept is defined as the totality of each person's beliefs about his or her inner self. It represents an integration of each individual's cultural heritage, environment, gender roles, ethnic and racial identity, spiritual beliefs and values, upbringing, education, basic personality traits, and cumulative life experiences.

This multidimensional construct mirrors an integration of individual's personal beliefs, values, attitudes, and behaviors. The self-concept has physical, emotional, social, and spiritual dimensions linked to functional well-being and health behaviors. It also incorporates feedback from others. How people perceive us helps to create or reinforce our self-perceptions.

Constructing the self-concept requires a cultural foundation (Shweder et al., 2006). Therefore self-identity usually incorporates ethnic identity (Bailey, 2003). Today globalization and increasing immigration have fostered the emergence of a hybrid ethnic identity as different and contrasting cultures become part of a multicultural identity (Arnett, 2013).

Closely intertwined with self-concept is **self-esteem**, defined as a person's personal sense of worth and well-being. The terms *self-image*, *self-concept*, and *self-perception* are often used interchangeably to refer to the way individuals view and assess themselves. Abundant essays have been written about self-esteem, especially regarding the importance of a high self-esteem among American teens,

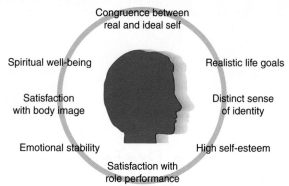

Fig. 9.1 Characteristics of a Healthy Self-Concept.

particularly young women (Gilligan et al., 1990). This tends to be a characteristically American phenomenon; for example, among traditional Asian cultures self-criticism is seen as a virtue and high self-esteem as a character flaw (Falk et al., 2009).

An important feature of self-concept *involves self-clarity,* which is defined as "the extent to which the facets of self-definition are stable and well defined, regardless of how many facets there are" (Vartanian, 2009, p. 99). *Self-concept clarity is clearly intertwined with healthy identity development.*

This relates to the individual's beliefs about his or her ability and capacity to accomplish a task and to deal with the challenges of life. This feature of the self-concept helps people to confront control issues and cope with the many facets of life. Self-efficacy plays a major part in determining our chances for success; in fact, some psychologists rate self-efficacy above talent in the recipe for success (Bandura, 1997).

A healthy self-concept including the above features, regardless of culture, reflects attitudes, emotions, and values that are realistic, congruent with each other, and consistent with a meaningful purpose in life. Fig. 9.1 identifies characteristics of a healthy self-concept. Each of these features is discussed further in the applications.

Significance of Self-Concept in Health Care

A strong sense of self has been described as a protective factor in coping with chronic illness (Mussato et al., 2014). When people experience a major health disruption, it alters the way they think, feel, value their sense of self, and the way they communicate with others.

Case Example

I once interviewed a patient with advanced cancer. Tears came to his eyes as he told me about how he had had to leave his job, could not run around with his grandchildren, could not do the things he loved,

---

not like he used to, nope, not anymore. A single diagnosis had inflicted such profound devastation. Note the pervasive nature of the impact on self-concept—it affects work, family, parental role, and social activities.

Self-concept reflects a person's personal reality, particularly in close relationships, careers, communication patterns, and life choices. Classically, adolescence was seen as the time of life during which individuals confronted the "self" developmentally. However, postmodern identity theory challenges the idea that these varied aspects of the self do not always form a unified consistent whole and that contradictions are bound to be encountered throughout life (Schachter, 2005). Nevertheless, choices congruent with the self-concept feel true, whereas those that are not consistent with one's personally determined self-concept create cognitive dissonance, doubt, uncertainty, and anxiety (Cooper, 2007, p. 6). Thus the clarity of self-concept becomes muddled.

Features and Functions of Self-Concept

Cunha and Goncalves (2009) refer to the self as an open *system;* fluid and dynamic. A person's self-concept consists of various coexisting self-images. Different aspects of the self-concept become visible, depending on the situation (Prescott, 2006). For example, a student might be a marginal student in English literature but a star in a mathematics course on differential equations. Which is the true self, or are both valid?

Self-concept helps people to make sense of their past and present; it helps them to communicate across varied situations and to imagine what they are capable of becoming physically, emotionally, intellectually, socially, and spiritually in relation to others in the future.

Over the course of a lifetime, self-concept changes and develops in complexity. Hunter (2008) noted, "As one ages, the 'self' develops and becomes a more and more unique entity formed by personal experiences and personally developed values and beliefs" (p. 318). Exercise 9.1 provides an opportunity for you to practice self-awareness by examining your self-concept.

Self-fulfilling prophecies. **Possible selves** is a term used to explain the future-oriented component of self-concept. Personal wishes and desires are valuable influences in goal setting and motivation, when they lead to realistic actions. For example, a nursing student might think, "I can see myself becoming vice president of nursing." Such thoughts help the novice nurse work harder to achieve professional goals. Negative possible selves can also become a self-fulfilling prophecy (Markus

EXERCISE 9.1   Simulation Exercise: Who Am I?

Purpose
To help students understand some of the self-concepts they hold about themselves.

Procedure
1. Spend 10–15 min reflecting about how you would have defined yourself during middle school or high school and how you would define yourself today.
2. What has changed in your sense of self, and if there were changes, why did they occur?
3. Using only **three one-word** descriptors, describe yourself today. There are no right or wrong answers.
4. Pick the one descriptor that you believe defines yourself best.
5. In small groups of four to six students, share your results.

Discussion
1. Were you surprised with the changes from your earlier descriptors as a teen or preteen?
2. Were you surprised with any of your choices as current descriptors?
3. How hard was it to pick the one best descriptor out of the five?
4. How did you describe yourself? Could your self-descriptors be categorized or prioritized in describing your overall self-concept?
5. What did you learn about the process of examining your self-concept from doing this exercise? What situational factors seemed to impact your descriptor choice?
6. How could you use this information in professional interpersonal relationships with patients?

Role of Self-Concept in Organizations/Request PDF. Available from: https://www.researchgate.net/publication/281175780_Role_of_Self-Concept_in_Organizations [accessed Oct 23 2018].

& Nurius, 1986). For example, Martha receives a performance evaluation indicating a need for improved self-confidence. Seeing this criticism as a negative commentary on her "self," she fulfills the attribution by performing awkwardly when she is being assessed in the clinical area.

Development of Self-Concept and Self-Esteem

Self-concept represents an interaction between the life experiences and challenges that occur and the individual's response to them. Consider the differences in the life experience and socialization of Prince George of Cambridge (oldest child of Prince William) versus a child born into poverty with both parents working to pay off a mortgage. What implications do you see for the development of each child's self-concept? Life experiences, social status, significant relationships, and opportunities influence how people define themselves throughout life. Interactions in the family environment were previously considered the primary source in the development of self-esteem (Robson, 1988). Recently, however, several studies have challenged this traditional view, demonstrating that genetic factors play a significant role in the etiology of self-esteem (Kendler & Gardner, 1998; Kamakura, Jukoando, & Ono, 2001; Neiss, Sedikes, & Stevenson, 2002), However, the external social context into which a child is born and personal caretaking relationships contribute to shaping the resulting self-concept.

Social environment plays an important role in shaping and supporting one's personal self-concept. Current research supports the idea that a nurturing home environment, sports participation, academic success, religious affiliation, professional opportunities, praise for successful accomplishments, and supportive mentors tend to encourage the development of a positive self-concept (Arnett, 2017). Factors such as poverty, a chaotic upbringing, loss of a parent, poor educational opportunities, and adverse life events contribute to the development of a negative self-concept. However, there are individuals who experience unfortunate social circumstances yet develop a dynamic self-concept as a reaction to their circumstances, creating a resiliency to the impact of negativity. They are interested in improving their environment and serve as role models to others about what is possible against all odds. Others with more fortunate life circumstances may develop negative self-concepts or overinflated positive self-concepts with little grounding in reality. At times these individuals may be at risk for having difficulty accepting negative events in life. This further illustrates how understanding an individual's self-concept assists nurses to individually determine which therapeutic intervention will help during health events. When life presents individuals with unpredictable trauma or devastation, nurses can play a critical role in helping patients to reframe a potentially incapacitating sense of self into one including more hope and broader options. In an effort to enhance resilience, nurses can help patients revisit personal strengths, consider new possibilities, incorporate new information, and seek out appropriate resources as a basis for making sound clinical decisions for themselves and taking constructive actions. Sometimes just a nurse's "supportive presence" can give a patient energy and reason to hope (Adler et al., 2014).

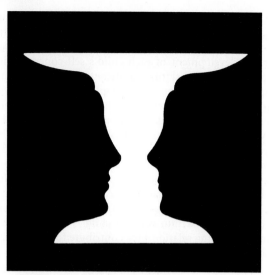

Fig. 9.2 The figure-ground phenomenon. Where you focus your attention makes a difference in your perception of the figures. (From the Westinghouse Learning Corporation: *Self-instructional unit 12: perception, 1970.* Reprinted with permission.)

Self-Concept in Interpersonal Relationships

Self-concept is formed in relation to others (Guerrero, Anderson, & Afifi, 2017). When two people communicate, each person's perceptions are influenced by his or her own self-concept and level of self-esteem. Sometimes referred to as an "affective margin of distortion," the factors presented in Fig. 9.2 can implicitly influence interpersonal interactions.

Language is influential in forming perceptions of the self and others and reflects society's values. Self-concept can easily be shaken by communication; therefore it is vital for nurses to be sensitive to the impact of language in interactions with patients (see Part II). Microaggressions involve communicating subtle and often unintentional discrimination pertaining to self-concepts of race, ethnicity, gender or any other demographic. This type of communication can be viewed as affecting self-concept by implying a negative slight or a blatant negative attribution. Derald Wing Sue (2007) clarifies that "microaggressions seem to appear in three forms: microassault, microinsult, and microinvalidation."

Sue's work (2007, p. 271) in professional communications identifies a *microassault* as an explicit negative verbal or nonverbal communication that offends an individual through criticism, slighting, or purposeful prejudicial actions. For example, identifying someone as a "Medicaid patient" when the cost of a generic drug is being discussed. This would clearly influence a patient's self-concept and might shut down further communication related to education about drug dosage.

Microinsults are subtle unintended rebuffs, but the insinuation would clearly offend the recipient. For example, during the nutritional assessment of a female patient with diabetes, a nurse comments that "all diabetics cheat on their diet." This not only demeans the patient's efforts to control her glucose levels but also reduces her identity to a diagnosis.

Microinvalidations are communications that discount or invalidate a person's values, feelings, or lifestyle (Sue, 2007). For example, stating to a single mother, "It must be difficult managing child rearing by yourself as a single mom." This message conveys that this patient represents a deficit model of child rearing. Rather than empowering the mother, the statement implies a lesser standard of parenting, which does not enhance the mother's self-esteem.

Although these nurse-patient communications seem harmless, they clearly communicate an expectation or attribution that can lead to increased levels of anger, mistrust, and loss of self-esteem.

It is critical for nurses to develop self-awareness. Attribution theory (Malle, 2011) holds that nurses' responses can compromise interaction with patients by unintentionally limiting a patient's sense of self-esteem. Therapeutic communication requires a well-defined, straightforward, unbiased approach, which allows nurses to more authentically connect with patients.

Cultural Identity

A clear cultural identity is positively related to a clear self-concept and self-esteem (Usborne & Taylor, 2010). An understanding of the fundamental differences in cultural worldviews within the context of globalization can help nurses to frame supportive interventions in ways that support ethnocultural variations and patients' self-concepts (see Chapter 7). In general, western cultures tend to be individualistic, whereas Asian cultures see the individual as part of a collective group. It is important to acknowledge that most cultures are not purely one or the other but rather a combination of the two in various proportions. Individual differences also exists within cultures, and each individual may have a combination of the two tendencies.

Case Example

"In individualist cultures, individual uniqueness and self-determination is valued. A person is all the more admirable if they are a 'self-made man' or 'make up their own mind' or show initiative or work well independently. Collectivist cultures, on the other hand, expect people to identify with and work well in groups, which protect them in exchange for loyalty and compliance"(Rutledge, 2013).

Gender

Gender refers to "socially constructed roles and behaviors that occur in a historical and cultural context, and that vary across societies and over time" (Leerdam, Rietveld, Teunissen, & Lagro-Janseen, 2014, p. 53). Self-perceptions regarding gender evolve from socially learned behaviors that are constructed by the prevailing culture. Historically, children in US kindergartens may distinguish between girls wearing dresses and liking dolls and boys liking rough play and playing active games (Martin & Ruble, 2010). Despite progressive feminist changes, subtle gender differences are still evidenced in the form of social expectations, career options, pay differentials, and so forth. They exist in how people are treated, what is important to them, and in how men and women are socialized to respond to verbal and nonverbal cues in communication.

This social construction has limitations. Many individuals do not fit into traditional gender categories and genuinely do not feel related to the socially constructed roles of society. Transgendered and intersexed people struggle with a society that may hold rigid boundaries around the constructs of sex and gender. Nurses working with patients need to approach gender identity as distinct from biology and consider the individual's subscribed gender identity.

Case Example

Having failed to complete the health intake questionnaire demographic information, Morgan tells the nurse, "If I go to the doctor, I'm labeled a 'female,' but in everyday life, most people think I'm a 'male'" (Wood et al., 2017). Nurses need to be supportive in this genuine aspect of identity and understand a patient's reluctance to refuse identification as male or female.

Theoretical Frameworks

Self-Concept Frameworks

The self is a central construct in theories of personality. These theories argue that our self-concept develops from and is influenced by social interactions with others. Sullivan (1953) refers to *self-concept* as a self-system that people develop to (1) present a consistent image of self, (2) protect themselves against feelings of anxiety, and (3) maintain their interpersonal security.

Humanism (Rogers, 1959) defines the *self* as "an organized, fluid, but consistent conceptual pattern of perceptions of characteristics and relationships or the 'I' and the 'me' together with values attached to these concepts" (p. 498). When the *"actual self"* (who we believe we are) and the *"ideal self"* (how a person would ideally like to be) are

similar, the person is likely to have a positive self-concept and self-esteem. Rogers equated having a coherent well-integrated self-concept with being mentally healthy and well adjusted (Diehl & Hay, 2007).

Cognitive approaches (Fattore, 2017) state that a child is born without a concept of self and must learn to differentiate the self from others in the intimate sphere of family, in friendships, and in cultural practices. This requires relating to others and having vast interaction in the environment.

Behaviorists believe that early childhood interactions foster self-concepts of a *good me* (resulting from reward and approval experiences), a *bad me* (resulting from punishment and disapproval experiences), and a *not me* (resulting from anxiety-producing experiences that are dissociated by the person as not being a part of his or her self-concept). These influences continue through adulthood and color a person's responses to life. Having a therapeutic relationship can help patients develop a different, more positive sense of self.

George Mead applies a sociological approach to the study of self-concept. The self-concept affects and is influenced by how people experience themselves in relation to others (Elliott, 2013). Mead's model emphasizes the influence of culture, moral norms, and language in framing self-concepts through interpersonal interactions (symbolic interactionism).

Erikson's Theory of Psychosocial Development

Erik Erikson's (1968, 1982) theory of psychosocial self-development is a well-known model. His theory emanated from his work as a therapist, and his theory has stimulated a wealth of research and application. Central to his framework is the concept of identity formation. He believed that "identity formation neither begins nor ends with adolescence: it is lifelong development" (Erikson, 1959, p. 122). Personality develops as a person responds to evolving developmental challenges (psychosocial crises) during the life cycle. As individuals pass through ascending stages of ego development, with mastery of each developmental task, a personal sense of identity evolves. This is most obvious during adolescence, when teens experiment with different roles as they seek to establish a strong, comfortable personal identity. This development is not linear, nor does it occur across physical, emotional, and social development in the same sequential order. This is seen in the physically mature adolescent who may behave in a less mature fashion socially and emotionally.

The first four stages of Erikson's model serve as building blocks for his central developmental task of establishing a healthy ego identity (identity vs. identity diffusion). Erikson's stages of ego development are outlined in Table 9.1.

TABLE 9.1   Erikson's Stages of Psychosocial Development, Clinical Behavior Guidelines, and Stressors

Stage of Personality Guidelines	Ego Strength or Virtue	Clinical Behavior Guidelines	Stressors
Trust versus mistrust	Hope	Appropriate attachment behaviors Ability to ask for assistance with an expectation of receiving it Ability to give and receive information related to self and health Ability to share opinions and experiences easily Ability to differentiate between how much one can trust and how much one must distrust	Unfamiliar environment or routines Inconsistency in care Pain Lack of information Unmet needs (e.g., having to wait 20 minutes for a bedpan or pain injection) Losses at critical times or accumulated loss Significant or sudden loss of physical function (e.g., a patient with a broken hip being afraid to walk)
Autonomy versus shame and doubt	Willpower	Ability to express opinions freely and to disagree tactfully Ability to delay gratification Ability to accept reasonable treatment plans and hospital regulations Ability to regulate one's behaviors (overcompliance, noncompliance, suggest disruptions) Ability to make age-appropriate decisions	Overemphasis on unfair or rigid regulation (e.g., putting patients in nursing homes to bed at 7 p.m.) Cultural emphasis on guilt and shaming as a way of controlling behavior Limited opportunity to make choices in a hospital setting Limited allowance made for individuality
Initiative versus guilt	Purpose	Ability to develop realistic goals and to initiate actions to meet them Ability to make mistakes without undue embarrassment Ability to have curiosity about health care Ability to work for goals Ability to develop constructive fantasies and plans	Significant or sudden change in life pattern that interferes with role Loss of a mentor, particularly in adolescence or with a new job Lack of opportunity to participate in planning of care Overinvolved parenting that does not allow for experimentation Hypercritical authority figures No opportunity for play
Industry vs. inferiority	Competence	Work is perceived as meaningful and satisfying Appropriate satisfaction with balance in lifestyle pattern, including leisure activities Ability to work with others, including staff Ability to complete tasks and self-care activities in line with capabilities Ability to express personal strengths and limitations realistically	Limited opportunity to learn and master tasks Illness, circumstance, or condition that compromises or obliterates one's usual activities Lack of cultural support or opportunity for training

TABLE 9.1 Erikson's Stages of Psychosocial Development, Clinical Behavior Guidelines, and Stressors—cont'd

Stage of Personality Guidelines	Ego Strength or Virtue	Clinical Behavior Guidelines	Stressors
Identity versus identity diffusion	Fidelity	Ability to establish friendships with peers Realistic assertion of independence and dependence needs Demonstration of overall satisfaction with self-image, including physical characteristics, personality, and role in life	Lack of opportunity Overprotective, neglectful, or inconsistent parenting Sudden or significant change in appearance, health, or status Lack of same-sex role models
Identity versus isolation	Fidelity	Ability to express and act on personal values Congruence of self-perception with nurse's observation and perception of significant others	Lack of opportunity to interact with others. Lack of guidance about socially proactive behaviors Loss of significant others Loss of memory Impaired hearing
Intimacy versus isolation	Love	Ability to enter into strong reciprocal interpersonal relationships Ability to identify a readily available support system Ability to feel the caring of others Ability to act harmoniously with family and friends	Competition Communication that includes a hidden agenda Projection of images and expectations onto another person Lack of privacy Loss of significant others at critical points of development
Generativity versus stagnation and self-absorption	Caring	Demonstration of age-appropriate activities Development of a realistic assessment of personal contributions to society Development of ways to maximize productivity Appropriate care of whatever one has created Demonstration of a concern for others and a willingness to share ideas and knowledge Evidence of a healthy balance among work, family, and self-demands	Aging parents, separately or concurrently with adolescent children Obsolescence or layoff in career "Me generation" attitude Inability or lack of opportunity to function in a previous manner Children leaving home Forced retirement
Integrity versus despair	Wisdom	Expression of satisfaction with personal lifestyle Acceptance of growing limitations while maintaining maximum productivity Expression of acceptance of certitude of death, as well as satisfaction with one's contributions to life Lack of opportunity	Rigid lifestyle Loss of significant other Loss of physical, intellectual, and emotional faculties Loss of previously satisfying work and family roles

Erikson believed that stage development is never final. Reworking of developmental stages can occur any time during the life span. Erikson's model can help nurses to analyze the age-appropriateness of behavior from an ego development perspective. For example, a teenager giving birth is still coping with issues of self-identity rather than generativity. Exercise 9.2 focuses on applying Erikson's concepts to patients' situations.

DEVELOPING AN EVIDENCE-BASED PRACTICE This study used a group comparison on self-report questionnaires to examine the multidimensional self-concept, global self-esteem, and psychological adjustment of an age- and gender-matched study sample of 41 individuals with traumatic brain injury (TBI) compared with 41 control participants. Three self-report questionnaires (Rosenberg Self-Esteem Scale, Tennessee Self-Concept Scale, and the Hospital Anxiety and Depression Scale) were administered to all study subjects.

Results: TBI patients showed significantly lower means of global self-esteem and self-concept on the Rosenberg Self-Esteem and Tennessee Self-Concept scales. TBI subjects rated themselves lower on self-dimensions related to social, family, academic/work, and personal self-concept as compared with controls. TBI survivors also reported higher mean levels on the Hospital Anxiety and Depression Scales.

Application to Your Clinical Practice: Recognition of self-concept and self-esteem as potential issues for TBI patients with negative emotional consequences may be an important underlying dynamic with these patients. Strategies to enhance self-esteem and strengthen self-concept should be components of effective care for TBI patients.

Modified from Ponsford, J., Kelly, A., & Couchman, G. (2014). Self-concept and self-esteem after acquired brain injury: a control group comparison. *Brain Injury*, 28(2), 146–154.

APPLICATIONS

Role of Self-Concept in Patient Centered Relationships

This Applications section identifies strategies to strengthen self-concept, self-efficacy, and self-esteem in health care relationships and communication. It is important to initiate caring relationships with the premise that each patient is a unique person with strengths, values, cultural beliefs, and experiential life concerns. What health providers say, how they say it, and what they do matters in establishing relationships supportive of patients' identities and patient-centered care (Drench, Noonan, Sharby, & Ventura, 2011).

EXERCISE 9.2 **Simulation Exercise: Erikson's Stages of Psychosocial Development**

Purpose
To help students apply Erikson's stages of psychosocial development to patient situations.

Procedure
This exercise may be done as a homework exercise with the results shared in class.

To set your knowledge of Erikson's stages of psychosocial development, identify the psychosocial crisis or crises each of the following patients might be experiencing:
1. A 14-year-old single female having her first child
2. A 50-year-old executive "let go" from his job after 18 years of employment
3. A 40-year-old stroke victim paralyzed on the left side
4. A 50-year-old woman caring for her 80-year-old mother, who has Alzheimer disease

Discussion
1. What criteria did you use to determine the most relevant psychosocial stage for each patient situation?
2. What conclusions can you draw from doing this exercise that would influence how you would respond to each of these patients?

Self-concept is an essential starting point for understanding patients' behaviors related to coping, engagement in meaningful activities, and improved mood (van Tuyl et al., 2014). Self-concept variables can act as facilitators or barriers to a patient's efforts to engage in healthier lifestyle behaviors and the self-management of chronic disorders (see also Chapter 10).

Patterns and Nursing Diagnosis Related to Self-Concept

Gordon (2007) identifies related functional health patterns as self-perception, self-concept, and value-belief patterns. Injury, illness, and treatment can challenge these functional health patterns regardless of specific medical diagnosis. As a person's perception of self-concept is disturbed, perception of the future becomes uncertain and unpredictable (Ellis-Hill & Horn, 2000).

Body Image Issues

Body image involves people's perceptions, thoughts, and behaviors associated with their appearance Bolton et al. (2010). Perception of one's body image changes throughout life, influenced by aging, the appraisals of others, cultural and social factors, and physical changes resulting from illness, injury, and even treatment effects. For example, the potential for impotence and incontinence with prostate surgery can, secondary to treatment, create a body image issue for men (Harrington, 2011). This body image issue may have further implications for nurses' assessment of self-esteem issues.

Body image refers to how people *perceive* their physical characteristics, not how they realistically appear to others. A critical dimension of body image is self-esteem, the value people place on their appearance, or biological or functional intactness (Slatman, 2011). For example, individuals with an eating disorder may see themselves as "fat" despite being dangerously underweight. Ideal body image reflects sociocultural norms and popular media portrayals. Research consistently finds that physical appearance is strongly related to overall high self-esteem (Harter, 2006); therefore nurses need to be cognizant of patients' perceptions of physical changes.

Cultures differ in their value of specific physical characteristics. In the United States, a trim figure in women and a lean, muscular body in men are admired (Vartanian, 2009). In other cultures, obesity may be viewed as a sign of prosperity, fertility, or the ability to survive (Boston Women's Health Book Collective, 1998). Sociocultural theories of body image suggest that body dissatisfaction results from a person's inability to meet unrealistic societal ideals. Any changes in physical appearance or function can challenge self-concept (Arnett, 2017; Dropkin, 1999)

Permanent and even temporary changes in appearance influence attributions that others may make, and how individuals perceive these responses. Discrimination can be subtle or overt, and the experience of a distorted body image can be long-lasting. In a study of overweight adolescents, a primary theme that emerged was "a forever knowing of self as overweight" (Smith & Perkins, 2008, p. 391), even after the study participants lost significant weight in later years.

Less overt body images disturbances—for example, infertility, loss of bladder function, and loss of energy from radiation treatments—affect the self-concept and require therapeutic care. Chronic pain or intermittent symptoms can also undermine a person's self-identity and self-confidence. People having these issues or conditions with fluctuating symptoms, such as epilepsy, can experience similar feelings of vulnerability and insecurity related to body image without validation from others.

Nursing Strategies

The *meaning* of body image is highly individual. Some, such as Helen Keller or Stephen Hawking, frame a potentially negative body image as a positive feature of their identities. Others let a physical deviation become their defining feature. Patients with the same medical condition

can have different body image issues (Bolton et al., 2010). Assessment should take the following into account:

- Negative communications about the body
- Preoccupation with or no mention of changes in body structure and function following medical interventions
- Reluctance to look at or touch a changed body structure
- Social isolation and loss of interest in friends and work after a change in body structure, appearance, or function
- Expressed concerns or fears about changes.

Patient-centered assessment includes the patient's strengths, expressed needs and goals, the nature and accessibility of the patient's support system, and the perception of the impact the changes have on lifestyle. Frequently deficits are magnified and compensatory personal resources are overlooked. Nurses can use a strengths-based approach by drawing on religious beliefs, supportive family and friends, autonomy efforts, persistence, life skills, talents, and hope. Simply listening to the patient's response to changes in health can provide insight into its effect on self-concept.

Case Example

A soldier who lost both legs in a roadside bomb attack in Afghanistan has declared that he would go back to the front line tomorrow. "Your life is not over. It is a new challenge. I am still me and that is the most important thing. I want to be out there. A lot of my friends are still out there and I just wish that I could be with them" (Harter, 2006).

Nurses can model acceptance for patients experiencing an altered body image. Acceptance is a process, and patients need time to reconcile body image issues. Open-ended questions about what the patient expects and helping patients identify social supports can facilitate acceptance. Talking with others who have similar changes can provide credible, practical advice. For example, a "Reach to Recovery" volunteer visit with a mastectomy patient and referrals to support groups can assist a client to accept help and advice.

Personal Identity

Identity is described as an intrapersonal psychological process consisting of a person's beliefs and values, characteristics and abilities, relationships with others, how they fit into the world, and personal growth potential (Arnett, 2017; Karademas et al., 2008). Spirituality is a significant resource and an essential component of persoal identty. The identity develops and changes over time in relation to stage of life, situations, and experiences. There are multiple dimensions to personal identity, just as there are in self-concept: gender and sexual identities, social role

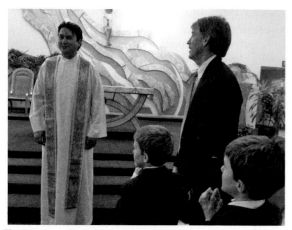

Fig. 9.3 Traditional religious practices and ceremonies strengthen value systems that are integral to personal self concepts.

identity (parent, student, widow, etc.), cultural and ethnic identity, economic contextual identity, and so forth. Each facet affects a person's world view, sense of self, and communication patterns with others.

Individuals pass through each life stage as outlined by Erikson; our perceptions of personal-identity change to reflect who we are in the present moment physically, psychologically, contextually, and spiritually. Jung (1960) contends that "The afternoon of life is just as full of meaning as the morning; only its meaning and purpose are different" (p. 138). Prior to midlife, the energy focus is outward; in midlife, the focus changes to a more selective inner reflection, thoughtful choices, and a more authentic reordering of priorities.

When a major and/or sudden change in health status forces a reappraisal of personal identity, its impact on a patient can be swift, life-altering, and compelling.

Case Example

"When I got up at last … and had learned to walk again, one day I took a hand glass and went to a long mirror to look at myself, and I went alone. I didn't want anyone … to know how I felt when I saw myself for the first time. But here was no noise, no outcry; I didn't scream with rage when I saw myself. I just felt numb. That person in the mirror couldn't be me. I felt inside like a healthy, ordinary, lucky person—oh, not like the ONE in the mirror! Yet when I turned my face to the mirror there were my own eyes looking back, hot with shame … when I did not cry or make any sound, it became impossible that I should speak of it to anyone, and the confusion and the panic of my discovery were locked inside me then and there, to be faced alone, for a very long time to come" (Goffman, 1963).

In this passage, note the speaker's expression of aloneness and reluctance to share the impact of bodily changes on personal identity.

Other individuals with cognitive impairment experience more complicated but shared alterations in identity. Sensory images enter the brain, but the neural cognitive connections people use to interpret meaning cannot occur. Lake (2014) speaks of dementia as a disorder that "slowly diminishes personhood and devastates the relationships that personhood enables" (p. 5). People with dementia lose their ability to set realistic goals, implement coherent patterns of behavior, maintain stable emotional responses, communicate clearly, and control basic elements of their lives. As the disease progresses, they may no longer recognize significant others, lose their sense of personal identity, experience hallucinations and paranoia, and demonstrate fluctuating awareness of the self. As one caregiver described it, "there are two deaths with Alzheimer's disease—the death of self and the actual death" (Capps, 2008). Interestingly however, in a study of adults with dementia, Fazio and Mitchell (2009) found that these patients could identify themselves in photographs taken with an instant camera despite forgetting the photo had been taken minutes earlier. This finding suggests a persistence of self even when memory is significantly impaired.

DEVELOPING AN EVIDENCED-BASED PRACTICE

Research into the initial stages of Alzheimer disease (AD), with the scope of developing some sort of "salvage therapy," is rather scarce.

Purpose: The purpose of this study was to extend knowledge about how subjects with a probable AD diagnosis or in a medium-low phase of the disorder maintain the continuity of self.

Method: This research was done from a psycholinguistic point of view with the goal of identifying how Alzheimer patients maintain the self through narrative.

Results: The structure of the narrative and the subsequent analysis of the transcribed material demonstrated the need to give shape to patients' stories. The analysis of this particular segment of the initial phase of the disease and how the disease progressively worsens seemed useful to understand how the patient's psyche reacts to the diagnosis and how he or she reorganizes his or her self-representation and, finally, if and in which way the subject's identity begins to deteriorate. Self-narrative may be effective in maintaining the self in AD patients if it is begun in the preliminary stages of AD (Toffle & Quattropani, 2015).

Application to Clinical Practice

Since self-narrative may be effective in maintaining the self in AD patients if begun in the preliminary stages of AD, caring for patients diagnosed with AD should include time for the sharing of narrative information that will allow the patient to continue to share memories and his or her self-representations with others. One therapeutic intervention is listening to stories and narratives that may be repeated and changed over time, but the activity supports the social self.

Nursing Strategies

Changes in self-perception occur with change in health status. Heijmans et al. (2004) suggest that in addition to accepting an illness and learning new self-management skills, many people have to adapt to an altered social identity and renegotiate relationships. This activity involves a degree of emotional discomfort because things are not the same for the patient or for those with whom the patient interacts. Renegotiating relationships can be awkward and anxiety-producing, and patients often need the nurse's support in determining how to respond.

Case Example

Linda is a registered nurse working in a busy surgery center. Returning to work after a hospitalization for major depression, she finds she has been relieved of her position as charge nurse. Other staff are highly protective of her. She is carefully watched to ensure that she is not going to relapse and she is given simpler tasks to avoid stressing her out. Linda cannot understand why her coworkers don't see her as the same person she was before. Although her depression is in remission, Linda has been "reclassified" as a mentally ill person in the eyes of her coworkers. Her colleagues' efforts are well intentioned, but they have a negative effect on Linda's sense of personal identity.

Blazer (2008) suggests that developing self-perceptions of achieving personal health and well-being may be as important as objective data for predicting health outcomes over time. Nurses can help patients reestablish a more positive self-identity by encouraging the patient and family to engage in open-ended questions in a spirit of mutual discovery related to the following:

- What is this patient coping with in relation to self-identity?
- What is this patient able to do in his or her current circumstances?
- What is needed to support this patient in reconnecting with the person that he or she is capable of being?

Including a significant family member in this discussion is essential. Family may not anticipate or have an awareness of a change in personal identity, as often the focus of return to health is more physically defined. Benner (2003) advocates exploring what matters to the patient and emphasizing a person's strengths as a basis for developing and enhancing creative meaning. This strengths-based approach creates a climate where patients *can* improve their situation and creates new possibilities for enhancing personal identity during illness. Even the smallest positive movement toward change can make a difference in a patient's self-image.

Box 9.1 describes patient-centered interventions to enhance personal identity.

BOX 9.1   Patient-Centered Interventions to Enhance Personal Identity: Perceptions and Cognition

- Explain to newly admitted patients their clinical environment, patient rights, and expected care routine.
- Actively listen and facilitate the patient's "story" of the present health care experience, including concerns about coping, impact on self and others, and hopes for the future.
- Remember that each patient is unique. Respect and tailor responses to support individual differences in personality, identity, responses, intellect, values, culture, and understanding of medical processes.
- Encourage as much patient input as is realistically possible into diagnostic and therapeutic regimens.
- Provide information as it emerges about changes in treatment, personnel, discharge, and after care. Include family members whenever possible and desired, particularly when giving difficult news.
- Explain treatment procedures including rationale and allow ample time for questions and discussion.
- Encourage family members to bring in familiar objects, pictures, or a calendar particularly if the patient is in the hospital or care facility for an extended period.
- Encourage as much independence and self-direction as possible.
- Avoid sensory overload and repeat instructions if the patient appears anxious.
- Use perceptual checks to ensure you and the patient have the same understanding of important material.
- Encourage older patients and seniors to maintain an active, engaged lifestyle in line with their interests, capabilities, and values.

Perception

Perception is a process through which we interpret sensory information and whereby a person transforms sensory data into connected personalized understanding. According to self-perception theory, we interpret our own actions in the same way as we interpret others' actions, and our actions are often socially influenced and not produced of our own free will, as we might expect (Bem, 1972) (consider the image in Fig. 9.3).

Depending on whether you focus on the background or the form, you can draw different conclusions. Which image do you see—a vase or two figures looking at each other? Any shift of focus, whether self-imposed or directed by others, can transform what you see as a perceptual image.

The same possibility applies to life situations. Helping patients to refocus their attention in contemplating difficult circumstances, or using a new perspective, can alter meaning and suggest different options. Perceptions differ because people develop mindsets that alter data in personal ways. Patients with delirium or psychoactive drug reactions experience global perceptual distortions, whereas those with mental illness can experience personalized perceptual distortions. Distorted perceptions influence interpretation of communication, whether sending, receiving, or interpreting verbal messages and nonverbal behaviors. Simple perceptual distortions can be challenged with compassionate questioning and sometimes targeted humor. Validation of perceptual data is needed because the nurse and the patient may not be processing the same reality.

Case Example

Grace Ann Hummer is a 65-year-old widow with arthritis, a weight problem, and failing eyesight. Admitted for a minor surgical procedure, Ms. Hummer tells the nurse she does not know why she is putting herself through all of this. Nothing can be done for her because she is too old and decrepit.

- *Nurse:* As I understand it, you came in today for removal of your bunions. Can you tell me more about your problem as you see it? *(Asking for this information separates the current situation from an overall assessment of ill health.)*
- *Patient:* Well, I've been having trouble walking, and I can't do some of the things I like to do that require extensive walking. I also have to buy "clunky" shoes that make me look like an old woman.
- *Nurse:* So you are not willing to be an old woman yet? *(Taking the patient's statement and challeng-*

ing the cognitive distortion presented in her initial comments with humor allows the patient to view her statement differently.)
- *Patient* (laughing): Right, there are a lot of things I want to do before I'm ready for a nursing home.

Questioning perceptions and active listening by the nurse help patients make sense of perceptual data in a more conscious way, and the patient feels heard. A cognitive appraisal of personal identity in the face of illness can contribute to treatment adherence and an enhanced sense of well-being. Keeping communication simple, delivering straightforward messages with compassion, and making interactions participatory with a back-and-forth dialogue reduce the potential for acting on perceptual distortions.

Cognition

Cognition represents the thinking processes people use in making sense of the world. What people *think* about their perceptions is the throughput that connects perceptions with associated feelings and directly influences clinical outcomes. According to Beck and Beck (2011), faulty perceptions of a situation can stimulate automatic negative thoughts, which may not be realistic. Referred to as cognitive distortions, automatic thoughts about self-constructed realities create negative feelings, which can have a powerful impact on communication and behavior. Conscious reality-based thought processes are essential to acquiring and sustaining an accurate interpretation of self. Nurses can use supportive strategies to assist patients to examine cognitive distortions so that they are better able to develop realistic solutions to difficult health problems. Examples of these strategies are outlined in the following paragraphs; they can help patients to reappraise their thinking, making it more conducive to effective functioning. Fig. 9.3 demonstrates the link between perceptions and behaviors.

Supportive Nursing Strategies

Cognitive behavioral approaches, originally developed by Aaron Beck, focus on encouraging patients to reflect on difficult situations from a broader respective. Beck refers to cognitive distortions as "thinking errors." Reflection on a variety of explanations provides patients with more options to realistically interpret the meaning of their perceptions. A sudden mood change suggests an automatic thought. Cognitive approaches help patients identify, reflect on, and challenge negative automatic thinking processes instead of

---

BOX 9.2   Examples of Cognitive Distortions

1. "All or nothing" thinking—the situation is all good or all bad; a person is trustworthy or untrustworthy.
2. Overgeneralizing—one incident is treated as if it happens all the time; picking out a single detail and dwelling on it.
3. Mind reading and fortune telling—deciding a person does not like you without checking it out; assuming a bad outcome with no evidence to support it.
4. Personalizing—seeing yourself as flawed instead of separating the situation as something you played a role in but did not cause.
5. Acting on "should" and "ought to"—deciding in your mind what is someone else's responsibility without perceptual checks; trying to meet another's expectations without regard for whether it makes sense to do so.
6. "Awfulizing"—assuming the worst, that every situation has a catastrophic interpretation and anticipated outcome.

EXERCISE 9.3   Simulation Exercise: What Matters to Me?

Purpose
To help students understand the relationship between self-concepts and what is valued.

Procedure
This exercise may be done as a homework exercise and shared with your small group.
- Spend 10–15 min reflecting about the three activities, roles, or responsibilities you value most in your life. (There are no right or wrong answers.)
- Now prioritize them and identify the one that you value the most. (This is never easy.)
- In one to two paragraphs, explain why the top contender is most important to you.
- In small groups of four to six students, share your results.

Discussion
1. Were you surprised by any of your choices or what you perceived as being most important to you?
2. In what ways do your choices affirm self-concept and self-esteem?
3. What are the implications of doing this exercise for your helping patients understand what they value and how this reflects self-esteem?

---

accepting them as reality. Common cognitive distortions are identified in Box 9.2.

Modeling cues to behavior and coaching patients to challenge cognitive distortions with positive self-talk and mindfulness is also helpful. Exercise 9.3 provides practice with recognizing and responding to cognitive distortions.

Self-Esteem

Self-esteem is defined as the *emotional* value a person places on his or her self-concept. People who view themselves as worthwhile and of value have high self-esteem. They challenge negative beliefs that are unproductive or interfere with successful functioning. With a positive attitude about self, an individual is more likely to view life as a glass half full rather than half empty. People with low self-esteem do not value themselves and do not feel valued by others. Self-esteem can be related to either a specific dimension of self, "I am a good writer," or it may have a more global meaning, "I am a good person who is worth knowing."

Self-esteem has a strong relation to happiness. Although the research has not clearly established causation, we are persuaded that high self-esteem does lead to greater happiness. Low self-esteem is more likely to lead to depression under some circumstances. Some studies support the buffer hypothesis, which is that high self-esteem mitigates the effects of stress, but other studies come to the opposite conclusion, indicating that the negative effects of low self-esteem are mainly felt in good times. Still others find that high self-esteem leads to happier outcomes regardless of stress or other circumstances (Baumeister et al., 2003). A person with high self-esteem views life's inevitable problems as challenges from which one can learn and grow. Table 9.2 identifies behaviors associated with high versus low self-esteem.

Self-esteem is closely linked to our emotions, particularly those of pride or shame (Brown & Marshall, 2001), and our sense of control (self-efficacy) over life events. Verbal and nonverbal behaviors presenting as frustration, inadequacy, anxiety, anger, or apathy suggest low self-esteem. This pattern tends to be defensive in relationships and seeks constant reassurance from others because of self-doubt. Instead of taking constructive actions that could raise self-esteem, people worry about issues they cannot control and see life's challenges as

TABLE 9.2   Behaviors Associated With High Versus Low Self-Esteem

People With High Self-Esteem	People With Low Self-Esteem
Expect people to value them	Expect people to be critical of them
Are active self-agents	Are passive or obstructive self-agents
Have positive perceptions of their skills, appearance	Have negative perceptions of their skills, appearance, sexuality, and behaviors
Perform equally well when being observed as when not being observed	Perform less well when being observed
Are nondefensive and assertive in response to criticism	Are defensive and passive in response to criticism
Can accept compliments easily	Have difficulty accepting compliments
Evaluate their performance realistically	Have unrealistic expectations about their performance
Are relatively comfortable relating to authority figures	Are uncomfortable relating to authority figures
Express general satisfaction with life	Are dissatisfied with their lot in life
Have a strong social support system	Have a weak social support system
Have a primary internal locus of control	Rely on an external locus of control

problems rather than opportunities. People with low self-esteem are less likely to correctly identify the informational value of their feelings (Harden, 2005). This is important, as they are easily influenced by what is referred to as "an affective margin of distortion" that can color communication (displayed in Fig. 9.3).

Self-esteem increases gradually throughout adulthood, peaking around the late sixties. (Robins et al., 2002) Over the course of adulthood, individuals increasingly occupy positions of power and status, which might promote feelings of self-worth. Many life span theorists have suggested that in midlife, people are concerned with trying to figure out how they want to spend their later years and what is important to them personally (Erikson, 1985).

Self-esteem declines in old age. The few studies of self-esteem in old age suggest that self-esteem begins to decline around age 70. This decline may be due to the dramatic confluence of changes that occur in old age, including changes in work (e.g., retirement), relationships (e.g., the loss of a spouse), and physical functioning (e.g., health problems) as well as a decline in socioeconomic status. The old-age decline may also reflect a shift toward a more modest, humble, balanced view of the self in old age (Erikson, 1985).

The experience of success or failure can also cause fluctuations in self-esteem (Crocker, Brook, & Niiya, 2006). Sources of situational challenges include loss of a job; loss of an important relationship; and negative changes in one's appearance, role, or status.

Long-standing issues of verbal or physical abuse, neglect, chronic illness, codependency, and criticism by significant others can result in lowered self-esteem. Illness, injury, and other health issues also challenge a person's self-esteem. Findings from a sizable number of research studies demonstrate an association with changes in health status, functional abilities, and emotional dysfunction, and lowering of self-esteem (Vartanian, 2009; Vickery, Sepehri, & Evans, 2008).

Case Example

Jenna was a professor at a major university when she was diagnosed with advanced metastatic breast cancer. All her life, Jenna had been a take-charge person and relished her capacity to run her life effectively and efficiently. People responded to her with high regard and respect because of her position and personality. Admitted to the hospital, Jenna brought her earlier expectation of being treated with deference along with her. She expected similar responsiveness from hospital staff. Her health care providers, unfamiliar with her background and personal identity issues, expected her to comply with treatment and not to challenge their authority. Angry at being unable to control her medical situation, Jenna became demanding and angry. The staff considered her a difficult, obstinate patient. Viewed from the context of being a "patient," Jenna's behavior seemed irrational; understood from the perspective of facing a sudden challenge to a lifelong self-concept of independence and deference, her seemingly "irrational" behavior made sense. Once the connection was made to Jenna's personal identity issues, a different dialogue emerged between staff and patient, with a deeper respect for Jenna's set of expectations and interpersonal needs. Provision of needed support for information and collaborative interpersonal responses resulted in a positive change in Jenna's attitude and full participation in her treatment. Interestingly, health professionals who become ill are often referred to as "difficult patients" because the shift in social roles from controlling care to being controlled shakes the foundation of the self.

Reed's (2014) middle-range theory of self-transcendence can help patients to expand their boundaries as a resource in difficult times. The theory encompasses the following four components:

- Intrapersonal (toward greater awareness of one's philosophy, values, and dreams)
- Interpersonal (to relate to others and one's environment)
- Temporal (to integrate one's past and future in a way that has meaning for the present)
- Transpersonal (to connect with dimensions beyond the typically discernible world), (p. 111)

Self-esteem can also be enhanced through social support. Rebuilding relationships with family, friends, teachers as well as participation in social activities and clubs can promote the process of achieving self-esteem. Exercise 9.4 introduces the role of social support in building self-esteem.

Nurses can help patients sort out and clarify the beliefs and emotions that get in the way of an awareness of their intrinsic value. Note how the patient describes achievements. Does the patient devalue accomplishments, project blame for problems onto others, minimize personal failures, or make self-deprecating remarks? Does the patient express shame or guilt? Does the patient seem hesitant to try new things or situations or express anxiety about coping with events? Observe defensive behaviors. Lack of culturally appropriate eye contact, poor hygiene, self-destructive behaviors, hypersensitivity to criticism, a need for constant reassurance, and the inability to accept compliments are behaviors associated with low self-esteem. Table 9.2 identifies characteristic behaviors related to self-esteem.

Therapeutic Strategies

When people have low self-esteem and low self-worth, notions that no one really cares predominate. By understanding these underlying feelings as a threat to self-esteem (e.g., intense fear, anguish about an anticipated loss, and lack of power in an unfamiliar situation), nurses can facilitate opportunities for sharing the patient's story. The nurse might identify a legitimate feeling by saying, "It must be frustrating to feel that your questions go unanswered," and then asking, "How can I help you?"

Nurses also help patients increase self-esteem by being psychologically present as sounding boards. The process of engaging with another human being who offers a different perspective and demonstrates control in responding to events can enhance self-esteem.

The implicit message the nurse conveys with personal presence and interest, information, and a guided exploration of the problem is twofold. The first is confirmation of the patient: "You are unique, you are important, and I will stay with you through this uncomfortable period."

The second is the introduction of the possibility of hope: "There may be some alternatives you haven't thought of that can help you cope with this problem. Would you ever consider…?" Once a person starts to take control over his or her responses to events, a higher level of well-being can result. Vital to implementation of this intervention is to

---

EXERCISE 9.4   Simulation Exercise: Social Support

Purpose
To help students understand the role of social support in significant encounters.

Procedure
1. Describe a "special" interpersonal situation that led to change, gave you direction, or had deep meaning for you.
2. Identify the person or people who helped make the situation meaningful for you.
3. Describe the actions taken by the people or person just identified that made the situation memorable.

Discussion
1. What did you learn about yourself from doing this exercise?
2. What do you see as the role of social support in making memories?
3. How might you use this information in your practice?

not minimize the energy required to change. As clear as the pathway to hope may be, the nurse needs to understand that it is not a simple road for the patient.

Using a strengths-based approach offers the patient some control. It is helpful to say, for example, "The thing that impresses me about you is…" or "What I notice is that although your body is weaker, it seems as if your spirit is stronger. Would you say this is true?" Such questions help the patient focus on positive strengths. Behaviors suggestive of enhanced self-esteem include the following:

- Taking an active role in planning and implementing self-care
- Verbalizing personal psychosocial strengths
- Expressing feelings of satisfaction with self and ways of handling life events

Self-Efficacy

Self-efficacy is "the belief in one's capabilities to organize and execute the courses of action required to manage prospective situations" (Bandura, 2007). In other words, self-efficacy is a person's belief in his or her ability to succeed in a particular situation. Self-efficacy is strongly associated with self-concept and self-esteem. People who believe that they can make changes and take control over their situation value their competence and ability to succeed. They are less likely to harbor self-doubts or dwell on personal deficiencies when difficulties arise. Successful self-management depends on developing self-efficacy (Marks, Allegrante, & Lorig, 2005; Simpson & Jones, 2013).

Support of self-efficacy is critical to helping people with mental illness live successfully in the community (Suzuki, Amagai, Shibata, & Tsai, 2011). Self-efficacy improves motivation and helps patients sustain their efforts in the face of temporary setbacks.

Self-management support should include specific problem-solving skills and processes patients need to cope. Breaking difficult tasks down into achievable steps and completing them reinforces self-efficacy. Explain why each step is important to the next and remind patients of progress toward a successful outcome.

Identify patient's strengths. Skills training in areas where patients have deficits while also sincerely noting patients' efforts and persistence will encourage patients to take their next steps. Work with patients to use solutions and resources within their means. For example, exercise may become an acceptable option if patients know of free or low-cost exercise programs for seniors living in the community. Encourage significant others in the patient's life to give support and approval. Families appreciate receiving specific suggestions and opportunities to give appropriate support.

Self-help and support groups can be useful adjuncts to treatment. Discovering that others with similar issues have found ways to cope encourages patients and reinforces self-efficacy that they too can achieve similar success. The understanding, social support, and reciprocal learning found in these groups can provide opportunities for valuable information sharing and role modeling (Humphreys, 2004).

Role Performance

Role performance requires self-efficacy with links to self-concept. Johnson, Cowin, Wilson, and Young (2012) suggest that professional identity can be conceptualized as a "logical consequence of self-identity" (p. 562). Quality of life, a priority goal in *Healthy People 2020*, and role performance are also interrelated. How effectively people are able to function within expected roles influences their value within society and affects personal self-esteem.

Role performance and associated role relationships matter to people, as evidenced in symptoms of depression, feelings of emptiness, and even suicide when a significant personal or professional role ceases to exist.

Case Example

"My values in life have changed completely. It was incredibly difficult to realize that as a 45-year-old man I was 'good for nothing.' I had been the rock that everybody relied on. Suddenly it was I who had to ask others for help. I'm prone to this disease and I know that one day I will fall ill again" (Raholm, 2008, p. 62).

Nurses need to be sensitive to the changes in role relationships that illness and injury produce for self, family, and relationships. An individual's social role can rapidly transform from independent self-sufficiency to vulnerability and dependence on others. New role behaviors may be uncomfortable and anxiety-producing. Asking open-ended and focused questions about the patient's relationships, across family, work, and social groups is a useful strategy for assessing role change. Box 9.3 presents suggestions that can be integrated into patient assessments.

Preconceived notions of role disruption for an ill or disabled person arise more commonly when the illness is protracted, recurrent, or seriously role-disruptive. Walker (2010) notes that when patients have to leave paid employment because of a chronic illness, it affects self-concept, because many people's social and personal identities are tied to their work roles. Nurses can coach patients about how to present themselves when they return to work. They can help patients learn how to respond to subtle and not-so-subtle discriminatory actions associated with others' lack of understanding of the patient's health situation.

Spiritual Aspects of Personal Identity

One's spiritual self-concept is concerned with one's relationship to a higher power and the vital life forces that support wholeness. When health fails or circumstances seem beyond control, it is often the spirit that sustains peoples' sense of self and helps to maintain a more balanced equilibrium. Baldacchino and Draper (2001) note that the presence of a spiritual force facilitates the patient's will to live, positive outlook, and sense of peace.

Spirituality is a unified concept, closely linked to a person's world view, providing a foundation for a personal belief system about the nature of a higher power, moral-ethical conduct, and reality. The term *spirituality* is often used synonymously with *religion*, but it is a much broader

---

BOX 9.3   Sample Assessment Questions Related to Role Relationships

Family

1. "Who do you see in your family as being supportive of you?," or "Who can you rely on to help you through any changes?"
2. "Who do you see in your family as being most affected by your illness (condition)?," or "Who do you think will need to adjust more than any other family member?"
3. "What changes do you anticipate as a result of your illness (condition) in the way you function in your family?," or "Will your health change how things get done in the family?"

Work

1. "What are some of the concerns you have about your job at this time?"
2. "Who do you see in your work situation as being supportive of you?"

Social

1. "How has your illness affected the way people who are important to you treat you?"
2. "Is there anyone outside of family you turn to for support?"
3. "If (name)_____ is not available to you, who else might you be able to call on for support?"

---

concept (Baldacchino & Draper, 2001). It signifies a positive approach, an accepting, embracing, loving attitude toward life, suffering, and death. A key difference is that religion involves beliefs and values within an organized faith community, whereas spirituality describes self-chosen beliefs and values that give personal meaning to one's life. It may or may not be associated with a particular faith (Tanyi, 2006).

Spirituality is associated with meaning and purpose in life (Sessana, Finnell, & Jezewski, 2007; Tanyi, 2006). A number of research studies link spirituality to health, quality of life, and well-being (Molzahn & Shields, 2008; Sapp, 2010). Spirituality helps people answer vital questions about what it is to be human, which human events have depth and value, and what are the imaginative possibilities of being. Steger and Frazier (2005) suggest that people derive a strong sense of well-being from their religious feelings and activities.

Over the course of a lifetime, spiritual beliefs change, deepen, or are challenged by life events. Spiritual strength allows nurses and other health care professionals to willingly stand with others in darkness yet remain whole—to deal with the everyday challenges and stresses of nursing in a spirit of peace and hope.

Spiritual aspects of self-concept can be expressed through the following:

1. Membership in a specific religious faith community
2. Mindfulness, meditation, or other personalized lifeways and practices
3. Cultural and family beliefs about forgiveness, justice, human rights, social justice
4. Crises or existential situations that stimulate a search for purpose, meaning, and values beyond the self

The Joint Commission (2017) mandates that health care agencies, including long-term hospice and home care services, assess patients' spiritual needs, provide for the spiritual care of them and their families, and supply appropriate documentation of that care. Health crises can be a time of spiritual renewal, when one discovers new inner resources, strengths, and capacities never before tested. Alternatively, it can signal a period of spiritual desolation, leaving the individual feeling abandoned, angry, and powerless to control or change important life circumstances.

Spiritual dimensions encompass people's spiritual beliefs, cultural practices, religious affiliation and level of participation, personal spiritual practices such as prayer, mindfulness, or meditation, feeling connected to a higher power, and the subjective importance of these practices and beliefs in a person's life (Blazer, 2012).

Assessment should take account of the patient's
- Willingness to talk about personal spirituality or beliefs

- Belief in a personal god or higher power
- Relevance of specific cultural or religious practices to the individual
- Changes in religious practices or beliefs
- Areas of specific spiritual concern activated by the illness, for example, is there an afterlife?
- Extent to which illness, injury, or disability has had an effect on the patient's spiritual beliefs
- Sources of hope and support
- Desire for visitation from clergy or pastoral chaplain

A patient's spiritual needs may be obvious and firmly anchored in positive relationships with clergy and a personal god, with a defined philosophical understanding of life and one's place in it. Alternatively, a spiritual sense of self can be expressed as a disavowal of a spiritual identity or allegiance to religious beliefs. Spiritual needs can reveal evidence of conflict or anger toward a higher power. For example, as he experienced his personal grief following the death of his wife, the noted author Lewis (1976) called his god "the cosmic sadist." Spiritual pain can be as severe as physical pain and often is closely accompanied by emotional pain.

Identifying a patient's current religious affiliations and practices is important, as is inquiry about his or her religious or cultural rituals. Josephson and Peteet (2007) suggest that the patient's words can be an entry into a discussion of spirituality; for example, if the patient uses a phrase such as "By the grace of God, I passed the final examination," you might ask something like, "It sounds like God plays a role in your life, is that true?" (p. 186).

Spiritual rituals and practices can be used to promote hope, support, and relieve anxiety for a patient experiencing spiritual pain. Inquire about current spiritual practices asking, "Are there any spiritual practices that are particularly important to you now?" Note that it is not unusual for the religion listed on the patient's chart to be different from the religious practices the patient currently follows. In addition, people who have never committed to a strong sense of religion previously may seek religious support in times of crisis (Baldacchino & Draper, 2001). Spiritual assessment information should be documented in the patient's record.

Miller (2007) suggests that "Hope is central to life and specifically is an essential dimension for successfully dealing with illness and for preparing for death" (p. 12). Spiritual well-being can be demonstrated in the face of adversity, in compassion for self and others, and in a sense of inner peace. Nurses see this in a patient's will to live or the complete serenity of some individuals in the face of life's most adverse circumstances.

Useful assessment questions might consist of "What do you see as your primary sources of strength at the present time?" and "In the past, what have been sources of strength for you in difficult times?" Miller (2007) identified several hope-inspiring strategies found in the literature, for example, helping patients and families to develop achievable aims, realize a sense of interpersonal connectedness, live in the present, and find meaning in their illness or situation. Sharing uplifting memories, affirmation of worth, and unconditional caring presence can stimulate a sense of hopefulness.

Case Example

Beatrice was diagnosed with breast cancer and given a planned treatment regime including chemotherapy and radiation. During her second session with chemotherapy, she commented to the nurse, "I can't handle any more of this. God has been unfair and let me suffer enough and it's time to just stop and let the disease kill me." The nurse recognized the feelings of despair and commented, "you have four more sessions and I understand you feel that this diagnosis is unfair. I agree it's unfair, but let's talk about this." Note that even when patient behaviors appear to be supportive of lifesaving efforts, the self can remain conflicted and hopeless.

Exercise 9.5 focuses on spiritual responses to distress. Spirituality can be a powerful resource in families and it is important to incorporate questions about the family's spirituality if they are involved in supporting the patient. Tanyi (2006) suggests nurses can incorporate spiritual assessment with the family, using questions such as the following:

- What gives the family meaning in their daily routines?
- What gives the family strength to deal with stress or crisis?
- How does the family describe their relationship with God, a higher power, or the universe?
- What spiritual rituals, practices, or resources do the family use for support?
- Are there any conflicts between family members related to spiritual views?
- If so, what might be the impact on the current health situation?

Nursing strategies. The compassionate presence of the nurse in the nurse-patient relationship is the most important tool the nurse has in helping the patient explore spiritual and existential concerns

EXERCISE 9.5 Simulation Exercise: Responding to Issues of Spiritual Distress

Purpose
To help students understand responses in times of spiritual distress.

Procedure
Review the following case situations and develop an appropriate response to each.

1. Mary is 16 years old and has just found out has a sexually transmitted disease. Her family belongs to a Christian church in which sex before marriage is not permitted. Mary feels guilty about her current status and sees it as "God punishing me for fooling around."
2. Kema is married to an abusive, alcoholic husband. She reads the Quran daily during Ramadan and prays for her husband's healing. She feels that God will turn the marriage around if she continues to pray for changes in her husband's attitude. "Praised be God...guide us to the right path" she implores.
3. Ari tells the nurse, "I feel that God has let me down. I was taught that those who follow the law or do good are rewarded while those who don't are punished. I have been a good rabbi, husband, father, and son. Now the doctors tell me I'm going to die and I am 50 years old. That doesn't seem fair to me."

Discussion
1. Share your answers with others in your group. Did you have to explore spiritual beliefs beyond your own?
2. Give and get feedback on the usefulness of your responses.
3. In what ways can you use this new knowledge in your nursing care?

(Carson & Koenig, 2008). Providing opportunities for patients to be self-reflective helps people sustain their beliefs, values, and spiritual sense of self in the face of tragedy. Gordon and Mitchell (2004) wrote, "Spiritual care is usually provided in a one-to-one relationship, is completely person centered and makes no assumptions about personal conviction or life orientation" (p. 646).

Providing privacy and quiet times for spiritual activities is important. An important component of nursing care is helping patients address their spiritual identity by providing time for spiritual practices and referral to chaplains or spiritual directors. This also includes advocating for the patient's spiritual practice related to dietary restrictions, mindfulness settings, holy day activities, meditating or praying, and end-of-life cultural practices. For example, in some forms of the Jewish religion, turning lights on or off or adjusting the position of an electric bed is not permitted on the Sabbath. There is no rule against these tasks being accomplished by the nurse.

Prayer and meditation. Praying with a patient, even when the patient is of a different faith, can be a soothing intervention. A spiritual care-based therapeutic relationship requires a personal perception of the nurse's own spirituality, which influences the degree to which the patient's spiritual needs are perceived (Vlasblom, Steen, Knol, & Jochemsen, 2011; Wu & Lin, 2011). There should be some evidence from the patient's conversation that praying or reading a holy book with a patient would be a desired support. According to some researchers (Daaleman, Usher, Williams, Rawlings, & Hanson, 2008; Sulmasy, 2006), spiritual support can be effectively provided through *indirect* means such as protecting patients' dignity, helping patients find meaning in their suffering, offering presence (sitting with patients and families), and talking about what is important to them.

Supporting Spirituality

Even in death, there are blessings as well as pain that have meaning for the person and enrich self-concept. Thomas describes his spiritual process of being "introduced, enticed, and sometimes dragged into the magnificent life of the soul" by the two soul mates he lost through death, as follows: Twice I have walked into the Valley of the Shadow of Death, lost my cherished mate, collapsed into the Canyon of Grief, and with their guidance managed to struggle out as a confident, spiritually embraced person. I live with a deep understanding of, and appreciation for, the meaning of God's grace and blessings.

Thomas (2011, p. 8)

Addressing spirituality is important in order to unify scientific knowledge, in practice, with an expression of human sensitivity and a deep awareness of the human being (Veloza-Gómez, Muñoz de Rodríguez, Guevara-Armenta, & Mesa-Rodríguez, 2017).

The self-concept is a dynamic construct, composed of many features, capable of developing new paths to help answer such question as, "Who am I?" "What is important to me in this situation or phase of life?" As a professional nurse, you will have many opportunities to help patients answer these questions.

SUMMARY

This chapter focuses on the self-concept as a key variable in the nurse-patient relationship. *Self-concept* refers to an acquired constellation of thoughts, feelings, attitudes, and beliefs that individuals have about the nature and organization of their personality. Self-concept develops through the interaction between experiences with the environment and personal characteristics.

Aspects of self-concept discussed in the chapter include body image, personal identity, role performance, self-esteem, self-efficacy, self-clarity, and spirituality. Disturbances in body image refer to issues related to changes in appearance and physical functions, both overt and hidden. Personal identity is constructed through cognitive processes of perception and cognition. Serious illnesses such as dementia and psychotic disorders threaten or crush a person's sense of personal identity. Self-esteem is associated with the emotional aspect of self-concept and reflects the value a person places on his or her personal self-concept and its place in the world. Self-efficacy pertains to the control individuals' feel they have to make changes in the face of challenges to self-clarity, which relates to the stability of the defined self. Self-esteem hopefulness and spirituality have been shown to be positively related to health related quality of life among pediatric oncology patients (Cantrell et al., 2016). Assessment of spiritual needs and corresponding spiritual care is a Joint Commission (2017) requirement for quality care. Understanding these elements of self-concept and the critical role they play in managing behavior is key to working effectively with patients of all ages. It is a core variable to consider in therapeutic communication, nurse-patient relationships, and interventions.

> **ETHICAL DILEMMA: What Would You Do?**
>
> Jimmy is a 68-year-old man with diabetes; he was brought to the emergency room in kidney failure. The doctor has indicated that he needs Jimmy to agree to dialysis, but Jimmy refuses, saying "this only prolongs the final result." He refuses to listen to any long-term plan of care, and his wife is confused about options beyond dialysis. The doctor wants you to get Jimmy's consent for immediate dialysis. As the nurse caring for this patient, what would you do?

DISCUSSION QUESTIONS

- What role do the various modalities of social media play in the development and/or validation of a person's self-concept?
- In what ways are spirituality and world view connected in defining self-concept?
- Drawing on your experience, what are some specific ways in which you can help another person develop a stronger sense of self?
- Describe a personal exchange with a patient or an observed clinical encounter with another provider in which you felt that you learned something important about the value of the health provider's presence in promoting self-esteem.

REFERENCES

Adler, R., Rosenfeld, L., & Proctor, R. (2014). *Interplay: The process of interpersonal communication*. New York: Oxford University Press.

Arnold, E. (2005). A voice of their own: Women moving into their fifties. *Health Care for Women International, 26*(8), 630–651.

Arnett, J. (2013). *Adolescence and Emerging Adulthood* (5th ed.). Pearson Publishing CO.

Bailey, J. (2003). Self-image, self-concept, and self-identity revisited. *Journal of the National Medical Association, 95*(5), 383–386.

Baldacchino, D., & Draper, P. (2001). Spiritual coping strategies: A review of the literature. *Journal of Advanced Nursing, 34*(6), 833–841.

Bandura, A. (1997). *Self-efficacy. The exercise of control*. New York: W.H. Freeman and Company.

Bandura, A. (2007). Self-efficacy in health functioning. In S. Ayers (Ed.), *Cambridge handbook of psychology, health and medicine* (2nd ed.) (pp. 191–193). New York: Cambridge University Press.

Baumeister, R. F., Campbell, J. D., Krueger, J. I., & Vohs, K. D. (2003). Does high self-esteem cause better performance, interpersonal success, happiness, or healthier lifestyles? *Psychological Science in the Public Interest, 4*(1), 1–44.

Beck, J., & Beck, A. (2011). *Cognitive conceptualization. Cognitive behavior therapy*. New York, NY: Guilford Press. chap. 3, pp. 29–46.

Bem, D. J. (1972). Self-perception theory. *Advances in Experimental Social Psychology, 6*, 1–62.

Benner, P. (2003). Reflecting on what we care about. *American Journal of Critical Care, 12*(2), 165–166.

Blazek, M., & Besta, T. (2012). Self-concept clarity and religious orientations: prediction of purpose in life and self-esteem. *Journal of Religion & Health*, 51(3), 947–960.

Blazer, D. (2008). How do you feel about…? Health outcomes late in life and self-perceptions of health and well-being. *Gerontologist*, 48(4), 415–422.

Blazer, D. (2012). Religion/spirituality and depression: What can we learn from empirical studies? *American Journal of Psychiatry*, 169, 10–12.

Bolton, M. A., Lobben, I., & Stern, T. A. (2010). The impact of body image on patient care. *Primary Care Companion to The Journal of Clinical Psychiatry*, 12(2).

Boston Women's Health Book Collective. (1998). *Our bodies, ourselves for the new century*. New York: Touchstone Simon & Schuster.

Brown, J., & Marshall, M. (2001). Self-esteem and emotion: Some thoughts about feelings. *Personality and Social Psychology Bulletin*, 27(5), 575–584.

Cantrell, M., Conte, T., Hudson, M., Ruble, K., & Herth, K., et al. (2016). Developing the evidence base in Pediatric nursing practice for promoting health-related quality of life in pediatric oncology patients. 34(2), 90–97.

Capps, D. (2008). Alzheimer's Disease and the Loss of Self. *Journal of Pastoral Care and Counseling*, 62(1–2), 19–28.

Carson, V., & Koenig, H. (2008). *Spiritual dimensions of nursing practice revised ed.* West Conshohocken, PA: Templeton Press.

Carson, V., & Stoll, R. (2008). Spirituality: Defining the indefinable and reviewing its place in nursing. In V. Carson, & H. Koenig (Eds.), *Spiritual Dimensions of Nursing Practice*. West Conshohocken, PA: Templeton Press. Revised ed.

Cooper, J. (2007). *Cognitive dissonance: 50 years of a classic theory*. London: Sage Publications.

Crocker, J., Brook, A. T., & Niiya, Y. (2006). The pursuit of self-esteem: contingencies of self-worth and self-regulation. *Journal of Personality*, 74(6), 1749–1771.

Cunha, C., & Goncalves, M. (2009). Commentary: Accessing the experience of a dialogical self: Some needs and concerns. *Culture Psychology*, 15(3), 120–133.

Daaleman, T., Usher, B. M., Williams, S., Rawlings, J., & Hanson, L. C. (2008). An exploratory study of spiritual care at the end of life. *Annals of Family Medicine*, 6(5), 406–411.

Diehl, M., & Hay, E. (2007). Contextualized self-representations in adulthood. *Journal of Personality*, 75(6), 1255–1283.

Drench, M., Noonan, A., Sharby, N., & Ventura, S. (2011). *Psychosocial aspects of health care* (3rd ed.). Englewood Cliffs, NJ: Prentice Hall.

Dropkin, M. J. (1999). Body image and quality of life after head and neck cancer surgery. *Cancer Practice*, 7, 309–313.

Elliott, A. (2013). *Concepts of the self*. Malden, MA: Polity Press.

Ellis-Hill, C., & Horn, S. (2000). Change in identity and self-concept: A new theoretical approach to recovery following a stroke. *Clinical Rehabilitation*, 14(3), 279–287.

Erikson, E. (1959). *Identity and the life cycle: Selected papers*. Oxford, UK: International Universities Press.

Erikson, E. (1968). *Identity: Youth and crisis*. New York: Norton.

Erikson, E. (1982). *The life cycle completed: A review*. New York: Norton.

Erikson, E. H. (1985). *The Life Cycle Completed*. New York: Norton.

Falk, C. F., Heine, S. J., Yuki, M., & Takemura, K. (2009). Why do Westerners self-enhance more than East Asians? *European Journal of Personality*, 23, 183–203.

Fattore, T., Mason, A. J., & Watson, E. (2017). "Self, Identity and well-being". *Children's Well-Being: Indicators and Research, vol 14*, 116.

Fazio, S., & Mitchell, D. (2009). Persistence of self in individuals with Alzheimer's disease. *Dementia*, 8, 39–59.

Gilligan, C., Brown, L., & Rogers, A. (1990). Psyche embedded: A place for body, relationships, and culture in personality theory. In A. Rabin, R. Zucker, R. Emmons, & S. Frank (Eds.), *Studying Persons and Lives* (pp. 86–147).

Goffman, E. (1963). *Stigma and social identity. Stigma: Notes on the management of spoiled identity*. Englewood Cliffs, NJ: Prentice Hall.

Gordon, M. (2007). *Self-perception-self-concept pattern. Manual of nursing diagnoses* (11th ed.). Chestnut Hill, MA: Bartlett Jones.

Gordon, T., & Mitchell, D. (2004). A competency model for the assessment and delivery of spiritual care. *Palliative Medicine*, 18(7), 646–651.

Guerrero, L., Anderson, P., & Afifi, W. (2017). *Close encounters: Communication in relationships* (4th ed.). Thousand Oaks, CA: Sage Publications.

Harden, K. (2005). Self-esteem and affect as information. *Personality and social psychology bulletin*, 31(2), 276–288.

Harter, S. (2006). The self. In N. Eisenberg (Ed.), *Handbook of child psychology* (pp. 505–571). Hoboken: Wiley.

Harrington, J. (2011). Implications of treatment on body image and quality of life. *Seminars in Oncology Nursing*, 27(4), 290–299.

Heijmans, M., Rijken, M., Foets, M., de Ridder, D., Schreurs, K., & Bensingt, J. (2004). The stress of being chronically ill: From disease-specific to task-specific aspects. *Journal of Behavioral Medicine*, 27, 255–271.

Humphreys, K. (2004). *Circles of recovery: Self-help organizations for addictions*. Cambridge: Cambridge University Press.

Hunter, E. (2008). Beyond death: Inheriting the past and giving to the future, transmitting the legacy of one's self. *Omega*, 56(40), 313–329.

Jackson, J. (2014). *Introducing language and intercultural communication*. New York: Routledge.

Johnson, M., Cowin, L. S., Wilson, I., & Young, H. (2012). Professional identity and nursing. Contemporary theoretical developments and future research challenges. *International Nursing Review*, 59(4), 562–569.

Joint Commission on Accreditation of Healthcare Organizations. (2017). *The Joint One Renaissance Blvd*. Oakbrook Terrace, IL 60181 https://www.jointcommission.org/.

Josephson, A., & Peteet, J. (2007). Talking with patients about spirituality and worldview: Practical interviewing techniques and strategies. *Psychiatric Clinics of North America*, 30, 181–197.

Jung, C. G. (1960). Collected works. *The psychogenesis of mental disease* (Vol. 3). Oxford, England: Pantheon.

Kamakura, T., Jukoando, & Ono, Y. (2001). Genetic and environmental influences on self-esteem in a Japanese twin sample. *Twin Research, 4*(6), 439–442.

Karademas, E., Bakouli, A., Bastouonis, A., Kallergi, F., Tamtami, P., & Theofilou, M. (2008). Illness perceptions, illness-related problems, subjective health and the role of perceived primal threat: preliminary findings. *Journal of Health Psychology, 13*(8), 1021–1029.

Kendler, K., & Gardner, K. (1998). A population-based twin study of self-esteem and gender. *Psychological Medicine, 28*(6), 1403–1409.

Konig, J. (2009). Moving experience: dialogues between personal cultural positions. *Culture & Psychology, 15*(1), 97–119.

Lake, N. (2014). *The caregivers: A support group's stories of slow loss, courage, and love.* New York, NY: Simon & Schuster, Inc.

Lee, S. J. & Oyserman, D. (2009). Possible selves theory. E. Anderman & L. Anderman (Eds). Psychology of Classroom Learning: An Encyclopedia. Detroit, Michigan: Macmillan Reference USA.

Leerdam, L., Rietveld, L., Teunissen, D., & Lagro-Janseen, A. (2014). Gender-based education during clerkships: A focus group study. *Advances in Medical Education and Practice, 26*(5), 53–60.

Lewis, C. S. (1976). *A grief observed.* New York: Bantam Books.

Lodi-Smith, J., & Roberts, B. (2010). Getting to know me: Social role experiences and age differences in self-concept clarity during adulthood. *Journal of Personality, 78*(5), 1383–1410.

Malle, B. (2011). Attribution theories: How people make sense of behavior. In C. Derck (Ed.), *Theories in Social Psychology* (pp. 72–95). Hoboken, NJ: Wiley Blackwell Publishing Ltd.

Marks, R., Allegrante, J., & Lorig, K. (2005). A review and synthesis of research evidence for self-efficacy-enhancing interventions for reducing chronic disability. Implications for health education practice (Part II). *Health Promotion Practice* (6), 148–156.

Markus, H., & Nurius, P. (1986). Possible selves. *American Psychologist, 41*, 954–969.

Martin, C., & Ruble, D. (2010). Patterns of gender development. *Annual Review of Psychology, 61*, 353–381.

McCormick, M., & Hardy, M. (2008). *Re-visioning family therapy: race, culture and gender in clinical practice* (2nd ed.). New York NY: The Guilford Press.

Miller, J. (2007). Hope: A construct central to nursing. *Nursing Forum, 42*(1), 12–19.

Molzahn, A., & Sheilds, L. (2008). Why is it so hard to talk about spirituality? *Canadian Nurses, 10*(4), 25–29.

Mussatto, K., et al. (2014). The importance of self-perceptions to psychosocial adjustment in adolescents with heart disease. *Journal of Pediatric Health Care, 28*(3), 251–261.

Myers, D. (2017). *Developing through the life span. Psychology in every day life.* (10th ed.). New York, NY: Worth Publishers.

NANDA International. (2014). *Nursing diagnoses: Definitions and classification 2012–2014.* Oxford UK: Wiley Blackwell.

Neiss, M. B., Sedikes, C., & Stevenson, J. (2002). Self-esteem: A behavioral genetic perspective. *European Journal of Personality, 16*, 351–367.

Oyserman, D., & Markus, H. (1998). (Chapter 7) Self as social representation. In U. Flick (Ed.), *The psychology of the social* (pp. 107–125). Cambridge, UK: Cambridge University Press.

Prescott, A. P. (2006). *The concept of self in education, family and sports.* New York NY: Nova Science Publishers.

Raholm, M. B. (2008). Uncovering the ethics of suffering using a narrative approach. *Nursing Ethics, 15*(1), 62–72.

Reed, P. G. (2014). Theory of self-transcendence. In M. J. Smith, & P. R. Liehr (Eds.), *Middle range theory for nursing* (3rd ed.) (pp. 109–140). New York: Springer.

Robins, R. W., Trzesniewski, K. H., Tracy, J. L., Gosling, S. D., & Potter, J. (2002). Global self-esteem across the lifespan. *Psychology and Aging, 17*, 423–434.

Robins, R. W., & Trzesniewski, K. (2005). Self-esteem development across the lifespan. *Current Directions in Psychological Science, 1*(3).

Robson, P. J. (1988). The British journal of psychiatry: The journal of mental science. *Self-Esteem - A Psychiatr View, 153*, 6–15 1988.

Rogers, C. (1959). A theory of therapy, personality and inter-personal relationships as developed in the client-centered framework. In S. Koch (Ed.), *psychology: a study of a science. Vol. 3: Formulations of the person and the social context.* New York: McGraw Hill..

Rutledge, C. M., Gilmor, K., & Gillen, M. (2013). Does this profile picture make me look fat? look and body image in college students. *Psychology of Popular Media Culture, 2*(4), 251–258.

Sapp, S. (2010). What have religion and spirituality to do with aging? three approaches. *Gerontologist, 50*(2), 271–275.

Schachter, E. (2005). Erikson meets the postmodern: can classic identity theory rise to the challenge. *Identity, 5–2*, 137–160.

Sessana, L., Finnell, D., & Jezewski, M. A. (2007). Spirituality in nursing and health related literature: A concept analysis. *Journal of Holistic Nursing, 25*(4), 252–262.

Shweder, R., Goodnow, J., Hatano, R., Levine, H., Markus, H., & Miller, P. (2006). The cultural psychology of development. One mind, many mentalities. In W. Damon (Ed.), *Hand of Child Psychology* (6th ed.). John Wiley and Sons.

Simpson, E., & Jones, M. C. (2013). An exploration of self-efficacy and self-management in COPD patients. *British Journal of Nursing, 13*(2219), 1105–1109.

Slatman, J. (2011). The meaning of body experience evaluation in oncology. *Health Care Analysis, 19*, 295–311.

Smith, M. J., & Perkins, K. (2008). Attending to the voices of adolescents who are overweight to promote mental health. *Archives of Psychiatric Nursing, 22*(6), 391–393.

Steger, M., & Frazier, P. (2005). Meaning in life: one link in the chain from religion to well-being. *Journal of Counseling Psychology, 52*, 574–582.

Stewart, A. J., Ostrove, J. M., & Helson, R. (2001). Middle aging in women: Patterns of personality change from the 30s to the 50s. *Journal of Adult Development, 8*, 23–37.

Stopa, L., Brown, M., Luke, M. A., & Hirsch, C. R. (2010). Constructing a self: The role of self-structure and self-certainty in social anxiety. *Behaviour Research and Therapy, 48*(10), 955–965.

Sue, D. W., Capodilupa, C., Torino, G., Bucceri, J., et al. (2007). Racial microagressions in everyday life. Implications for clinical practice. *American Psychologist, 62*(4), 271–286.

Sullivan, H. S. (1953). *The interpersonal theory of psychiatry.* New York: Norton.

Sulmasy, D. P. (2006). Spiritual issues in the care of dying patients. *JAMA: The Journal of the American Medical Association, 296*(11), 1385–1392.

Suzuki, M., Amagai, M., Shibata, F., & Tsai, J. (2011). Participation related to self-efficacy for social participation of people with mental illness. *Archives of Psychiatric Nursing, 25*(5), 359–365.

Tanyi, R. (2006). Spirituality and family nursing: Spiritual assessment and interventions for families. *Journal of Advanced Nursing, 53*(3), 287–294.

Thomas, J. (2011). *My saints alive: reflections on a journey of love, loss and life.* Charlottesville VA: Create space independent publishing platform.

Toffle, M. E., & Quattropani, M. C. (2015). The Self in the Alzheimer's patient as revealed through psycholinguistic-story based analysis 6th world conference on psychology counseling and guidance. *Society Behavioral Science, 205*, 361–372.

van Tuyl, L. H. D., Hewlett, S., Sadlonova, M., et al. (2014). The patient perspective on remission in rheumatoid arthritis: 'You've got limits, but you're back to being you again'. *Annals of the Rheumatic Diseases. 74*(6), 1004–1010.

Usborne, E., & Taylor, D. (2010). The role of cultural identity clarity for self-concept, clarity, self-esteem, and subjective well-being. *Personality and Social Psychology Bulletin, 36*(7), 883–897.

Vartanian, L. (2009). When the body defines the self: Self-concept clarity, internalization, and body image. *Journal of Social Clinical Psychology, 28*(1), 94–126.

Veloza-Gómez, M., Muñoz de Rodríguez, L., Guevara-Armenta, C., & Mesa-Rodríguez, S. (2017). The importance of spiritual care in nursing practice. *Journal of Holistic Nursing, 35*(2), 118–131.

Vlasblom, J. P., Steen, J. V., Knol, D. L., & Jochemsen, H. (2011). Effects of a spiritual care training for nurses. *Nurse Education Today, 31*, 790–796.

Vickery, C., Sepehri, A., & Evans, C. (2008). Self-esteem in an acute stroke rehabilitation sample: A control group comparison. *Clinical Rehabilitation, 22*, 179–187.

Walker, C. (2010). Ruptured identities: Leaving work because of chronic illness. *International Journal of Health Services, 40*(4), 629–643.

Wood, J., & Fixmer, N. (2017). *Gendered lives: Communication, gender, and culture* (12th ed.). Cenage Learning.

Wu, L.-F., & Lin, L.-Y. (2011). Exploration of clinical nurses' perceptions of spirituality and spiritual care. *The Journal of Nursing Research, 19*, 250–256.

10

Developing Patient-Centered Therapeutic Relationships

Elizabeth C. Arnold

OBJECTIVES

At the end of this chapter, the reader will be able to:

1. Define a patient-centered care (PCC) relationship in health care.
2. Explain the differences between social and therapeutic relationships.
3. Identify theoretical relationship models used in nursing practice.
4. Discuss the core concepts of patient-centered relationships in health care.
5. Discuss therapeutic use of self in patient-centered relationships.
6. Discuss the main features of each relationship phase.
7. Explain how patient-centered communication is embedded in contemporary health care professional relationships.

INTRODUCTION

The Institute of Medicine (IOM, 2001) identifies patient centeredness as one of "six pillars of quality health care," and the World Health Organization (WHO, 2007) calls for health care delivery, "which takes into account the preferences and aspirations of individual service users, and the cultures of their communities" (p. 9).

Over the past two decades, chronic, noncommunicable health conditions have replaced infectious diseases as the dominant health care burden (Palmer et al., 2017, p. 1). Patient- and family-centered care are new models of care delivery, which support the inclusion of the patient and the patient's family as essential members of the interprofessional care team. Patients are expected to take an active role in self-managing the care of their chronic diseases.

Effective PCC/PFCC relationships are critical to patient healing and satisfaction. Whether caring for the patient individually, or as an interprofessional team member, nurses are in a unique position to gather, provide, and explain essential data throughout a care experience. They function as crucial professional resources, to provide ongoing support in the care and compassionate coaching that patients and families need when they are feeling vulnerable in health care situations.

Whereas patients and families cannot always defeat a health disorder or injury, with help, they can learn to succeed in spite of it, to achieve a meaningful life. Chapter 10 explores core concepts, and the essential features of PCC relationships.

BASIC CONCEPTS

The importance of PCC relationships as a major constituent component of safe quality health care delivery cannot be overemphasized. Research indicates that effective PCC relationships are a significant predictor of positive health outcomes (Hibbard, 2017).

Definitions

A patient-centered relationship is categorized as a "therapeutic alliance," linked to helping patients achieve identifiable health goals. The National Council of State Boards of Nursing (NCSBN, 2014) defines a ***therapeutic relationship*** as "one that allows nurses to apply their professional knowledge, skills, abilities, and experiences towards meeting the health needs of the patient" (p. 3). ***Patient-centered care (PCC) relationships*** represent a subset of professional therapeutic relationships, in which nurses and other health professionals engage with their patients specifically related to

- understanding the patient experience of an illness,
- effective self-management of chronic health problems,
- development of healthy lifestyle behaviors to prevent or minimize the development of chronic disorders,
- increased satisfaction with clinical outcomes and well-being.

Patient-centered care (PCC) relationships begin with the expectation that patients will take an active participatory role in self-managing their chronic health condition(s) (Locatelli, 2015). They are characterized as a clinical partnership between a patient and selected providers. "Recognizing the patient, or designee as a source of control, and a full partner in providing compassionate and coordinated care based on respect for patient's preferences, values and needs" is a new and critical dimension of PCC (Dolansky & Moore, 2013).

Professional and personal roles are not interchangeable in a PCC relationship; Both roles are relevant to achievent of clinical outcomes but they complement rather than replace one another. Both roles are relevant to successfully achieving desired clinical care outcomes. The patient is the best informant about the personalized nature of the patient's illness, and its impact on the patient's life. Current understandings of PPC relationships incorporate patient needs, values, and preferences in all aspects of care. "Indicators of a strong therapeutic alliance include mutual trust among all parties, coordinated and continuous health care, and the patient's perception of feeling respected and cared for" (Street, Makoul, Arora, & Epstein, 2009, p. 298). The correlation between therapeutic relationship and patient centeredness is portrayed in Fig. 10.1.

The continuum of PCC relationships found in contemporary health care settings range from those found

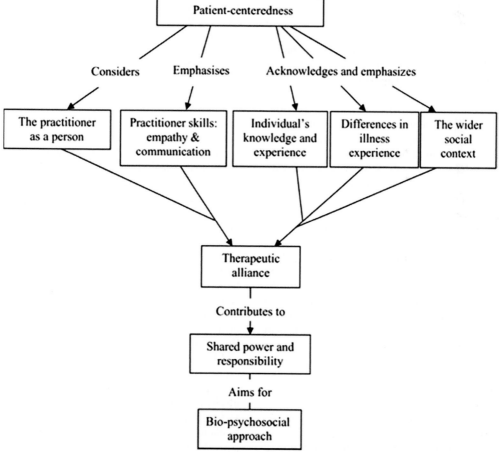

Fig. 10.1 Model of Patient Centeredness in Nurse-Patient Relationships. (From Lhussier, M., Eaton, S., Forster, N., Thomas, M., Roberts, S., & Carr, S. M. [2015]. Care planning for long-term conditions—a concept mapping. *Health Expectations, 18*(5), 605–624.)

in critical care, to relationships supporting primary care self-management of chronic conditions, in preventive and urgent care settings. Home-based and long-term care settings involve documentation of person-centered care at a higher level of intervention than ever before.

PCC relationships are time limited, subject to treatment, and other regulatory concerns. A PCC relationship can span an 8-hour shift. It can occur episodically, or at regularly scheduled times; as a single encounter, or as an emergency care contact. Longer term relationships can last over a period of days, weeks, or months as in a mental health inpatient setting or rehabilitation center. Regardless of the amount of time spent, each PCC relationship can, and should, be meaningful. The relationship typically terminates when identified clinical objectives are achieved, or the patient is transferred to a different care setting.

Patient-Centered Care Relationships

PCC relationships are based on the premise that each person's experience of an illness, injury, or disease is a total human experience, and much more than simply a biomedical process. "Patient and family centered care applies to patients of all ages and can be practiced in any health care setting" (Mitchell, Chaboyer, Baumeister, & Foster, 2009, p. 543).

Relational connections in patient-centered relationships offer supportive intervention that is *holistic, respectful, individualized, and empowering* (Morgan & Yoder, 2012). Each relationship is based on the importance of understanding the patient as a unique individual with a health need, or functional capacity that interferes with one or more aspects of his/her life in a meaningful way. In addition to a patient's physical and clinical needs, nurses need to consider each patient's cognitive, sociocultural, and emotional context, as these data frame the patient's personalized experience of health issues. Addressing situational, cultural, religious, and family circumstances allows for a more inclusive *holistic* targeted understanding of the patient's preferences and life goals. These data allow nurses to individualize, support, and understand the fuller dimensions of a patient's health issues. Listening to what a patient identifies as primary concerns provides stronger information about the patient's values and preferences.

Respectful care starts with careful listening and emphasizes the patient's strengths, abilities, wishes, and goals. Respect assumes, until proven otherwise, that patients are interested in bettering their health, and are willing to make positive efforts, even when those efforts are not clearly visible. Nurses demonstrate respectful care when they support patient autonomy and realistic care goals.

PCC is *individualized care*. Listening to what the patient identifies as his or her main concern provides contextual data about patient values and preferences within the family and community. Once you have a composite picture of each patient, and of what matters to the patient and family, it becomes easier to develop a care plan based on individual patient goals and values. Motivation and interest are significant contributors to relevant goal development and continued efforts to achieve personally relevant life and health goals.

A patient-centered assessment seeks an integrated understanding of each patient's contextual world—including emotional needs and life issues. These data form a relational informational platform that "fits" the patient and provides a common ground for developing mutually agreed upon self-management and health-related clinical strategies.

Developing a PCC Plan

A PCC plan is designed to encourage patient autonomy, and to develop self-efficacy in all aspects of care. Accurately assessing the patient's knowledge base and personal need for information as you search for common ground about each patient's life issues and bio-psychosocial health needs is critical. Self-efficacy plays an important role in personal motivation (Bandura, 2012). Self-efficacy is defined as the confidence that a person holds about personal ability to achieve goals or to complete a task. Self-efficacy beliefs affect the quality of human functioning through cognitive, motivational, affective, and decisional processes. Specifically, people's beliefs in their efficacy will influence whether they have confidence in their abilities to achieve the goals they set for themselves.

Barlow et al. (2002) defines self management as a "individual's ability to manage symptoms, treatment, physical and psychosocial consequences and lifestyle changes inherent in living with a chronic condition" (p. 178). An important patient-centered focus of the relationship is on considering options and making choices in consultation with the patient and other team providers. Nurses and other professional care providers contribute evidence-based data and professional expertise to the clinical plan. The patient provides individualized personal data. Knowledge of a patient's coping strategies, strengths, and limitations, plus joint perceptions about symptoms, expectations, and previous life experiences, are significant contextual contributors to a PCC plan. Patient care plans ideally revolve around each patient's primary reasons for seeking health care, personal and family concerns, and available resources. Shared decision making, in which patients and providers strive to "make health care decisions together," strengthens the patient–provider bond that allows the clinical relationship to move forward toward successful management of chronic disorders.

RELATIONAL PROCESSES IN PATIENT-CENTERED CARE

The experience of "becoming a patient" varies from person to person. In a professional health relationship, neither clinician nor patient exists independently of the other. A patient-centered relationship seeks to understand the patient as a person with emotional, physical, and spiritual needs coping with health-related life issues. What happens within this relationship becomes the shared product of their interaction. Patient-centered interactions take place within the context of the nurse/patient culture, personal worldviews, previous life experiences, the nature of the illness and its impact on other relationships, and personal values—all of which are important to the patient.

Relevant *content* that emerges in the assessment phase of a PCC relationship becomes the basis for shared decision making between patients and their clinical providers. These data support will influence the specific step progression toward identified therapeutic goals. Gaining information about your patient's culture and other life roles provides supporting data regarding what is important to understanding the full picture of an individual health care situation. While nursing practice necessarily requires an evidence-based foundation, its natural home lies in understanding and responding to the full *human* experience of individuals in need of health care (Lazenby, 2013).

Once a patient and clinician(s) agree on a workable action plan, applicable patient education, compassionate coaching, and informed support of targeted self-management strategies become an important focus of the care partnership. These communication strategies are specifically designed to incorporate patient values and preferences as an essential component of care, to whatever extent is possible.

Professional relationships and informational transfer are major communication tools used to meet one or more of the following care goals:

- Understanding the patient's experience of an illness,
- Helping patients to effectively self-manage chronic health problems,
- Encouraging patients to develop healthy lifestyle behaviors to prevent or minimize the development of chronic disorders.

Collaborative Patient-Centered Relationships

Collaborative interprofessional care approaches embedded in designated health care teams, rather than single practitioners assuming responsibility for the patient-centered health care of patients have become the new norm in health care delivery. This paradigm shift is based on the premise that no single health care discipline can provide complete care for a patient with today's multiple chronic health care needs (Batalden, Ogrinc, & Batalden, 2006; IOM, 2003). Interprofessional collaborative relationships bring together the sophisticated medical, nursing, pharmacy, rehabilitative, psychological, and social work skills needed to support desired patient-centered outcomes. The relationship aspect develops from mutual respect and power sharing among all team members, including the patient, to achieve clinical outcomes (see also Chapter 23).

Care coordination among multiple care providers is an essential component of interprofessional patient-centered relationships (WHO, 2010). Contemporary practice requires that nurses lead, coordinate, and integrate their professional nursing skills with those of other health team members (depending on the circumstances) for maximum effectiveness.

Therapeutic Relationships

The NCSBN (2014) defines a *therapeutic relationship* as "one that allows nurses to apply their professional knowledge, skills, abilities, and experiences toward meeting the health needs of the patient" (p. 3). Therapeutic relationships in health care can take place in a variety of venues, ranging from preventive care through intensive care management of an acute medical or psychological condition, and follow-up care of patients, post hospitalization.

Time spent with patients varies. A patient-centered relationship can span an 8-hour full shift in a hospital. They occur at regularly scheduled times, as a single encounter, or as an emergency care contact. Longer term relationships can last over a period of days, weeks, or months in a mental health inpatient setting, or in a rehabilitation center. Patient-centered relationships increasingly take place in community-based medical homes, in the patient's home, or as a one-time encounter in an urgent care center.

Depending on the geographic area, some PCC relationships can take place digitally. Patients have a new capability to communicate with providers through secure patient portals, and to receive copies of patient records. Patients can communicate directly, make appointments, ask questions, request refills on medications, and report new symptoms.

Elements of Patient-Centered Relationships

PCC is basically examining health care from the patient perspective of their care and their relationships with the health professionals caring for them (Ferguson, Ward,

Card, Sheppard, & McMurty, 2013). A **patient-centered relationship** considers each individual patient as a *person* first and foremost; with distinctive personally held values, beliefs, and life goals. Second, this person is a "patient with a medical or psychiatric diagnosis," requiring treatment and tangible professional support to resolve a chronic illness, or to improve preventive care. In crisis situations, immediate life-sustaining issues take precedence. Personal factors, especially those related to patient dignity and individuality, should still be incorporated.

Contemporary patient-centered relationships represent a new paradigm in health care delivery. Although nurses continue to have an intimate relationship on many levels with their patients, more patients than not suffer from one or more chronic illnesses. These conditions require careful monitoring and personalized clinical attention over significant periods of time, and possibly a lifetime, long-term. Self-management of chronic disorder(s) requirements led to development of a new model, The Chronic Care Model, developed by Dr. Edward Wagner and colleagues (2001). This model proposes "a patient-professional partnership, involving collaborative care, and self-management education" (Bodenheimer, Lorig, Holman, & Grumbach, 2002, p. 2469). The chronic care model is presented below. Fig. 10.3 displays nursing diagnoses associated with Maslow's hierarchy of needs (Fig. 10.4).

A major value of the PCC model is its integrated utility across multiple care settings. The inclusion of transitional care initiatives helps offset potential gaps in service. In addition to patient education and traditional care provision, nurses work with patients and families to help them develop the self-management skills and strategies they need to cope with chronic disorders such as diabetes, arthritis, and cardiac issues. "Self management" refers to the daily decisions and behaviors patients

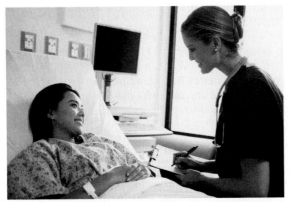

Fig. 10.2 Patient-Centered Assessments Should Include Your Patient's Strengths, Abilities, Goals, and Preferences Related to Health Issues. (Copyright © monkeybusinessimages/iStock/Thinkstock.)

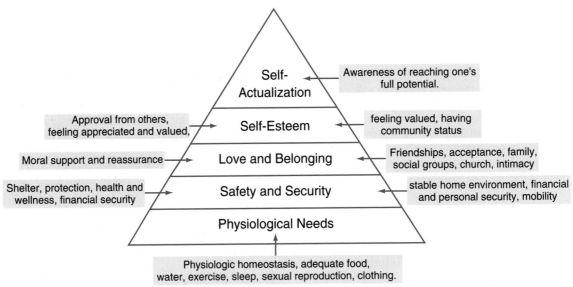

Fig. 10.3 Behavioral Examples Reflecting Maslow's Need Hierarchy Corresponding With Maslow's Hierarchy of Needs.

must take to manage their long term conditions, and their lives (Lhussier et al., 2015). Nurses also support and coach patients in developing problem-solving skills and other self-management skills to support healthy lifestyle behaviors. Having confidence to self-manage a chronic health condition is consistent with the triple aim of improved clinical outcomes, better quality of life, and lower costs.

Each PCC represents a unique relational encounter that validates the assumption that "a core value of nursing is that the people we serve are uniquely valuable as human beings" (Porter, O'Halloran, & Morrow, 2011, p. 107). Patients and nurses have different personalities. Their ways of relating with others, and the circumstances surrounding each relationship, differ. What is supportive to one patient or family may not be to another.

Caring as a Core Value in Therapeutic Relationships

Caring represents a core foundational value in professional nursing relationships. It is this component of professional relationships that is best remembered by patients, families, and nurses. Think about a significant relationship you have had with a patient, or experienced yourself as a patient. What made it special or meaningful to you?

The caring involved in patient-centered relationships is not so much about the words themselves, or about specific tasks. Rather, it is about a sustained connection, and the meaning that caring connection holds for the recipient(s) (Crowe, 2000). Caring as a key characteristic of professional nursing should be embodied as a visible component of each nurse's relationship, with patients and families, and with each other.

Patient-Centered Versus Social Relationships

Therapeutic patient-centered relationships share many characteristics of social relationships. All relationships work better when participants are actively engaged, when each participant listens carefully, and when each person respects the other as an equal partner. Communication strengths, such as authenticity, presence, acceptance, positive regard, empathy, respect, self-awareness, and competence, when deliberately employed contribute to the success of therapeutic professional relationships.

The differences relate to purpose, the type of involvement, and the privacy protections. Social relationships are established and maintained to meet mutual need, and/or friendship purposes. Therapeutic relationships are established for professional health-related purposes within a specific time setting. The focus of attention is always on patient health concerns, and the actions needed to help patients identify and resolve issues related to health and well-being. This is a major distinction between the two types of relationship.

Therapeutic relationships are subject to ethical and legal standards. Unlike social relationships, they are purposefully linked to supporting patients in meeting health-related goals. Professional relationships have a defined beginning and ending. There are rules governing the structure, interpersonal behaviors, and topics developed within the relationship. Table 10.1 outlines the differences between social and therapeutic relationships.

Theoretical Frameworks

Theoretical frameworks that support the study of patient-centered relationships in nursing practice include Peplau's interpersonal nursing theory, Carl Rogers' person-centered theory, and Maslow's needs theory.

Hildegard Peplau's Interpersonal Nursing Theory

Hildegard Peplau's (1997) interpersonal nursing theory is a well-known theory of interpersonal relationships in nursing. She identifies four sequential phases of a nurse-patient relationship: *pre-interaction, orientation, working phase* (problem identification and exploitation), and *termination*. These phases are an overlapping part of a holistic relationship. Each phase serves to broaden as well as deepen the emotional connection between nurse and patient (Reynolds, 1997). Peplau identified six professional roles the nurse can assume during the course of the nurse-patient relationship. (see box 10-1 on page (pg. 186) of this chapter.)

Carl Rogers' Client-Centered Model

Carl Rogers' model states that each person has within him/herself the capacity to heal if given support and treated with respect and unconditional positive regard in a caring, authentic, therapeutic relationship. Rogers presents a person-centered approach to the study of therapeutic relationships, and the relevant concepts supporting it. He identifies three major provider attributes of person-centered relationships in therapeutic setting, as:

- authenticity (being "real" in a relationship without artificial facades),
- prizing (trust and respect),
- empathetic understanding.

Abraham Maslow's Needs Theory

The International Council of Nurses (ICN) declares, "human needs guide the work of nursing" (2010). Abraham Maslow's (1970) needs theory offers a motivational

TABLE 10.1   Differences Between Helping Relationships and Social Relationships

Helping Relationships	Social Relationships
Health care provider takes responsibility for the conduct of the relationship and for maintaining appropriate boundaries	Both parties have equal responsibility for the conduct of the relationship
Relationship has a specific health-related purpose and goals	Relationship may or may not have a specific purpose or goals
Meeting the professional health-related needs and goals of the patient determine the duration of the relationship	Relationship can last a lifetime or terminate spontaneously at any time
Focus of the relationship is on the needs of the patient	The needs of both partners can receive equal attention
Relationship is entered into because of a patient's health care need	Relationship is entered into spontaneously for a wide variety of purposes
Choice of who to be in relationship is not available to either the helper or the helpee	Behavior for both participants is spontaneous; people choose companions
Self-disclosure by the nurse is limited to data that facilitates the health-related relationship. Self-disclosure by the patient is expected and encouraged	Self-disclosure for both parties in the relationship is expected and encouraged

framework that nurses use to prioritize patient needs in planning their care. Fig. 10.2 shows Maslow's (1970) model as a pyramid, with need requirements occurring in an ascending fashion from basic survival needs through to self-actualization.

Maslow defines first-level needs as *deficiency* needs, meaning that these are fundamental needs required for human survival. First-level *basic physiological needs* include hunger, thirst, sexual appetites, and sensory stimulation. Maslow's second-level, *safety and security needs*, describe basic physical safety and emotional security; for example, financial safety, freedom from injury, safe neighborhood, and freedom from abuse. Until basic deficiency needs are met, people cannot attend to personal growth needs.

Satisfaction of basic deficiency needs allows for attention to the fulfillment of growth needs. *Love and belonging needs* relate to emotionally connecting with, and experiencing, oneself as being a part of a family, and/or community. The next level, *self-esteem needs*, refers to a person's need for recognition and appreciation. A sense of dignity, respect, and approval by others for oneself is a hallmark of successfully meeting self-esteem needs. Maslow's highest level of need satisfaction, *self-actualization*, refers to a person's need to achieve his or her (self-defined) human potential. Self-actualized individuals are not superhuman; they are subject to the same feelings of insecurity that all individuals experience. The difference is that they accept this vulnerability as part of their human condition. Not everyone reaches this developmental stage.

Nurses use Maslow's theory with patients and families to prioritize nursing interventions that best match with patient needs and priorities. Simulation Exercise 10.1 provides practice using Maslow's model in clinical practice.

Elements of Patient-Centered Care

McCormack and McCance (2010) describe PCC as "an approach to practice established through the formation and fostering of therapeutic relationships between all care providers, patients, and others significant to them in their lives" (p. 13).

The IOM (2001) landmark report *Crossing the Quality Chasm: A New Health System for the 21st Century* identified patient centeredness to be one of the six aims for improvement of the US Health Care System. This document defines PCC as "care that is respectful of and responsive to individual patient preferences, needs, and values, and ensures that patient values guide all clinical decisions" (IOM, 2001). What each of these reports has in common is an insistence upon the primacy of the patient in all aspects of care decision making and clinical care.

APPLICATIONS

The term "patient-centered care" was initially developed by the Picker Institute in 1988. The model represents a significant shift in focus from a disease model to one emphasizing inclusion of the patient and family as full partners in planning and implementing meaningful health care. A *healing* relationship consists of an honest connection between the health professional and the patient, marked with respect for the dignity of the patient, and a genuine desire to support the patient to achieve maximum health and well-being through an action plan tailored to patient needs, values, and preferences.

SIMULATION EXERCISE 10.1   Introductions in the Nurse-Patient Relationship

Purpose

To provide simulated experience with initial introductions.

Procedure

The introductory statement forms the basis for the rest of the relationship. Effective contact with a patient helps build an atmosphere of trust and connectedness with the nurse. The following statement is a good example of how one might engage the patient in the first encounter:

"Hello, Mr. Smith. I am Sally Parks, a nursing student. I will be taking care of you on this shift. During the day, I may be asking you some questions about yourself that will help me to understand how I can best help you." Role-play the introduction to a new patient with one person taking the role of the patient; another, the nurse; and a third person, an involved family member, with one or more of the following patients:

1. Mrs. Dobish is a 70-year-old patient admitted to the hospital with a diagnosis of diabetes and a question about cognitive impairment.
2. Thomas Charles is a 19-year-old patient admitted to the hospital following an auto accident in which he broke both legs and fractured his sternum.
3. Barry Fisher is a 53-year-old man who has been admitted to the hospital for tests. The physician believes he may have a renal tumor.
4. Marion Beatty is a 9-year-old girl admitted to the hospital for an appendectomy.
5. Barbara Tangiers is a 78-year-old woman living by herself. She has multiple health problems including chronic obstructive pulmonary disease and arthritis. This is your first visit.

Discussion and Reflective Analysis

1. In what ways did you have to modify your introductions to meet the needs of the patient and/or circumstances?
2. What were the easiest and hardest parts of doing this exercise?
3. How could you use this experience as a guide in your clinical practice?

DEVELOPING AN EVIDENCE-BASED PRACTICE

Purpose: The purpose of this scoping review of the research was to identify the core elements of PCC approaches. Specifically, this review focused on communication, partnership, and health promotion, which were found across PCC models included in this review study.

Method: This scoping review explored articles published since 1990, using Medline, Cinahl, and Embase. The key terms "patient-centered or client-centered care" and "framework or model" were used to identify relevant studies.

Findings: This study retrieved 101 articles, of which 19 met inclusion criteria. From these articles, 25 different patient-centered frameworks/models were identified. All identified studies incorporated communication, partnership, and health promotion. The authors noted that much empiric evidence was sourced for the most consistently defined component of PCC: "communication" (p. 271).

Application to Your Clinical Practice: This scoping review affirms the importance of communication, partnership, and health promotion as primary components of patient-centered approaches in contemporary health care.

Modified from Constand, M. K., MacDermid, J. C., Dal Bello-Hass, V., & Law, M. (2014). Scoping review of patient-centered care approaches in health care. *BMC Health Services Research, 14*, 271–281.

- coordinated and integrated care;
- clear, high-quality information and education for the patient and family;
- physical comfort, including pain management;
- emotional support and alleviation of fear and anxiety;
- involvement of family members and friends, as appropriate;
- continuity, including through care-site transitions; and
- access to care (Barry & Edgman-Levitan, 2012, p. 780).

STRUCTURE OF PATIENT-CENTERED RELATIONSHIPS

Boundaries

The emotional integrity of the nurse-patient relationship depends "on maintaining relational boundaries" (LaSala & O'Brien, 2009, p. 424). **Professional boundaries** represent invisible structures imposed by legal, ethical, and professional standards of nursing that respect the rights and privacy of the patient, and protect the functional integrity of the alliance between nurse and patient.

The Picker Institute (2017) confirms eight characteristics of care as significant indicators of quality and safety in patient-centered relationships. They include the following:
- respect for the patient's values, preferences, and expressed needs;

Professional boundaries spell out the parameters of the health care relationship. They define how nurses should relate to patients as a helping person: not as a friend, not as a judge, but as a skilled professional partner committed to helping the patient achieve mutually defined health care goals (Fronek et al., 2009)). Examples of professional relationship boundaries include the setting, time, purpose, focus of conversation, and length of contact.

Unlike social relationships, therapeutic relationships incorporate a particular type of communication responsibility and role function throughout the relationship. Boundaries in a therapeutic relationship act in a similar way, as do guard rails at important sites that are put in place to protect the public from danger when observing a tourist attraction. When patients seek health care, they look to their health care providers as skilled responsible guides to help them achieve optimum health and well-being. The NCSBN (2011) conceptualize professional boundaries as "the spaces between the nurse's position and power, and patient vulnerability." Nurses are the keepers of the guard in professional relationships as well as key informants and professional guides.

Boundary violations take advantage of a patient's vulnerability and represent a conflict of interest, capable of compromising the goals of the therapeutic relationship. They are subject to ethical and legal constraints (Sheets, 2001).

The nurse, not the patient, is responsible for creating and maintaining professional boundaries. **Boundary crossings** give the appearance of impropriety and can lead to boundary violations. Examples of boundary crossings include meetings outside of the relationship, or disclosing personal intimate details about aspects of the nurse's life that would not be common knowledge (Bruner & Yonge, 2006).

LEVEL OF INVOLVEMENT

Professional behaviors exist on a continuum. To be effective, nurses must maintain an emotional objectivity, while remaining human and present to patients and families. The level of involvement on the professional behavior continuum can fluctuate, depending on patient needs. It should never compromise the boundaries of professional behavior, nor minimize the nature of the helping relationship. An important feature of a therapeutic relationship is the nurse's level of involvement, as presented in Fig. 10.1.

The professional level of involvement becomes a problem when a nurse limits involvement to minimum care tasks (under-involvement), or becomes emotionally over-involved in a patient's care. Over-involvement can be associated with *countertransference*, which occurs when something in the patient activates a nurse's unconscious

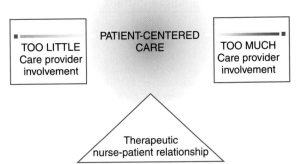

Fig. 10.4 Levels of Involvement: A Continuum of Professional Behavior. (From National Council of State Boards of Nursing (NCSBN). (2009). *A nurse's guide to professional boundaries.* Chicago: NCSBN. Retrieved from https://www.ncsbn.org/ProfessionalBoundaries_Complete.pdf.)

unresolved feelings from previous relationships or life events (Scheick, 2011). Over-involvement results in the nurse's loss of the essential objectivity needed to support the patient in meeting health goals. Additionally, over-involvement can compromise one or more of the following: the nurse's obligation to the service agency, collegial relationships with other health team members, and professional responsibilities to other patients (Morse, 1991).

Warning signs that the nurse is becoming over-involved can include:

- giving extra time and attention to certain patients,
- visiting patients during off-duty hours,
- doing things for patients that they could do for themselves,
- discounting the actions of other professionals,
- keeping secrets with a patient,
- believing that they are the only one who understands the patient's needs.

The opposite of over-involvement is *disengagement,* which occurs when a nurse emotionally or physically withdraws from having more than a superficial contact with a patient. Disengagement can be related to either the patient's behavior or intensity of suffering. It can be a symptom of burnout or heightened stress for the nurse. For example, an increased number of deaths or high stress levels on a unit can create compassion fatigue, which can lead to disengagement as a self-protective mechanism (Hofmann, 2009). Signs of disengagement include withdrawal, limited perfunctory contacts, minimizing the patient's suffering, and engaging in defensive or judgmental communication. Regardless of the reason, the outcome of disengagement is that a patient feels isolated and sometimes abandoned when care is mechanically delivered with limited human connection.

Maintaining a Helpful Level of Involvement

Maintaining a helpful level of involvement is always the responsibility of the professional nurse. To sustain a helpful level of professional connection and/or to regain perspective in a relationship, Carmack (1997) suggests that nurses take the following actions:

- Focus on the process of care while acknowledging that the outcome may or may not be within your control.
- Focus on the things that you can change while acknowledging that there are things over which you have no control.
- Be aware and accepting of your professional limits and boundaries.
- Monitor your reactions and seek assistance when you feel uncomfortable about any aspect of the relationship.
- Balance giving care to a patient with taking care of yourself, without feeling guilty.

Emotional reactions will occur in clinical situations. Debriefing after a highly emotional event helps nurses resolve and put strong feelings into perspective. Support groups for nurses working in high-acuity nursing situations and for the mentoring of new nurses are recommended.

PHASES OF A PATIENT-CENTERED RELATIONSHIP

A patient-centered relationship consists of three phases: orientation, working, and termination. Prior to meeting a patient for the first time, there is a short window of time (referred to as the pre-interaction phase) to think about your own professional goals for the interaction, and what you hope to achieve. Included in this process is a brief examination of your own personal biases, perhaps based on past experiences.

Pre-Interaction Phase

The pre-interaction phase is the only phase of the relationship in which the patient is not directly involved. Prior to meeting your patient, you should review what is known about them from the chart or report. Having a quick overview of a patient's status before your first meeting can make a difference in your initial approach. Knowing that your patient has had a sleepless night prior to your meeting him, or is newly aware of another diagnosis, or that this is a first hospitalization can influence your initial approach. Obstacles are easier to handle when they are anticipated. For example, two young women admitted to the hospital for the delivery of a first baby—one happily married, the other a single woman who is not planning on keeping her baby—might have very different interpersonal needs. Having knowledge of the difference in demographics affords the nurse greater interpersonal sensitivity in approaching each of these patients for the first time.

The pre-interaction phase is a time for you to reflect briefly on your own professional goals, and to address any gaps in easily correctable knowledge or potential bias such that you can work with your patient without judgment. Miller (2001) notes, "As you become more clear about who you are and why you do what you do, you will become more receptive to whomever you are with" (p. 23).

Orientation Phase

Nurses enter a PCC therapeutic relationship in the "stranger" role. The orientation phase shares some characteristics of getting to know someone you have just met in a new relationship. The expectation is that this "introductory" phase will lead to developing a conversational ease, and the trust needed to move communication to a deeper level.

Creating a comfortable setting where you and the patient can sit facing each other at eye level with a comfortable distance between you is essential. The setting should be as private as possible. Assessments and other care interviews should be scheduled at times when the patient is alert and not in pain. If a family member is to be involved, seating for that person should be accommodated as a principal contributor to the dialogue.

Establishing Rapport

Establishing rapport is an essential prerequisite for engaging the patient and family in committing to self-maintenance strategies. Developing a working alliance with your patients and their families starts with your first encounter. First impressions count. Start with an introduction of yourself as a professional nurse, the time frame you will be working with the patient, and your role in caring for the patient. This can be followed by a simple statement like, "I'd like to get to know you better. Can you tell me about what concerns you most at this time?" Listen actively, and ask fewer, rather than more, questions.

Listen to the patient's story with as few interruptions as possible. People make sense of things by talking about them. As the patient shares his or her personal story, keep in mind that your patient may be experiencing a broad spectrum of health issues with emotional as well as cognitive challenges to full understanding. Your initial response should be to give undivided attention to what the patient is saying, to use minimum encouragers, and to frame any initial comments, or open-ended questions in neutral, nonjudgmental language. You can use the suggestions for integrating empathy into listening responses that are presented in Box 10.2.

Each patient's experience of illness or injury is unique, despite similarities in diagnosis, or personal characteristics (McCance et al., 2011). Basic understanding of your patient's experience should relate to a systematic exploration of the questions, "What is this person's human experience of living with this illness, or injury?" and "How can I, as a health care professional, help you at this point in time?" Patient preferences and values will become visible as the patient shares the story of a personal illness. Putting a painful situation into words places boundaries on it, which enhances the processing of its meaning.

Empathy acts as a human echo in acknowledging that the helper understands and is interested in the patient's perspectives and concerns (Egan, 2014). Guiding principles (e.g., presence, purpose, positive regard, authenticity, active listening, and respect for the dignity of the patient) strengthen the establishment and healing influence of each therapeutic relationship (McGrath, 2005). Ask for validation of patient concerns frequently to confirm understanding, especially if you have trouble following the dialogue. This also indicates interest and helps build a common understanding.

Developing a Collaborative Relationship

Engaging the Patient

The goal of engaging the patient is a first step in developing a collaborative working relationship to achieve patient-centered health and health promotion goals. Both the patient and the nurse have rights and responsibilities in today's SDM. Trust is essential to patient engagement and to effective decision making in PCC (Ferguson et al., 2013). The American Hospital Association (AHA, 2003) has developed a brochure outlining the rights and responsibilities of patient care partnerships. The document is accessible in multiple languages on the AHA web site. Hospitals today have copies of comprehensive patient rights posted on their web sites. Written copies are given to patients on admission. A sample listing of common patient rights and responsibilities is provided in Box 10.3.

Your assessment meeting with the patient should have two outcomes. First, the patient should emerge from the encounter(s) feeling that the nurse is interested in him or her as a person separate from their diagnosis. Second, both the nurse and the patient should have a better picture of the patient's health needs and issues, and a beginning idea of what will be needed to resolve them.

Collaborative Partnership in Developing Patient-Centered Care Goals

An initial integrated assessment strategy allows the nurse and patient to jointly and authentically construct the personalized meaning of a health experience into a meaningful whole. The next step in the assessment process is to develop a shared understanding of potential options related to these data. PCC goals and action plans of therapeutic relationships usually relate to some, or all, of the following activities:

- Supporting patients and families to accurately understand the patient's personalized experience of an illness
- Helping patients and their families develop practical strategies to effectively self-manage chronic health conditions
- Linking patients and families with appropriate health care team professionals for relevant information, guidance, and support

BOX 10.3 Patient Rights and Responsibilities

All patients have the following rights:

- Impartial access to the most appropriate treatment regardless of race, age, sexual preference, national origin, religion, handicap, or source of payment for care
- To be treated with respect, dignity, and personal privacy in a safe, secure environment
- Confidential treatment of all communication and other records related to care or payment, except as required by law or signed insurance contractual arrangements (all patients should receive Notice of Privacy Practices)
- Active participation in all aspects of decision making regarding personal health care
- To know the identity and professional status of each health care provider
- To have treatments and procedures explained to them in ways they can understand
- To receive competent interpreter services, if required, to understand care or treatment
- To refuse treatment, including life-saving treatment, after being told of the potential risks associated with such refusal
- To receive appropriate pain management
- To express grievances regarding any violation of patient rights internally and/or to the appropriate agency

All patients have the following responsibilities:

- To treat their care providers with respect and courtesy, including timely notification for appointment cancellations
- To provide accurate, complete information about all personal health matters
- To follow recommended treatment plans
- To assume responsibility for personal actions, if choosing to refuse treatment
- To follow hospital regulations regarding safety and conduct

Patient-centered approaches to health care: A systematic review of randomized controlled Trials. Retrieved from https://www.researchgate.net/publication/253335907_Patient-Centered_Approaches_to_Health_Care_A_Systematic_Review _of_Randomized_Controlled_Trials?tab=overview.

- Providing emotional and informational support to help patients and their families understand options and make realistic decisions about the best options
- Assisting patients/families to cope with, and find meaning in, difficult personal health circumstances

- Helping patients discover new directions in line with their interests, values, and capabilities
- Helping patients access community-based health care resources and rehabilitative services, as needed
- Empowering patients with the knowledge and tools they need to be successful negotiators in working with their health care team

SHARED DECISION MAKING

Shared responsibility for decision making and integrating multiple perspectives in health care management across a continuum of care that extends into the community has become a new norm in health care delivery. *Shared decision making* refers to an interactive process between clinicians and patients, which "promotes defining problems, presenting options, and providing high-quality information so patients can participate more actively in care" (Epstein & Peters, 2009, p. 195). It is patient specific. Collaborative patient-centered treatment planning begins with jointly developed patient data, which serves as the basis for SDM between patients and their providers about realistic achievable health goals (Elwyn et al., 2012; Mead & Bower, 2000). Patient decision aids include written materials, videos, and interactive electronic presentations. Content should include information about different options and clinical outcomes, related clinical benefits, and possible side effects.

SDM is patient specific. Coupled with the concept of SDM is the concept of autonomy in which decisions need to be made about care interventions (Entwistle, Carter, Cribb, & McCaffery, 2010). The inclusion of patient values and preferences, as well as the reality of the clinical facts, is essential. Specific opportunities to determine the relevance of patient priorities in the SDM process include:

- Delivering shift reports at the bedside,
- Reviewing care plans for the day early in the shift with patients,
- Asking directly about patient/family priorities, and
- Close collaboration with other health team members to deliver quality care (Jasovsky, Morrow, Clementi, & Hindle, 2010).

Simulation Exercise 10.2 offers an opportunity to better understand the process of SDM.

SELF-MANAGEMENT IN PATIENT-CENTERED RELATIONSHIPS

Today's patients are charged to take a prominent role in their own care process, to whatever extent is possible. Barlow, Wright, Sheasby, Turner, and Hainsworth (2002) define *self-management* as "the individual's ability to manage the symptoms and the consequences of living

SIMULATION EXERCISE 10.2   Shared Decision Making

Purpose

To develop awareness of shared decision making in treatment planning.

Procedure

1. Read the following clinical situation.
2. Mr. Singer, aged 48 years, is a white, middle-class professional recovering from his second myocardial infarction. After his initial attack, Mr. Singer resumed his 10-hour workday, high-stress lifestyle, and usual high-calorie, high-cholesterol diet of favorite fast foods, alcohol, and coffee. He smokes two packs of cigarettes a day and exercises once a week by playing golf. Mr. Singer is to be discharged in 2 days. He expresses impatience to return to work, but also indicates that he would like to "get his blood pressure down and maybe drop 10 pounds."
3. Role-play this situation in dyads, with one student taking the role of the nurse, and another student taking the role of the patient.
4. Develop treatment goals that seem realistic and achievable, considering Mr. Singer's preferences, values, and health condition.
5. After the role-playing is completed, discuss some of the issues that would be relevant to Mr. Singer's situation and how they might be handled.
6. What are some concrete ways in which you could engage Mr. Singer's interest in changing his behavior to facilitate a healthier lifestyle?

with a chronic condition, including treatment, physical, social, and lifestyle changes" (p. 177). Self-management strategies are designed to enable and strengthen a patient's competence and self-efficacy in managing one or more chronic disorders. The desired outcome is to promote the active involvement of the patient in developing lifestyle habits consistent with achieving maximum health and well-being.

"Respecting and responding to patient preferences—the hall-mark of patient-centered care—means eliciting, exploring, and questioning preferences and helping patients construct them" (Epstein & Peters, 2009, p. 197). Health counseling has the potential to empower patients with the information, skills, and resources to support themselves in maintaining healthy lifestyles, continuing with treatment regimens, and/or recovering from illness or injury.

Self-Management Strategies

Patients are more motivated when the goals are clear and are important to them. They view the steps needed as being achievable and meaningful. They are not as meaningful if they are not compatible with the patient's values, or the patient does not believe he or she has the resource support to achieve or sustain self-management strategies.

Setting Realistic Goals

Exploring a patient's interest in and motivation for changing behaviors is the starting point. Self-management strategies work best when they are linked to a patient's values, interests, capabilities, and resources. The patient has to believe that a goal is both meaningful and achievable. Nurses need to get an idea about patient and family motivation to make changes. The following questions can be helpful.

How important is it for you to lose the weight?

(Learning about the patient's perspective)

"Are you interested in learning more about …?"

Patients are expected to be active agents in supporting their own health care processes. Contemporary health relationships are designed to empower patients and families to assume as much a person responsibility as possible for the self-management of chronic illness. Both nurse and patient have responsibilities to work toward agreed-on goals. Shared knowledge, negotiation, joint decision-making power, and respect for the capacity of patients to actively contribute to their health care to whatever extent is possible are essential components of the partnership required of PCC (Gallant, Beaulieu, & Carnevale, 2002).

Patient-centered relationships contribute both directly and indirectly to patient outcomes, including patient self-efficacy, empowerment, and high-quality evidence-based clinical decisions aligned with patient values and preferences (Reeve et al., 2017). Simulation Exercise 10.2 looks at SDM.

A patient-centered partnership honors the patient's right to self-determination. It gives the patient and family maximum control over health care decisions. The patient always has the autonomous right to choose personal goals and courses of action, even if they are at odds with professional recommendations. A collaborative partnership between nurse and patient leads to enhanced self-management, better health care utilization, and improved health outcomes (Hook, 2006). The tasks involved include

- discussing care management alternatives
- SDM
- development of realistic action plans.

Therapeutic Use of Self

The therapeutic relationship is not simply about what the nurse does, but who the nurse *is* in relation to patients and their families. Perhaps the most important tools nurses have at their disposal is their use of self. LaSala and O'Brien (2009) uses the words of Florence Nightingale. Nurses achieve "the moral ideal" whenever they use "the whole self" to form relationships with "the whole of the person receiving care" (p. 423). This use of self describes an optimal connection of nurse and patient in a therapeutic relationship.

Authenticity (Realness or Genuineness)

Authenticity is recognized as a precondition for the therapeutic use of self in the nurse–patient relationship. Being genuine or authentic is closely aligned with honesty. The concept builds on a person's values and is influenced by a person's culture (Van den Heever, Poggenpoel, & Myburgh, 2015).

Self-awareness is an intrapersonal process, which allows nurses to self-reflect on aspects of their personal feelings and beliefs. A common definition of self-awareness include the nurse's conscious recognition of personal thoughts, motivations, strengths and emotions, and how each can influence their behavior in the professional relationship (Monat, 2017). This gives the nurse more options to be therapeutic. For example, in a situation when a nurse realized that the respiratory therapist would be better equipped to explain the process of weaning the patient from a ventilator, she arranged for the therapist to provide the explanation, while providing her presence and support by staying with the patient during the explanation and the weaning process (Levigne & Kautz, 2010). To remain authentic, nurses need to be clear about their personal values, beliefs, stereotypes, and personal perspectives, because of their potential influence on patient decisions (McCormack & McCance, 2006; Morse, Havens, & Wilson, 1997).

Self-awareness allows nurses to engage with a patient when parts of the relationship may be painful, distasteful, or uncomfortable. Self-awareness helps identify the interpersonal space and draws the line between the nurse and patient, separating the reality of one from the other.

Self-awareness of bias or value conflicts is important to acknowledge because these factors can sabotage relationship goals. The reality is that there are some patients who are difficult to work with productively (Erlen & Jones, 1999). Much of the time, patients who are difficult are also in psychological pain, which colors how they feel about themselves and about life. Being calm, interested, but not pushy helps to make for a better interpersonal encounter. A useful strategy in such situations is to seek further understanding of the patient as a person.

Nurses need to acknowledge over-involvement, avoidance, anger, frustration, or detachment from a patient when it occurs.

Case Example

Brian Haggerty is a homeless individual who tells the nurse, "I know you want to help me, but you can't understand my situation. You have money and a husband to support you. You don't know what it is like out on the streets."

Instead of responding defensively, the nurse responds, "You are right; I don't know what it is like to be homeless, but I would like to know more about your experiences. Can you tell me what it has been like for you?"

With this listening response, the nurse invites the patient to share his experience. The data might allow the nurse to appreciate and address the loneliness, fear, and helplessness the patient is experiencing, which are universal feelings.

Presence

Being "present" in a professional relationship requires a nurse's full attention. Bridges et al. (2013) define presence as the "nurse's ability to be 'present' in the relationship (rather than adopting a work persona), to expose themselves fully to understanding the patient's and their own experiences, to be open and truthful in their dealings, and to be generous in committing to the patient's best interests" (p. 764). *Presence* involves the nurse's capacity to know when to provide help and when to stand back; when to speak frankly and when to withhold comments because the patient is not ready to hear them.

McDonough-Means and Kreitzer (2004) describe *presence* as having two dimensions: "being there" and "being with" (p. S25). Nursing presence is evidenced through active listening; relevant caring communication; and the sharing of skills, knowledge, and competencies related to patient-specific problems (McCormack & McCance, 2006; Morse et al., 1997). The gift of presence enriches the sense of self and the lives of the nurse and patient in ways that are unique to each person and situation (Covington, 2003; Easter, 2000; Hawley & Jensen, 2007).

DEVELOPING AN EVIDENCE-BASED PRACTICE

Purpose: The purpose of this scoping review of the research was to describe the inclusion of three core elements of PCC approaches: communication, partnership, and health promotion across PCC models.

Method: This scoping review explored articles published since 1990, using Medline, Cinahl, and Embase. The key terms "patient-centered" or "client-centered care," "framework" or "model," were used to identify relevant studies.

Findings: This study retrieved 101 articles, of which 19 met inclusion criteria. From these articles, 25 different patient-centered frameworks/models were identified. All identified studies incorporated communication, partnership, and health promotion. The authors noted that much empiric evidence was sourced for the most consistently defined component of PCC: communication (p. 271).

Application to Your Clinical Practice: This scoping review affirms the importance of communication, partnership and health promotion as essential components of patient-centered approaches in contemporary health care.

Modified from Constand, M. K., MacDermid, J. C., Dal Bello-Hass, V., & Law, M. (2014). Scoping review of patient-centered care approaches in health care. *BMC Health Services Research, 14,* 271–281.

APPLICATIONS

Although professional relationships in clinical settings share many characteristics with social relationships, there are structural and functional distinctions. Table 10.1 presents the differences between a (therapeutic) patient-centered relationship and a social relationship. The goal of a therapeutic relationship is ultimately promotion of the patient's health and well-being.

Having an idea of potential patient issues before meeting with the patient and family gives direction to the best clinical approach. For example, you would use a different opening approach with a patient whose infant is in the neonatal intensive care unit, and one who is "rooming in" with her healthy infant.

Valuing the Patient's Experience

"Relationship-centered care recognizes that the clinician-patient relationship is the unique product of its participants and its context" (Beach & Inui, 2006). Technology can be off-putting if it becomes the primary focus of the interaction. It is important to demonstrate during patient interviews that you value the person as a human being over technology. This is an area commented on by patients.

Preparing to Meet the Patient and Family

Awareness of your professional goals is important when initiating your first contact. This reflection allows you to select concrete and specific nursing actions that are purposeful and aligned with individualized patient needs. For example, a patient with a new diagnosis or first hospitalization has different issues than someone with a long history of similar data points in personal patient care.

Specific patient needs dictate the most appropriate interpersonal setting. In hospital settings, if the door is closed, you need to knock before entering the room. A private space in which the nurse and patient can talk without being uninterrupted is essential. When an assessment interview takes place at the bedside in a hospital setting, the door should be closed, and the curtain drawn in a two-bed room. This area is the patient's "space." Each time a nurse is sensitive to the environment in a nurse–patient relationship, the nurse models thoughtfulness, respect, and empathy. One-on-one relationships with psychiatric patients commonly take place in a designated private space away from the patient's bedroom. In the patient's home, the nurse is always the patient's guest. If the relationship is to be ongoing, for example, in a subacute, rehabilitation, or psychiatric setting, it is important to share initial plans related to time, purpose, and other details with staff. This simple strategy can avoid scheduling conflicts.

Orientation Phase

Peplau's developmental phases parallel the nursing process. The orientation phase correlates with the assessment phase of this process. The identification component of the working phase corresponds to the planning phase, whereas the working phase parallels the exploitation component of the implementation phase. The final resolution phase of the relationship corresponds to the evaluation phase of the nursing process.

Key Concepts

Nurses enter interpersonal relationships with patients in the *"stranger" role.* The patient does not know you, and you do not know the patient as a person. Nurses have an advantage as the care environment is familiar to them. This is not necessarily true for patients. Many patients not only need an introduction to the nurse, but also need an orientation to the setting, and what to expect in the assessment phase.

You can begin the process of developing trust by providing the patient with basic information about yourself (e.g., name and professional status) (Peplau, 1997). This can be a simple introduction: "Good morning, Mrs. Kenney, I am Susan Smith, a registered nurse, and I am going to be your nurse on this shift." Nonverbal supporting behaviors of a handshake, eye contact, and a smile can reinforce your words.

Introductions are important even with patients who are confused, aphasic, comatose, or unable to make a cogent response because of mental illness or dementia. Starting with the first encounter, patients begin to assess the trustworthiness of each nurse who cares for them. Sustained attention is probably the single most important indicator of relationship interest.

After introducing yourself, the next query should be: "How would you prefer to be addressed?" Simulation Exercise 10.1 is designed to give you practice in making introductory statements.

Clarifying the Purpose of the Relationship.
Clarity of purpose related to identifiable health needs is an essential dimension of the nurse-patient relationship (LaSala & O'Brien, 2009). It is difficult to fully participate in *any* working partnership without understanding its purpose and expectations. Patients need basic information about the purpose and nature of the assessment interview, including what information is needed, how the information will be used, how the patient can participate in the treatment process, and what the patient can expect from the relationship. To understand the importance of orientation information, consider the value of your having a clear syllabus and expectations for your nursing courses. It can make all the difference in actively engaging your interest.

The length and nature of the relationship dictate the depth of the orientation. An orientation given to a patient by a nurse assigned for a shift would be different from that given to a patient when the nurse assumes the role of primary care nurse over an extended period. When the relationship is of longer duration, the nurse should discuss its parameters (e.g., length of sessions, frequency of meetings, and role expectations of the nurse and patient). It is important to give the patient sufficient orientation information to feel comfortable, but not so much that it overloads the initial getting-to-know-you process.

Assessment interview meetings should have two outcomes. First, the patient should feel that the nurse is interested in him or her as a person, apart from their diagnosis. Second, the patient and nurse should emerge from the encounter with a better understanding of the most relevant health issues, and know what will happen next. At the end of the contact, the nurse should thank the patient for his or her participation, and provide the patient with easy ways to access professional help, if needed.

Establishing trust.
Carter (2009) defines **trust** as "a relational process, one that is dynamic and fragile, yet involving the deepest needs and vulnerabilities of individuals" (p. 404). Patients intuitively assess the nurse's trustworthiness through their "presence," focused attention, and actions. "Impression" data regarding the level of the nurse's interest, knowledge base, and competence are factored into the patient's decision to trust and to engage actively in the relationship. Kindness, competence, and a willingness to be actively involved get communicated through the nurse's words, tone of voice, and actions. Does the nurse seem to know what he or she is doing? Is the nurse tactful and respectful of cultural differences? Confidentiality, sensitivity to patient needs, and honesty help to confirm your trustworthiness and to strengthen the relationship. As your patient experiences you as a "person" they can depend on, their sense of vulnerability decreases (Dinc & Gastmans, 2012).

Assessing Patients' Emotional Needs in Communication.
A patient's level of trust can fluctuate with illness, age, and the influence of past successful or unsuccessful encounters with others (Carter, 2009). Modifications in your approach make a difference. For example, you would hold a different conversation with an adolescent than you would with an elderly patient. The acutely ill patient will need short contacts that are to the point, empathic, and related to providing comfort and care. Patients with mental illness typically require more time and patience to engage in a trusting relationship. The idea of having a professional person care about them—in fact, any person—in any "real way" can be incomprehensible. Having this awareness helps the nurse look beyond the bizarre behaviors that some patients present in response to their fears about helping relationships.

Case Example With a Psychiatric Patient
Nurse (with eye contact and enough interpersonal space for comfort): "Good morning, Mrs. O'Connell. My name is Karen Martin. I will be your nurse today." (Patient looks briefly at the nurse, and looks away, then gets up and moves away.)

Nurse: "This may not be a good time to talk with you. Would you mind if I checked back later with you?" (The introduction coupled with an invitation for later communication respects the patient's need for interpersonal space and allows the patient to set the pace of the relationship.)

Later, the nurse notices that Mrs. O'Connell circling around the area the nurse is occupying, but she does not directly approach the nurse. The nurse smiles encouragingly and repeats nondemanding invitations to the patient, which give the patient the time and space to become more comfortable.

Continued

Schizophrenic patients often enter and leave the space occupied by the nurse, almost circling around a space that is within visual distance of the nurse. With patience and tact, the nurse engages the patient slowly with a welcoming look and brief verbal contact. Over time, brief meetings that involve an invitation and a statement as to when the nurse will return help reduce the patient's anxiety, as indicated in the dialogue in the following case example. Many mentally ill patients respond better to shorter, frequent contacts until trust is established.

Participant observation. Peplau describes the role of the nurse in all phases of the relationship as being that of a "participant observer." This means that the nurse simultaneously actively participates in and observes the progress of the relationship as it unfolds. Observations about changes in the patient's behavior, and feedback, help direct subsequent dialogue and actions in the relationship. According to Peplau, observation includes self-awareness on the part of the nurse. This self-reflection is as critical to the success of the relationship as is the assessment of the patient's emerging responses in the relationship (McCarthy & Aquino-Russell, 2009).

Case Example

Terminally ill patient (to the nurse): "It's not the dying that bothers me as much as not knowing what is going to happen to me in the process."

Nurse: "It sounds as though you can accept the fact that you are going to die, but you are concerned about what you will have to experience. Tell me more about what worries you."

By linking the emotional context with the content of the patient's message, the nurse enters into the patient's world, and demonstrates a desire to understand the situation from the patient's perspective. Nurses need to be aware of the different physical and nonverbal cues that patients give with their verbal messages. Noting facial expressions and nonverbal cues with "You look exhausted" or "You look worried" acknowledges the presence of these emotional factors and normalizes them. Simulation Exercise 10.3 is designed to help you to critically observe a person's nonverbal cues.

Self-awareness is a critical component of participant observation. Peplau (1997) states: Nurses must observe their own behavior, as well as the patient's, with "unflinching self-scrutiny and total honesty in assessment of their behavior in interactions with

patients" (p. 162). In some ways, nurses act as a mirror for the patient, reflecting back to the patient a fuller picture of the human experience of illness and its contextual dimensions.

Self-awareness in therapeutic relationships is a reflective intrapersonal process. This introspective process helps nurses get in touch with their personal values, feelings, attitudes, motivations, strengths, and limitations—and how these reflections might color or affect the relationship with individual patients. Critically examining their own behaviors and the impact on the relationship helps nurses create a safe, trustworthy, and caring relational structure (Lowry, 2005).

Orientation phase: where to start with assessment. The patient's current health situation is a good starting place for choice of topic. Some fundamental differences such as age and first experience with a medical diagnosis are self-evident from observation and chart review, but should be verified for accuracy. Other less obvious differences may emerge as the patient tells his or her story. Framing questions based on your knowledge of developmental and

---

SIMULATION EXERCISE 10.3   Nonverbal Messages

Purpose

To provide practice in validation skills in a nonthreatening environment.

Procedure

1. Each student, in turn, tries to communicate the following feelings to other members of the group without words. They may be written on a piece of paper, or the student may choose one directly from the following list.
2. The other students must guess what behaviors the student is trying to enact.

Pain	Anxiety	Shock	Disinterest
Anger	Disapproval	Disbelief	Rejection
Sadness	Relief	Disgust	Despair
Confidence	Uncertainty	Acceptance	Uptightness

Discussion and Reflective Analysis

1. Which emotions were harder to guess from their nonverbal cues? Which ones were easier?
2. Was there more than one interpretation of the emotion?
3. How would you use the information you developed today in your future care of patients?

social determinants of health communication is important, even at this stage of the relationship. For example, individual perceptions of personal health needs, values, supportive relationships, and social concerns of adolescents, parents, older adults, etc. are quite different. A homeless patient has different life issues and concerns than a patient with a similar health condition who has good health insurance and a supportive family.

Sharing Information. Open, honest communication, and two-way sharing of information is essential for effective SDM and planning. The trust that develops within the relationship is incremental, based on mutual respect for what each person brings to the therapeutic alliance.

It is important to keep in mind that SDM "is shaped by the entire encounter—not just the point where a decision is made—and even more broadly, by the nature of the patient-provider relationship" (Matthias, Salyers, & Frankel, 2013, p. 176). Therapeutic relationships should directly revolve around the patient's needs and preferences.

You can begin to elicit data about the patient by simply asking why he or she is seeking treatment at this time. Using questions that follow a logical sequence, when there is something you do not understand, and asking only one question at a time helps a patient feel more comfortable. This strategy is likely to elicit more complete data. You can periodically check in with the patient with a simple statement such as, "I wonder if you have any questions so far…," or "is there anything you would like to add?"

An open, trusting relationship is important to the development of a realistic, committed outcome. The questions you ask should be part of a conversation, not an inquisition. Taking time to know the patient as a person means understanding the patient's thoughts and feelings about the nature of his or her health issues. It is important to assess patient strengths as these can bolster the patient's resolve and focus attention on potential new initiatives. It is important to inquire about the patient's fears and concerns about the impact of the illness or injury on their life and on important relationships. How patients perceive their health status, their reasons for seeking treatment at this time, and their expectations for health care are critical data. It is important to identify patient strengths, as these can be important in choosing and implementing targeted treatment goals. Success breeds success! Similarities and differences between patient and family perceptions of illness, and patient strengths and treatment preferences, constitute relevant supportive data.

Using empathetic responses. Empathetic responses are as critical as the information you provide, as they encourage patients and families to more fully experience the health alliance as an equal partnership. Linking statements from you, such as "I can only imagine how hard this must be for you" or, "it must have been quite a shock when this happened" acknowledge that coping with an ongoing chronic disease process can produce a serious assault to a person's sense of well-being. Most people are very concerned with a significant medical change.

If there is any reason to suspect the reliability of the patient as a historian, interviewing significant others assumes greater importance. For example, if a patient has one perception about his/her management and personal self-care, and family members have a significantly different awareness, these differences can become a nursing concern if they can't be reconciled. Differences in expectations can facilitate or hinder the treatment process. They should be discussed and documented in the patient's medical record.

Defining the problem(s). Nurses can act as a sounding board, asking questions about parts of the communication that are not understood, and helping patients to describe their problems in concrete terms. You can facilitate this process by asking for specific details to bring the patient's needs into sharper focus. For example, you can ask, "Could you describe for me what happened next," or "Tell me something about your reaction to (your problem)," or "How do you feel about…?" Time should be allowed between questions for the patient to respond fully. Commonly, such questions are asked, but sometimes not enough time is allowed for the patient to fully respond.

Feelings are essential components of any health problem. Patients usually find it easier to talk about factual data related to a problem rather than to express the feelings associated with their issue. Feelings are typically more personal reflections. Nurses can help patients connect important personal feelings with significant situations. For example, saying, "It sounds as if you feel _____ because of _____" helps the patient to express the relationship between situational data and its emotional impact. You can also ask directly "what worries you the most about your diagnosis (or what we have talked about so far?)" related to clinical issues and other patient concerns.

Understanding the Patient's Perspective. PCC requires understanding each patient's illness experience with the broader framework of

- life history, including unique personal and developmental issues;
- family history and level of social support;
- employment, school, and community background;
- cultural background and spiritual connections;
- quality of life, financial resources, and knowledge of support services (Scholl, Zill, Harter, & Dirmaier, 2014).

All involved care providers have a legal and ethical responsibility to participate in helping patients understand the nature of an illness as a basis for developing meaningful options in resolving it. Once the nurse and patient develop a working definition of the problem, the next step is to brainstorm the best ways to meet treatment goals. The brainstorming process occurs more easily when you as a nurse are relaxed, and are willing to understand views different from your own. Brainstorming involves generating multiple ideas, while suspending judgment until all possibilities are presented. However, having evidence-based knowledge of potential treatment goals, risk/benefit ratios, and other options are essential components of effective SDM.

The next step is to look realistically at ideas that could work, given the resources that the patient has available right now, and patient preferences. Resistance can be worked through with the empathetic reality testing of various options. Peplau (1997) suggests that a general rule of thumb in working with patients is to "struggle with the problem, not with the patient" (p. 164).

The last component of the assessment process relates to determining the kind of help needed, and who can best provide it. Careful consideration of the most appropriate sources of help is an important, but often overlooked, part of the assessment process needed in the planning phase.

Defining goals. Self-management goals should be based on the patient's values, preferences, and capabilities in relation to personalized goal achievement. Chosen health goals should have meaning to the patient. For example, modifying the exchange lists with a diabetic adolescent's input so that they include substitutions that follow normal adolescent eating habits can facilitate acceptance of unwelcome dietary restrictions. The nurse conveys confidence in the patient's capacity to solve his or her own problems by expecting the patient to provide data, to make constructive suggestions, and to develop realistic goals. This strategy also helps ensure that the patient's preferences and values are discussed and incorporated.

Working (Exploitation/Active Intervention) Phase

With relevant patient-centered goals to guide nursing interventions and patient actions, the conversation turns to active problem solving related to assessed health care needs. Patients are better able to discuss deeper, more difficult issues, and to experiment with new roles and actions in the working phase, and the relationship with provider nurses is judged to be trustworthy as a guide to action. Corresponding to the *implementation phase* of the nursing process, the working phase focuses on self-directed actions related to personal health goals, the self-monitoring of changes, and the self-management of personal health care, to whatever extent is possible in promoting the patient's health and well-being.

Supporting Patient Self-Management Strategies

Helping patients develop realistic self-management strategies is a key concept in caring for patients experiencing chronic disorders. Johnson, McMorris, MapelLentz, and Scal (2015) note: "***Effective self-management*** requires autonomous action, and active participation in health-related decision making and behaviors," (p. 666). Asking, "what is the most important outcome you hope to accomplish in managing your health issues?" is a good lead in to this discussion. Avoid taking more responsibility for actions than the patient or situation requires. For example, it may seem more efficient time-wise to give a bath to a stroke victim, but what happens when this patient goes home and lacks either the confidence or the skills to complete this task safely?

Self-management is defined as a patient's ability to manage the symptoms and consequences of living with a chronic condition, including treatment, physical, social, and lifestyle changes (Barlow et al., 2002). Self-management strategies identify the focus of action plans for health problems in contemporary health care. Nurses should provide enough structure and guidelines for patients to explore problem issues and to develop realistic solutions—but no more than is needed. Lorig and Holman (2003) developed a classic, thorough article on the history, meaning, tasks, and outcomes of self-management. Breaking a seemingly insoluble problem down into simpler chunks is a nursing strategy that makes doing difficult tasks more manageable. For example, a goal of eating three meals a day may seem overwhelming to a person suffering from nausea and loss of appetite associated with gastric medical issues. A smaller goal of having small amounts of applesauce or chicken soup and a glass of milk three times a day may sound more achievable, particularly if the patient can choose the times and the food. In difficult nursing situations, there are options, even if the choice is to die with dignity or to change one's attitude toward an illness or a family member. The patient's right to make decisions, provided they do not violate self or others, needs to be accepted by the nurse, even when it runs contrary to the nurse's thinking. This action protects the patient's right to autonomy.

Tuning in to the patient's response patterns. Tuning in to the patient's response patterns emphasizes shared information, and joint actions that connect, collaborate, and create new possibilities for health and well-being. In the process of shared inquiry about the issues at hand, new possibilities can emerge, even in brief encounters. Nurses are in a position to be able to discuss and affirm the unique integration of biological and social processes that can influence a successful recovery process.

The art of nursing requires that nurses recognize differences in individual patient response patterns. Elderly adults may need a slower pace. People in crisis usually respond better to a simple structured level of support and may need repetition. It is not unusual for patients and families to completely forget what has been said in a stressful situation (Gaston & Mitchell, 2005).

Throughout the working phase, nurses need to be sensitive about whether the patient is still responding at a useful level. Looking at difficult problems and developing strategies to resolve those problems is not an easy process, especially when resolution requires significant behavioral changes. If the nurse is perceived as inquisitive, rather than facilitative, communication breaks down.

Nurses have a responsibility to pace interactions in ways that offer support as well as challenge. Deciding whether to proceed or to pause to consider issues that may have arisen is a clinical judgment. This decision should be based on the patient's verbal responses and overall body language. Warning signs that the pace may need adjustment include changes in facial expression, loss of eye contact, fidgeting, abrupt changes in subject, or asking to be left alone.

Strong emotion should not necessarily be interpreted as reflecting a level of interaction stretching beyond the patient's tolerance. Tears or an emotional outburst may reflect honestly felt emotion. A well-placed comment, such as, "I can see that this is difficult for you," acknowledges the feeling, and may stimulate further discussion.

Health disruptions create distress and usually require adaptive changes in more than one life domain. In addition to providing direct care, nurses need to help patients and families cope with unique emotional and reality challenges associated with the patient's health disruption (see Chapter 16).

Most problems, should they arise, should be treated as temporary setbacks that provide new information about what needs to happen next. Helping patients develop alternative strategies to successfully cope with unexpected responses can strengthen a patient's problem-solving abilities. Alternative options (i.e., a Plan B) when an original plan does not bring about the desired results can be empowering.

Shared Decision Making. Barry and Edgman-Levitan (2012) identify SDM as the "pinnacle of patient-centered care" (p. 780). Effective decision making represents both a cognitive and an interpersonal process. This concept requires transparent communication because of the active involvement of patients and families that is needed to consider the pros and cons of treatment options. Decisions should reflect patient priorities, preferences, and values, as well as the reality of the clinical situation. In addition to providing patients with information about their disease process or injury, patients need to have a clear understanding of treatment options related to the side effects and the potential consequences of each option, including what happens if no treatment is given.

Elwyn et al. (2012) outline three key steps in an effective SDM process model. They label these as:

- *Choice talk*: consists of finding out what information the patient has, how much information the patient wants, and who should be involved in the decision-making process. Inquiry into patient goals and concerns can help frame the option talk in the next step. Choice talk also requires assessing whether or not the information a patient already has is the correct information.
- *Option talk*: consists of providing sufficient and relevant information about potential treatment options, the risks involved, the pros and cons of one option versus another. This discussion should consider what the health provider knows about the patient's values, preferences, priorities, and concerns. The extent of risk, and the potential for outcome uncertainty should be included in the discussion. It is important to check in with patients about their potential fears, expectations, and other ideas that they may have about different options.
- *Decision talk*: involves participatory active engagement, because this is when the patient needs to make a decision. Whenever possible, patients should not be forced to make a choice without being ready to make one. It is helpful to ask, "Are you ready to make a decision, or do you need more time to think about it?" Some patients need not only time, but also more information. They may want to consult with others who would be affected. This is particularly true for patients from a high context culture. It is critical that the decision be based on each patient's informed choice. Having additional opportunities to revisit what led to the decision helps to confirm that the patient is comfortable with the decision.

Defusing challenging behaviors. Challenging behaviors can sabotage a therapeutic relationship. There is no unique way to approach a difficult patient, and no single interpersonal strategy that works equally well with every patient. Some patients clearly are more emotionally accessible and attractive to work with than others, but virtually every patient is anxious and many times what a nurse encounters as anger or despondency is covering anxiety. When a patient seems unapproachable or is hostile, it may not be easy to maintain an empathetic response pattern. However, it is important because so often the patient is projecting his/her anxiety onto a person he/she knows is less likely to retaliate. Other times, the patient may appear disinterested in meaningful conversation, but the same patient factors of anxiety or powerlessness may be operative.

Case Example

I tried, but he just wasn't interested in talking to me. I asked him some questions, but he didn't really answer me. So, I tried to ask him about his hobbies and interests. It didn't matter what I asked him, he just turned away. Finally, I gave up because it was obvious that he just didn't want to talk to me. Although, from this nurse's perspective, the behavior of the patient in this case example may represent a lack of desire for

Continued

a relationship, in many cases the rejection is not personal. It can reflect boredom, insecurity, or physical discomfort. Anxiety expressed as anger or unresponsiveness may be the only way a patient can control fear in a difficult situation. Rarely does it have much to do with the interpersonal approach used by the nurse, unless the nurse is truly insensitive to the patient's feelings or the needs of the situation. In this situation, the nurse might say, "It seems to me that you just want to be alone right now, but I would like to help you, so if you don't mind, I'll check back later with you. Would that be okay?" Most of the time, patients appreciate the nurse's willingness to stay involved.

For novice nurses, it is important to recognize that all nurses have experienced some form of patient rejection at one time or another. It is helpful to explore whether the timing was right, whether the patient was in pain or was feeling overwhelmed without being able to process the reasons why, and—potentially—what other circumstances might have contributed to the patient's attitude. Behaviors that initially seem maladaptive may appear quite adaptive when the full circumstances of the patient's situation are understood. A question you might want to consider is: Are you at your best, from any perspective, when you are feeling angry or anxious?

Before confronting a patient, you should anticipate possible outcomes. You will be more successful if you take the time to appreciate the impact of the confrontation on a patient's self-esteem. Calling a patient's attention to a contradiction in behavioral response is usually threatening. Preserving the patient's personal dignity is a basic human right that nurses should always keep in mind, irrespective of the patient's external behaviors (Stievano, Rocco, Sabatino, & Alvaro, 2013).

Giving constructive feedback. Constructive feedback involves drawing the patient's attention to the existence of unacceptable behaviors or contradictory messages while respecting the fragility of the therapeutic alliance, and the patient's need to protect the integrity of his/her self-concept. To be effective, constructive confrontations are best attempted when the following criteria have been met:
- The nurse has established a firm, trusting bond with the patient.
- The timing and environmental circumstances are appropriate.
- The confrontation is delivered in a private setting, in a nonjudgmental, calm, and empathetic manner.
- Only those behaviors capable of being changed by the patient are up for discussion.

- The nurse supports the patient's autonomy and right to self-determination as long as it does not interfere with the rights of others.

Case Example

Mary Kiernan is 5 feet 2 inches tall and weighs 260 pounds. She has attended weekly weight management sessions for the past 6 weeks. Although she lost 8 pounds the first week, 4 pounds in week 2, and another 4 pounds by week 5, her weight loss seems to have hit a plateau. Jane Tompkins, her primary nurse, notices that Mary seems to be able to stick to the diet until she gets to dessert, then she cannot resist temptation. Mary is very discouraged about her lack of further progress. Consider the effect of each response on the patient.

Response A
Nurse: You're supposed to be on a 1200-calorie-a-day diet, but instead you're sneaking dessert. If you eat dessert when you are on a diet, you are kidding yourself that you will lose weight.

Response B
Nurse: I can understand your discouragement, but you have done quite well in losing 16 pounds. It seems as though you can stick to the diet until you get to dessert. Do you think we need to talk a little more about what hooks you when you get to dessert? Do you want to consider finding some alternatives that would help you get back on track?

The first statement is direct, valid, and concise, but it is likely to be disregarded or experienced as being unfeeling by the patient. The patient already knows the information the nurse has shared. In the second response, the nurse reframes a behavioral inconsistency as a temporary setback. By initially introducing an observed strength of the progress achieved so far, the nurse reaffirms trust in the patient's resourcefulness, while proposing that the problem might be resolved in a different way. Both responses require similar amounts of time and energy on the part of the nurse; however, the patient is likely to accept the nurse's second comment as being more supportive if constructive criticism is paired with an acknowledgment of the patient's strong points.

Self-disclosure. **Self-disclosure** refers to an intentional (limited) sharing of relevant personal data used to enhance the nurse-patient relationship. Deering (1999) suggests that appropriate self-disclosure can facilitate the relationship, providing the patient with information that is both immediate and personalized.

The following are guidelines for keeping *self-disclosure* at a therapeutic level:

1. Keep your disclosure brief and relevant to the patient's situation.
2. Do not imply that your lived experience is exactly the same as the patient's experience.
3. Do not share intimate details of your life.

The nurse, not the patient, is responsible for regulating the amount of disclosure needed to facilitate the relationship. If the patient asks a nonoffensive, superficial question, the nurse may answer briefly with a minimum of information, and return to a patient focus. Simple questions such as, "Where did you go to nursing school?" and "Do you have any children?" may simply represent the patient's effort to establish common ground for conversation (Morse, 1991).

Answering the patient briefly but returning the focus to the patient is a good guideline. You can make a simple statement such as, "This is your time, and I think I can help you best by hearing more about …" (identify the patient's medical concern, clinical question, or reason for seeking care). Simulation Exercise 10.4 provides an opportunity to explore self-disclosure in the nurse-patient relationship.

Termination Phase

Unlike social relationships, therapeutic relationships have a predetermined ending. They typically end when treatment outcomes have been achieved, the patient has been discharged, or the number of visits authorized by insurance has been achieved. In the termination phase, the nurse and patient jointly evaluate the patient's responses to treatment and explore the meaning of the relationship and what goals have been achieved. Discussing patient achievements and patient-centered plans for the future are activities with relevance for the termination phase.

Termination is a significant issue in long-term settings such as skilled nursing facilities, bone marrow transplant units, rehabilitation hospitals, and state psychiatric facilities. Meaningful long-term relationships can and do develop in these settings. If the relationship has been effective, real work has been accomplished. Nurses need to be sufficiently aware of their own feelings so that they may use them constructively without imposing them on the patient. It is appropriate for nurses to share some of the meaning the relationship held for them, as long as such sharing fits the needs of the interpersonal situation and is not excessive or too emotionally intense.

Termination of a PCC relationship should be final. To provide the patient with even a hint that the relationship will continue is unfair. Continuing to communicate with a patient through social media can be an inadvertent boundary

---

SIMULATION EXERCISE 10.4   Self-Disclosure Assessing Nurse Role Limitations in Self-Disclosure

Purpose

To help students differentiate between a therapeutic use of self-disclosure and spontaneous self-revelation.

Procedure

1. Make a list of **three phrases** that describe your own personality or the way you relate to others, such as the following:

I am shy.
I get angry when criticized.
I'm nice.
I'm smart.
I'm sexy.
I find it hard to handle conflicts.
I'm interested in helping people.

2. Mark each descriptive phase with one of the following:

A = Too embarrassing or intimate to discuss in a group.
B = Could discuss with a group of peers.
C = If disclosed, this behavior characteristic might affect my ability to function in a therapeutic manner.

3. Share your responses with the group.

Discussion and Reflective Analysis

1. What criteria did you use to determine the appropriateness of self-disclosure?
2. How much variation was there in what each student would feel comfortable sharing with others in a group or clinical setting? And why?
3. Were there any behaviors commonly agreed on that would never be shared with a patient?
4. What interpersonal factors or behaviors of a patient would facilitate or impede self-disclosure by the nurse in the clinical setting?
5. What did you learn from doing this exercise that could be used in future encounters with patients?

---

violation" (Ashton, 2016). It keeps the patient emotionally involved in a relationship that no longer has a health-related goal. This is a difficult issue for nursing students who see no harm in telling the patient they will continue to keep in contact. However, this perception underestimates the positive things that the patient received from the relationship, and limits your time for other patient responsibilities. For the current patient, it is important to help him or her move to the next step of their journey. When the patient is unable to express feelings about endings, the nurse may recognize them in the patient's nonverbal behavior.

Case Example

A teenager who had spent many months on a bone marrow transplant unit had developed a real attachment to her primary nurse, who had stood by her during the frightening physical assaults to her body and appearance occasioned by the treatment. The patient was unable to verbally acknowledge the meaning of the relationship with the nurse directly, despite having been given many opportunities to do so by the nurse. The patient said she could not wait to leave this awful hospital and that she was glad she did not have to see the nurses anymore. Yet, this same teenager was found sobbing in her room the day she left, and she asked the nurse whether she could write to her. The relationship obviously had meaning for the patient, but she was unable to express it verbally.

Gift giving. Patients sometimes wish to give nurses gifts at the end of a constructive relationship because they value the care provided by the nurse. Accepting gifts from patients requires careful reflection and professional judgment by the nurse. Nurses should consider two questions: what meaning does the gift have for the relationship, and in what ways might acceptance change the dynamics of the therapeutic alliance? Token gifts, such as chocolates or flowers, may be acceptable. In general, nurses should not accept money or gifts of significant material value. Should this become an issue, you might suggest making the gift to the health care agency, or a charity. It is always appropriate to simply thank the patient for their generosity and thoughtfulness (Lambert, 2009). Simulation Exercise 10.5 is designed to help you think about the implications of gift giving in the nurse-patient relationship.

Evaluation. Objective evaluation of clinical outcomes achieved in the nurse-patient relationship should focus on the following:
- Was the problem definition adequate and appropriate for the patient?
- Were the interventions chosen adequate, consistent with patient preferences, and appropriate to resolve the patient's problem?
- Were the interventions implemented effectively and efficiently to both the patient's and the nurse's satisfaction within the allotted time frame?
- Is the patient progressing toward maximum health and well-being?
- Is the patient satisfied with his or her progress and care received?
- What type of follow-up care or self-monitoring is needed?

SIMULATION EXERCISE 10.5
Understanding Applications of Maslow's Hierarchy of Needs

Purpose
To help students understand the usefulness of Maslow's theory in prioritizing patient needs. Identify one student as group scribe for each small group of students.

Procedure
1. Divide the class into small groups, with each group assigned to a step of Maslow's hierarchy. Each group will then brainstorm examples of different ways a patient need at each level might be expressed in clinical practice.
2. Identify potential responses from the nurse that might address each need.
3. Share examples with the larger group and discuss the concept of prioritization of needs using Maslow's hierarchy.

Reflective Discussion Analysis
1. In what ways is Maslow's hierarchy helpful to the nurse in prioritizing patient needs?
2. What limitations, if any, do you see with the theory?
3. How could you apply Maslow's hierarchy to patients in your clinical setting?

- If follow-up care is indicated, is the patient satisfied with the recommendation and able to carry forward his or her treatment plan in the community?

Adaptation for Brief Relationships

Hagerty and Patusky (2003) have argued the need to reconceptualize brief therapeutic relationships. Here are some suggestions for relating to patients in brief therapeutic relationships. Four essential qualities are needed to establish relatedness in short-term relationships: "sense of belonging, reciprocity, mutuality and synchrony" (Moser, Houtepen, Spreeuwenberg, & Widdershoven, 2010, p. 218). Developing a brief relationship with patients represents a *working alliance with active support.* The same recommendations for self-awareness, empathy, therapeutic boundaries, active listening, competence, mutual respect, partnership, and level of involvement hold true as key elements of even the briefest therapeutic relationships.

Orientation Phase

Following introductions and initial comments, the therapeutic alliance begins with a "here and now" focus on

SIMULATION EXERCISE 10.6   Identifying Patient Strengths

Purpose

To identify personal strengths in patients with serious illness.

Procedure

1. Think about a patient you have had with a serious or prolonged chronic illness.
2. What personal strengths does this person possess that could have a healing impact? For example, strengths can be courage, patience, fighting spirit, family, and so on.
3. Write a one-page description of the patient and the personal strengths observed, despite the patient's medical or psychological condition.

Discussion and Reflective Analysis

1. If you didn't have to write the description, would you have been as aware of the patient's strengths?
2. How could you help the patient maximize his or her strengths to achieve quality of life?
3. What did you learn from this exercise that you can use in your future clinical practice?

problem identification, and an emphasis on quickly understanding the context in which the problem is embedded. Start with the patient's chief concern, followed by the patient's symptoms and the personal and emotional context in which they occur. Allowing the patient to tell his or her personalized story of an illness or injury with minimum interruptions, conveys respect and interest (Nicholson et al., 2010).

Listen for what is left out, and pay attention to what the patient's story elicits in you. Acknowledge the patient's feelings with a statement such as "Tell me more about..." (with a theme picked up from the patient's choice of words, hesitancy, or nonverbal cues), which usually prompts further explanations.

Anderson (2001) echoes Rogers' belief that all people have potential for self-constructive behaviors. As you interact with the patient, there will be opportunities to observe patient strengths, and to comment on them. Every patient has healthy aspects of his or her personality and personal strengths that can be drawn on to facilitate individual coping responses. Building on personal strengths a person already has feels more familiar. Simulation Exercise 10.6 provides an opportunity to explore the value of acknowledging personal strengths.

Even the briefest therapeutic encounter should be patient-centered with an emphasis on understanding the patient's personalized experience of an illness and its social context (Bardes, 2012). A simple statement posed at the beginning of each shift, such as, "What is your most important need today?" or "What is the most important thing I can do for you today?" helps focus the relationship on immediate concerns that are important to the patient (Cappabianca, Julliard, Raso, & Ruggiero, 2009). This type of concern allows the patient and you to develop a shared understanding of what is uniquely important to the patient in the present moment. Researchers consider PCC as being "defined by a focus on outcomes that people notice and care about including, not only survival, but function, symptoms and modifiable aspects of quality of life (QOL)" (Rodriguez, Mayo, & Gagnon, 2013, p. 1795).

Focusing on Essential Information

The nurse's goal as a health provider is to gather accurate, reliable information. Because the time frame for a patient-centered relationship may last only a few hours or days, nurses need to focus on what is absolutely essential, rather than on everything that might be nice to know.

Finding out how much the patient already knows can save time. You also can ask the patient directly: "What is your greatest concern at this moment?" Another view involves looking at the patient's needs from a broader contextual perspective, one that takes into consideration which problems, if treated, would also help correct other health problems. This has a double benefit in terms of patient success and satisfaction.

The more actively engaged your patient is in the assessment and planning process, the easier it is to find common ground. Planning will be smoother if you and your patient choose problems critical to moderating their illness experience. Choose goals first that are of interest to the patient as these offer the best return on your investment. Two basic questions are, what does this illness's symptoms mean to the patient and what is your patient's primary concern?

Ask about the patient's daily routine. Tailoring your coaching and support to a patient's level of activation and encouraging small achievable steps are actions that help maximize interest and the effectiveness of self-management strategies (Greene & Hibbard, 2012).

Engaging the patient's family early in the treatment process is also essential. Nurses must be familiar enough with the patient's symptoms and behaviors so they can accurately communicate the meaning of symptoms and suffering to family members, or other health care colleagues and team members. This data allow nurses to advocate for their patients (Bridges et al., 2013). This is also important from the perspective of discharge as most patients have to manage their recovery in home environments with less supervision and coaching.

As nurses increasingly move from a bedside role into a managerial coordination role, they become responsible for clarifying, integrating, and coordinating different aspects of the patient's care as part of an interprofessional team (see Chapter 22). An important component of this responsibility is ensuring that the patient and the family understand and are able to negotiate treatment initiatives with health care team providers. The nurse is frequently the liaison resource between the team and the patient/family for follow-up explanations.

Working Phase

Brief relationships should be solution-focused right from the start. Giving patients your undivided attention, and using concise active listening responses is essential to understanding the complexity of issues facing patients.

Adapting one's lifestyle to compensate for the demands of a chronic disease is difficult (Friesen-Storms, Bours, Van der Weijdn, & Beurskens, 2015). A central focus, agreed on by nurse and patient, promotes the small behavioral changes, and related coping skills needed to meet patient goals. Patients tend to work best with nurses who appear confident and empathetic. One way of helping patients discover the solutions that fit them best is by engaging them in determining and implementing activities to meet therapeutic goals at every realistic opportunity. Conveying a realistic hopeful attitude that the goals developed with the patient are likely to be achieved is important.

Action plans should be as simple and specific as possible. Changes in the patient's condition or other circumstances may require treatment modifications that should be expected in short-term relationships. Keeping patients and families informed, and working with them on alternative solutions, is essential to maintaining trust in short-term relationships.

Termination Phase

The termination phase in short-term relationships can include discharge planning, agency referrals, and arranging follow-up appointments in the community for the patient and family. Anticipatory guidance in the form of simple instructions or a review of important skills is appropriate. Coordination of post discharge plans with other health care disciplines, families, and communities

---

SIMULATION EXERCISE 10.7   What Is Patient-Centered Care?

Purpose

To stimulate a reflective discussion of the dimensions of PCC.

Procedure

1. Watch the World Health Organization video "what is people-centered care?" (Short video, <3 min, available on YouTube.)
2. Write a one-page descriptor of a patient in which you discuss his/her personal strengths, for example, fighting spirit, family, and patient preferences or values.
3. How can you specifically implement PCC in your clinical setting?
4. What fundamental changes would you need to implement to advance the purposes of PCC for your patient?

---

to support positive patient health changes should be the norm, not the exception. It is important to check with the patient's family about the level of support they will be able to provide. Usually, the nurse has never seen the patient's home and knows little about the patient's family life. Check with the hospitalist or discharging physician; share the expected departure time with the staff, and ensure the patient has everything in order before leaving the facility.

The importance of the relationship, no matter how brief, should not be underestimated. Simulation Exercise 10.7 Sudden illness or exacerbations of a chronic illness dramatically change a person's life—often in unexpected ways. Although your patient may be one of several persons you have taken care of during a shift, the relationship may represent the only interpersonal or professional contact available to a lonely and frightened person. Even if contact has been brief, you should stop by to say goodbye, and to check that everything is in order before you leave. The dialogue in such cases can be simple and short: "Mr. Jones, I will be going off duty in a few minutes. I enjoyed working with you. Miss Smith will be taking care of you this evening. Is there anything I can do for you before I go?" Check to see if the patient has the call button. If the patient has a white board with caregiver names on it, you should put the names of the next nurse and ancillary staff person who will care for the patient. If you will not be returning at a later date, you should briefly share this information with the patient.

SUMMARY

The nurse-patient relationship represents a purposeful use of self in all professional relations with patients and other people involved with the patients. Respect for the dignity of the patient and self, person-centered communication, and authenticity in conversation are process threads underlying all communication responses.

Therapeutic relationships have professional boundaries, purposes, and behaviors. Boundaries keep the relationship safe for the patient. They spell out the parameters of the therapeutic relationship, and the nurses are ethically responsible for maintaining them throughout the relationship. Effective relationships enhance the well-being of the patient and the professional growth of the nurse. The professional relationship goes through a developmental process characterized by four overlapping yet distinct stages: pre-interaction, orientation, working phase, and termination phase. The pre-interaction phase is the only phase of the relationship the patient is not part of. During the pre-interaction phase the nurse develops the appropriate physical and interpersonal environment for an optimal relationship in collaboration with other health professionals and significant others in the patient's life.

The orientation phase of the relationship defines the purpose, roles, and rules of the process, and provides a framework for assessing patient needs. The nurse builds a sense of trust through consistency of actions. Data collection forms the basis for developing relevant nursing diagnoses. The orientation phase ends with a therapeutic contract mutually defined by nurse and patient.

The working phase is the problem-solving phase of the relationship, paralleling the planning and implementation phases of the nursing process. As the patient begins to explore difficult problems and feelings, the nurse uses a variety of interpersonal strategies to help the patient develop new insights and methods of coping.

The final phase of the nurse-patient relationship occurs when the essential work of the intervention phase is complete. The ending should be thoroughly and compassionately defined early enough in the relationship so that the patient can process it appropriately. Primary tasks associated with the termination phase of the relationship include summarization and evaluation of completed activities and referrals when indicated. Short-term relationships incorporate the same skills and competencies as traditional nurse-patient relationships, but with a sharper focus on the here and now. The action plan needs to be as simple and specific as possible.

ETHICAL DILEMMA: What Would You Do? LaSala and O'Brien (2009) presents a case example (courtesy Lindsey O'Brien) in which a patient with lymphoma refused a blood transfusion after her first round of chemotherapy. Her physician was upset that she would not accept this logical treatment. The nurse in this case example said, "I explained to him what her beliefs were and why she refused blood. He continued to look confused, and I said, 'We may not understand it fully, but we have to respect her decision and not let our personal opinions impede our care.' He looked at me and said I was absolutely right" (LaSala & O'Brien, 2009, p. 425 [quote from O'Brien]).

Reflective Analysis Discussion Questions
1. In what ways do organizational structure and expectations in your clinical setting enhance or impede development of therapeutic relationships in nursing care?
2. What does the phrase "being present in health care relationships" mean?
3. How does a relational partnership support effective patient and family decision-making processes?
4. What do you see as the most important attribute of PCC? What is the basis for your choice?

REFERENCES

American Hospital Association (AHA). (2003). *The Patient care partnership: Understanding expectations, rights and responsibilities.* Retrieved from: http://www.aha.org/content/00-10/pcp_english_030730.pdf.

American Nurses Association. (2010). *Nursing: scope and standards of practice* (2nd ed.). Silver spring, MD: Author.

Anderson, H. (2001). Postmodern collaborative and person-centered therapies: What would Carl Rogers say? *Journal of Family Therapy, 23*(4), 339–360.

Bandura, A. (2012). On the functional properties of perceived self-efficacy revisited. *Journal of Management, 38*, 9–44.

Bardes, C. (2012). Defining patient-centered medicine. *Journal of Nursing Education, 366*, 782–783.

Barlow, J., Wright, C., Sheasby, J., Turner, A., & Hainsworth, J. (2002). Self-management approaches for people with chronic conditions: A review. *Patient Education and Counseling, 48,* 177–187.

Barry, M., & Edgman-Levitan, S. (2012). Shared decision making—The pinnacle of patient centered care. *Journal of Nursing Education, 366*(9), 780–781.

Bartz, C. (2010). International Council of Nurses and person-centered care. *International Journal of Integrated Care, 10*(Suppl.), e010.

Batalden, P., Ogrinc, G., & Batalden, K. (2006). From one to many. *Journal of Interprofessional Care, 20*(5), 549–551.

Beach, M. C., & Inui, T. (2006). Relationship-centered care research network, relationship-centered care: A constructive reframing. *Journal of General Internal Medicine, 21*(Suppl. 1), S3–S8.

Benbow, D. (2013). Professional boundaries: when does the nurse–patient relationship end? *Journal of Nursing Regulation, 4*(2), 30–33.

Bodenheim, T., Wagner, E., & Grumbach, K. (2002). Improving primary care for patients with chronic illness: the chronic care model. *The Journal of the American Medical Association, 288,* 1775–1779.

Bridges, J., Nicholson, C., Maben, J., Pope, C., Flatley, M., Wilkinson, C., et al. (2013). Capacity for care: meta-ethnography of acute care nurses' experiences of the nurse patient relationship. *Journal of Advanced Nursing, 69*(4), 760–772.

Bruner, B., & Yonge, O. (2006). Boundaries and adolescents in residential treatment centers: What clinicians need to know. *Journal of Psychosocial Nursing and Mental Health Services, 44*(9), 38–44.

Cappabianca, A., Julliard, K., Raso, R., & Ruggiero, J. (2009). Strengthening the nurse-patient relationship: What is the most important thing I can do for you today. *Creative Nursing, 15*(3), 151–156.

Carmack, B. (1997). Balancing engagement and disengagement in caregiving. *Image (IN), 29*(2), 139–144.

Carter, M. (2009). Trust, power, and vulnerability: A discourse on helping in nursing. *Nursing Clinics of North America, 44,* 393–405.

Committee on Quality Care in America. (2001). *Crossing the quality chasm: A new health system for the 21st century.* Washington, DC: Institute of Medicine.

Covington, H. (2003). Caring presence: Delineation of a concept for holistic nursing. *Journal of Holistic Nursing, 21*(3), 301–317.

Crowe, M. (2000). The nurse-patient relationship: A consideration of its discursive content. *Journal of Advanced Nursing, 31*(4), 962–967.

Deering, C. G. (1999). To speak or not to speak? Self-disclosure with patients. *American Journal of Nursing, 99*(1 Pt 1), 34–38.

Dinc, L., & Gastmans, C. (2012). Trust and trustworthiness in nursing: An argument-based literature review. *Nursing Inquiry, 19*(3), 223–237.

Dolansky, M., & Moore, S. (2013). Quality and safety education for nurses (QSEN). The key is systems thinking. *Online Journal of Issues in Nursing, 18*(3), 1.

Easter, A. (2000). Construct analysis of four modes of being present. *Journal of Holistic Nursing, 18*(4), 362–377.

Egan, G. (2014). *The skilled helper: A problem-management and opportunity-development approach to helping* (10th ed.). Belmont, CA: Brooks Cole, Cengage Learning.

Elwyn, G., Frosch, D., Thompson, R., Joseph-Williams, N., Lloyd, A., Kinnersley, P., et al. (2012). Shared decision making: A model for clinical practice. *Journal of General Internal Medicine, 27,* 1361–1367.

Entwistle, V., Carter, S., Cribb, A., & McCaffery, K. (2010). Supporting patient autonomy: The importance of clinician-patient relationships. *Journal of General Internal Medicine, 25*(7), 741–745.

Epstein, R. M., & Peters, E. (2009). Beyond patients' preference. *Journal of the American Medical Association, 302*(2), 195–197.

Erlen, J. A., & Jones, M. (1999). The patient no one liked. *Orthopedic Nursing, 18*(4), 76–79.

Ferguson, L., Ward, H., Card, S., Sheppard, S., & McMurty, J. (2013). Putting the 'patient' back into patient-centered care: An education perspective. *Nurse Education in Practice, 13,* 283–287.

Friesen-Storms, J., Bours, G., Van der Weijedn, T., & Beurskens, A. (2015). Shared decision making in chronic care in the context of evidence based practice in nursing. *International Journal of Nursing Studies, 52,* 393–402.

Fronek, P., Kendall, M., Ungerer, G., Malt, J., Eugarde, E., & Geraghty, T. (2009). Towards healthy professional-patient relationships: The value of an interprofessional training course. *Journal of Interprofessional Care, 23*(10), 16–29.

Gallant, M., Beaulieu, M., & Carnevale, F. (2002). Partnership: An analysis of the concept within the nurse-patient relationship. *Journal of Advanced Nursing, 2,* 149–157.

Gaston, C., & Mitchell, G. (2005). Information giving and decision-making in patients with advanced cancer. *Social Science & Medicine, 61*(10), 2252–2264.

Greene, J., & Hibbard, J. (2012). Why does patient activation matter? An examination of the relationships between patient activation and health-related outcomes. *Journal of General Internal Medicine, 27,* 520–526.

Hagerty, B., & Patusky, K. (2003). Reconceptualizing the nurse-patient relationship. *Journal of Nursing Scholarship, 35*(2), 145–150.

Hawley, M. P., & Jensen, L. (2007). Making a difference in critical care nursing practice. *Qualitative Health Research, 17*(5), 663–674.

Hibbard J. (2017). Patient activation and the use of information to support important health decisions.

Hofmann, P. (2009). Addressing compassion fatigue. The problem is not new, but it requires more urgent attention. *Healthcare Executive, 24*(5), 40–42.

Hook, M. (2006). Partnering with patients—A concept ready for action. *Journal of Advanced Nursing, 56*(2), 133–143.

Institute of Medicine (IOM). (2001). *Crossing the quality chasm: A new health system for the 21st century.* Washington, DC: National Academies Press.

IOM. (2003). *Institute of Medicine (IOM) health professions education: A bridge to quality.*

Jasovsky, D., Morrow, M., Clementi, P., & Hindle, P. A. (2010). Theories in action and how nursing practice changed. *Nursing Science Quarterly, 23*(1), 29–38.

Johnson, K., McMorris, B., MapelLentz, S., & Scal, P. (2015). Improving self-management through patient-centered communication. *Journal of Adolescent Health, 57*(6), 666–672.

Lambert, K. (2009). Gifts and gratuities for the case manager. *Professional Case Management, 14*(1), 53–54.

Lazenby, M. (2013). On the humanities of nursing. *Nursing Outlook, 61*(1), e9–e14.

Levigne, D., & Kautz, D. D. (2010). The evidence for listening and teaching may reside in our hearts. *Medsurg Nursing, 19*, 194–196.

Lhussier, M., Eaton, W., Forster, N., Thomas, M., Roberts, S., & Carr, S. M. (2015). Care planning for long term conditions—A concept mapping. *Health Expectations, 18*, 605–624.

Lorig, K., & Holman, H. (2003). Self-management education: History, definition, outcomes, and mechanisms. *Annals of Behavioral Medicine, 26*(1), 1–7.

Lowry, M. (2005). Self-awareness: Is it crucial to clinical practice? Confessions of a self-aware-aholic. *American Journal of Nursing, 105*(11), 72CCC–72DDD.

Maslow, A. (1970). *Motivation and personality* (2nd ed.). New York: Harper & Row.

Matthias, M., Salyers, M., & Frankel, R. (2013). Re-thinking shared decision-making: Context matters. *Patient Education and Counseling, 91*, 176–179.

McCance, T., McCormack, B., & Dewing, J. (2011). An exploration of person-centeredness in practice. *Online Journal of Issues in Nursing, 16*(2), 1.

McCarthy, C., & Aquino-Russell, C. (2009). A comparison of two nursing theories in practice: Peplau and Parse. *Nursing Science Quarterly, 22*(1), 34–40.

McCormack, B., & McCance, T. V. (2006). Development of a framework for person-centred nursing. *Journal of Advanced Nursing, 56*(5), 472–479.

McCormack, B., & McCance, T. (2010). *Person-centered nursing: Theory and practice.* Oxford: Wiley Blackwell.

McDonough-Means, M., & Kreitzer, I. (2004). Bell: Fostering a healing presence and investigating its mediators. *Journal of Alternative and Complementary Medicine, 10*(Suppl. 1), S25–S41.

McGrath, D. (2005). Healthy conversations: Key to excellence in practice. *Holistic Nursing Practice, 19*(4), 191–193.

Mead, N., & Bower, P. (2000). Patient-centredness: A conceptual framework and review of empirical literature. *Social Science & Medicine, 51*, 1087–1110.

Miller, J. (2001). *The art of being a healing presence.* Ft. Wayne: Willowgreen Publishing.

Mitchell, M., Chaboyer, W., Baumeister, E., & Foster, M. (2009). Positive effects of a nursing intervention on family-centered care in adult critical care. *American Journal of Critical Care, 18*(6), 543–552.

Monat, J. (2017). The emergence of humanity's self-awareness. *Futures, 86*, 27–35.

Morse, J. (1991). Negotiating commitment and involvement in the nurse-patient relationship. *Journal of Advanced Nursing, 16*, 455–468.

Morse, J. M., Havens, G. A., & Wilson, S. (1997). The comforting interaction: Developing a model of nurse-patient relationship. *Scholarly Inquiry for Nursing Practice, 11*(4), 321–343.

Moser, A., Houtepen, R., Spreeuwenberg, C., & Widdershoven, G. (2010). Realizing autonomy in responsive relationships. *Medicine, Health Care, and Philosophy, 13*, 215–223.

National Council of State Boards of Nursing (NCSBN). (2011). *A nurse's guide to the use of social media.* Retrieved from: https://www.ncsbn.org/NCSBN_SocialMedia.pdf.

National Council of State Boards of Nursing (NCSBN). (2014). *A nurse's guide to professional boundaries.* Retrieved from: https://www.ncsbn.org/ProfessionalBoundaries_Complete.pdf.

Nicholson, C., Flatley, M., Wilkinson, C., Meyer, J., Dale, P., & Wessel, L. (2010). Everybody matters 2: Promoting dignity in acute care through effective communication. *Nursing Times, 106*(21), 12–14.

Quoted in, LaSala, C., & O'Brien, L. (2009). Moral accountability and integrity in nursing practice. *Nursing Clinics of North America, 44*, 423–434.

Palmer, K., Marengoni, A., Forjaz, M. J., Jureviciene, E., Laatikainen, T., Mammarella, F., et al. (2017). Multimorbidity care model: Recommendations from the consensus meeting of the joint action on chronic diseases and promoting healthy ageing across the life cycle. *Health Policy, 122*(1), 4–11.

Peplau, H. E. (1997). Peplau's theory of interpersonal relations. *Nursing Science Quarterly, 10*(4), 162–167.

Peplau, H. E. (1992). Interpersonal relations: a theoretical framework for application in nursing practice. *Nursing Science Quarterly, 5*(1), 13–18.

Picker Institute. (2017). *Principles of patient-centered care.* Retrieved from: http://pickerinstitute.org/about/picker-principles/.

Porter, S., O'Halloran, P., & Morrow, E. (2011). Bringing values back into evidenced based nursing: Role of patients in resisting empiricism. *Nursing Science Quarterly, 34*(2), 106–118.

Reeve, J., Thissen, D., Bann, C., Mack, N., Treiman, K., Sanoff, H. K., et al. (2017). Psychometric evaluation and design of patient-centered communication measures for cancer care settings. *Patient Education and Counseling, 100*, 1322–1328.

Reynolds, W. (1997). Peplau's theory in practice. *Nursing Science Quarterly, 10*(4), 168–170.

Rodriguez, A., Mayo, N., & Gagnon, B. (2013). Independent contributors to overall quality of life in people with advanced cancer. *British Journal of Cancer, 108*, 1790–1800.

Scheick, D. (2011). Developing self-aware mindfulness to manage countertransference in the nurse-patient relationship: An evaluation and developmental study. *Journal of Professional Nursing, 27*(2), 114–123.

Scholl, I., Zill, J. M., Harter, M., & Dirmaier, J. (2014). An integrative model of patient-centeredness a systematic review and concept analysis. *PLoS One, 9*(9) e107828.

Sheets, V. (2001). Professional boundaries: Staying in the lines. *Dimensions of Critical Care Nursing, 20*(5), 36–40.

Stievano, A., Rocco, G., Sabatino, L., & Alvaro, R. (2013). Dignity in professional nursing: Guaranteeing better patient care. *Journal of Radiology Nursing, 32*(3), 120–123.

Street, R. L., Makoul, G., Arora, N. K., & Epstein, R. M. (2009). How does communication heal? Pathways liking clinician-patient communication to health outcomes. *Patient Education and Counseling, 74*, 295–301.

Van den Heever, A., Poggenpoel, M., & Myburgh, C. P. H. (2015). Nurses perceptions of facilitating genuineness in a nurse-patient relationship. *Health SA Gesondheid, 20*, 109–117.

Wagner, E. H., Austin, B. T., Davis, C., Hindmarsh, M., Schaefer, J., & Bonomi, A. (2001). Improving chronic illness care: Translating evidence into action. *Health Affairs, 20*(6), 64–78.

World Health Organization (WHO). (2007). *People centred health care. A policy framework.* Geneva: WHO Press.

WHO. (2010). *World health organization: Framework for action on interprofessional education and collaborative practice.* Geneva Switzerland.

SUGGESTED READING

Ashton, K. (2016). Teaching nursing students about terminating professional relationships, boundaries and social media. *Journal of Nursing Education, 37*, 170–172.

Ballou, K. (1998). A concept analysis of autonomy. *Journal of Professional Nursing, 14*(2), 102–110.

Bernabeo, E., & Holmboe, E. (2013). Patients, providers and systems need to acquire a specific set of competencies to achieve truly patient centered care. *Health Affairs, 32*(2), 250–258. Retrieved from: https://doi.org/10.1377/hlthaff.2012.1120.

Berwick, D. M. (2002). A user's manual for the IOM's 'quality chasm' report. *Health Affairs, 21*, 80–90.

Bodenheimer, T., Lorig, K., Holman, H., & Grumbach, K. Patient self-management of chronic disease in health care. *The Journal of the American Medical Association, 288*(19), 2469–2475.

Brunero, S., Lamont, S., & Coates, M. (2010). A review of empathy education in nursing. *Nursing Inquiry, 17*(1), 65–74.

Buber, M. (1957). Distance and relation. *Psychiatry, 20*, 97–104.

Buber, M. (1958). *I and thou.* New York: Charles Scribner's Sons.

Castro, E., Regenmortel, T., Vanhaecht, K., Sermeus, W., & Hecke, A. (2016). Patient empowerment, patient participation and patient-centeredness in hospital care: A concept analysis based on a literature review. *Patient Education and Counseling, 99*, 1923–1939.

Clark, A. (2010). Empathy: An integral model in the counseling program. *Journal of Counseling and Development, 88*(3), 348–356.

Cronin, C. (2004). *Patient centered care: An overview of definitions and concepts.* Washington, DC: National Health Council.

Daniels, L. (1998). Vulnerability as a key to authenticity. *Image—Journal of Nursing Scholarship, 30*(2), 191–193.

De Boer, D., Delnoij, D., & Rademakers, J. (2013). The importance of patient-centered care for various patient groups. *Patient Education and Counseling, 90*, 405–410.

Elwyn, G., Dehlendorf, C., Epstein, R., Marrin, K., White, J., & French, D. (2014). Shared decision making and motivation: Achieving patient-centered care across the spectrum of health care problems. *Annals of Family Medicine, 12*(3), 270–275.

Epstein, R. M., & Street, R. L. (2011). The values and value of patient centered care. *Annals of Family Medicine, 9*(2), 100–103.

Epstein, R. M., & Street, R. L., Jr. (2007). *Patient-centered communication in cancer care: Promoting healing and reducing suffering.* Bethesda, MD: National Cancer Institute.

Erikson, A., & Davies, B. (2017). Maintaining integrity: How nurses navigate boundaries in pediatric palliative care. *Journal of Pediatric Nursing, 35*, 42–49.

Errasti-Ibarrondo, B., Pérez, M., Carrasco, J. M., Lama, M., Zaragoza, A., & Arantzamendi, M. (2015). Essential elements of the relationship between the nurse and the person with advanced and terminal cancer: A meta-ethnography. *Nursing Outlook, 63*(3), 255–268.

Fasulo, A., Zinken, J., & Zinkin, K. (2016). Asking 'what about' questions in chronic self-management meetings. *Patient Education and Counseling, 99*, 917–923.

French, K. (2015). Transforming nursing care through health literacy acts. *Critical Care Nursing Clinics of North America, 50*, 87–98.

Frist, W. H. (2005). Shattuck lecture: Health care in the 21st century. *New England Journal of Medicine, 352*(3), 267–272.

Fumagalli, L., Radaelli, G., Lettieri, E., Bertele, P., & Masella, C. (2015). Patient empowerment and its neighbours: Clarifying the boundaries and their mutual relationships. *Health Policy, 119*, 384–394.

Greene, J., Hibbard, J., Sacks, R., & Overton, V. (2015). When patient activation levels change, health outcomes and costs change too. *Health Affairs, 34*, 431–437.

Halldorsdottir, S. (2008). The dynamics of the nurse-patient relationship: Introduction of a synthesized theory from the patient's perspective. *Scandinavian Journal of Caring Sciences, 22*(4), 643–652.

Hartley, S. (2002). Drawing the lines of professional boundaries. *Renalink, 3*(2), 7–9.

Holstrom, I., & Roing, M. (2010). The relation between patient-centeredness and patient empowerment: A discussion on concepts. *Patient Education and Counseling, 79*, 67–172.

Interprofessional Education Collaborative Expert Panel. (2011). *Core competencies for interprofessional collaborative practice: Report of an expert panel.* Washington, DC: Interprofessional Education Collaborative.

Kitson, A., Marshall, A., Bassett, K., & Zeitz, K. (2013). What are the core elements of patient centered care? A narrative review and synthesis of the literature from health policy, medicine and nursing. *Journal of Advanced Nursing, 69*(1), 4–15.

Krau, S. (2015). Patient centered care and lifelong learning. *Nursing Clinics of North America, 50*(4) xi–xii.

Légaré, F., & Witteman, H. O. (2013). Shared decision making: Examining key elements and barriers to adoption into routine clinical practice. *Health Affairs (Millwood), 32*(2), 276–284.

Lyles, J., Dwamena, F., Lein, C., & Smith, R. (2001). Evidence-based patient-centered interviewing. *Journal of Clinical Outcomes Management, 8*(7), 28–34.

Mazor, K., Street, R. L., Sue, V. M., Williams, B., & Rabin, N. K. (2016). Assessing patients' experiences with communication across the cancer center continuum. *Patient Education and Counseling, 99*, 1343–1348.

McCorkle, R., Ercolano, E., Lazenby, M., Schulman-Green, D., Schilling, L. S., Lorig, K., et al. (2011). Self-management: Enabling and empowering patients living with cancer as a chronic illness. *CA: A Cancer Journal for Clinicians, 61*, 50–62.

Mead, N., & Bower, P. (2002). Patient centred consultations and outcomes in primary care: A review of the literature. *Patient Education and Counseling, 48*, 51–61.

Morgan, S., & Yoder, L. (2012). A concept analysis of person centered care. *Journal of Holistic Nursing, 30*(1), 6–15.

Murray, E., Pollack, L., White, M., & Lo, B. (2007). Clinical decision-making: Patients' preferences and experiences. *Patient Education and Counseling, 65*(2), 189–196.

Oshima Lee, E., & Emanuel, E. J. (2013). Shared decision making to improve care and reduce costs. *Journal of Nursing Education, 368*(1), 6–8.

Pew Health Professions Commission, & Tresolini, C. P. (1994). *Health professions education and relationship-centered care: Report.* San Francisco, CA: Pew Health Professions Commission.

Pulvirenti, M., McMillan, J., & Lawn, S. (2014). Empowerment, patient centered care and self-management. *Health Expectations, 17*, 303–310.

QSEN Institute. (2014). *QSEN competencies.* Retrieved from: http://qsen.org.competencies/prelicensure-kas/.

Rogers, C. (1958). The characteristics of the helping relationship. *Personnel and Guidance Journal, 37*(1), 6–16.

Shively, M. J., Gardetto, N. J., Kodiath, M. F., Kelly, A., Smith, T. L., Stepnowsky, C., et al. (2013). Effect of patient activation on self-management in patients with heart failure. *Journal of Cardiovascular Nursing, 28*, 20–34.

Sidani, S. (2008). Effects of patient-centered care on patient outcomes: An evaluation. *Research and Theory for Nursing Practice, 22*, 24–37.

Small, D., & Small, R. (2011). Patients first! Engaging the hearts and minds of nurses with a patient-centered practice model. *Online Journal Issues in Nursing, 16*(2) Manuscript 2.

Sommerfeldt, S. (2013). Articulating nursing in an interprofessional world. *Nurse Education in Practice, 13*, 519–523.

Spector, N., & Kappel, D. M. (2012). Guidelines for using electronic and social media: The regulatory perspective. *Online Journal of Issues in Nursing, 17*(3), 1. Retrieved from: https://doi.org/10.3912/OJIN.

Street, R. L. (2013). How clinician-patient communication contributes to health improvement: Modeling pathways from talk to outcome. *Patient Education and Counseling, 92*, 286–291.

Street, R. L. (2017). The many "Disguises" of patient-centered communication: Problems of conceptualization and measurement. *Patient Education and Counseling, 100*(11), 2131–2134.

The Joint Commission. (2001). *The health care at the crossroads: Strategies for addressing the evolving nursing crisis.* Washington, DC: Author.

Wagner, E. H., Austin, B. T., & Von Korff, M. (1996). Organizing care for patients with chronic illness. *Milbank Quarterly, 74*(4), 511–544.

Windover, A., Boissy, A., Rice, T., Gilligan, T., Velez, V., & Merlino, J. (2014). The REDE model of health care communication: Optimizing relationship as a therapeutic agent. *Journal of Patient Experience, 1*(1), 8–13.

World Health Organization (WHO). (2006). *Quality of care: A process for making strategic choices in health systems.* Geneva: WHO Press.

World Health Organization (WHO). (n.d.). WHO: What is people-centred care? YouTube.com.

11

Bridges and Barriers in Therapeutic Relationships

Kathleen Underman Boggs

OBJECTIVES

At the end of the chapter, the reader will be able to:

1. Analyze which nursing actions can promote patient-centered communication using respect, caring, empowerment, trust, empathy, mutuality, veracity, and confidentiality.
2. Describe personal and organizational barriers to the development of effective communication.
3. Analyze which nursing actions best reduce barriers to communication.
4. Identify research-supported relationships between communication outcomes, such as patient empowerment and improvements in self-care.
5. Apply findings from research studies to foster communication in clinical practice.

Health communication is a multidimensional process. It includes aspects from the sender and the receiver of a message. This chapter focuses on the communication components of the nurse-patient relationship acting as bridges to promote patient health and safety outcomes. Effective communication improves patient satisfaction, facilitates patient decision-making, and promotes adherence to treatment protocols. Types of nursing communications have been shown to affect patient participation (Tobiano, Marshall, Bucknall, & Chaboyer, 2016). We apply the concepts of respect, caring, empowerment, trust, empathy, and mutuality, as well as confidentiality and veracity. We actively engage patient participation in health decisions, a right recognized by the World Health Organization (WHO) 2015.

Implementing actions that convey feelings of respect, caring, warmth, acceptance, and understanding to the patient is an interpersonal skill that requires practice (Fig. 11.1). Novice students may encounter interpersonal situations that leave them feeling helpless and inadequate. Feelings of sadness, anger, or embarrassment, although overwhelming, are common. Through practice, discussion of these feelings in peer groups, and experiential learning activities, you gain skills to deal with these feelings.

BASIC CONCEPTS

Bridges to the Relationship

Accurate nursing communication about the patient's condition is crucial to the efficient provision of high-quality, safe care. It improves patient outcomes (Koo et al., 2016). Safety issues and related communication tools are discussed in Chapters 2 and 23. Communication also affects us as providers in terms of our job satisfaction and stress levels. The following concepts describe methods to help you improve your communication and barriers to avoid.

Respect

Conveying genuine respect for your patients assists in building professional relationships. Because your mutual goal is to maximize your patient's health status, you need to convey respect for their values and opinions. Asking them what they prefer to be called and always addressing them as such is a correct initial step. Of course, you avoid the sort of casual addresses portrayed in bad television shows, such as "How are you feeling, honey?" "Mom, hold your baby," or "How are we feeling today?" We try to remember that hospitalized patients feel a loss of control in relation to interpersonal relationships with staff.

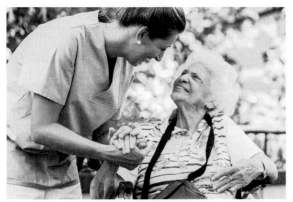

Fig. 11.1 Touch adds in communication. (Copyright © kzenon/iStock/Thinkstock.)

Lack of Respect

Patients report feeling devalued when they perceived that staff were avoiding talking with them or were unfriendly; they felt comforted when a little "chit-chat" was exchanged.

Collaborative Communication

In a true collaborative model, each team member conveys respect and assumes responsibility for initiating clear communication (TeamSTEPPS webinar, 2017). Lack of respect among team members is associated with poor communication, leading to adverse patient outcomes. In establishing patient-centered care, we should treat every patient as a respected member of the team (a QSEN competency), as suggested in Mr. Syds' case.

Case Example: Mr. Syds

Mr. Syds is recovering from pulmonary distress in an intensive care unit. This morning as the team gathers at his bed for rounds, he confides in his nurse about feeling a "sense of doom." Noting his anxious expression, falling oxygenation levels, and slight temperature, the nurse uses the CUS TeamSTEPPS communication tool, saying "I am concerned about these changes." Mr. Syds feedback taken together with physiological data prompts pattern recognition among team members. They explore the possibility that his pressure ulcer (local infection) may be evolving into sepsis (a systemic infection). In patient-centered care, this type of patient-nurse-team feedback loop might correlate with what Trainer, Liske, and Nenadovic (2016) identifies as flow of information crucial to patient outcome.

Caring

Caring is an intentional human action characterized by commitment and a sufficient level of knowledge and skill to allow you to support basic integrity. You offer caring to your patient by means of the therapeutic relationship. Nursing theorists, especially Watson, describe the need to develop and sustain a helping, trusting, caring relationship. Your ability to care develops from a natural response to help those in need, from the knowledge that caring is a part of nursing ethics, and from respect for self and others. As a caring nurse, you give patient-centered care, recognizing and assisting the patients in their struggle for health and well-being rather than simply doing things for them. They detect care and empathy from your behaviors (Richardson, Perry, & Hughes, 2015).

Provision of a caring relationship that facilitates health and healing is identified as an essential feature of contemporary nursing practice in the Social Policy Statement of the American Nurses Association (ANA, 2010). In the professional literature, the focus of the caring relationship is clearly placed on meeting patient needs. Patient-centered care is a QSEN competency. The behavior of "caring" is not an emotional feeling. Rather, it is a chosen response to need. You willingly give of yourself as an ethical responsibility.

Patients want us to understand why they are suffering. Health care workers tend to speak in a medical language that values facts and events. In contrast, patients tend to value associations and causes. To bridge this potential gap, you need to convey a sense that you truly care about their perspective. Families also need to experience a sense of caring from the nurse. Many families do not believe health care workers have a clear understanding of the problems they are encountering while caring for their ill family member. "Caring" interventions in the form of conferences where family members could express emotions and talk with experts, in conjunction with being given written materials, may help decrease anxiety. Refer to Table 16.2 for interventions to reduce family anxiety.

Lack of Caring

Although nursing has had a long-standing commitment to patient-focused care, sometimes you may observe a situation in which you feel a nurse is apathetic, trying to meet his or her own needs rather than the patient's needs. Some nurses develop a detachment that interferes with expressions of caring behaviors. At other times, nurses can be so rushed to meet multiple demands that they seem unable to focus on the patient. Simulation Exercise 11.1 will help you focus on the concept of caring.

Empowerment

Empowerment is defined as assisting patients to take charge of their lives. Our nursing goal is to use communication skills to build bridges to form partnerships, a QSEN competency. We use the interpersonal process to provide information, tools, and resources that help patients build skills to reach their health goals. Empowerment is an

---

SIMULATION EXERCISE 11.1 **Application of Caring**

Purpose
To help you apply caring concepts to nursing.

Procedure
Identify some aspect of caring that might be applied to nursing practice. Work in a group to compile a list.

Reflective Discussion
Discuss examples of how this form of caring could be implemented in a nurse-patient situation.

---

important aim in every nurse-patient relationship and is addressed by nursing theories such as Orem's view of the patient as an agent of self-care. Empowered patients feel valued and are more likely to adopt successful coping methods Studies demonstrate that the more involved people are in their own care, the better the health outcome.

Lack of Empowerment

Unempowered patients do not take responsibility for their own health. In the past, many providers exhibited a paternalistic attitude toward their patients characterized by the attitude of "I know what is best for you or I can do it better." Empowerment should extend to families. Lack of information about giving care, managing medicines, or recognizing approaching crises can be a major impediment to those who care for sick relatives. Failure to assist patients and their families to assume personal responsibility, or failure to provide appropriate resources and support, undermines empowerment.

Trust

Establishing **trust** is the foundation in all relationships. The development of a sense of interpersonal trust, a sense of feeling safe, is the keystone in the nurse-patient relationship. Trust provides a nonthreatening interpersonal climate in which people feel comfortable revealing their needs. The nurse is perceived as dependable. Establishment of this trust is crucial toward enabling you to make an accurate assessment of needs.

Trust is also the key to establishing effective work team relationships. Lack of trust in the workplace has detrimental effects for the organization and coworkers, undermining performance and commitment. According to Erikson (1963), trust is developed by experiencing consistency, sameness, and continuity during care by a familiar caregiver. Trust develops based on past experiences. In the nurse-patient relationship, maintaining an open exchange of information contributes to trust. For the patient, trust implies a willingness to place oneself in a position of vulnerability, relying on health providers to perform as expected. Honesty is a basic building block in establishing trust. Studies show that patients or their surrogates want

---

BOX 11.1 **Techniques Designed to Promote Trust**

- Convey respect.
- Consider the patient's uniqueness.
- Show warmth and caring.
- Use the patient's proper name.
- Use active listening.
- Give sufficient time to answer questions.
- Maintain confidentiality.
- Show congruence between verbal and nonverbal behaviors.
- Use a warm, friendly voice.
- Use appropriate eye contact.
- Smile.
- Be flexible.
- Provide for allowed preferences.
- Be honest and open.
- Give complete information.
- Provide consistency.
- Plan schedules.
- Follow through on commitments.
- Set limits.
- Control distractions.
- Use an attending posture: arms, legs, and body relaxed; leaning slightly forward.

"complete honesty," and most prefer complete disclosure. Box 11.1 lists interpersonal strategies that help promote a trusting relationship.

Mistrust

Mistrust has an effect not only on communication but on healing-process outcomes. Trust can be replaced with mistrust, as might occur if the nurse violates patient confidentiality. Just as some agency managers treat employees as though they are not trustworthy, some nurses treat some patients as though they are misbehaving children. An example might be a community health nurse who is inconsistent about keeping patient appointments or a pediatric nurse who indicates falsely that an injection will not hurt.

SIMULATION EXERCISE 11.2 **Techniques that Promote Trust**

Purpose
To provide practice in using trust promoting skills.

Procedure
1. Read the list of interpersonal techniques designed to promote trust (see Box 11.1).
2. Individual: Describe the relationship with your most recent patient. Was there a trusting relationship? How do you know? Which techniques did you use? Which ones could you have used?
3. Small group: Break class up into groups of three. Have

students interview another group member to obtain a brief health history. The third member observes and records trusting behaviors. Interviews should last 5 min; then share findings.

Reflective Analysis
Share findings in class with a focus on techniques and outcomes observed. Consider relative effectiveness. Alternative exercise: Have dyads do the BACKWARD FALL in which one student falls backward and the student behind catches him or her.

Such behaviors create mistrust. It is hard to maintain trust in any situation when one person cannot depend on another. Having confidence in the nurse's skills, commitment, and caring allows the patient to place full attention on the health situation requiring resolution. Of course, patients can also jeopardize the trust a nurse has in them. Sometimes patients "test" a nurse's trustworthiness by sending the nurse on unnecessary errands or talking endlessly on superficial topics. As long as nurses recognize testing behaviors and set clear limits, it is possible to develop trust. Simulation Exercise 11.2 is designed to help students become more familiar with the concept of trust.

Empathy

Empathy is the ability to be sensitive to and communicate understanding of the patient's feelings. Empathy is the ability to put yourself into another's position. Empathy and empathetic communication are crucial to the practice of nursing, characteristic of a helping relationship. Empathy is an important element of a therapeutic relationship. The ability to effectively communicate empathy is associated with improved satisfaction and patient adherence to treatments. A policy statement from the American Academy of Pediatrics extends this communication component to your patient's family (Levetown, 2008).

An empathetic nurse perceives and *understands* the patient's emotions *accurately*. Some nurses might term this as *compassion*, which has been identified by staff nurses as being crucial to the nurse-patient relationship. Communication skills are used to convey respect and empathy. Although expert nurses recognize the emotions a patient feels, they hold on to their objectivity, maintaining their own separate identities. As a nurse, you try not to overidentify with or internalize the feelings of your patient. If internalization occurs, objectivity is lost, together with the ability to help the patient move through their feelings. It is important to recognize that these feelings belong to them, not to you.

Communicate your understanding of the meaning of a patient's feelings by using both verbal and nonverbal communication behaviors. Maintain direct eye contact, use attending open body language, and keep a calm tone of voice. Acknowledging your patients' message about their feelings, difficulties, or pain helps create a positive connection (Williams, Brown, McKenna, Beovich, & Etherington, 2016). Remember to validate accuracy by restating what you understand the patient to be conveying, and have them confirm verbally that this is accurate. If you need more information about their feelings, ask them to expand on their message, perhaps asking, "Are there other things about this that are bothering you?" Now that you have full information, you can directly make interventions to address their needs.

Lack of Empathy

A failure to understand patient needs may lead you to fail to provide essential education or to provide needed emotional support. Major *organizational* barriers to empathy exist in the clinical environment, including a lack of time *associated with heavy workloads*. Several studies suggest that a lack of empathy will affect the quality of care, result in less favorable health outcomes, and lower patient satisfaction. As providers, we can consciously choose to express empathy.

Mutuality

Mutuality is the recognition of reciprocity in which we value and support the well-being of patients (Berezin & Lamont, 2016). It means that the nurse and patient agree on the patient's health problems and the means for resolving them. Both parties are committed to enhancing the patient's well-being. This is characterized by mutual respect for the autonomy and value system of the other. In developing mutuality, you maximize your patient's involvement in all phases of the nursing process. Mutuality is collaboration

SIMULATION EXERCISE 11.3   Evaluating Mutuality

Purpose

To identify behaviors and feelings on the part of the nurse and the patient that indicate mutuality.

Procedure

Complete the following questions by answering yes or no after terminating with a patient; then bring it to class. Discuss the answers. How were you able to attain mutuality, or why were you unable to attain it?

1. Was I satisfied with the relationship?
2. Did the patient express satisfaction with the relationship?

3. Did the patient share feelings with me?
4. Did I make decisions for the patient?
5. Did the patient feel allowed to make his or her own decisions?
6. Did the patient accomplish his or her goals?
7. Did I accomplish my goals?

Reflection and Discussion

In groups, analyze vignettes for mutuality.

---

in problem solving and drives the communication at the initial encounter. Evidence of mutuality is seen in the development of individualized patient goals and nursing actions that meet identified, unique health needs. Simulation Exercise 11.3 provides practice in evaluating mutuality.

As nurses, we respect interpersonal differences. We involve our patients in the decision-making process. We accept their decisions even if we do not agree with them. Effective use of values clarification a assists patients in decision making. Those who clearly identify their own personal values are better able to solve problems effectively. Decisions then have meaning to the patient. There is a greater probability that they will work to achieve success. When a mutual relationship is terminated, both parties experience a sense of shared accomplishment and satisfaction.

Veracity

Veracity or truthfulness in communication is the most important aspect in upholding a high standard of ethical nursing (ANA, 2015). Legal and ethical standards mandate specific nursing behaviors, such as confidentiality, beneficence, and respect for patient autonomy. These behaviors are based on professional nursing values that stem from ethical principles. By adhering to these "rules," nurses build their therapeutic relationships. When patients know they can expect the truth, the development of trust is promoted and helps build your relationship.

Barriers to Veracity

Sometimes it is not as easy to maintain truthfulness as we would hope. For example, the physician or the family may not have told the patient all that you know. Any deception (lies or omissions) erodes trust in care providers, but there may be a need to balance truth-telling with the need

to preserve some hope. Avoiding demeaning comments about other health providers, which will damage trust, has been found to aid in establishing a trusting relationship (Babatsikou & Gerogianni, 2012). When questioned by a patient, you can support their desire to seek a second medical opinion.

Patient-Centered Communication

Within conversations between patient and nurse, the patient should remain the focus. We should focus our energy on what our patient is trying to tell us. We strive to use the "unconditional regard" advocated by Carl Rogers, accepting our patient's comments as we do a valued person.

In social conversations, it is common to take turns. When the other person speaks, we may mentally rehearse our response. However, in professional patient-nurse communication, this means that we are not listening with 100% attention directed toward what the patient is trying to tell us.

Acceptance

Everyone has biases. We need to make it a goal to reduce bias by recognizing a patient as a unique individual, both different from and similar to self. Acceptance of the other person needs to be total. The authors believe unconditional acceptance, as described by Rogers (1961), is essential in the helping relationship. It does not imply agreement or approval; acceptance occurs without judgment. Mr. Fred Rogers, the children's television show host, ended his programs by telling his audience, "I like you just the way you are." How wonderful if we, as nurses, could convey this type of acceptance through our words and actions. Simulation Exercise 11.4 examines ways of reducing clinical bias.

Stereotyping acts as a communication barrier. This is the process of attributing characteristics to a group of

---

SIMULATION EXERCISE 11.4   Reducing Clinical Bias by Identifying Stereotypes

Purpose

To identify and reduce nursing biases. Practice identifying professional stereotypes and how to reduce them is one component of maintaining high-quality nursing care.

Procedure

Each of the following describes a stereotype. Identify the stereotype and how it might affect nursing care. As a nurse, what would you do to reduce the bias in the situation? Are there any individuals or groups of people for whom you would not want to provide care (e.g., homeless women with foul body odor and dirty nails)?

Situation A

Mrs. Daniels, an obstetric nurse who believes in birth control, comments about her client, "Mrs. Gonzales is pregnant again. You know the one with six kids already! It makes me sick to see these people on welfare taking away from our tax dollars. I don't know how she can continue to do this."

Situation B

Mrs. Brown, a registered nurse on a medical unit, is upset with her 52-year-old female patient. "If she rings that buzzer one more time, I'm going to disconnect it. Can't she understand that I have other patients who need my attention more than she does? She just lies in bed all day long. And she's so fat; she's never going to lose any weight that way."

Situation C

Mrs. Waters, a staff nurse in a nursing home, listens to the daughter of a 93-year-old resident, who says, "My mother, who is confused most of the time, receives very little attention from you nurses, while other patients who are lucid and clear-minded have more interaction with you. It's not fair! No wonder my mother is so far out in space. Nobody talks to her. Nobody comes in to say hello."

---

people as though all persons in the identified group possessed them. People may be stereotyped according to ethnic origin, culture, religion, social class, occupation, age, and other factors. Even health issues can be the stimulus for stereotyping individuals. For example, alcoholism, mental illness, and sexually transmitted diseases are fertile grounds for the development of stereotypes. Stereotypes have been shown to be consistent across cultures and somewhat across generations, although the value placed on a stereotype changes. Stereotypes are learned during childhood and reinforced by life experiences.

Stereotypes are never completely accurate. No attribute applies to every member of a group. All of us like to think that our way is the correct way, and that everyone else thinks about life experiences just as we do. The reality is that there are many roads in life, and one road is not necessarily any better than another. Emotions play a role in the value we place on negative stereotypes. Stereotypes based on strong emotions are called prejudices. Highly emotionally charged stereotypes are less amenable to change. In the extreme, this can result in discrimination.

Confidence

TeamSTEPPS talks about the need for each team member to practice competently. Nursing competence comes from education and experience. So practice those skills, but also be aware of communicating confidence in your competence to patients. In the second most watched TED talk, Amy Cuddy says, "fake it until you make it." She is discussing nonverbal behaviors that convey confidence. Seek out opportunities to hone your competence. A mild level of **anxiety** heightens one's awareness of the surrounding environment and fosters learning and decision making. Therefore, it may be desirable to allow a mild degree of anxiety. It is not prudent, however, to prolong even a mild state of anxiety. Speakers at the QSEN Nation Conference (2017) emphasized that asking for help is not a sign of weakness, but rather is a sign of strength.

Anxiety

Such feelings can become a personal barrier to communication in a patient-centered relationship. Anxiety is a vague, persistent feeling of impending doom. It is a universal feeling; no one fully escapes it. The impact on the self is always uncomfortable. It occurs when a threat (real or imagined) to one's self-concept is perceived. Lower satisfaction with communication is associated with increased patient anxiety. Anxiety is usually observed through the physical and behavioral manifestations of the attempt to relieve the anxious feelings. Although individuals experiencing anxiety may not know they are anxious, specific behaviors provide clues that anxiety is present. Simulation Exercise 11.5 identifies behaviors associated with anxiety. Table 11.1 shows how an individual's sensory perceptions, cognitive abilities, coping skills, and behaviors relate to the intensity and level of anxiety experienced. Suggestions for reducing your anxiety or for de-stressing are listed in Box 11.2. Some of these can be taught to patients.

SIMULATION EXERCISE 11.5   Identifying Verbal and Nonverbal Behaviors Associated With Anxiety

Purpose

To broaden the learner's awareness of behavioral responses indicating anxiety.

Procedure

List as many anxious behaviors as you can think of. Each column has a few examples to start. Discuss the lists in a group, and then add new behaviors to your list.

Verbal	Nonverbal
Quavering voice	Nail biting
Rapid speech	Foot tapping
Mumbling	Sweating
Defensive words	Pacing

Reflective Analysis: Construct other examples.

TABLE 11.1   Levels of Anxiety With Degree of Sensory Perceptions, Cognitive and Coping Abilities, and Manifest Behaviors

Level of Anxiety	Sensory Perceptions	Cognitive and Coping Ability	Behavior
Mild	Heightened state of alertness; increased acuity of hearing, vision, smell, touch	Enhanced learning, problem solving; increased ability to respond and adapt to changing stimuli; enhanced functioning*	Walking, singing, eating, drinking, mild restlessness, active listening, attending, questioning
Moderate	Decreased sensory perceptions; with guidance, able to expand sensory fields	Loss of concentration; decreased cognitive ability; cannot identify factors contributing to the anxiety-producing situation; with directions can cope, reduce anxiety, and solve problems; inhibited functioning	Increased muscle tone, pulse, respirations; changes in voice tone and pitch, rapid speech, incomplete verbal responses; engrossed with detail
Severe	Greatly diminished perceptions; decreased sensitivity to pain	Limited thought processes; unable to solve problems even with guidance; cannot cope with stress without help; confused mental state; limited functioning	Purposeless, aimless behaviors; rapid pulse, respirations; high blood pressure; hyperventilation; inappropriate or incongruent verbal responses
Panic	No response to sensory perceptions	No cognitive or coping abilities; without intervention, death is imminent	Immobilization

*Functioning refers to the ability to perform activities of daily living for survival purposes.

Proxemics

Proxemics is the study of an individual's use of space. Intrusion potentially *impacts negatively on patient-centered communication*. Personal space is an invisible boundary around an individual. The emotional personal space boundary provides a sense of comfort and protection. It is defined by past experiences, current circumstances, and our culture. The optimal territorial space needed by most individuals living in Western culture is 86 to 108 square feet of personal space. Other research has found that 60 square feet is the minimum needed for each client in multiple-occupancy rooms, and 80 square feet is the minimum for private rooms in hospitals and institutions. Critical care units offer even less square footage.

Among the many factors that affect the individual's need for personal distance are cultural dictates. In some cultures, people approach each other closely, whereas in others, more personal space is required. In most cultures, men need more space than women do. People generally need less space in the morning. The elderly need more control over their space, whereas small children generally like to touch and be touched by others. Although the elderly appreciate human touch, they generally do not like it to be applied indiscriminately. Situational anxiety causes a need for more space. Persons with low self-esteem prefer more space, as well as some control over who enters their space and in what manner. Usually people will tolerate a person standing close to them at their side more readily

BOX 11.2 Nursing Strategies to Reduce Anxiety

For Patient:
- Use active listening to show acceptance.
- Be honest; answer all questions at the patient's level of understanding.
- Explain procedures, surgery, and policies, and give appropriate reassurance based on data.
- Act in a calm, unhurried manner.
- Speak clearly, firmly (but not loudly).
- Give information regarding laboratory tests, medications, treatments, and rationale for restrictions on activity.
- Set reasonable limits and provide structure.
- Encourage self-affirmation through positive statements such as "I will" and "I can."
- Use drawings or play therapy with dolls, puppets, and games with youth.
- Use a therapeutic touch.
- Initiate recreational activities, such as physical exercise, music, card games, board games, crafts, and reading.
- Teach deep breathing and relaxation exercises.
- Use guided imagery.

For Nurses:
- Treat sleep as a precious medicine.
- Eat healthy, fuel up.
- Exercise daily.
- Meditate daily (even if only for 5 min).
- Use guided imagery, positive attitude, and positive affirmations.
- Listen to music.
- Do chair yoga.
- Download the Breathe app, and have it remind you to do deep breathing periodically.
- Take your assigned breaks to do some of the above!

Modified from Gerrard, B., Boniface, W., & Love, B. (1980). *Interpersonal skills for health professionals.* Reston, VA: Reston Publishing; TeamSTEPPS National Conference, June 2017; and others.

than directly in front of them. Direct eye contact causes a need for more space. Placing oneself at the same level (e.g., sitting while patients are sitting, or standing at eye level when they are standing) allows more access to the patient's personal space because such a stance is perceived as less threatening.

Violations of Personal Space

Hospitals are not home. Many nursing-care procedures are a direct intrusion into your patient's personal space.

Commonly, procedures that require tubes (e.g., nasal gastric intubation, administration of oxygen, catheterization, and intravenous initiation) restrict mobility, resulting in loss of control over personal territory. When more than one health professional is involved, the impact of the intrusion on the patient may be even stronger. In many instances, personal space requirements are an integral part of a person's self-image. When patients lose control over personal space, they may experience a loss of identity and self-esteem. It is recommended that you maintain a social physical body distance of 4 feet when not actually giving care.

When institutionalized patients are able to incorporate parts of their rooms into their personal space, it increases their self-esteem and helps them to maintain a sense of identity. This feeling of security is evidenced when a patient asks, "Close my door, please." Freedom from worry about personal space allows the patient to trust the nurse and fosters a therapeutic relationship. When invasions of personal space are necessary while performing a procedure, you can minimize the impact by explaining why a procedure is needed. Conversation at such times reinforces their feelings that they are human beings worthy of respect and not just objects being worked on. Advocating for patient personal space needs is an aspect of the nursing role. This is done by communicating the patients' preferences to other members of the health team and including them in the care plan.

Home is not quite home when the home health nurse, infusion nurse, or other aides invade personal space. Some modification of "take-charge" behavior is required when giving care in a patient's home.

Cultural Barriers

Cross-cultural communication is discussed extensively in Chapter 7. Every interaction encounters a basic challenge of communication when the culture of your patient differs from your own. Barriers include health literacy problems or cultural definitions of the sick role. For example, in some cultures, the sick role is no longer valid after symptoms disappear, so when your patient's diabetes is under control, family members may no longer see the need for a special diet or medication. As we move into a more multicultural society, all health care providers need to work to become culturally competent communicators. *Culturally competent communication* is characterized by a willingness to try to understand and respond to your patient's beliefs. Knowledge of cultural preferences helps you avoid stereotyping and allows you to adapt your communication.

Gender Differences

Gender is defined as the culture's attributions of masculine or feminine. Recently, more attention has been given to gender role, communication barriers, and health inequalities. Research results give mixed findings, though some studies suggest patient perceptions differ according to the nurse's gender. The authors believe gender need not be a factor in developing therapeutic communication with patients. Research does support the need for communications training for all health care workers. It takes practice for us to master communication skills.

Organizational System Barriers

Communication barriers inherent in health care system agencies are commonly discussed in the professional literature. Frequent interruptions and lack of time are cited by Flick (2012) and many others. Often such barriers to communication stem from cost-containment measures.

Heavy Workload

This is often mentioned as a barrier to communication and to opportunities to engage patients. Lack of time can result from low staff-to-patient ratios or financial pressure for early discharge. Tobiano et al. (2016) suggests including patients as we develop care plans as a means to increase dialogue. In our care for patients with increasingly complex health problems and heavier workloads, we may think we lack the time to spend communicating. Developing quality communication using team rounds may be a solution. This method of reporting at the bedside includes the patient as a team partner in the day's care goals. However, Rehder et al. found that becomes a barrier to communication if the nurse tries to multitask (2012).

Production Expectations

The primary care literature describes agency demand for minimal appointment time with patients. Primary care providers, such as nurse practitioners, are often constrained to focus just on the chief complaint to maximize the number of patients seen, leading to "the 15-minute office visit." These system barriers limit the nurse's ability to develop substantial rapport with patients. Adequate time is essential to develop therapeutic communication to achieve effective care responsive to patient needs.

Inconsistent Caregivers

Along with workload barriers, another characteristic of organizations that creates communication barriers is lack of consistent nurse assignment and increased use of temporary staff known as agency nurses, casual nurses, or floaters. To overcome system barriers to communication, we need to work as a team to deliver consistent care. Working to develop open communications in our agencies leads to better communication and improved patient safety (TeamSTEPPS Webinar, July 12, 2017).

DEVELOPING AN EVIDENCE-BASED PRACTICE
A higher level of evidence-based practice (EBP) results from meta-analysis of multiple research findings to determine the actual "best practice." The Agency for Healthcare Research and Quality (AHRQ, n.d.) has published many online articles for you to access.

The chapter on "Promoting Engagement by Patients and Families to Reduce Adverse Events" cites more than 30 studies. Review *results*, among which are those listed below:

Application to Your Practice
As we engage our patients' help in reducing adverse occurrences, we use communication skills that might promote trust, caring, and empowerment, such as asking patients to:
- remind or ask every health care worker touching them and their equipment to wash their hands;
- have the nurse provide a personalized list of hospital medications, which the patient can check each time someone gives him or her a medication; and
- bring a written list of questions to each health care visit.

APPLICATIONS

Behaviors described in this chapter can be learned and are fundamental to your nursing role (Richardson et al., 2015). Many nursing actions recommended here are mandated by the ANA Code of Ethics for Nurses discussed in Chapter 3. The actions specified include confidentiality, autonomy, beneficence, veracity, and justice. Mutuality is addressed in the ANA position statement on human rights. Providers with good communication skills have greater professional satisfaction and experience less job-related stress. Studies of patient perceptions generally show a correlation between good nurse communicators and good quality of care. Practice simulations and exercises provide you with opportunities to improve your skills. Part of any simulation exercise to strengthen nursing communication is the offering of feedback.

Steps in the Caring Process

Several articles identify four steps to help you communicate C.A.R.E. with your patient:

C = First, *connect* with your patient. *Offer your attention.* Here you introduce your purpose in developing a professional relationship (i.e., meeting his or her health needs). Use the patient's formal name, and avoid terms of endearment, such as "sweetie" or "honey." Show intent to care. Attentiveness is a part of communication skill training that is probably decreased by work-related stress, time constraints, and so forth.

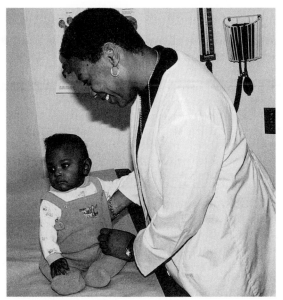

Fig. 11.2 Infants lack verbal communication skills. The nurse's comforting touch and pleasant vocal tone help overcome this barrier. (Courtesy Adam Boggs.)

A = The second step is to *appreciate* the patient's situation. Although the health care environment is familiar to you, it is a strange and perhaps frightening situation for the patient. Acknowledge your patient's point of view and express concern.

R = The third step is to *respond* to what your patient needs. What are his or her priorities? What are his or her expectations for health care?

E = The fourth step is to *empower* the patient to problem-solve with you. The patient gains strength and confidence from interactions with providers, enabling the patient to move toward achievement of goals (Fig. 11.2).

The ability to become a caring professional is influenced by your previous experiences. A person who has received caring is more likely to be able to offer it to others. Caring should not be confused with caretaking. Although caretaking is a part of caring, it may lack the necessary intentional giving of self. Self-awareness about feelings, attitudes, values, and skills is essential for developing an effective, caring relationship.

Strategies for Empowerment

In the coming years, there will be a highly increased focus on assisting patients to assume more responsibility for their health conditions. We will increasingly teach them new roles and skills to manage their illnesses. We may never fully understand the decisions some patients make, but we support their right to do so. Your method for **empowering** should include the following key strategies:

- *Accept* them as they are by refraining from any negative judgments.
- Assess their level of understanding, *exploring their perceptions and feelings* about their conditions and discussing issues that may interfere with self-care.
- Establish mutual goals for health care by forming an alliance, *mutually deciding* about their care.
- Find out how much information they want to know.
- Reinforce *autonomy,* for example, by allowing them to choose the content in the teaching plan.
- *Offer information* in an environment that enables them to use it.
- Make sure your patients *actively participate* in their care plans.
- Encourage networking with a support group and the use of m-Health apps (see Chapter 26).
- Clarify with them that they hold the major *responsibility* for both the health care decisions they make and their consequences.

Application of Empathy to Levels of Nursing Actions

Nursing actions that facilitate empathy can be classified into three major skills: (a) recognition and classification of requests, (b) attending behaviors, and (c) empathetic responses.

Processing requests: Two types of requests are for information and action. These requests do not involve interpersonal concerns and are easier to manage. Another form of request is for understanding involvement, which entails the patient's need for empathetic understanding. Use attending behaviors: *Attending behaviors* facilitate empathy and include an attentive, open posture; responding to verbal and nonverbal cues through appropriate gestures and facial expressions; using eye contact; and allowing patient self-expression. Verbally acknowledging nonverbal cues shows you are attending, as does offering time and attention, showing interest in the patient's issues, offering helpful information, and clarifying problem areas. These responses encourage patients to participate in their own healing.

Make empathetic responses: You communicate *empathy* when you show your patients that you understand how they are feeling. This helps them identify emotions that are not readily observable and connect them with the current situation. For example, observing nonverbal cues, such as a worried facial expression, and verbalizing this reaction with an empathetic comment, such as "I understand that this is very difficult for you," validates what they are feeling and tells them you understand them. Using the actions listed in Table 11.2, the nurse applies attending behaviors and nursing actions

TABLE 11.2 Levels of Nursing Communication Behavior

Level	Category	Nursing Communication Behavior
1. **Pro**cess	Gathers data Accepts	Becomes aware of goals & patient care plan Uses patient's correct name Maintains eye contact Adopts open posture
2. **A**ct	Listens	Responds to cues Nods head Smiles Encourages responses Uses therapeutic silence
	Clarifies	Asks open-ended questions Restates the problem Validates perceptions Acknowledges confusion
	Informs	Provides honest, complete answers Assesses patient's knowledge Confronts conflict Summarizes teaching points
3. **R**eflect	Analyzes	Identifies unknown emotions Interprets underlying meanings Evaluates outcomes Communicates with team to revise care plan

BOX 11.3 Tips to Reduce Relationship Barriers

- Establish trust.
- Demonstrate caring and empathy.
- Empower your patient.
- Recognize and reduce anxiety.
- Maintain appropriate personal distance.
- Practice cultural sensitivity, and work to be bilingual.
- Use therapeutic relationship-building activities such as active listening.
- Avoid medical jargon.

to express empathy. Verbal prompts, such as "Hmm," "Uh-huh," "I see," "Tell me more," and "Go on," facilitate expression of feelings. The nurse uses open-ended questions to validate perceptions. Using informing behaviors listed in Table 11.2 enlarges the database by providing new information and gives feedback to your patient. Remember, demonstrating empathy as a communication behavior has been shown to positively affect the outcome of your care.

Reduction of Barriers in Nurse-Patient Relationships

Recognition of barriers is the first step in eliminating them, and thus enhancing the therapeutic process. Practice with exercises in this chapter should increase your recognition of possible barriers. Findings from many studies have emphasized the crucial importance

of honesty, cultural sensitivity, and caring, especially in listening actively to suggestions and complaints from the patient and family. Refer to Box 11.3 for a summary of strategies to reduce communication barriers in nurse-patient relationships.

Respect for Personal Space

We need to assess a patient's personal space needs. Assessment includes cultural and developmental factors that affect perceptions of space and reactions to intrusions. In some situations, if you need to increase your patient's sense of personal space, you can decrease direct eye contact or position your body at an angle. Examples might be when bathing, changing dressings, etc. At the same time, it is important for you to talk gently during such procedures and to elicit feedback, if appropriate.

There is a discrepancy between the minimum amount of space an individual needs and the amount of space hospitals are able to provide in multiple-occupancy rooms. Actions to ensure private space and show respect include:

- closing the door to the room to allow rest;
- providing privacy when disturbing matters are to be discussed;
- explaining procedures before implementation;
- entering another person's personal space with warning (e.g., knocking or calling the patient's name) and, preferably, waiting for permission to enter;
- providing an identified space for personal belongings and treating them with care;
- encouraging the inclusion of personal and familiar objects on the nightstand;
- decreasing direct eye contact during hands-on care;
- minimizing bodily exposure during care;
- using only the necessary number of people during any procedure; and
- using touch appropriately.

SUMMARY

This chapter focuses on essential concepts that act as bridges in constructing a meaningful, effective nurse-patient relationship, including caring, empowerment, trust, empathy, mutuality, and confidentiality. Respect for the patient as a unique person is a basic component of each concept.

Caring is described as a commitment by the nurse that involves profound respect and concern for the unique humanity of every patient and a willingness to confirm their personhood.

Empowerment is assisting patients to take charge of their own health.

Trust represents an individual's emotional reliance on the consistency and continuity of experience. The patient perceives the nurse as trustworthy, a safe person with whom to share difficult feelings about health-related needs.

Empathy is the ability to accurately perceive another person's feelings and to convey their meaning to the patient. Nursing behaviors that facilitate the development of empathy are accepting, listening, clarifying and informing, and analyzing. Each of these behaviors implicitly recognizes the patient as a unique individual worthy of being listened to and respected.

Mutuality is characterized by reciprocity in setting goals and collaborating in methods. To foster mutuality within the relationship, nurses need to remain aware of their own feelings, attitudes, and beliefs.

Barriers described include anxiety, stereotyping, over familiarity, and personal space violations. Organizational system demands, such as a heavy workload, limit time for nurse-patient communication. Solutions focus on open communication among all team members caring for the patient.

ETHICAL DILEMMA: What Would You Do?

There are limits to your professional responsibility to maintain confidentiality. Any information that, if withheld, might endanger the life or physical and emotional safety of the patient or others needs to be communicated to the health team or appropriate people immediately.

Consider the teen who confides his plan to shoot classmates. Can you breach confidentiality in this case? How about when you notice genital warts (from sexually transmitted human papilloma virus) on a 5-year-old child, but who shows no other signs of sexual abuse?

QUESTIONS FOR REFLECTIVE ANALYSIS AND DISCUSSION

1. How would you teach a nurse to apply the strategies for anxiety reduction and de-stressing provided in Box 11.2?

2. Reflect on which behaviors in Simulation Exercise 11.4 demonstrated empathy. Could you add the phrase, "That must have been difficult," to what the nurse role-player said?

3. Contrast stereotypes you have heard about in a health care setting. Discuss them in a group.

4. Analyze how proxemics changes in different situations. What is your own preferred space distance? To what do you attribute this preference? Under what circumstances do your needs for personal space change?

REFERENCES

Agency for Healthcare Research and Quality [AHRQ]. (n.d.). www.ahrq.gov. Accessed 26.9.18.

American Nurses Association (ANA). (2010). *Nursing's social policy statement: The essence of the profession.* Silver Spring, MD/Washington, DC: Author. http://nursingworld.org/social-policy-statement/.

American Nurses Association (ANA). (2015). Code of ethics for nurses with interpretive statements. http://nursingworld.org/Documentvault/Ethics-1/Code-of-Ethics-for-Nurses/html/ .

Babatsikou, F. P., & Gerogianni, G. K. (2012). The importance of role-play in nursing practice. *Health Science Journal* 6(1):4–10, 2012. A Nursing Department Technological Educational Institute of Athens online publication. Available at www.hsj.gr.

Berezin, M., & Lamont, M. (2016). Mutuality, mobilization, and messaging for health promotion: Toward collective cultural change. *Social Science & Medicine, 165,* 201–205.

Erikson, E. (1963). *Childhood and society* (ed 2). New York, Norton.

Flick, C. L. (2012). Communication: A dynamic between nurses and physicians. *MedSurg Nursing, 21*(6), 385–387.

Koo, L. W., Horowitz, A. M., Radice, S. D., Wang, M. Q., Wang, M. Q., & Kleinman, D. V. (2016). Nurse practitioners use of communication technologies: Results of a Maryland oral health literacy survey. *PLOS ONE,* 1–16.

Levetown, M. (2008). American Academy of Pediatrics Committee on Bioethics: Communicating with children and families: From everyday interactions to skill in conveying distressing information. *Pediatrics, 121*(5), e1442–e1460.

QSEN Institute: QSEN competencies. http://qsen.org or www.qsen.org/about-qsen. Accessed 20.9.18.

Rehder, K. J., Uhl, T. L., Meliones, D. A., Turner, D. A., Smith, P. B., & Mistry, K. P. (2012). Targeted interventions improve shared agreement of daily goals in the pediatric intensive care unit. *Pediatr Crit Care Med, 13*(1), 6–10.

Richardson, C., Perry, M., & Hughes, J. (2015). Nursing therapeutics: Teaching student nurses care, compassion, & empathy. *Nurse Education Today, 35,* e1–e5.

Rogers, C. (1961). *On becoming a person.* Boston: Houghton-Mifflin.

Team. (June 14–16, 2017). *STEPPS National Conference.* Cleveland, Ohio.

TeamSTEPPS Webinar (July, 2017). www.ahrq.gov/team-stepps/webinars/index.html. Accessed 20.9.18.

Tobiano, G., Marshall, A., Bucknall, T., & Chaboyer, W. (2016). Activities patients and nurses undertake to promote patient participation. *Journal of Nursing Scholarship, 48*(4), 362–370.

Trainer, R., Liske, L., & Nenadovic, V. (2016). Critical care nursing: Embedded complex systems. *The Canadian Journal of Critical Care, 27*(1), 11–16.

Williams, B., Brown, T., McKenna, L., Beovich, B., & Etherington, J. (2016). *Attachment and empathy in Australian undergraduate paramedic, nursing, and occupational therapy students: A cross-sectional study,* 1–7. Collegian https://doi.org/10.1016/j.colegn.2016.11.004.

World Health Organization (WHO). (2015). *Patient participation in decisions.* http://www.who.int/mediacentre/news/statements/.

12

Communicating With Families

Shari Kist, Elizabeth Arnold

OBJECTIVES

At the end of the chapter, the reader will be able to:

1. Define family and identify its components.
2. Apply family-centered concepts to the care of the family in clinical settings, using standardized family-assessment tools.
3. Apply the nursing process to the care of families in clinical settings.

4. Identify nursing interventions for families in the intensive care unit (ICU).
5. Identify nursing interventions for families in the community.

INTRODUCTION

The purpose of this chapter is to describe family-centered relationships and communication strategies that nurses can use to support family integrity in health care settings. Chapter 12 identifies family theory frameworks and ways to maximize productive communication with family members. Practical assessment and intervention strategies address family issues that affect a patient's recovery and support self-management of chronic health conditions or peaceful death in clinical practice.

BASIC CONCEPTS

Definition of Family

The term *family* can have several definitions, particularly in today's society. The legal definition describes the family as individuals related through marriage, blood ties, adoption, or guardianship. As a biological unit, *family* describes the genetic connections among people. The US Census Bureau (2013) defines *family* in the following way: "A family is a group of two people or more (one of whom is the householder) related by birth, marriage, or adoption and residing together; all such people (including related subfamily members) are considered as members of one family. A household consists of all people who occupy a housing unit regardless

of relationship. A household may consist of a person living alone, or multiple unrelated individuals or families living together." However, as health care providers, it is more appropriate to use the Wright and Leahey (2013) definition, that "a family is who they say they are." Identified family members may or may not be blood related. Strong emotional ties and durability of membership characterize family relationships regardless of how uniquely they are defined. Even when family members are alienated or distanced geographically, they "can never truly relinquish family membership" (Goldenberg & Goldenberg, 2013, p. 3). During times of crisis, such as a seriously ill family member, family members react to the situation and one another with a wide range of reactions. Each family member responds in unique ways. Communication, even when reactive, is designed to maintain the integrity of the family.

Understanding the family as a system is relevant in today's health care environment, as the family is an essential part of the health care team. Families have a profound influence on ill family members as advisors, caretakers, supporters, and sometimes irritants. Patients who are very young, very old, and those requiring assistance with self-management of chronic illness are particularly dependent on their families.

Support from the health care team during times of stress and crisis are necessary to provide information and empowerment to successfully adapt. Both resources and supports are essential for family empowerment (Trivette, Dunst, & Hamby, 2010). Resources and supports include beliefs, past experiences, help-giving and receiving practices, strengths, and capabilities; and they are pieces of information that help explain patient and family responses to health disruptions.

Conducting a family assessment is essential "to (1) assure that the needs of the family are met, (2) uncover any gaps in the family plan of action, (3) offer multiple supports and resources to the family" (Kaakinen, Gedaly-Duff, Coehlo, & Hanson, 2010, p. 104).

Family Composition

There is significant diversity in the composition of families, family beliefs and values, how they communicate with one another, ethnic heritage, life experiences, commitment to individual family members, and connections with the community (Goldenberg & Goldenberg, 2013, p. 2). Families today are much more complex than in past generations. Box 12.1 identifies different types of family compositions (Fig. 12.1).

The "typical American family" today has many variations (Goldenberg & Goldenberg, 2013, p. 3). Single-parent families must accomplish the same developmental tasks as two-parent families, but in many cases they do it without the support of the other partner or sufficient financial resources. Blended families have a different life experience than those in an intact family because their family structure is often more complex. Children may be members of more than one family unit, linked biologically, physically, and emotionally to people who may or may not be a part of their daily lives. Parents, step- or half-brothers and sisters, two or more sets of grandparents, and multiple aunts and uncles may make up a blended family (Kaakinen et al., 2010, p. 135). The child may spend extended periods in separate households, each with a full set of family expectations that may, or may not, be similar. Initially, the parents in blended families may cohabitate, making for a sense of uncertainty for all involved (Jensen & Schafer, 2013). Blended families can offer a rich experience for everyone concerned, but they are more complex because of multiple connections. Table 12.1 displays some of the differences between biological and blended families. Issues for blended families include discipline, money, use of time, birth of an infant, death of a stepparent, inclusion at graduation, and marriage and health care decisions.

Theoretical Frameworks

Theoretical frameworks are used to provide a means for understanding certain processes and relationships between and among essential concepts. Numerous theoretical frameworks exist that can be used to understand family composition. Ludwig von Bertalanffy's (1968)

BOX 12.1   Types of Family Composition

- Nuclear family: a father and mother, with one or more children, living together as a single family unit
- Extended family: nuclear family unit's combination of second- and third-generation members related by blood or marriage but not living together
- Three-generational family: any combination of first-, second-, and third-generation members living within a household
- Dyad family: husband and wife or other couple living alone without children
- Single-parent family: divorced, never married, separated, or widowed man or woman and at least one child; most single-parent families are headed by women
- Stepfamily: family in which one or both spouses are divorced or widowed with one or more children from a previous marriage who may not live with the newly reconstituted family
- Blended or reconstituted family: a combination of two families with children from one or both families and sometimes children of the newly married couple
- Common law family: an unmarried couple living together with or without children
- No kin: a group of at least two people sharing a nonsexual relationship and exchanging support who have no legal, blood, or strong emotional ties to each other
- Polygamous family: one man (or woman) with several spouses
- Same-sex family: a homosexual couple living together with or without children
- Commune: groups of individuals (may or may not be related) living together and sharing resources
- Group marriage: all individuals are "married" to one another and are considered parents of all the children

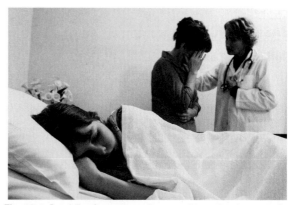

Fig. 12.1 Providing frequent updates, and emotional support for family members is an important part of patient centered care. (Copyright © Hemera Technologies/AbleStock.com/Thinkstock.)

TABLE 12.1 Comparing Differences Between Biological and Blended Families

Biological Families	Blended Families
Family is created without loss.	Family is born of loss.
There are shared family traditions.	There are two sets of family traditions.
One set of family rules evolves.	Family rules are varied and complicated.
Children arrive one at a time.	Instant parenthood of children at different ages occurs.
Biological parents live together.	Biological parents live apart.

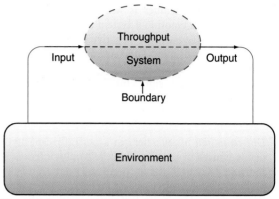

Fig. 12.2 Systems Model: Interaction With the Environment.

general systems theory provides a conceptual foundation for family system models (Barker, 1998). Having a systems perspective allows one to examine the interdependence among all parts of the system to see how they support the system as a functional whole. Systems' thinking maintains that the whole is greater than the sum of its parts with each part reciprocally influencing its function. If one part of the system changes or fails, it affects the functioning of the whole. A clock is a useful metaphor. It displays time correctly, but only if all parts work together. If any part of the clock breaks down, the clock no longer tells accurate time.

A system interacts with other systems in the environment. An interactional process occurs when inputs are introduced into the system in the form of information, energy, and resources. Within each system, the information is processed internally as the system actively processes and interprets its meaning. The transformation process of raw data into desired outputs is referred to as *throughput*. The *output* refers to the result or product that leaves the system. Each system is separated from its environment by boundaries that control the exchange of information, energy, and resources into and out of the system. Evaluations of the output and feedback loops from the environment inform the system of changes needed to achieve effective outputs. Fig. 12.2 identifies the relational components of a human system's interaction with the environment, using von Bertalanffy's model.

Systems theory can be applied to the human system. Individuals take in food, liquids, and oxygen to nourish the body (inputs). Within the body, a transformational process occurs through enzymes and other metabolic processes (throughputs), so the body can use the inputs. This interactional process results in the human organism's growth, health, and capacity to interact with the external environment (outputs). Nonusable outputs excreted from the body include urine, feces, sweat, and carbon dioxide. A person's skin represents an important boundary between the environment and the human system.

Family systems have boundaries that regulate information coming into and leaving the family system. Family systems theory describes how families strive for harmony and balance (homeostasis), how the family is able to maintain its continuity despite challenges, (morphostasis), and how the family is able to change and grow over time in response to challenges (morphogenesis). Feedback loops describe the patterns of interaction that facilitate movement toward morphogenesis or morphostasis. These feedback loops impact goal setting in behavioral systems. The systems principle of equifinality describes how the same outcome or end state can be reached through different pathways. This principle helps explain why some individuals at high risk for poor outcomes do not develop maladaptive behaviors (Cicchetti & Blender, 2006). *Hierarchy* is the term used to describe the complex layers of smaller systems that exist within a system. Communication can also be thought of as a complex system in which the message or output must be interpreted within an appropriate context.

Bowen's Systems Theory

Murray Bowen's (1978) family systems theory conceptualizes the family as an interactive emotional unit. He believed that family members assume reciprocal family roles, develop automatic communication patterns, and react to one another in predictable, connected ways, particularly when family anxiety is high. Once anxiety heightens within the system, an emotional process gets activated (Nichols & Schwartz, 2009), and dysfunctional communication patterns can emerge. For example, if one person is overly responsible, another family member may become less likely to assume normal responsibility.

Until one family member is willing to challenge the dysfunction of an emotional system by refusing to play his or her reactive part, the negative emotional energy fueling a family's dysfunctional communication pattern persists.

Bowen developed eight interlocking concepts to explain his theoretical construct of the family system (Bowen Center for the Study of the Family, 2013; Gilbert, 2006).

- *Differentiation of self* refers to a person's capacity to define himself or herself within the family system as an individual having legitimate needs and wants. It requires making "I" statements based on rational thinking rather than emotional reactivity. Self-differentiation takes into consideration the views of others but is not dominated by them. Poorly differentiated people are so dependent on the approval of others that they discount their own needs (Hill, Hasty, & Moore, 2011). Individuals with a well-differentiated sense of self exhibit a balanced, realistic dependence on others and can accept conflict and criticism without an excessive emotional reaction. Self-differentiation serves as the fundamental means of reducing chronic anxiety within the family system and enhancing effective problem solving. Self-differentiation emphasizes thinking rather than feeling in communication.
- *Multigenerational transmission* refers to the emotional transmission of behavioral patterns, roles, and communication response styles from generation to generation. It explains why family patterns tend to repeat behaviors in marriages, child rearing, choice of occupation, and emotional responses across generations without understanding why it happens.
- *Nuclear family emotional system* refers to the way family members relate to one another within their immediate family when stressed. Family anxiety shows up in one of four patterns: (1) dysfunction in one spouse, (2) marital conflict, (3) dysfunctional symptoms in one or more of the children, or (4) emotional distancing.
- *Triangles* refer to a defensive way of reducing, neutralizing, or defusing heightened anxiety between two family members by drawing a third person or object into the relationship (MacKay, 2012). If the original triangle fails to contain or stabilize the anxiety, it can expand into a series of "interlocking" triangles, for example, into school issues or an extramarital affair.
- *Family projection process* refers to an unconscious casting of unresolved anxiety in the family on a particular family member, usually a child. The projection can be positive or negative, and it can become a self-fulfilling prophecy as the child incorporates the anxiety of the parent as part of his or her self-identity.

- *Sibling position*, a concept originally developed by Walter Toman (1992), refers to a belief that sibling positions shape relationships and influence a person's expression of behavioral characteristics. Each sibling position has its own strengths and weaknesses. This concept helps explain why siblings in the same family can exhibit very different characteristics. For example:
  - Oldest or only children more serious, assume leadership roles, and like to be in control. They may experience more trouble with staying connected with others or depending on them.
  - Youngest siblings are characterized as being followers, spontaneous, and fun loving, with a stronger sense of humor. They are more likely to be interested in quality of life and relationships.
  - Middle child positions embrace characteristics of both the oldest and the youngest; they are likely to be adventuresome and independent, but not leaders. The child in the middle position may feel neglected, or may take on the role of peacemaker.
  - Although sibling position is a factor in explaining different relational behaviors, it is not useful as a descriptor of life functioning because a person occupying any sibling position can be either successful or unsuccessful (Gilbert, 2006).
- *Emotional cutoff* refers to a person's withdrawal from other family members as a means of avoiding family issues that create anxiety. Emotional cutoffs range from total avoidance to remaining in physical contact, but in a superficial manner. All persons have unresolved emotional attachments, but the extent varies widely among individuals.
- *Societal emotional process* refers to parallels that Bowen found between the family system and the emotional system operating at the institutional level in society. As anxiety grows within a society, many of the same polarizations, lack of self-differentiation, and emotion-based thinking dominate behavior and system outcomes.

Family Legacies

Family legacies have a powerful influence on family relationships and in shaping parenting practices. Families of one generation tend to function in a similar manner to the previous generation. Knowledge of family relationships helps explain behaviors that would not be clear without having a family context. Helping families gain clarity about how their family heritage can be used as an asset in health care and/or what areas need work strengthens the potential for effective family-centered care.

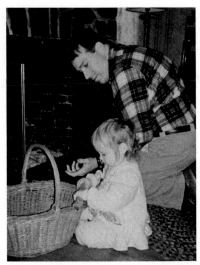

Shared family traditions strengthen family bonds.

Many theoretical frameworks exist that support understanding of family structure and function. Other family theories fall into three groupings related to structure, development, and resiliency theories. Table 12.2 identifies major characteristics of family theories. Other family-related theoretical frameworks based on the social sciences, family therapy, and nursing also exist (Kaakinen et al., 2010, p. 9).

The challenge for health care providers is to be able to apply a theoretical understanding of family structure and function to an actual patient-care situation (Segaric & Hall, 2005). In many settings, nurses have a tendency to focus care on the individual. This is important, but the nurse must also understand that the family is impacted by even minor health deviations of a family member. Thus, understanding individuals as members of families from a theoretical perspective is necessary.

DEVELOPING AN EVIDENCE-BASED PRACTICE This article describes a quality-improvement initiative to allow family members to be present during dressing changes in the adult burn intensive care unit. The impetus for this project was a hospital-wide patient- and family-centered care (PFCC) initiative. The traditional practice of not allowing family members to be present during dressing changes was inconsistent with the aims of PFCC. Previously, family members had been excluded from dressing changes because they were considered to increase the risk for infection and because it was thought family members would not be able to tolerate viewing the procedure. It was believed that the lack of family involvement contributed to lower patient and family satisfaction scores and a lack of preparation for care upon discharge.

Following a comprehensive literature review and discussion with members of the health care team, the decision was made to permit family presence during dressing changes. Either the patient or their designee (if unable to make decisions) had to agree to allow other family members to be present during dressing changes. Family members who wished to participate were educated on what would happen during the entire dressing-change process. In addition, family members were instructed on handwashing and the use of personal protective equipment. They were also instructed on what to do in the event that they became faint, weak, or nauseated. Following the dressing change, family members had the opportunity to provide their reactions to the experience and to ask questions related to the procedure.

The outcome measures included patient satisfaction and rates of infection. More than 2 years of data both before and after implementation of family presence were used for comparison. Family members who were present during dressing changes reported greater satisfaction with being informed and involved, discharge planning, and perception of staff attitudes when compared with the time period without family presence. Infection rates demonstrated a decrease during the implementation of family presence during dressing changes. Limitations were identified as low response rates and the fact that multiple practice changes were simultaneously implemented.

Application to Your Clinical Practice: The results of this quality-improvement initiative demonstrate the positive effects of PFCC. It was not just family members seeing the dressing change being performed, but additional benefits included an increased interaction with family members that helps to improve family members' comfort in interacting with staff members. By allowing family members to be more involved in multiple aspects of patient care, the nurse-family relationship is enhanced, which can contribute to improved patient outcomes.

Modified from Bishop, S. M., Walker, M. D., & Spivak, I. M. (2013). Family presence in the adult burn intensive care unit during dressing changes. *Critical Care Nurse, 33*(1), 14–22.

TABLE 12.2   Key Features of Other Family Theories

Theory	Key Elements	References
Structural family theory	Emphasizes how the family unit is structured (subsystems, hierarchies, and boundaries). Function is assessed in relation to instrumental functioning (completing tasks during times of health and illness) and expressive functioning (communication patterns, problem solving, and power structures). Families strive to maintain homeostasis.	Fivaz-Depeursinge, Lopes, Python, and Favez (2009); Minuchin (1974)
Developmental family theory	Eight specific developmental tasks are outlined starting with a childless couple and ending with retirement. Traits that demonstrate successful family development are identified.	Antle, Christensen, van Zyl, and Barbee (2012); Duvall (1958)
Family stress theory	Family response to and coping with stressful events are explained. Factors associated with positive resolution include family system resources, flexibility, and problem-solving skills.	Frain, Berven, Chan, and Tschopp (2008); Lavee (2013)

Antle, B. F., Christensen, D. N., van Zyl, M. A., Barbee, A. P. (2012). The impact of the Solution Based Casework (SBC) practice model on federal outcomes in public child welfare, *Child Abuse & Neglect 36*(4), 342–353; Duvall, E. (1958). *Marriage and family development*. Philadelphia: JB Lippincott; Fivaz-Depeursinge, E., Lopes, F., Python, M., Favez, N. (2009). Coparenting and toddler's interactive styles in family coalitions, *Family Process 48*(4), 500–516. https://doi:10.1111/j.1545-5300.2009.01298.x; Frain, M., Berven, N., Chan, F., Tschopp, M. (2008). Family resiliency, uncertainty, optimism, and the quality of life of individuals with HIV/AIDS, Rehabil Counsel Bull *52*(1), 16–27; Lavee, Y. (2013). Stress processes in families and couples. In G. W. Peterson, K. R. Bush (Eds). *Handbook of marriage and the family* (p. 159–176). New York, Springer. McCubbin, H. I., McCubbin, M. A., Thompson, A. (1993). Resiliency in families: the role of family schema and appraisal in family adaptation to crisis. In T. H. Brubaker, ed. *Family relations: challenges for the future*. Newbury Park, CA, Sage; Minuchin, S. (1974). *Families and family therapy*. Boston: Harvard University Press.

APPLICATIONS

Family-Centered Care

Family-centered care allows health care providers to have a uniform understanding of the patient and family's knowledge, preferences, and values as the basis for shared decision making. This provides consistent information to all involved in the patient's care and allows the family to identify any barriers that might arise with the care plan.

Health events of one family member have the potential to affect the whole family. Trotter and Martin (2007) note, "Families share genetic susceptibilities, environments, and behaviors, all of which interact to cause different levels of health and disease" (p. 561). They are instrumental in helping patients appreciate the need for diagnosis and treatment and in encouraging the patient to seek treatment. Family members are involved in a patient's health care decisions, ranging from treatment options to critical decisions about end-of-life care. Families play a pivotal advocacy role in treatment by monitoring and insisting on quality care for a family member.

The nurse in family-centered care are to:
- understand the impact of a medical crisis on family functioning, dynamics and health

- appreciate and respond empathetically to the emotional intensity of the experience for the family, and
- determine the appropriate level of family involvement in holistic care of the patient, based on an understanding of fundamental family system concepts (Leon & Knapp, 2008).

Assessment

As defined at the beginning of this chapter, nurses should consider that "a family is who they say they are" (Wright & Leahey, 2009, p. 70). Regardless of how it occurs, any health disruption becomes a family event. For immediate health care purposes, *family* is defined as the significant people in the patient's environment who are capable and willing to provide family-type support. However, even when the family is not directly involved in the family member's care, they will have feelings and opinions about the situation. Nonsupportive family responses have been associated with negative patient outcomes, while supportive positive family responses are associated with positive patient outcomes (Rosland, Heisler, & Piette, 2012). Simulation Exercise 12.1 allows you to analyze positive and negative family responses. Box 12.2 provides examples of situations that could warrant family assessment and nursing intervention.

SIMULATION EXERCISE 12.1   Positive and Negative Family Interactions

Purpose
To examine the effects of functional versus dysfunctional communication.

Procedure
Answer the following questions in a brief essay:
1. Recall a situation in dealing with a patient's family that you felt was a positive experience? What characteristics of that interaction made you feel this way?
2. Recall a situation in dealing with a patient's family that you felt was a negative experience? What characteristics of that interaction made you feel this way?

Discussion
Compare experiences, both positive and negative. What did you see as the most striking differences? In what ways were your responses similar or dissimilar from those of your peers? What do you see as the implications of this exercise for enhancing family communication in your nursing practice?

BOX 12.2   Indicators for Family Assessment

- Initial diagnosis of a serious physical or psychiatric illness or injury in a family member
- Family involvement and understanding needed to support recovery of patient
- Deterioration in a family member's condition
- Illness in a child, adolescent, or cognitively impaired adult
- A child, adolescent, or adult child having an adverse response to a parent's illness
- Discharge from a health care facility to the home or an extended-care facility
- Death of a family member
- Health problem defined by family as a family issue
- Indication of threat to relationship (abuse), neglect, or anticipated loss of family member

Assessment Tools

Initially, the nurse may not have the opportunity to complete a thorough family assessment. However, throughout the initial assessment and during ongoing nurse-patient interactions, the nurse must be attentive to cues indicating potential family-related concerns. The nurse should take into consideration the anticipated health needs of the individual patient upon discharge. For example, a 30-year-old patient who had major reconstructive knee surgery and cannot bear weight on the affected leg for 4 weeks will require consistent personal assistance for a period of time. Family members are often called into action in such circumstances. However, if some type of family discord previously existed, the patient may not feel comfortable requesting assistance from family members and may feel uncomfortable asking even close friends for assistance. In this case, the nurse acts as intermediary to facilitate conversations among potential caregivers.

Other situations (see Box 12.2) require a more in-depth assessment of family structure and function. Wright and Leahey's (2013) 15-minute interview, consisting of the genogram, ecomap, therapeutic questions, and commendations, provides a comprehensive look at family relationships. Assessment tools, such as the genogram, ecomap, and family time lines, are used to track family patterns. The structured format of these tools focuses on getting relational data quickly and can sensitize clinicians to systemic family issues that affect patterns of health and illness (Gerson, McGoldrick, & Petry, 2008).

Genograms

A *genogram* is defined as a diagram, which uses a standardized set of connections to graphically record basic information about family members and their relationships over three generations. Genograms can be updated and/or revised as new information emerges. A genogram can be used to identify patterns of inheritable medical conditions, but when used as part of a family psychosocial assessment, it provides information about family relationships and the personal perspective of the individual providing the information (Chrzastowski, 2011). Such information may be used to guide in-depth family assessment and future interventions.

There are three parts to genogram construction: mapping the family structure, recording family information, and describing the nature of family relationships. Fig. 12.3 identifies the symbols used to map family structure, with different symbols representing pregnancies, miscarriages, marriages, deaths, and other family events. Male family members are noted with a square and females with a circle. The oldest sibling is placed on the left, with younger siblings following from left to right, in order of birth. In the case of multiple marriages, the earliest is placed on the left and the most recent on the right. Lines drawn between significant family members identify the strength of relational patterns that are overly close, close, distant, cut off, or conflicted. An example of a family genogram is presented in Fig. 12.4.

The genogram explores the basic dynamics of a multigenerational family. Its multigenerational format, which traces family structure and relationships through three generations is based on the assumption that family relationship patterns are systemic, repetitive, and adaptive. Data about ages, birth and death dates, miscarriages, relevant illnesses, immigration, geographical location of current members, occupations and employment status, educational levels, patterns of family

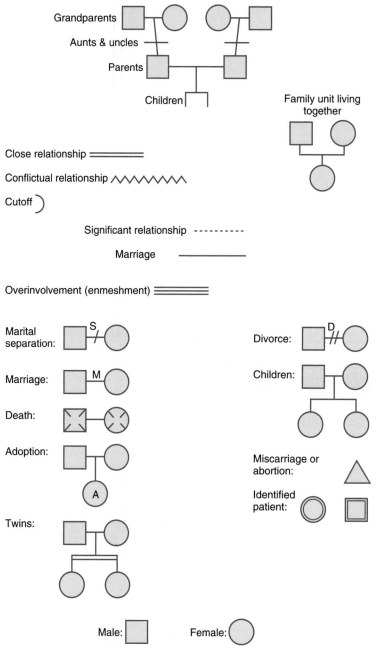

Fig. 12.3 Symbols for a Genogram.

members entering or leaving the family unit, religious affiliation or change, and military service are written near the symbols for each person. The recorded information about family members allows families and health professionals to simultaneously analyze complex family interaction patterns in a supportive environment. The impact of multiple generations on family relationships is more readily visible.

The genogram offers much more than a simple diagram of family relationship. Formal and informal learning about appropriate social behaviors and roles takes place within the family of origin. People learn role behaviors and responsibilities expected in different life stages experientially, by way of role modeling, and through direct instruction. Simulation Exercise 12.2 provides practice with developing a family genogram.

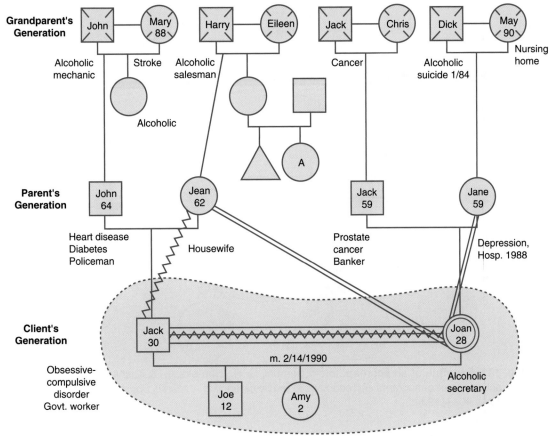

Fig. 12.4 Basic Family Genogram.

SIMULATION EXERCISE 12.2   Family Genograms

Purpose

To practice creating a family genogram.

Procedure

Students will break into pairs and interview one another to gain information to develop a family genogram. The genogram should include demographic information, occurrence of illness or death, and relationship patterns for three generations. Use the symbols for diagramming in Fig. 12.3 to create a visual picture of the family information. Validate your genogram for accuracy with your informant.

Discussion

Each person will display the genogram they developed and discuss the process of obtaining information. Discuss strategies for obtaining information expediently yet sensitively and tactfully. Consider additional questions that could be used to gather additional information. Were you able to identify patterns that could be helpful in assisting individuals to cope with a health crisis? Discuss how genograms can be used by a nurse in a clinical setting.

Ecomaps

An ecomap visually illustrates relationships between family members and the external environment (Kaakinen et al., 2010, p. 112). Beginning with an individual family unit or patient, the diagram extends to include significant social and community-based systems with which they have a relationship.

The diagram provides a quick visual of friends and community resource utilization. Adding the ecomap is an important dimension of family assessment, providing awareness of community supports that could be or are not being used to assist families. Ecomaps can point out resource deficiencies and conflicts in support services that can be corrected.

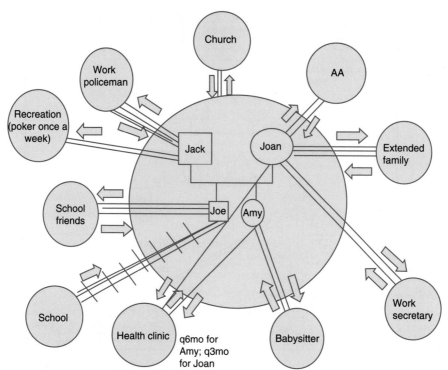

Fig. 12.5 Example of an Ecomap. (From Rempel, G. R., Neufeld, A., & Kushner, K. E. (2007). Interactive use of genograms and ecomaps in family caregiving research. *Journal of Family Nursing, 13*(4), 403–419.)

An ecomap starts with an inner circle representing the family unit, labeled with relevant family names. Smaller circles outside the family circle represent significant people, agencies, and social institutions with whom the family interacts on a regular basis. Examples include school, work, church, neighborhood friends, recreation activities, health care facilities or home care, and extended family. Lines are drawn from the inner family circle to outer circles indicating the strength of the contact and relationship. Straight lines indicate relationship, with additional lines used to indicate the strength of the relationship. Dotted lines suggest tenuous relationships. Stressful relationships are represented with slashes placed through the relationship line. Directional arrows indicate the flow of the relational energy. Fig. 12.5 shows an example of an ecomap. Simulation Exercise 12.3 provides an opportunity to construct an ecomap.

Family Time Lines

Time lines offer a visual diagram that captures significant family stressors, life events, health, and developmental patterns throughout the life cycle. Family history and patterns developed through multigenerational

transmission are represented as vertical lines. Horizontal lines indicate the timing of life events occurring over the current life span. These include such milestones as marriages, graduations, and unexpected life events, such as disasters, war, illness, death of person or pet, moves, births, and so forth (Fig. 12.6). Time lines are useful in looking at how the family history, developmental stage, and concurrent life events might interact with the current health concern.

By completing a family assessment, the nurse is able to develop a personalized plan of care for both the patient and the family. The findings of a family assessment should be documented for use by other members of the health care team and to avoid redundant collection of data.

Applying a Family-Centered Framework
Orienting the Family

The nurse-family relationship depends on reciprocal interactions between nurses and family members in which both are equal partners. Nurses should begin offering information to the family as soon as the patient is admitted to the hospital or service agency. Orientation to the facility,

SIMULATION EXERCISE 12.3 Family Ecomaps

Purpose

To practice creating a family ecomap.

Procedure

Using the interview process, students will break into pairs and interview one another to gain information to develop a family ecomap. The ecomap should include information about resources and stressors in the larger community system, such as school, church, health agencies, and interaction with extended family and friends for each student's family.

Discussion

Each person will display his or her ecomap and discuss the process of obtaining information. Discuss strategies for obtaining information expediently yet sensitively and tactfully. Explain how additional information obtained from an ecomap improves understanding of a family. Analyze the ecomap for areas that could be problematic if the informant were faced with a serious health issue. Describe how ecomaps can be used by a nurse in a clinical setting.

Note: Simulation Exercises 12.3 and 12.4 can be carried out during the same interview.

location of the cafeteria and restrooms, parking options, nearby lodging, and access to the hospitalist or physician are important points to include in early family interactions.

The initial family encounter sets the tone for the relationship. How nurses interact with each family member may be as important as what they choose to say. Begin with formal introductions, and explain the purpose of gathering assessment data. Even this early in the relationship, you should listen carefully for family expectations and general anxiety or expressed concerns about the patient, which may be revealed more through behavior than through words.

When interacting with families, the nurse must ensure the patient's right to privacy. With the implementation of the Health Insurance Portability and Accountability Act (HIPAA), family members may receive information regarding patient status only with the permission of either the patient or their designee (US Department of Health and Human Services, 2008). This means that as a nurse, you cannot give out information regarding your patient's health status either over the phone or in person without the patient's consent. Most facilities have developed strategies to ensure that staff members do not

disclose unauthorized information. For example, some facilities have adopted the use of a "code word" that is established upon admission. The code word is shared with only those family members who the patient wishes to receive information (McCullough & Schell-Chaple, 2013). If the person inquiring about the patient does not know the code word, then the nurse should politely inform the individual that for privacy reasons information cannot be provided.

Gathering Assessment Data

Determining the association/relationship of the family member to the patient is an initial step nurses can take in establishing a relationship. You might say, "I would like to hear what you think is the impact of your child's illness on the entire family." This statement guides your assessment, but also reminds the family that each family member is of concern to the health care team (Ylven & Granlund, 2009). Box 12.3 illustrates a framework for a family assessment with a patient entering cardiac rehabilitation. Family participation in the assessment process enhances the therapeutic relationship and completeness of the data. It is important to inquire about the family's cultural identity, rituals, values, level of family involvement, decision making, spiritual beliefs, and traditional behaviors as they relate to the health care of the patient (Leon & Knapp, 2008).

Knowledge of a family's past medical experiences, concurrent family stressors, and family expectations for treatment are essential pieces of family assessment data. Suggested questions include:

- How does the family view the current health crisis?
- What is each family member's most immediate concern?
- Has anyone else in the family experienced a similar problem?
- Are there any other recent changes or sources of stress in the family that make the current situation worse (pile up of demands)?
- How has the family handled the problem to date?
- Can you tell me what you expect from the health care team?
- As you close the session, ask, "Is there anything else I should know about your family and this experience?" Simulation Exercise 12.4 looks at assessment of family coping strengths.

Problem Identification

Based on assessment data (initial and ongoing), the nurse identifies if problems related to family communication and functioning exist. Even if no problem is identified, the nurse must be alert for cues that indicate potential problems in family communication and function. Some problems related to family function may require referral

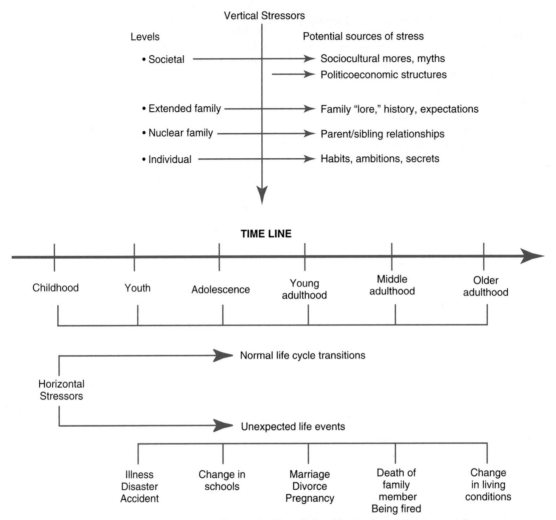

Fig. 12.6 Time-Line Assessment Example Identifying Vertical and Horizontal Stressors.

to a social worker, family therapist, or other member of the health care team. In other instances, it may be appropriate for the nurse to provide assistance to the family. Health related communication issues can involve: unexpressed fears or anger management of uncertainty, or finding common ground for shared decision making.

Planning

The more the family can be involved in the planning process, the greater is the likelihood of successful adaptation (Kaakinen et al., 2010, p. 116). The development of appropriate nursing actions should be based on mutually established goals. For the bedside nurse,

these goals are often short term, focusing on improving awareness of areas to improve communication (see the following subsection regarding interventive questioning). Resources are available to help ensure family engagement.

The Agency for Healthcare Research and Quality (AHRQ) has developed the Guide to Patient and Family Engagement in Hospital Quality and Safety. This document has a multidisciplinary focus with four specific strategies:

Strategy 1: Working with patients and families as advisors
Strategy 2: Communicating to improve quality
Strategy 3: Nurse bedside shift report
Strategy 4: IDEAL discharge planning (AHRQ, 2013)

BOX 12.3 Family Assessment for Patient Entering Cardiac Rehabilitation

Coping and Stress
- Who lives with you? _____
_____
- How do you handle stress? _____
_____
- Have you had any recent changes in your life (e.g., job change, move, change in marital status, loss)? _____
_____
- On whom do you rely for emotional support? _____
- Who relies on you for emotional support? _____
_____
- How does your illness affect your family members or significant others? _____
- Are there any health concerns of other family members? _____
- If so, how does this affect you? _____

Communication and Decision Making
- How would you describe the communication pattern in your family? _____
- How does your family address issues and concerns? _____
- Can you identify strengths and weaknesses within the family? _____
- Are family members supportive of each other? _____
- How are decisions that affect the entire family made? _____
- How are decisions implemented? _____
_____

Role
- What is your role in the family? _____
_____
- Can you describe the roles of other family members? _____

Value Beliefs
- What is your ethnic or cultural background? _____
_____
- What is your religious background? _____
_____

- Are there any particular cultural or religious healing practices in which you participate? _____
_____

Leisure Activities
- Do you participate in any organized social activities? _____
- In what leisure activities do you participate? _____
_____
- Do you anticipate any difficulty with continuing these activities? _____
- If so, how will you make the appropriate adjustments? _____
- Do you have a regular exercise regimen? _____
_____

Environmental Characteristics
- Do you live in a rural, suburban, or urban area? _____
_____
- What type of dwelling do you live in? _____
_____
- Are there stairs in your home? _____
- Where is the bathroom? _____
_____
- Are the facilities adequate to meet your needs? _____
- If not, what adjustments will be needed? _____
_____
- How do you plan to make those adjustments? _____
_____
- Are there any community services provided to you at home? (explain) _____
- Are there community resources available in your area? _____
- Do you have any other concerns at this time? _____
_____
- Is there anything that we have omitted? _____
_____
- Signature _____ (must be completed by RN) Date/Time

Developed by Conrad J, University of Maryland School of Nursing, 1993.

The preceding resources provide overall guidelines for patient- and family-centered care. As part of the overall plan of care, the nurse makes the most of communication skills to provide care to patients and families.

Interventive Questioning

Wright and Leahey (2009) identify questioning as a nursing intervention that nurses can use with families to identify family strengths; help family members sort out their personal fears, concerns, and challenges in health care

SIMULATION EXERCISE 12.4 Family Coping Strategies

Purpose

To broaden awareness of coping strategies among families.

Procedure

Each student is to recall a time when his or her family experienced a significant health crisis and how they coped. (Alternative strategy: Pick a health crisis you observed with a family in clinical practice.) Respond to the following questions:

1. Did the crisis cause a readjustment in roles?
2. Did it create tension and conflict, or did it catalyze members into turning to one another for support? Look at the behavior of individual members.
3. What would have helped your family in this crisis? Write a descriptive summary about this experience.

Discussion

Each student shares his or her experience. Discuss the differences in how families respond to crisis. Compile a listing of coping strategies and helpful interventions on the board. Discuss the nurse's role in support of the family.

BOX 12.4 Examples of Therapeutic Questions

- Who in the family is best at encouraging your mother to comply with her diet?
- What information do you still need to understand the prognosis of your disease? Who else would benefit from this information?
- Who is suffering the most?
- What do you feel when you see your family member in pain?
- If there were one question you could have answered now, what would it be?
- How can we best help you and your family?
- If your family member's treatment does not go well, who will be most affected?

Adapted from Wright, L. M., & Leahey, M. (2009). *Nurses and families: A guide to family assessment and intervention* (5th ed.). Philadelphia: F. A. Davis.

situations; and provide a vehicle for exploring alternative options. Family-centered interventions relate to: "(1) providing direct care, (2) removing barriers to needed services, and (3) improving the capacity of the family to act on its own behalf and assume responsibility" (Kaakinen et al., 2010, p. 117).

Interventive questioning can be either linear or circular. Linear questions are questions that facilitate understanding of a situation by both the nurse and family members. Circular questions are questions that lead to introspection, greater depth of understanding, and behavioral change. Circular questions focus on family interrelationships and the effect a serious health alteration has on individual family members and the equilibrium of the family system. Examples of therapeutic questions are found in Box 12.4. Both linear and circular questioning should be used as part of effective nursing care. The nurse uses information the family provides as the basis for additional questions.

The following case example demonstrates the use of circular questioning when the nurse asks a family, "What has been your biggest challenge in caring for your mother at home?"

In this example, each family member's concern is related, but different. The therapeutic circular question opens a discussion about each person's anxiety. As family members hear the concerns of other family members and as they hear themselves respond, their perspective broadens. The resulting conversation forms the basis for developing strategies that are mutually acceptable to all family members.

Case Example

Daughter: My biggest challenge has been finding a balance between caring for my mother and also caring for my children and husband. I have also had to learn a lot about the professional and support resources that are available in the community.

Son-in-law: For me, the biggest challenge has been convincing my wife that I can take over for a while, in order for her to get some rest. I worry that she will become exhausted.

Mother: I have appreciated all the help that they give me. My biggest challenge is to continue to do as much as possible for myself so that I do not become too much of a burden on them. Sometimes I wonder about moving to a palliative care setting or a hospice (Leahey & Harper-Jaques, 1996, p. 135).

Meaningful involvement in the patient's care not only differs from family to family, it differs among individual family members (Ylven & Granlund, 2009). Individual family members have different perspectives. Hearing each family member's perspective helps the family and nurse develop a unified understanding of significant treatment goals and implications for family involvement.

SIMULATION EXERCISE 12.5   Developing a Family Nursing Care Plan

Purpose

To practice skills needed with difficult family patterns.

Procedure

Read the case study, and think of how you could interact appropriately with this family.

Mr. Monroe, age 43 years, was chairing a board meeting of his large, successful manufacturing corporation when he developed shortness of breath, dizziness, and a crushing, viselike pain in his chest. An ambulance was called, and he was taken to the medical center. Subsequently, he was admitted to the coronary unit with a diagnosis of an impending myocardial infarction (MI).

Mr. Monroe is married with three children: Steve, age 14; Sean, age 12; and Lisa, age 10. He is the president and majority stockholder of his company. He has no history of cardiovascular problems, although his father died at the age of 38 of a massive coronary occlusion. His oldest brother died at the age of 42 from the same condition, and his other brother, still living, became a semi-invalid after suffering two heart attacks, one at the age of 44 and the other at 47.

Mr. Monroe is tall, slim, suntanned, and very athletic. He swims daily; jogs every morning for 30 min; plays golf regularly; and is an avid sailor, having participated in every yacht regatta and usually winning. He is very health-conscious and has had annual physical checkups. He watches his diet and quit smoking to avoid possible damage to his heart. He has been determined to avoid dying young or becoming an invalid like his brother.

When he was admitted to the coronary care unit, he was conscious. Although in a great deal of pain, he seemed determined to control his own fate. While in the unit, he was an exceedingly difficult patient, a trial to the nursing staff and his physician. He constantly watched and listened to everything going on around him and demanded complete explanations about any procedure,

equipment, or medication he received. He would sleep in brief naps and only when he was totally exhausted. Despite his obvious tension and anxiety, his condition stabilized. The damage to his heart was considered minimal, and his prognosis was good. As the pain diminished, he began asking when he could go home and when he could go back to work. He was impatient to be moved to a private room so that he could conduct some of his business by telephone.

When Mrs. Monroe visited, she approached the nursing staff with questions regarding Mr. Monroe's condition, usually asking the same question several times in different ways. She also asked why she was not being "told everything."

Interactions between Mr. Monroe and Mrs. Monroe were noted by the staff as Mr. Monroe telling Mrs. Monroe all the things she needed to do. Little intimate contact was noted.

Mr. Monroe denied having any anxiety or concerns about his condition, although his behavior contradicted his denial. Mrs. Monroe would agree with her husband's assessment when questioned in his company.

Discussion

1. What questions would you ask the patient and family to obtain data regarding their adaptation to crisis?
2. What family nursing diagnosis would apply with this case study?
3. What nursing interventions are appropriate to interact with this patient and his family?
4. What other members of the health care team should be involved with this family situation?
5. How would you plan to transmit the information to the family?
6. What outcomes and measures would you use to determine success or failure of the nursing care plan?

Developed by Conrad, J. (1993). University of Maryland School of Nursing, Baltimore, MD.

Although treatment plans should be tailored around personal patient goals, acknowledging family needs, values, and priorities enhances compliance, especially if they are different. Shared decision making and the development of realistic, achievable goals makes it easier for everyone concerned to accomplish them with a sense of ownership and self-efficacy about the process. Taking small achievable steps is preferred to attempting giant steps that misjudge what the family can realistically do. Simulation Exercise 12.5 provides practice with developing a family nursing care plan.

Implementation

Nurses can only offer interventions; it is up to the family to accept them (Wright & Leahey, 2013). Suggested nursing actions to promote positive change in family functioning include the following:

- encouraging the telling of illness narratives,
- commending family and individual strengths,
- offering information and opinions,
- validating or normalizing emotional responses,
- encouraging family support,

- supporting family members as caregivers, and
- encouraging respite.

Encouraging Family Narratives

Families need to tell their story about the experience of their loved one's illness or injury; this may be quite different from how the patient is experiencing it. The differences can lead to a more complete understanding. Such sharing can help build mutual support and empathy (Walsh, 2002). Nurses play an important role in helping families understand, negotiate, and reconcile differences in perceptions without losing face.

Case Example

Frances is a patient with a diagnosis of breast cancer. When she sees her oncologist, Frances reports that she is feeling fine, eating, and able to function in much the same way as before receiving chemotherapy. Her husband's perception differs. He reports that her appetite has declined such that she only eats a few spoonfuls of food and she spends much of the day in bed. What Frances is reporting is true. When she is up, she enjoys doing what she did previously, although at a slower pace, and she does eat at every meal. Frances is communicating her need to feel normal, which is important to support. What her husband adds is also true. Her husband's input allows Frances to receive the treatment she needs to stimulate her appetite and give her more energy.

Incorporating Family Strengths

Otto (1963) introduced the concept of family strengths as potential and actual resources that families can use to make their lives more satisfying and fulfilling when health care changes are required, and they usually are with patients suffering from serious illness or injury, working through family strengths rather than focusing on deficits is useful. Viewing the family as having strengths to cope with a problem rather than being a problem is a healing strategy. The intent is not that the family comes away from a stressful event or period without blemish, but instead that the existing skills and coping strategies are used in a healthy manner (Walsh, 2002). While each family's experience with illness varies, commonalities exist. The nurse should share strategies that families in similar situations have found effective.

Giving Commendations

Commendations involve "recognizing capabilities, skills and competencies" (Poor, 2013). Commendations are particularly effective when the family seems dispirited or

---

SIMULATION EXERCISE 12.6   Offering Commendations

Purpose
To practice using commendation skills.

Procedure
Students will work in groups of three students. Each student will develop a commendation about the two other students in the group. The commendation should reflect a personal strength that the reflecting student has observed over a period of time. Examples might include kindness, integrity, commitment, persistence, goal-directedness, tolerance, or patience. Write a brief paragraph about the trait or behavior that you observe in this person. If you can, give some examples of why you have associated this particular characteristic with the person. Each student, in turn, should read his or her reflections about the other two participants, starting the conversation with good eye contact, the name of the receiving student, and a simple orienting statement (e.g., "Kelly, this is what I have observed in knowing you...").

Discussion
Class discussion should focus on the thought process of the students in developing particular commendations, the values they focused on, and any consideration they gave to the impact of the commendation on the other students. The students can also discuss the effect of hearing the commendations about themselves and what it stimulated in them. Complete the discussion by considering how commendations can be used with families and how they can be used to counteract family resistance to working together.

---

confused about a illness or accident. More than a simple compliment, commendations should reflect patterns of behavior observed in the family unit over time. Wright and Leahey (2013) differentiate between a commendation ("Your family is showing much courage in living with your wife's cancer for 5 years.") and a compliment ("Your son is so gentle despite feeling so ill.") (p. 270). They suggest giving at least one commendation per interview. There may be situations that seem extremely dire, but by identifying even one positive factor, a family may feel empowered to push through the difficult situation. Simulation Exercise 12.6 provides practice with giving commendations.

Informational Support

Helping a family become aware of information from the environment and how to access it empowers families. By showing interest in the coping strategies that have and have not worked, the nurse can help the family recognize progress in their ability to cope with a difficult situation.

You can offer family members support related to talking with extended family, children, and others about the patient's illness. You can help family members prepare questions for meeting with physicians and other health professionals. Encouraging family members to write down key points to be addressed with other family members and physicians can be helpful. Written instructions should also be provided upon discharge.

The statement that discharge planning begins at admission is very true when it comes to providing families with information. The nurse should anticipate assistance that will be needed upon discharge that will require family involvement. Because family members are not available consistently, the nurse should plan family teaching sessions prior to the time of discharge to create an environment more conducive to learning (Kornburger, Gibson, Sadowski, Maletta, & Klingbeil, 2013). The use of the "teach-back" method can be used with families and individual patients. Review Chapter 15 regarding health teaching.

If the patient is more seriously ill, and is receptive, the nurse should see this as an opportunity to provide information regarding end-of-life decision making. Decisions regarding end-of-life care are best carried out when families are not in a crisis mode. Thus, you can engage with families in discussions about the cultural, ethical, and physical implications of using or discontinuing life-support systems. This is nursing's special niche, as these conversations are rarely one-time events, and nurses can provide informal opportunities for discussing them during care provision. Refer to Chapter 21 for additional information regarding advanced directives and end-of-life care planning.

Meeting the Needs of Families With Critically Ill Patients

Having a family member in an intensive care unit (ICU) represents a serious crisis for most families. Eggenberger and Nelms (2007) suggest, "Patients enter a critical care unit in physiological crisis, while their families enter the hospital in psychological crisis" (p. 1619). Box 12.5 identifies the care needs of the families of critically ill patients. Family-centered relationships are key dimensions of quality care in the ICU.

Proximity to the Patient

The need to remain near the patient is a priority for many family members of patients in the ICU (Perrin, 2009). Although the family may appear to hover too closely, it is

---

BOX 12.5 Caring for Family Needs in the Intensive Care Unit

Families of critically ill patients need to:
- Feel there is hope
- Feel that hospital personnel care about the patient
- Have a waiting room near the patient
- Be called at home about changes in the patient's condition
- Know the prognosis
- Have questions answered honestly
- Know specific facts about the patient's prognosis
- Receive information about the patient at least once a day
- Have explanations given in understandable terms
- Be allowed to see the patient frequently

Perrin, K. (2009). *Understanding the essentials of critical care nursing* (pp. 40–41). Upper Saddle River, NJ: Pearson Prentice Hall.

---

usually an attempt to rally around the patient in critical trouble (Leon, 2008). Viewed from this perspective, nurses can be more empathetic. As the family develops more confidence in the genuine interest and competence of the staff, the hovering tends to lessen.

Visitation policies may need to be adjusted based on the availability of family members and patient needs (Hart, Hardin, Townsend, Ramsey, & Mahrle-Henson, 2013). Staff need to be aware that family members may have obligations that prevent visits at expected times of day. When families visit loved ones in the ICU, the nurse should acknowledge them and provide any updated information that is available.

Families can be a primary support to patients, but they usually need encouragement and concrete suggestions for maximum effect and satisfaction. Family members feel helpless to reverse the course of the patient's condition and appreciate opportunities to help their loved one. Suggesting actions that family members can take at the bedside include doing range-of-motion exercises, holding the patient's hand, positioning pillows, and providing mouth care or ice chips. Talking with and reading to the patient, even if the person is unresponsive, can be meaningful for both the family and patient.

Helping families balance the need to be present with the patient's needs to conserve energy and have some alone time to rest or regroup is important. Family members also need time apart from their loved one for the same reasons. Tactfully explaining the need of critically ill patients to have family presence without feeling pressure to interact can be supportive. Encouraging families to take respite breaks is equally important. Providing information regarding dining and lodging can facilitate periods of rest for family members.

At the same time, nurses need to be sensitive to and respect a family member's apprehension or emotional state about their critically ill family member. Individual family members may need the nurse's support in talking about difficult feelings. Nurses can role model communication with patients, using simple caring words and touch. Families are quick to discern the difference between nurses who are able to connect with a critically ill patient in this way and those who are not, as evidenced in a family member's comment that "some seem to have a way with him and they talk to him like he is awake" (Eggenberger & Nelms, 2007, p. 1623).

Breaking Bad News to Families

The physician is the provider who most often delivers life-threatening critical information to patients and families. It is often the nurse at the bedside who ensures adequate patient and family understanding of information that has been provided. Additionally, nurses often notify patients and family members of significant changes in patient status, such as poor wound healing, transfers, a need for further testing, and so forth (Edwards, 2010). Sometimes, this occurs over the telephone, which further complicates the communication process. In each instance, well-planned communication can facilitate positive coping and adaptation.

The situation, background, assessment, recommendation (SBAR) format (see Chapter 2) can be adapted to guide the communication of bad news to families. The nurse should plan for notifying patients and families of bad news in a similar manner to communicating with other health team members. Making notes of key points can assist the nurse to remember items, which need to be addressed during a conversation. If the bad news is to be delivered in person, then the nurse should plan for a private, quiet setting (Pirie, 2012). If the news is to be delivered over the phone, the nurse should ask if it is a good time for a conversation. Present some background information, and alert the person that bad news is coming. The bad news should be presented in a factual, concise manner. Then the nurse should allow for a period of silence to show respect for the individual and to allow the person to process the information. In follow-up, the nurse should ask if the person understands the information that has been presented and ask for questions. The interaction should close with a summary of the treatment plan and when further communication can be expected (Pirie, 2012).

Providing Information

Families with family members in the ICU have a fundamental need for information, particularly if the patient is unresponsive. Many families have stated, "Not knowing is the worst part." Providing updated information as a clinical situation changes is critical. This information is particularly critical when family members must act as decision makers for patients who cannot make them on their own (Perrin, 2009). The use of a "Family Supportive Care Algorithm" that guided communication among family members and the health care team demonstrated families' improved sense of participation in decision making and perception of staff working as a team (Huffines et al., 2013).

Families of a patient in the ICU need ongoing information on the patient's progress, modifications in care requirements, and any changes in expected outcomes, opportunities to ask questions and clarify information empower families. Identifying one family member to act as the primary contact helps ensure continuity between staff and family. A short daily phone call when family members cannot be present maintains the family connection and reduces family stress (Leon, 2008). Nurses in the ICU often serve as mediators between patient, family, and other health providers to ensure that data streams remain open, coordinated, and relevant.

How health care providers deliver information is important. Even if the patient's condition or prognosis leaves little room for optimism, the family needs to feel some hope and that the staff genuinely cares about what is happening with the patient and family (Perrin, 2009).

Caring for Families in the Pediatric Intensive Care Unit

Most parents of hospitalized children, particularly those in the pediatric intensive care unit (PICU), want to be with their children as often as possible (Kaakinen et al., 2010, p. 361). Parents of children in the PICU need frequent reassurance from the nurse about why things are being done for their child and about treatment-related tubes and equipment. They want to actively participate in their child's care and have their questions honestly answered.

Families act as the child's advocate during hospitalization, either informally, by insisting on high-quality care, or formally, as the legal surrogate decision maker designated to make health care decisions on behalf of the patient. The nurse is a primary health care provider agent in working with families facing these issues. A critical intervention for the family as a whole and its individual members is to help them recognize their limitations and hidden strengths and to maintain a balance of health for all members.

Family-Centered Relationships in the Community

Nearly half of all adult US citizens are affected by at least one chronic disease (Centers for Disease Control and Prevention [CDC], 2012). Four modifiable risk factors (physical activity, obesity, smoking, and alcohol consumption) contribute substantially to the financial and emotional burden associated with chronic disease. Community-based nurses have many opportunities to educate and assist individuals to decrease risk factors and self-manage existing diseases. Many individuals are able to self-manage their disease, but an increasing number require family support with coping, self-management, and palliative care.

Nurses in nonacute care settings have multiple opportunities to provide screening and health teaching to newly insured families. A major portion of these interactions should focus on encouraging families to adopt a healthy lifestyle to decrease the incidence of disease and illness. Concurrently, the concept of patient-centered care is becoming widely adopted throughout health care. For community-dwelling individuals, the concept of patient-centered care focuses on empowering individuals to not only self-manage chronic diseases, but also to make appropriate lifestyle modifications with the intent of either preventing disease or minimizing the effects of disease. The combination of PPACA and patient-centered care should stimulate nurses to consider what constitutes effective communication when providing health education to families. Families need to feel empowered to take responsibility for their health state (Kaakinen et al., 2010, p. 478). Family empowerment develops when well-designed interventions are appropriate to the needs and resources of the family unit. The concepts presented in Chapter 15 can be used within the context of family health teaching.

Family caregivers are common as more people live with chronic illness on a daily basis; the level of assistance required varies on a person-by-person basis. Healthy family members have concurrent demands on their time from their own nuclear families, work, church, and community responsibilities.

A significant change in health status can exacerbate previously unresolved relationship issues, which may need advanced intervention, in addition to the specific health care issues. When individual family members are experiencing a transition, for example, ending or entering a relationship or a job change, they may not be as available to provide support and can experience unnecessary guilt. Nurses need to consider the broader family responsibilities people have as an important part of the context of health care in providing holistic care to a family.

Meeting Family Informational Needs

Providing information to family caregivers often starts when the patient is discharged from an acute-care facility. With the passage of time, the individual's needs for assistance may change, but the caregiver may lack the ability to adequately modify the care being provided. A sense of "preparedness" was identified as a factor in contributing to the hope and anxiety of caregivers (Henriksson & Arestedt, 2013). As a result, nurses in clinics and community-based centers should be responsive to cues from caregivers indicating deficient knowledge. Nurses can offer suggestions about how to respond to these changes and offer support to the family caregiver as they emerge. Helping family members access services, support groups, and natural support networks at each stage of their loved one's illness empowers family members because they feel they are helping in a tangible way.

Supporting the Caregiver

Discharge planning requires attention to caring for the caregiver as well as the patient (Walton, 2011). Providing emotional support is crucial to helping families cope. Remaining aware of one's own values and staying calm and thoughtful can be very helpful to a family in crisis. Remember that your words can either strengthen or weaken a family's confidence in their ability to care for an ill family member. Focus initially on issues that are manageable within the context of home caregiving. This provides a sense of empowerment. The nurse can encourage the family to develop new ways of coping or can list alternatives and allow the family to choose coping styles that might be useful to them. Focus on what goes well, and ask the family to share their ideas about how to best care for the patient. You can help normalize feelings of resentment and help family members set reasonable limits on overly dependent behavior.

Many families will need information about additional home care services, community resources, and options needed to meet the practical, financial, and emotional demands of caring for a chronically ill family member. There are support groups available for family caregivers of patients with chronic illnesses. These are extremely helpful supports for family members. Not only can they provide practical ideas, but the support of being able to talk about your feelings, and finding that you are not alone, is healing for family members and indirectly beneficial for patients.

Encouraging families to use natural helping systems increases the network of emotional and economic support available to the family in a time of crisis. Examples of natural helping systems include contact with other relatives, neighbors, friends, and churches. Promoting effective coping strategies and minimizing barriers to providing care should be implemented by community-based nurses (Leeman, Skelly, Burns, Carlson, & Soward, 2008).

Validating and Normalizing Emotions

Families can experience many conflicting emotions when placed in the position of providing protracted care for a loved one. Compassion, protectiveness, and caring can be intermingled with feelings of helplessness and being trapped. Major role reversals can stimulate anger and resentment for both patient and family caregiver.

Sibling or family position or geographic proximity may put pressure on certain family members to provide a greater share of the care. Criticism or advice from less-involved family members can be disconcerting, and conflicts about care decisions can create rifts in family relationships. Some caregivers find themselves mourning for their loved one, even though the person is still alive, wishing it could all end, but feeling guilt about having such thoughts.

These emotions are normal responses to abnormal circumstances. Listening to the family caregiver's feelings and struggles without judgment can be the most healing intervention you can provide. Nurses can normalize negative feelings by offering insights about common feelings associated with chronic illness. Family members may need guidance and permission to get respite and recharge their commitment by attending to their own needs. Support groups can provide families with emotional and practical support and a critical expressive outlet.

Psychosocial concerns for parents with chronically ill children can cover many relationship issues, for example, how to respond and discipline children with chronic illness. Parents must balance caring for their chronically ill child along with parenting other children (Kaakinen et al., 2010, p. 255). Healthy siblings may experience feelings of resentment, worry that they might contract a similar illness, or have unrealistic expectations of their part in the treatment process. Siblings need clear information about the sick child's diagnosis and care plan and the opportunity to experience their own childhood as fully as possible. Simulation Exercise 12.7 provides practice with using intervention skills with families.

Pitfalls to Avoid

While we, as nurses, strive to be effective in all communication, there are times that our communication efforts are less than ideal. Wright and Leahey (2013) identified three common errors that occur in family nursing.

1. Failure to create context for change. In such instances, the nurse does not establish a therapeutic environment for open discussion of family concerns. Another

---

SIMULATION EXERCISE 12.7   Using Intervention Skills With Families

Purpose
To practice using intervention skills with families.

Procedure
Describe a situation in which you have worked with a family. This may be from a clinical experience or other personal experience. Think about how you talked with the family regarding a specific problem.
Consider the following:

- Did you talk with the family about the problem and learn how they have dealt with the problem, their perception of the problem, and its impact on their family?
- What would be some approaches identified in the text to help them explore the problem in more depth and begin to develop viable options?
- Did you feel you were too intrusive or not assertive enough?
- Did you validate all members' perceptions and perspectives? Did you clarify information and feelings? Did you remain nonjudgmental and objective?
- Did you respect the family's values and beliefs without imposing your own? Did you assist the family in clarifying and understanding the problem in a way that could lead to resolution?

Discussion
In small groups, discuss your responses to the questions above. Be attentive to the experiences of others. Did they have similar experiences? Discuss strategies to facilitate goal-directed communication and problem resolution. How can nurses best provide support to families? How could families learn to use honest communication most of the time? How does one influence this in one's own family?

---

example would be a plan of care that would not be effective in light of the family situation (resources, distance, health state). To avoid this pitfall, the nurse should be respectful of each family member, obtain as much information about the family and its members as possible, and acknowledge the difficulty of the situation.

2. Avoid taking sides. To minimize the risk of taking sides, the nurse should use questioning skills that help family members develop insight into the depth and scope of the problem. The use of circular questions, as discussed earlier, can be helpful.

3. Giving too much advice prematurely. Nurses inherently are in a position to provide patients and families with information and advice. However, it must be well timed and appropriate to the particular situation. To avoid this pitfall, obtain as much information from family members as possible before providing suggestions. Advice should be framed so that it is expressed as a suggestion, rather than a set of rules. Follow up with family members to get their reaction to your suggestion.

Using Technology to Enhance Family Communication

The use of the Internet and other mobile technologies has progressed dramatically. Many community-dwelling individuals use electronic communication devices on a daily basis, whether via a cellular phone or the Internet. The utilization of electronic communication with patients and families is less common but increasing rapidly. Federal regulations as outlined in HIPAA apply to all modes of communication and must be considered when communicating with family members in an electronic format.

Families today are often geographically separated. Encouraging and assisting patients to send e-mail or call using a wireless phone can decrease that distance. Simply hearing the voice of a patient can help to allay fear for distant relatives. Caring Bridge (caringbridge.org) is an organization that offers free personalized websites for individuals undergoing serious health concerns. Online support groups are becoming more prevalent for those experiencing health issues and for families and caregivers (van der Eijk et al., 2013). The nurse should assess the comfort level of family members with the use of technology. Learning to use a smart phone, e-mail, or other technology-based communication can add to the stress of an already anxious situation, and there are other educational modalities if the family member is not really interested. However, if there is interest, the web and YouTube offer good information, and seeing a skill presented on a video may be more useful than simple verbal instructions.

Evaluations

Evaluation should include both determining effectiveness of nursing interventions and self-reflection by the nurse regarding personal effectiveness. The nurse at the bedside may not see long-term benefits from family interactions due to the episodic nature of contemporary health care. It is important that the nurse provide closure to patient interactions in any setting. You can accomplish this task by summarizing the interaction, asking the family if they have any questions, and providing information regarding follow-up. Bereaved families have reported that the support received from nurses played an important role in how they were able to cope (MacConnell, Aston, Randel, & Zwaagstra, 2012). No matter how brief family interactions are, your impact may be substantial.

Referrals should include a summary of the information gained to date and should be communicated by the health team member most knowledgeable about the patient's condition. Patients and families should be provided with information related to referrals and next steps.

Self-evaluation and self-reflection by the nurse can be used to identify which communication strategies were successful in a given situation and which were not (Kaakinen et al., 2010, p. 119). By identifying effective and ineffective family communication techniques, a repertoire of skills can be developed, thus enhancing the overall effectiveness of nurses' communication and practice.

SUMMARY

This chapter provides an overview of family communication and the complex dynamics inherent in family relationships. Families have a structure, defined as the way in which members are organized. Family function refers to the roles people take in their families, and family process describes the communication that takes place within the family. Family-centered care is developed through a combination of strategies designed to gather information in a systematic, efficient manner starting with the genogram, ecomap, and timeline. Therapeutic questions and giving commendations are interventions nurses can use with families. Families with critically ill members need continuous updated information and the freedom to be with their family member as often as possible. Involving the family in the care of the patient is important. Parents want to participate in the care of their acutely ill patient. Nursing interventions are aimed at strengthening family functioning and supporting family coping during hospitalization and in the community.

ETHICAL DILEMMA: What Would You Do?

Terry Connors is a 90-year-old woman living alone in a two-story house. She has two daughters, Maria and Maggie. Maria lives 90 miles away, but works two jobs because her husband has been laid off for 9 months. Her other daughter Maggie lives in another state. So far, Terry has been able to live by herself, but within the past 2 weeks, she fell down a few stairs in her house and she has trouble hearing the telephone. Terry has very poor vision, walks with a cane, and relies on her neighbors for assistance several times a week. Maria and her husband visit every 2 weeks to bring groceries. Both Maria and Maggie worry about her and would like to see her in a nursing home. Terry will not consider this option. As the nurse working with this family, how would you address your ethical responsibilities to Terry, Maria, and Maggie?

DISCUSSION QUESTIONS

1. Identify family communication situations (e.g., end of life, family discord) that you believe would be professionally challenging. Describe strategies that you, as a nurse, could use to be prepared to better manage those situations.

2. How would you personally feel as a nurse delivering bad news to a family?

REFERENCES

Ackley, B. J., & Ladwig, G. B. (2011). *Nursing diagnosis handbook: An evidence-based guide to planning care.* St. Louis, MO: Mosby.

Agency for Healthcare Research and Quality (AHRQ). (2013). *Guide to patient and family engagement in hospital quality and safety.* Retrieved from http://www.ahrq.gov/professionals/systems/hospital/engagingfamilies/guide.html.

Antle, B. F., Christensen, D. N., van Zyl, M. A., & Barbee, A. P. (2012). The impact of the Solution Based Casework (SBC) practice model on federal outcomes in public child welfare. *Child Abuse & Neglect, 36*(4), 342–353.

Barker, P. (1998). Different approaches to family therapy. *Nursing Times, 94*(14), 60–62.

Bishop, S. M., Walker, M. D., & Spivak, I. M. (2013). Family presence in the adult burn intensive care unit during dressing changes. *Critical Care Nurse, 33*(1), 14–22.

Bowen Center for the Study of the Family. (2013). Bowen theory: societal emotional process. Retrieved from http://www.thebowencenter.org/pages/conceptsep.html.

Bowen, M. (1978). *Family Therapy in Clinical Practice.* Northvale, NJ: Jason Aronson.

Centers for Disease Control and Prevention (CDC). (2012). *Chronic diseases and health promotion.* Retrieved from http://www.cdc.gov/chronicdisease/overview/index.htm.

Chrzastowski, S. K. (2011). A narrative perspective on genograms: Revisiting classical family therapy methods. *Clinical Child Psychology and Psychiatry, 16*(4), 635–644. https://doi.org/10.1177/1359104511400966.

Cicchetti, D., & Blender, J. A. (2006). A multiple levels of analysis perspective on resilience: Implications for the developing brain, neural plasticity, and preventive interventions. *Annals of the New York Academy of Sciences, 1094,* 248–258.

Duvall, E. (1958). *Marriage and family development.* Philadelphia: J. B. Lippincott.

Edwards, M. (2010). How to break bad news and avoid common difficulties. *Nursing & Residential Care, 12*(10), 495–497.

Eggenberger, S., & Nelms, T. (2007). Being family: The family experience when an adult member is hospitalized with a critical illness. *Journal of Clinical Nursing, 16*(9), 1618–1628.

Fivaz-Depeursinge, E., Lopes, F., Python, M., & Favez, N. (2009). Coparenting and toddler's interactive styles in family coalitions. *Family Process, 48*(4), 500–516. https://doi.org/10.1111/j.1545-5300.2009.01298.x.

Frain, M., Berven, N., Chan, F., & Tschopp, M. (2008). Family resiliency, uncertainty, optimism, and the quality of life of individuals with HIV/AIDS. *Rehabilitation Counseling Bulletin, 52*(1), 16–27.

Gerson, R., McGoldrick, M., & Petry, S. (2008). *Genograms: Assessment and intervention* (3rd ed.). New York, NY: W. W. Norton & Co.

Gilbert, R. (2006). *The eight concepts of Bowen theory.* Falls Church, VA: Leading Systems Press.

Goldenberg, H., & Goldenberg, I. (2013). *Family therapy: An overview.* Belmont, CA: Cengage Brooks/Cole.

Hart, A., Hardin, S. R., Townsend, A. P., Ramsey, S., & Mahrle-Henson, A. (2013). Critical care visitation: Nurse and family preference. *Dimensions of Critical Care Nursing: DCCN, 32*(6), 289–299. https://doi.org/10.1097/01.DCC.0000434515.58265.7d.

Henriksson, A., & Arestedt, K. (2013). Exploring factors and caregiver outcomes associated with feelings of preparedness for caregiving in family caregivers in palliative care: A correlational, cross-sectional study. *Palliative Medicine, 27*(7), 639–646.

Henry, J., & Kaiser Family Foundation (2011). *Focus on health reform: Summary of the affordable care act.* Washington, DC: Author. Retrieved from http://kaiserfamilyfoundation.files.wordpress.com/2011/04/8061-021.pdf.

Hill, W. J., Hasty, C., & Moore, C. (2011). Differentiation of self and the process of forgiveness: A clinical perspective for couple and family therapy. *Australian and New Zealand Journal of Family Therapy, 32*(1), 43–57.

Huffines, M., Johnson, K. L., Smitz Naranjo, L. L., Lissauer, M., Fishel, M. A., D'Angelo Howes, S. M., et al. (2013). Improving family satisfaction and participation in decision making in an intensive care unit. *Critical Care Nurse, 33*(5), 56–68.

Jensen, T., & Schafer, K. (2013). Stepfamily functioning and closeness: Children's views on second marriages and stepfather relationships. *Social Work, 58*(2), 127–136.

Kaakinen, J. R., Gedaly-Duff, V., Coehlo, D. P., & Hanson, S. M. H. (2010). *Family health care nursing: Theory practice and research.* Philadelphia, PA: F. A. Davis.

Kornburger, C., Gibson, C., Sadowski, S., Maletta, K., & Klingbeil, C. (2013). Using "Teach-Back" to promote a safe transition from hospital to home: An evidence-based approach to improving the discharge process. *Journal of Pediatric Nursing, 28*, 282–291.

Lavee, Y., (2013). Chapter 8: Stress processes in families and couples. In G. W. Peterson, & K. R. Bush (Eds.), *Handbook of marriage and the family* (pp. 159–176). New York: Springer.

Leahey, M., & Harper-Jaques, S. (1996). Family-nurse relationships: core assumptions and clinical implications. *Journal of Family Nursing, 2*(2), 133–152.

Leeman, J., Skelly, A. H., Burns, D., Carlson, J., & Soward, A. (2008). Tailoring a diabetes self-care intervention for use with older, rural African American women. *Diabetes Educator, 34*(2), 310–317.

Leon, A. (2008). *Involving family systems in critical care nursing: Challenges and opportunities, Dimensions of Critical Care Nursing: DCCN, 27*(6), 255–262.

Leon, A., & Knapp, S. (2008). Involving family systems in critical care nursing: Challenges and opportunities. *Dimensions of Critical Care Nursing: DCCN, 27*(6), 255–262.

MacConnell, G., Aston, M., Randel, P., & Zwaagstra, N. (2012). Nurses' experiences providing bereavement follow-up: An exploratory study using feminist poststructuralism. *Journal of Clinical Nursing, 22*, 1094–1102.

MacKay, L. (2012). Trauma and Bowen family systems Theory: working with adults who were abused as children. *Australian and New Zealand Journal of Family Therapy, 33*(3), 232–241.

McCullough, J., & Schell-Chaple, H. (2013). Maintaining patients' privacy and confidentiality with family communications in the intensive care unit. *Critical Care Nurse, 33*(5), 77–79.

Minuchin, S. (1974). *Families and family therapy.* Boston, MA: Harvard University Press.

Nichols, M., & Schwartz, R. (2009). *Family therapy: Concepts and methods* (9th ed.). Upper Saddle River, NJ: Prentice Hall.

Otto, H. (1963). Criteria for assessing family strength. *Family Process, 2*, 329–338.

Perrin, K. (2009). *Understanding the essentials of critical care nursing.* Upper Saddle River, NJ: Pearson Prentice Hall.

Pirie, A. (2012). Pediatric palliative care communication: Resources for the clinical nurse specialist. *Clinical Nurse Specialist, 26*(4), 212–215.

Poor, C. J. (2013, Dec. 10). Important interactional strategies for everyday public health nursing practice. *Public Health Nursing,* 1–7. https://doi.org/10.1111/phn.12097. [Epub ahead of print].

Rempel, G., Neufeld, A., & Kushner, K. (2007). Interactive use of genograms and ecomaps in family caregiving research. *Journal of Family Nursing, 13*(4), 403–419.

Rosland, A., Heisler, M., & Piette, J. (2012). The impact of family behaviors and communication patterns on chronic illness outcomes: A systematic review. *Journal of Behavioral Medicine, 35*(2), 221–239.

Segaric, C. A., & Hall, W. A. (2005). The family theory-practice gap: a matter of clarity? *Nursing Inquiry, 12*(3), 210–218.

Toman, W. (1992). *Family therapy and sibling position.* New York: Jason Aronson Publishers.

Trivette, C. M., Dunst, C. J., & Hamby, D. W. (2010). Influences of family-systems intervention practices on patent-child interactions and child development. *Topics in Early Childhood Special Education, 30*(1), 3–19.

Trotter, T., & Martin, H. M. (2007). Family history in pediatric primary care. *Pediatrics, 120*(Suppl), S60–S65.

US Census Bureau. (2013). *Current population survey: Definitions.* Retrieved from http://www.census.gov/cps/about/cpsdef.html.

US Department of Health and Human Services. (2008). *Health information privacy.* Retrieved from http://www.hhs.gov/ocr/privacy/hipaa/faq/disclosures_to_friends_and_family/523.html.

van der Eijk, M., Faber, M., Aarts, J., Kremer, J., Munneke, M., & Bloem, B. (2013). Using online health communities to deliver patient centered care to people with chronic conditions. *Journal of Medical Internet Research, 15*(6), e115. https://doi.org/10.2196/jmir.2476.

von Bertalanffy, L. (1968). *General systems theory.* New York: George Braziller.

Walsh, F. (2002). A family resilience framework: Innovative practice applications. *Family Relations, 51*(2), 130–136.

Walton, M. (2011). Communicating with family caregivers. *American Journal of Nursing, 111*(12), 47–53.

Wright, L. M., & Leahey, M. (2009). *Nurses and families: A guide to family assessment and intervention* (5th ed.). Philadelphia: F. A. Davis.

Wright, L., & Leahey, M. (2013). *Nurses and families: A guide to family assessment and intervention* (6th ed.). Philadelphia PA: FA Davis Company.

Ylven, R., & Granlund, M. (2009). Identifying and building on family strength: A thematic analysis. *Infants & Young Children, 22*(4), 253–263.

13

Resolving Conflicts Between Nurse and Patient

Kathleen Underman Boggs

OBJECTIVES

At the end of the chapter, the reader will be able to:

1. Define conflict and contrast the functional with the dysfunctional role of conflict in a therapeutic relationship.
2. Recognize personal styles of response to conflict situations and discriminate among passive, assertive, and aggressive responses to conflict situations.
3. Specify the characteristics of assertive communication

strategies to promote conflict resolution in nurse-patient relationships.
4. Practice strategies to de-escalate violence in the workplace.
5. Analyze findings from research studies and evidenced-based practice and discuss how they can be applied to communicating with patients holding differing values in your clinical practice.

Patient-centered care is one of the six Quality and Safety Education for Nurses (QSEN, n.d.) competencies described in Chapter 3. Our goal is to fully partner with our patients so that they are active participants in the management of their care (Agency for Healthcare Research and Quality [AHRQ], 2016). According to QSEN, one desired "Attitude" is that we respect our patient as a central, core member of the health team. However, even when nurse-patient goals are mutual, our values or viewpoints may differ. Collaboration is our focus but, as in all interactions among human beings, some disagreements are inevitable.

Conflict is a natural part of human relationships. We all have times when we experience negative feelings about a situation or person, but in nursing this can compromise patient safety. When this occurs, direct communication is needed. This chapter emphasizes the dynamics of conflict and the problem-solving skills needed for successful resolution between you and your patients. Effective nurse-patient communication is critical. According to nurses, open communication is a key factor in avoiding threatening situations (Avander, Heikki, Bjersa, & Ergstrom, 2016). When conflict occurs, knowing how to respond calmly allows you to use feelings as a positive force. Some patients approach their initial encounter with a nurse with verbal hostility or even physical aggression, as when we admit an intoxicated patient to the emergency department. Maintaining safety

for self and patient is paramount. To listen and to respond creatively to intense emotion when your first impulse is to withdraw or to retaliate demands a high level of skill, empathy, and self-control. Many of these skills can also be applied to the workplace conflicts discussed in Chapters 22 and 23.

BASIC CONCEPTS

Definition

Conflict is defined as disagreement arising from differences in attitudes, values, or needs in which the actions of one party frustrate the ability of the other to achieve his or her expected goals. This results in stress or tension. Conflict serves as a warning that something in the relationship needs closer attention. Conflict is not necessarily a negative; it can become a positive force leading to growth in relationships. Conflict resolution is a learned process.

Nature of Conflict

All conflicts have certain things in common: (1) a concrete *content problem issue* and (2) relationship or *process issues,* which involves our emotional response to the situation. It is immaterial whether the issue makes realistic sense to you. It feels real to your patient and needs to be dealt with.

Unresolved, such issues will interfere with your and your patient's success in meeting goals. Most people experience conflict as discomfort. Previous experiences with conflict situations, the importance of the issue, and possible consequences all play a role in the intensity of our reactions. For example, a patient may have great difficulty asking questions of the physician regarding treatment or prognosis but experience no problem asking similar questions of the nurse or family. The reasons for the discrepancy in comfort level may relate to previous experiences. Alternatively, it may have little to do with the actual persons involved. Rather, the patient may be responding to anticipated fears about the type of information the physician might give.

Causes of Conflict

Poor communication is the main cause of misunderstanding and conflict. Psychological causes of conflict include differences in values or personality and multiple demands causing high levels of stress. If your nursing care does not fit in with your patient's cultural belief system, conflict can result. Recognize that our culture has moved toward greater incivility in mainstream society. This is reflected within the health care system.

Workplace Violence

A safe work environment is a prerequisite for providing good-quality care (Longo, Cassidy, & Sherman, 2016). Violence in the workplace is defined as an expression of anger by others manifested as threats or attacks either physical or psychological. Behaviors include negative dysfunctional aggression expressed as verbal abuse, derogatory speech, harassment, bullying, pushing, hitting, or even attacks with weapons. Violence is classified as an occupational hazard. Globally nurses are at higher risk owing to their direct contact with distressed people (International Council of Nurses [ICN], 2006; Nowrouzi & Huynh, 2016; Waschgler, Ruiz-Hernandez, Llor-Esteban, & Garcia-Izquierdo, 2013). At the same time the incidence of violence is greatly underreported (Campbell & Burg, 2015; Phillips, 2016).

Conflict can escalate to violent threats or actions. Nurses need to be aware that the stressful nature of illness can aggravate factors that lead to violent behavior on the part of patients or their family members.

Incidence of Violence

Statistics show that violence against health care workers is increasing in every country and in every health care setting (Llor-Esteban, Sanchez-Munoz, Ruiz-Hernandes, & Jimenez-Barbero, 2016; NICE Guideline #10, 2015; Wei, Chiou, Chien, & Huang, 2016; World Health Organization [WHO], 2012). Nurses and social workers are at three times greater risk for experiencing violence in the workplace than are other professionals. The highest risk exists in emergency departments, psychiatric settings, and nursing homes (American Association of Critical Care Nurses [AACN], 2004; American Nurses Association [ANA], 2002, 2012; NICE Guideline #10, 2015; US Department of Labor Occupational Safety and Health Administration [OSHA], 2004). Approximately 80% of nurses will experience violence, often physical violence, at some time during their careers (Brann & Hartley, 2016; Hahn et al., 2013; Llor-Estaban et al., 2016). The Joint Commission's (TJC, 2010) *Sentinel Event Alert*, Issue 45, addresses prevention specifying controlling access to health care agencies and advocating staff education. TJC notes that communication failures were inherent in 53% of reported acts of violence. Violence against health care workers ranges from threats to assaults to murder, yet it is estimated that about 80% of these occurrences remain unreported. (ANA, 2012; NICE Guideline #10, 2015; OSHA, 2004).

Outcomes

Adverse outcomes for nurses include increased stress, job dissatisfaction, somatic illness, emotional trauma, increased absenteeism, posttraumatic stress disorder, self-medication abuse, and death (Avander et al., 2016). In addition to physical harm to the worker, *Healthy People 2020* (US Department of Health and Human Services, 2014) and other sources have identified problems for the health system, such as increased agency costs due to lost work days, job turnover, and occasionally litigation. Nurses educated in violence prevention and management will be better prepared. Consider the case of Mr. Dixon.

Case Example: Mr. Dixon

Experienced staff nurse Elaine Kaye RN works in a busy emergency department where access to the treatment rooms is blocked by a locked security door. Staff do not wear necklaces or neck chains, nor do they carry implements, but Ms. Kaye does wear an ID badge (per the US Department of Labor Occupational Safety and Health Administration [OSHA] recommendations). While Dr. Hughes is treating Donny, age 12, who appears to be suffering from convulsions related to overdosing on methylphenidate (Ritalin), Ms. Kaye notices that Mr. Dixon is becoming increasingly agitated in the waiting room.

Mr. D: "Why aren't you people doing more?"

Nurse (in a low tone of voice): "My name is Ms. Kaye and I am helping with your son. I'll be keeping you up to date with information as soon as we know anything. I know this is a stressful..."

Continued

Mr. D (interrupting in a louder voice): "I demand to know why you people won't tell me what is going on."

Nurse: "I see that you are really upset and feeling angry. Let's move over here to the conference area for privacy."

Mr. D: "You guys are no good."

Nurse: "I want to understand your point of view. You…"

Mr. D throws a chair.

Nurse: "This is an upsetting time for you, but violence is not acceptable. Please calm down and we will sit down. Let's both take a deep breath, and then you can explain to me what you need…"

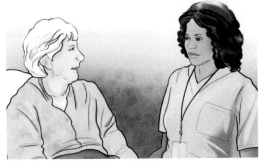

Fig. 13.1 Principles of conflict resolution:
- Identify the conflict issue
- Listen to the patient's perspective
- Acknowledge you have heard by validating, using "I" sentences, avoiding "you"
- Stay focused on this issue; know and control your own responses
- Use the "no blame" approach and discuss options, alternative solutions
- Negotiate and agree on a solution
- Summarize
- Follow through.

Strategies to prevent escalation of violent behavior are discussed in the "Applications" section of this chapter. Suggestions for physical and organizational safeguards are available from the Occupational Safety and Health Administration (www.osha.gov).

Stage of Anger

- **Mild:** Feels some tension, irritability. Acts argumentative, sarcastic, or is difficult to please
- **Moderate:** Observably angry behaviors such as motor agitation and loud voice
- **Severe:** Shows acting out behaviors, cursing, using violent gestures but is not yet out of control
- **Rage:** Behaving in an out-of-control manner, physically aggressive toward others or self

Goal: Work for Conflict Resolution

Unresolved nurse-patient conflict impedes the quality and safety of patient care. It not only undermines your therapeutic relationship but can also result in your emotional exhaustion, leading to **burnout**. Energy is transferred to conflict issues instead of being used to build the relationship.

As nurses, our goal is to collaborate with patients to maximize their health. To accomplish this we need to communicate clearly to prevent or reduce levels of conflict. We know that resolving a long-standing conflict is a gradual process in which we may have to revisit the issue several times to fully resolve it.

Conflict-Resolution Principles

It goes without saying that professionals always demonstrate respect for patients. Gender and cultural factors that influence responses are described elsewhere. Fig. 13.1 lists some principles of conflict resolution. These may also be applied to conflicts with colleagues.

Understand Your Own Personal Responses to Conflict

Conflicts between nurse and patient are not uncommon. First gain a clear understanding of your own personal responses, since conflict creates anxiety that may prevent you from behaving in an effective, assertive manner. No one is equally effective in all situations. Completing Simulation Exercise 13.1 may help you identify your personal responses.

Recognize your own "triggers" or "hot buttons." What words or patient actions trigger an immediate emotional response in you? These could include having someone yelling at you or speaking to you in an angry tone of voice. Once you recognize the triggers, you can better control your own responses. It is imperative that you focus on the current issue. Put aside past history. Listing prior problems will raise emotions and prevent resolution. Identify *available options*. Rather than immediately trying to solve the problem, look at the range of possible options. Create a list of these options and work with the other party to evaluate the feasibility of each option. By working together, you shift expectations from adversarial conflict to an expectation of a win-win outcome. After discussing possible solutions, select the best one to resolve the conflict. Evaluate the outcome based on fair, objective criteria.

Know the Context

Second, understand the context or the circumstances in which the situation occurs. Most interpersonal conflicts involve some threat to one's sense of control or self-esteem. Nurses have been shown to respond to the stress of not having enough time to complete their work by imposing

SIMULATION EXERCISE 13.1   Personal Responses to Conflict

Purpose:
To increase awareness of how students respond in conflict situations and the elements in situations (e.g., people, status, age, previous experience, lack of experience, or place) that contribute to their sense of discomfort.

Procedure:
Break the class up into small groups of two. You may do this as homework or create an Internet discussion room. Think of a conflict situation that could be handled in different ways.

The following feelings are common correlates of interpersonal conflict situations that many people say they experienced in conflict situations that they have not handled well.

Anger	Competitiveness	Humiliation
Annoyance	Defensiveness	Inferiority
Antagonism	Devaluation	Intimidation
Anxiousness	Embarrassment	Manipulation
Bitterness	Frustration	Resentment

Although these feelings generally are not ones we are especially proud of, they are a part of the human experience. By acknowledging their existence within ourselves, we usually have more choice about how we will handle them.

Reflective Analysis and Discussion
Construct different responses and then explain how the different responses might lead to different outcomes.

BOX 13.1   Behaviors of a Nurse That Create Anger in Others

- Violating one's personal space
- Speaking in a threatening tone
- Providing unsolicited advice
- Judging, blaming, criticizing, or conveying ideas that try to create guilt
- Offering reassurances that are not realistic
- Communicating using "gloss it over" positive comments
- Speaking in a way that shows you do not understand your patient's point of view
- Exerting too much pressure to make a person change his or her unhealthy behavior
- Portraying self as an infallible "I know best" expert
- Using an authoritarian, sarcastic, or accusing tone
- Using "hot button" words that have heavy emotional connotations
- Failing to provide health information in a timely manner to stressed individuals

more controls on their patients, who then often react by becoming more difficult. Other behaviors of nurses that may lead to anger in patients or families are listed in Box 13.1. Patients who feel listened to and respected are generally receptive.

Situations that may cause nurses to become frustrated or angry include working with patients who dismiss what they say or who ask for more personal information than nurses feel comfortable sharing, patients who sexually harass or target a nurse in a personal attack, or family members who make demands that nurses are unable to fulfill.

Develop an Effective Conflict Management Style

Five distinct **styles of response** to conflict have been documented. In the past, nurses were found to commonly use avoidance or accommodation when they were faced with a conflict situation (Sayer, McNeese-Smith, Leach, & Phillips, 2012). Many felt that any conflict was destructive and needed to be suppressed. Current thinking holds that conflict can be healthy and can lead to growth when, with conflict-resolution training, we develop a collaborative problem-solving approach.

Avoidance is a common response to conflict. Nurses using avoidance distance themselves from their patients or provide less support. Sometimes an experience makes you so uncomfortable that you want to avoid the situation or person at all costs, so you withdraw. This style is appropriate when the cost of addressing the conflict is higher than the benefit of resolution. Sometimes you just have to "pick your battles," focusing your energy on the most important issues. However, use of avoidance postpones the conflict, leads to future problems, and damages your relationship with your client, making it an *I lose, you lose* situation.

Accommodation is another common response. We surrender our own needs in a desire to smooth over the conflict. This response is cooperative but nonassertive. Sometimes this involves a quick compromise or giving false reassurance. By giving into others, we maintain peace but do not actually deal with the issue, so it will likely resurface in the future. It is appropriate only when the issue is more important to the other person. This is an *I lose, you win* situation. Harmony results. Good will may be earned that can be used in the future (McElhaney, 1996).

Competition is a response style characterized by domination. You exercise power to gain your own goals at the expense of the other person. It is characterized by aggression and lack of compromise. Authority may be used to suppress the conflict in a dictatorial manner. This leads to increased stress. It is an effective style only when there is a need for a quick decision, but leads to problems in the long term, making it an *I win now but then lose and you lose* situation.

Compromise is a solution still commonly found to be employed by nurses. By compromising, each party gives a little and gains a little. It is effective only when both parties hold equal power. Depending on the specific work environment and the issue in dispute, it can be a good solution, but since neither party is completely satisfied, it can eventually become an *I lose, you lose* situation.

Collaboration is a solution-oriented response in which we work together cooperatively to solve problems. To manage the conflict, we commit to finding a mutually agreeable solution. This involves directly confronting the issue, acknowledging our feelings, and using open communication. Steps for productive confrontation include identifying concerns of each party, clarifying assumptions, communicating honestly to identify the real issue, and working collaboratively to find a solution that satisfies everyone. Collaboration is considered to be the most effective style for genuine resolution. This is an *I win, you win* situation.

Structure Your Response

In mastering assertive responses, it may be helpful initially to use these steps:

1. Express empathy: "I understand that_____"; "I hear you saying _____." *Example:* "I understand that things are difficult at home."
2. Describe your feelings or the situation: "I feel that _____"; "This situation seems to me to _____." *Example:* "But your 8-year-old daughter has expressed a lot of anxiety, saying, 'I can't learn to give my own insulin shots.'"
3. State expectations: "I want _____"; "What is required by the situation is _____." *Example:* "It is necessary for you to be here tomorrow when the diabetic teaching nurse comes so you can learn how to give injections and your daughter can, too, with your support."
4. List consequences: "If you do this, then _____ will happen" (state positive outcome); "If you don't do this, then _____ will happen" (state negative outcome). *Example:* "If you get here on time, we can be finished and get her discharged in time for her birthday on Friday." Focus on the present

- The focus should always be on the present. Focus only on the present issue. The past cannot be changed, so "stay in the moment."
- Limit your discussion to *one topic issue* at a time to enhance the chance of success. Usually it is impossible to resolve a conflict that is multidimensional with a single solution. By breaking the problem down into simple steps, you will allow enough time for a clear understanding. You might paraphrase the patient's words, reflecting the meaning back to the him or her to validate its accuracy. Once the issues have been delineated clearly, the steps needed for resolution may appear quite simple.

Being assertive in the face of an emotionally charged situation demands thought, energy, and commitment. Assertiveness also requires the use of common sense, self-awareness, knowledge, tact, humor, respect, and a sense of perspective. Although there is no guarantee that the use of assertive behaviors will produce the desired interpersonal goals, the chances of a successful outcome are increased because the information flow is optimally honest, direct, and firm. Often the use of assertiveness brings about changes in ways that could not have been anticipated. Changes occur because the nurse offers a new resource in the form of objective feedback with no strings attached.

Use "I" Statements

Statements that begin with "You…" sound accusatory. When statements point a finger or imply judgment, most people respond defensively. "We" statements should be used only when you actually mean to look at an issue collaboratively. Use of "I" statements is one of the most effective conflict management strategies you can use. Assertive statements that begin with "I" suggest that the person speaking accepts full responsibility for his or her own feelings and position in relation to the conflict. "I" statements feel clumsy at first and take a little practice to use. The following is one suggested format:

"I feel_____ (use a name to claim the emotion you feel)

when_____ (describe the behavior nonjudgmentally)

because_____ (describe the tangible effects of the behavior)."

Example: "I feel uncomfortable when a patient's personal problems are discussed in the cafeteria because someone might overhear confidential information."

Make Clear Statements

Statements rather than questions set the stage for assertive responses to conflict. When you do use a question, "how" questions are best because they are neutral, seek more information, and imply a collaborative effort. Avoid "why" questions as they put other people on the defensive, asking them to explain their behavior. Use a strong, firm, tactful manner and state the situation clearly. Consider the case of Mr. Gow.

Case Example: Mr. Gow

Mr. Gow is a 35-year-old executive who has been hospitalized with a myocardial infarction. He has been acting seductively toward some of the young nurses but he seems to be giving Miss O'Hara an especially hard time.

Mr. Gow: Come on in, honey, I've been waiting for you.

Nurse (using appropriate facial expression and eye contact, and replying in a firm, clear voice): Mr. Gow, I would rather you called me Miss O'Hara.

Mr. G.: Aw, come on now, honey. I don't get to have much fun around here. What's the difference what I call you?

Nurse: I feel that it does make a difference, and I would like you to call me Miss O'Hara.

Mr. G.: Oh, you're no fun at all. Why do you have to be so serious?

Nurse: Mr. Gow, you're right. I am serious about some things, and being called by my name and title is one of them. I would prefer that you call me Miss O'Hara. I would like to work with you, however, and it might be important to explore the ways in which this hospitalization is hampering your natural desire to have fun.

In this interaction the nurse's position is defined several times, using successively stronger statements before the shift is made to refocus on Mr. Gow's needs. Notice that the nurse labeled the behavior, not the patient, as unacceptable. Persistence is essential when initial attempts at assertiveness appear too limited.

Use Moderate Pitch and Vocal Tone

The strength of a forceful assertive statement depends on the nature of the conflict situation as well as the degree of confrontation needed to resolve the conflict successfully. Starting with the least amount of assertiveness required to meet the demands of the situation conserves energy and does not place you in an "overkill" bind. It is not necessary to use all your resources at one time or to express your ideas too strongly. We sometimes lose effectiveness by becoming too long-winded. Long explanations detract from the spoken message. Get to the main point quickly, saying what is necessary in the simplest, most concrete way possible. This cuts down on the possibility of misinterpretation.

SIMULATION EXERCISE 13.2 Pitching the Assertive Message

Purpose:
To increase awareness of how the meaning of a verbal message can be significantly altered by changing one's tone of voice.

Procedure:
Break class up into groups of five. Write on a slip of paper one of the following five vocal pitches: whisper, soft tone with hesitant delivery, moderate tone and firm delivery, loud tone with agitated delivery, and screaming. Have each person in turn pick one of five pieces of paper and demonstrate that tone while the others in the group try to identify in which tone the assertive message is being delivered.

Reflective Analysis:
Using information learned from the text to support your answer, justify how tone can affect perceptions of a message's content.

Pitch and tone of voice contribute to another person's interpretation of the meaning of your assertive message. A soft, hesitant, passive presentation can undermine an assertive message. The same is true if a harsh, hostile, aggressive tone is used. Try a firm but moderate presentation to effectively convey your message by doing Simulation Exercise 13.2.

Outcome: Positive Growth

Traditionally conflict was viewed as a destructive force to be eliminated. Actually conflicts that are successfully resolved lead to stronger relationships. The critical factor is the willingness to explore and resolve it mutually. Appropriately handled, conflict can provide an important opportunity for growth. Practice to develop conflict management skills is essential and effective.

Outcome: Dysfunction, Such as Unresolved Conflict

As mentioned, unresolved conflicts tend to resurface later, impeding your ability to give quality care. If the emotional aspect of the conflict is expressed too strongly, the nurse can feel attacked.

Nature of Assertive Behavior

Assertive behavior is defined as setting goals, acting on those goals in a clear, consistent manner, and taking responsibility for the consequences of those actions. Assertive communication is conveying this objective in a

---

BOX 13.2   Characteristics Associated With the Development of Assertive Behavior

- Express your own position, using "I" statements.
- Make clear statements.
- Speak in a firm tone, using moderate pitch.
- Assume responsibility for personal feelings and wants.
- Make sure verbal and nonverbal messages are congruent.
- Address only issues related to the present conflict.
- Structure responses so as to be tactful and show awareness of the client's frame of reference.
- Understand that undesired behaviors, not feelings, attitudes, and motivations, are the focus for change.

SIMULATION EXERCISE 13.3 Assertive Responses

Purpose:
To increase awareness of assertiveness.

Procedure:
Role-play the following scenario:
  You are working full time, raising a family, and taking 12 credits of nursing classes. The teacher asks you to be a student representative on a faculty committee. You say the following:
1. "I don't think I'm the best one. Why don't you ask Karen? If she can't, I guess I can."
2. "Gee, I'd like to, but I don't know. I probably could if it doesn't take too much time."
3. "I do want students to have some input to this committee, but I am not sure I have enough time. Let me think about it and let you know in class tomorrow."

Reflective Analysis and Discussion:
1. Critique the options, describing how they could be altered.
2. Select the most assertive response. Defend your choice using the text.

---

direct manner, without anger or frustration. The assertive nurse is able to stand up for his or her personal rights and the rights of others.

Components of assertive communication include the ability (1) to say no, (2) to ask for what you want, (3) to appropriately express both positive and negative thoughts and feelings, and (4) to initiate, continue, and terminate the interaction. This honest expression of yourself does not violate the needs of others but does demonstrate self-respect rather than deference to the demands of others. Conflict creates anxiety, which may prevent you from behaving assertively. Assertive behaviors range from making a direct, honest statement about your beliefs to taking a very strong, confrontational stand about what will and will not be tolerated. Assertive responses contain "I" statements that take responsibility. This behavior is in contrast with **aggressive behavior**, which has a goal of dominating while suppressing the other person's rights. Aggressive responses often consist of "you" statements that fix blame on the other person. Box 13.2 lists characteristics of assertive behavior. Remember that assertiveness is a learned behavior and assertive responses need to be practiced!

Nonassertive behavior in a professional nurse is related to lower levels of autonomy. Continued patterns of nonassertive responses have a negative influence on you and on the standard of care you provide. Practice your own assertiveness in Simulation Exercise 13.3.

Safety

It is your responsibility to maintain your own safety and that of patients. Mindfully be aware. Team STEPPS suggests the use of "situation monitoring" to recognize emergent conflicts. When you are confronted by an angry patient or family member, use your skills to defuse the situation, addressing their concerns. If anger enters the *rage stage*, leave and get help. Do not stay in a dangerous situation. It cannot be overemphasized that if you feel in danger, LEAVE! Each agency should have a resource team to call for intervention assistance. Don't be a hero, CALL FOR HELP!

DEVELOPING AN EVIDENCE-BASED PRACTICE
It is well documented that conflict in the workplace occurs more in health care than elsewhere. Conflict management and de-escalation strategies are also documented. Ameliorating the effects of stress from workplace conflict was studied by Hersch and colleagues (2016), among others. They studied effects of an online stress management program on 106 staff nurses and managers from six hospitals using a randomized pretest-posttest trial. Stress was measured by the "Nursing Stress Scale."

Results
Nurses in the experimental group, who accessed the web-based program BREATHE: Stress Management for

Nurses, over a 3-month period reported significantly better handled [less] perceived stress. The BREATHE program was effective in moderating stress associated with conflict with doctors and other nurses, with workload issues, with inadequate preparation issues and with stress stemming from caring for dying patients.

Application to Your Clinical Practice
An extensive literature review highlights the following effective strategies for coping with conflict:
- Paying attention to your own responses (emotional reactions may escalate conflict to aggression)
- Managing your own responses by staying calm, not overreacting, communicating nonverbal nonthreatening messages, speaking softly, and using cognitive restructuring to replace negative ways of thinking
- Using relaxation and other coping strategies, including the online BREATHE program or downloading relaxation Apps, and practicing deep breathing immediately before responding
- Seeking to create a supportive work environment
- Identifying early risk factors in patients, such as difficulty sleeping and concentrating, hostility or anger, and expression of threats
- Focusing on the patient to discern the underlying problem
- Implementing de-escalation steps, confronting conflict immediately to prevent escalation to violence, and setting limits in a nonconfrontational way
- Showing respect to all, remaining empathetic and nonjudgmental, and not dictating choices

Compiled from References: Cheng (2016), CPI [OSHA] (2017), Dwarswaard and van de Bovenkamp (2015), Haugvaldstad and Husum (2016), Hersch et al. (2016), Watkins et al. (2017).

APPLICATIONS

It is essential to recognize the potential for conflict. And Team STEPPS reminds us to use situation monitoring, continually scanning our environment to understand what is going on around us. Practicing the following strategies can help you to improve your conflict-resolution skills. By doing so we demonstrate that we are developing the **QSEN attitude** of continuously improving our own communication and conflict-resolution skills.

Preventing Conflict

In addition to managing your own responses to patient provocations, model behavior by adopting a professional, "calm" demeanor and low tone of voice. Use conflict-prevention strategies: Signal your readiness to listen with attending behaviors such as good body position, eye contact, and a receptive facial expression. Give your undivided attention to a patient or visitor whom you identify as potentially becoming aggressive. Multiple studies show that nurses' anticommunication attitudes act as a barrier. Increasing your positive appreciation of your patient does facilitate communication. As nurses, we hold the belief that all patients have value as human beings. Try some of the strategies described in this chapter to help prevent or resolve conflict.

Assessing the Presence of Conflict in the Nurse-Patient Relationship

To get resolution, you need to acknowledge the presence of conflict. Often the awareness of our own feelings of discomfort is an initial clue. Evidence of the presence of conflict may be *overt*, that is, observable in the patient's behavior and expressed verbally. For example, a patient might criticize you. No one likes to be criticized and a natural response might be anger, rationalization, or blaming others. But as a professional nurse, you recognize your response, recognize the conflict, and work toward resolution so that constructive changes can take place.

More often, conflict is *covert* and not so clear-cut. The conflict issues are hidden. Your patient talks about one issue, but talking does not seem to help and the issue does not get resolved. He or she continues to be angry or anxious. Subtle behavioral manifestations of covert conflict might include a reduced effort by your patient to engage in self-care; frequent misinterpretation of your words; and behaviors that are out of character for your patient, such as excessive anger. For example, your patient might become unusually demanding, have a seemingly insatiable need for your attention, or be unable to tolerate reasonable delays in having his or her needs met. Such problems may represent anxiety stemming from conflicting feelings. Behaviors are often negatively affected by feelings of pain, loss, helplessness, frustration, or fear. As nurses, we affect the behavior of our patients through our actions. This can lead to positive or negative outcomes. See Simulation Exercise 13.4 for practice in defining conflict issues.

Sometimes the feelings themselves become the major issue, so that valid parts of the original conflict issue are hidden; consequently, conflict escalates. Consider how to respond to Ms. Dentoni.

SIMULATION EXERCISE 13.4   Defining Conflict Issues: Case Analyses

Purpose:
To help organize information and define the problem in interpersonal conflict situations.

Procedure:
In each conflict situation, look for specific behaviors (including words, tone, posture, and facial expression); feeling impressions (including words, tone, intensity, and facial expression); and need (expressed verbally or through actions).

Identify the behaviors, your impressions of the behaviors, and needs that the client is expressing in the following situations. Suggest an appropriate nursing action. Situation 1 is completed as a guide.

Situation 1
Mrs. Patel, a patient from India, does not speak much English. Her baby was just delivered by cesarean section, and it is expected that Mrs. Patel will remain in the hospital for at least 4 days. Her husband tells the nurse that Mrs. Patel wants to breastfeed, but she has decided to wait until she goes home to begin because she will be more comfortable there and she wants privacy. The nurse

knows that breastfeeding will be more successful if it is initiated soon after birth.

Behaviors: The client's husband states that his wife wants to breastfeed but does not wish to start before going home. Mrs. Patel is not initiating breastfeeding in the hospital.

Your impression of behaviors: Indirectly, she is expressing physical discomfort, possible insecurity, and awkwardness about breastfeeding. She may also be acting in accordance with cultural norms of her country or family.

Underlying needs: Safety and security. Mrs. Patel probably will not be motivated to attempt breastfeeding until she feels safe and secure in her home environment.

Suggested nursing action: Provide family support and guarantee total privacy for feeding.

Situation 2
Mrs. Moore is brought back to the unit from surgery after a radical mastectomy. The doctor's orders call for her to ambulate, cough, and deep breathe and to use her arm as much as possible in self-care activities. Mrs. Moore asks the nurse in a very annoyed tone, "Why do I have to do this? You can see that it is difficult for me. Why can't you help me?"

Case Example: Mrs. Dentoni

Mrs. Dentoni is scheduled for surgery at 8 a.m. tomorrow. As the student nurse assigned to care for her, you have been told that she was admitted to the hospital 3 hours ago and that she has been examined by the house resident. The anesthesia department has been notified of her arrival. Her blood work and urine have been sent to the laboratory. As you enter her room and introduce yourself, you notice that Mrs. Dentoni is sitting on the edge of the bed and appears tense and angry.

Mrs. D.: I wish people would just leave me alone. Nobody has come in and told me about my surgery tomorrow. I don't know what I'm supposed to do—just lie around here and rot, I guess.

At this point, you can probably sense the presence of conflicting feelings, but it is unclear whether this patient's emotions relate to anxiety about the surgery or to anger about some real or imagined invasion of privacy because of the necessary laboratory tests and physical examination. Your patient might also be annoyed by you or by a lack of information from the surgeon. She may feel the need to know that hospital personnel see her as a person and care about her feelings. Before you can respond empathetically to

the patient's feelings, they will have to be decoded.

Nurse (in a concerned tone of voice): You seem really upset. It's rough being in the hospital, isn't it?

Notice that the reply is nonjudgmental and tentative and does not suggest specific feelings beyond those the patient has shared. There is an implicit request for her to validate your perception of her feelings and to link the feelings with a concrete issue. You process verbal as well as nonverbal cues. Concern is expressed through your tone of voice and words. The content focus relates to the patient's predominant feeling tone, because this is the part of the conflict that is shared with you. It is important to maintain a nonanxious, relaxed presence.

Techniques for Conflict Resolution

Remember that your goal is to *de-escalate* the conflict. We need to be modeling respect. Use the strategies for conflict resolution described in this section. Mastery takes practice. Although this seems like a lot of information, an incident can occur in only a few minutes. Stay calm. Use *The 3 Ps of Crisis De-escalation*:

- *Position* (face patient but remain closer to the exit, making eye contact only 60% of the time)

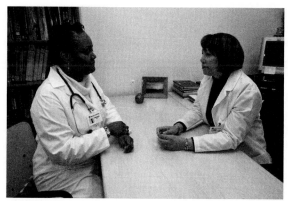

Fig. 13.2 Reaching a common understanding of the problem in a direct, tactful manner is the first step in conflict resolution.

- **Posture** (relax your stance with uncrossed arms; rotate and relax your shoulders)
- **Proximity** (stay 1.5 to 3 feet away)

Reaching a common understanding of the problem in a direct, tactful manner is the first step in conflict resolution, moving you toward a goal of reaching a resolution acceptable to both parties (Fig. 13.2).

Prepare for the Encounter

Careful preparation often makes the difference between being successful or failing to assert yourself when necessary. Mentally visualize yourself responding assertively. Clearly identify the issue in conflict. For communication to be effective, it must be carefully thought out in terms of certain basic questions, such as the following:

- *Purpose.* What is the purpose or objective of this information? What is the central idea, the one most important statement to be made?
- *Organization.* What are the major points to be shared, and in what order?
- *Content.* Is the information to be shared complete? Does it convey who, what, where, when, why, and how?
- *Word choice.* Has careful consideration been given to the choice of words?
- If you wish to be successful, you must consider not only what is important to you in the discussion but what is important to the other person. Bear in mind the other person's viewpoint. The case featuring about Mr. Pyle illustrates this idea.

Case Example: Mr. Pyle

Mr. Pyle is an 80-year-old bachelor who lives alone. He has always been considered a proud and stately gentleman. He has a sister, 84 years old, who lives in Florida. His only other living relatives, a nephew and his wife, also live in another state. Mr. Pyle recently changed his will so that it excludes his relatives, and he refuses to eat. When his neighbor brings in food, he eats it, but he won't fix anything for himself. He tells his neighbor that he wants to die and that he read in the paper about a man who was able to die in 60 days by not eating. As the visiting nurse assigned to his area, you have been asked to make a home visit and assess the situation.

The issue in this case example is not one of food intake alone. Any attempt to talk about why it is important for him to eat or expressing your point of view in this conflict immediately on arriving is not likely to be successful. Mr. Pyle's behavior suggests that he feels that there is little to be gained by living any longer. His actions suggest further that he feels lonely and may be angry with his relatives. Once you correctly ascertain his needs and identify the specific issues, you may be able to help Mr. Pyle resolve his intrapersonal conflict. His wish to die may not be absolute or final because he eats when food is prepared by his neighbor and he has not yet taken a deliberate, aggressive move to end his life. Each of these factors needs to be assessed and validated with him before an accurate nursing diagnosis can be made.

Organize Information

Plan your approach for a time and place conducive to collaborative discussion. Do not respond in the heat of the moment. Organizing your information and validating the appropriateness of your intervention with another knowledgeable person who is not directly involved is useful. Sometimes it is wise to rehearse out loud what you are going to say. Remember to adhere to the principle of focusing on the conflict issue. Avoid bringing up the past.

Manage Your Own Anxiety or Anger

Recognizing and controlling your own natural emotional response to upsetting behavior may be one key factor in managing conflict. Refer to Box 11.2 and use some immediate de-stressing behaviors, such as taking three deep breaths. Conflict produces anxiety and creates feelings of helplessness. You should see this discomfort as a signal that you need to deal with the situation. As mentioned earlier, part of an initial assessment of an interpersonal conflict includes recognition of the nurse's intrapersonal contribution to the conflict as well as that of the patient. It is not wrong to have ambivalent feelings about taking care of people with different lifestyles and values; however, you must acknowledge this to yourself. Remember that these feelings are about themselves, not about you.

Confronting the behavior now should keep you from losing control later as the problem escalates. Most people experience some variation of a physical response when taking interpersonal risks. A useful strategy for managing your own anger is to vent to a friend using "I" statements as long as this does not become a complaining, whining session. Another strategy to manage your own anger is to "take a break." A cooling-off period, doing something else for a few minutes or hours until your anger subsides, is acceptable. Take care that you reengage, however, so that this does not become just an avoidance response style. Communicate with the correct person; do not take out your frustration on someone else. Focus on the one issue involved. Try saying, "I would like to talk something over with you before the end of shift/before I go." Before you actually enter the patient's room, do the following:

- Cool off. Wait until you can speak in a calm, friendly tone.
- Take a few deep breaths. Inhale deeply and count "1-2-3" to yourself. Hold your breath for a count of 2 and exhale, counting again to 3 slowly.
- Fortify yourself with positive statements (e.g., "I have a right to respect."). Anticipation is usually far worse than the reality.
- Defuse your own anxiety or anger before confronting the patient.
- Focus discussion on one issue.

Time the Encounter

Timing is a determinant of success. Know specifically the behavior you wish to have the patient change. Make sure that they are capable physically and emotionally of changing the behavior. Select a time when you both can discuss the matter privately and use neutral ground, if possible. Select a time when the patient is most likely to be receptive.

Timing is also important if an individual is very angry. The key to assertive behavior is choice. Sometimes it is better to allow someone to let off some "emotional steam" before engaging in conversation. In this case, the assertive thing to do is to choose silence accompanied by a calm, relaxed body posture. These nonverbal actions convey acceptance of feeling and a desire to understand. Validating the anger and reframing the conflict are useful steps. Comments such as, "I'm sorry you are feeling so upset" recognize the significance of the emotion being expressed without getting into the cause.

Put Situation into Perspective

Do not play the blame game. Put the issue into perspective. How urgent is it to resolve this issue? How important is the issue? Will the issue be significant in a year? In 10 years? Will there be a significant situational change with resolution?

This is another way of saying "pick your battles." Not every situation is worth expending your time and energy. Remind yourself that anger may be caused by a problem in communicating; patients who are frustrated may become angry when they cannot make staff understand.

Use Therapeutic Communication Skills

Refer to the discussion on therapeutic communication in Chapter 10. Particularly useful is *active listening*. Really trying to understand what the patient is upset about requires more skill than just listening to his or her words. Listening closely to what they are saying may help you understand their point of view. This understanding may decrease the stress. Repeat what the patient said to make sure communication is crystal clear.

Nursing Communication Interventions: Following the CARE Steps

Riley (2017) adapted a CARE acronym to help nurses confront conflict situations. Refer to Box 13.3. Use the therapeutic nursing communication skills described in Chapter 10. Particularly useful in dealing with conflict situations is use of active listening and paraphrasing.

C = Clarify.

Choose direct, declarative sentences. Use objective words and avoid mixed messages. Make sure verbal and nonverbal communication is congruent. Maintain an open stance and omit any gestures that might be interpreted as criticism, such as rolling your eyes or sighing heavily. Avoid mixed messages. One example of inappropriate communication might be found in the case of Larry, a staff nurse who works the 11 p.m. to 7 a.m. shift. Larry needs to get home to make sure his children get on the bus to school. A geriatric patient routinely asks for a breathing treatment while Larry is reporting off. Instead of setting limits, Larry uses a soft voice and smiles as he tells her that he cannot be late in reporting off. Another example is Mr. Carl, the 29-year-old patient who constantly makes sexual comments to a young student nurse. She laughs as she tells him to cut it out. Directly state the behavior that is a problem.

A = Articulate why the behavior is a problem

Acknowledge the feelings associated with conflict, because it is emotions that escalate conflict.

R = Request a behavior change

Avoid blaming. This would only make your patient feel defensive or angry. Clearly *request that he or she change* the behavior. Rather than just stating your position, try to use some objective criterion to examine the situation.

BOX 13.3	**Nursing Communication Interventions: Following the CARE Steps**	
C	Clarify the be-havior that is a problem	Use communication skills, especially active listening skills, to identify issues of concern to the patient.
		• Use a calm tone and avoid conveying irritation.
		• Paraphrase patient's message to be sure you understand.
		• Ask for clarification if needed.
		• Suggest simple interventions to decrease anxiety (deep breathing relaxation and guided imagery).
		• Factually state the problem, focusing only on the current issue.
A	Articulate why the behavior is a problem	Explain the institution's policies.
		• Explain the limits of your role.
		• Set limits firmly.
R	Request a change in the problem behavior	Work with the entire health team so all use the same uniform approach to the patient's demands.
		• Develop a mutual health care plan: involve patient in care and set goals.
		• Review and reevaluate whether you and patient have same goals.
E	Evaluate progress	Provide education: explain all options, with outcomes.
		• Verbalize incentives and withdrawal of privileges to modify unacceptable behavior.
		• Promote trust by providing immediate feedback.

Saying, "I understand your need to…, but the hospital has a policy intended to protect all our patients" might help you talk about the situation without escalating into anger. Psychiatric units have known rules against verbal abuse, violence such as throwing objects, violence against others, and so on. You can restate these "rules" together with their known violation outcomes (medication, seclusion, manual restraint), in a calm but firm voice.

There obviously will be situations in which such a thorough assessment is not possible, but each of these variables affects the success of the confrontation. For example, a patient with dementia who makes a pass at a nurse may simply be expressing a need for affection in much the same way that a small child does; this behavior needs a caring response rather than a reprimand. A 30-year-old patient with all his cognitive faculties who makes a similar pass needs a more confrontational response.

Mutually generate some options for resolution. Focus on ways to resolve the problem by listing possible options. You are familiar with the "fight-or-flight" response to stress: Many people can respond to conflict only by either fighting or avoiding the problem. But brainstorming possible options and discussing pros and cons can turn the "fight" response into a more mutual "seeking a solution" mode of operations. Set mutual goals. Every member of the health care team needs to be "on the same page," presenting a similar approach to this patient.

Readiness is vital. The behavior may need to be confronted, but the manner in which the confrontation is approached and the amount of preparation or groundwork that has been done beforehand may affect the outcome.

For longer-term behavioral problems consider the use of a written contract, spelling out alternative behaviors, unacceptable ones, and their consequences.

E = Evaluate the conflict resolution.

Encourage behavior change by stating the outcomes, the positive consequences of changing, or the negative implications for failing to change. Evaluate the degree to which the interpersonal conflict has been resolved. Sometimes a conflict cannot be resolved in a short time, but the willingness to persevere is a good indicator of a potentially successful outcome. Accepting small goals is useful when the attainment of large goal is not possible. Your goal is open communication, with frequent **feedback** leading to successful problem solving.

For a patient, perhaps the strongest indicator of conflict resolution is the degree to which he or she is actively engaged in activities aimed at accomplishing tasks associated with the treatment goals. Here are some questions that you, as the nurse, you might want to address if modifications are necessary:

- What is the best way to establish an environment that is conducive to conflict resolution? What else needs to be considered?

- What self-care behaviors can be expected if these changes are made? These need to be stated in ways that are measurable.

Consider how to manage the case of Mr. Plotsky.

Case Example: Mr. Plotsky

Mr. Plotsky, age 29, has been employed for 6 years as a construction worker. About 4 weeks ago, while operating a forklift, he was struck by a train, leaving him paraplegic. After 2 weeks in intensive care, he was transferred to a neurological unit. When staff members attempt to provide physical care, such as changing his position or getting him up in a chair, Mr. Plotsky throws things, curses angrily, and sometimes spits at the nurses. Staff members become very upset; several nurses have requested assignment changes. Some staff members try bribing him with food to encourage good behavior; others threaten to apply restraints. The manager schedules a behavioral consultation meeting with a psychiatric nurse or clinical specialist. The immediate goal of this staff conference is to bring staff feelings out into the open and facilitate increased awareness of the staff's behavioral responses when confronted with Mr. Plotsky's behavior. The outcome goal is to use a problem-solving approach to develop a behavioral care plan so that all staff members respond to Mr. Plotsky in a consistent manner.

The Anger-Management Process: Nursing Behaviors to Avoid Violent Patient Behavior

Table 13.1 details nursing behaviors to avoid violence when you are dealing with an angry patient or family member.

Maintain Self-Control

Once you identify that a patient in a conflict situation may be so angry that he or she could be at risk for acting-out or violent behavior, your initial step is to maintain your self-control. Remember, you are modeling self-control! Early recognition is the key to preventing escalation. Illness generates feelings of powerlessness where your patients may feel they have little control. Anger is more powerful, so by focusing on their anger, they can feel more in

TABLE 13.1	Five Steps for Nursing Behaviors With an Angry Patient to Avoid Violence	
Step	**Nurse**	**Angry Patient or Family Member**
1. Control self	Appear calm, relax, and take two deep breaths. Remember to talk in low tone, monotone. Focus only on defusing anger or potential for violence. Remove any necklaces, cords around neck (risk of being strangled). Do not respond to insults to self or team; do not become defensive. Avoid arguing, saying no, or hurrying.	Assess for unusually stressed individual and potential for violence. Does the patient appear out of control? If so, *leave*! Remember, showing your anxiety will increase the patient's anxiety and anger. Reasoning with an enraged individual is impossible; *focus on de-escalation.* Devote only 3–5 minutes in attempting to de-escalate! (If it takes longer, it is not working.) Skip to the last step!
2. Nonthreatening body posture	Never touch an angry person; respect his or her personal space. Relax facial muscles; do not smile. Assume a neutral position, hands down by your side, one foot in front of the other in a relaxed posture. Stay at same eye level; try to get the patient to sit. If standing, do not position yourself face to face; be at an angle (so you can sidestep). Never turn your back. If standing, stay four times farther away than usual: Do not "crowd" the patient. Do not gesture; never point finger. Always be closest to the door (so you can escape if necessary).	Allow the patient to move around or pace (movement can help control stress). Allow the patient to break eye contact; avoid a constant stare. Monitor the patient's body position; watch for escalation in gestures.

TABLE 13.1	Five Steps for Nursing Behaviors With an Angry Patient to Avoid Violence—cont'd	
Step	**Nurse**	**Angry Patient or Family Member**
3. Verbal de-escalation	Be nonconfrontational, nonjudgmental. Use the communication skills in Box 13.3 and therapeutic skills such as active listening and paraphrasing. Introduce yourself; call the patient by name while making occasional eye contact. Communicate clearly and simply. Respond in a low, calm, gentle tone of voice; do not raise your voice. Be empathetic. Be neutral; avoid being defensive. Do not argue. Always be respectful. Do not dismiss any concern but always answer a request for information. Appeal to the patient's cognitive rather than emotional self in trying to identify the underlying problem. Help the patient verbalize his or her anger. Offer to work with the patient to help him or her deal with the issue. Answer selectively, ignore generalized ranting comments, and focus on just giving the information requested. Set limits (empathize with the patient's underlying feelings but not with his or her behavior). State clearly that violence is **not** acceptable. Give the patient options for alternative behavior (e.g., "Let's take a break and have a [paper] cup of water"). If the patient has a weapon, ask permission to move; do NOT be a hero.	Allow the patient to ventilate some of his or her anger and discuss problem. Help the patient identify his or her own anger (e.g., "I notice you are clenching your fists and talking more loudly than usual. These are things people do when angry. Help me to understand"). Help the patient identify the source of his or her anger. Have the patient use a relaxation technique such as deep breathing. Give the patient permission to feel angry, but set limits on acting out and violent behavior (e.g., "It's okay to feel angry about...but not okay to act on it" or "It's natural to feel angry about... but throwing things isn't okay..."). Support the patient's attempts to control his or her feelings. The patient needs to know the consequences of his or her continued acting out behavior.
4. Containment	Be aware of backup resources (orderlies, call to security, etc.). You can choose to leave. Use physical restraints if necessary. Place patient in seclusion or locked isolation room in psychiatric setting. Use enforced chemical restraint (medication). Report all threats.	Implement agency violence code. Allow or ask the patient to leave. Represent containment as a policy of the institution, not "I will restrain you." For some patients with brain damage or mental illness, it is appropriate to remove them from the source of their irritation to a calm environment, such as a lock room, to give them a sort of a time-out.
5. Debrief immediately: analyze and report	Reflect on the incident. What can be done to prevent a recurrence? Can you identify the trigger? Sometimes too long a wait, too little information, or even an insensitive or hostile comment from staff can be a trigger.	After calming down, the patient needs assistance to reflect on alternative ways of behaving and to plan for the future. Activate the patient's support system.

control. This coping mechanism may work for them temporarily, but when you are the target, it can be difficult. Understanding this dynamic may help you to not take their behavior personally.

To maintain the situation you attempt to reduce strong emotion to a workable level by providing a neutral, accepting, interpersonal environment. Within this context, you can acknowledge their emotion as a necessary component of adaptation to life. You convey acceptance of the individual's legitimate right to have feelings. Say, "I'm not surprised that you are angry about..." or simply stating, "I'm sorry you are hurting so much." Such statements acknowledge your patients' uncomfortable emotions, convey an attitude of acceptance, and encourage them to express themselves. Once a feeling can be put into words, it becomes manageable because it has concrete boundaries. Remember, there is a continuum:

Anxiety → Anger → Aggression

Talk About It

The second strategy in defusing a strong emotion is to talk the emotion through. For the patient, this someone is often the nurse. For the nurse, this might be a nursing supervisor or a trusted colleague. Unlike complaining, the purpose of talking the emotion through is to help the person bring the feeling up to a verbal level, which helps him or her to gain control. Verbalization helps the individual to connect with the personal feelings surrounding the incident.

Use Tension-Reducing Actions and Therapeutic Communication Skills

The third strategy is intervention. The specific needs expressed by the emotion suggest actions that might help the patient deal with his or her emotion. Convey mutual respect and avoid any "put-down" type of comment. Sometimes the most effective action is simply to listen. Active listening in a conflict situation involves concentrating on what the other person is upset about. Listening can be so powerful that it alone may reduce feelings of anxiety and frustration.

Physical activity can also reduce tension. For example, taking a walk can help control anxiety and defuse an emotionally tense situation. If your patient is so upset that he or she constitutes a danger, talk softly in a calm tone; face the patient but allow maximum space and an exit for yourself should it become necessary. Many hospitals and psychiatric units have a "code word" that is used to summon trained help.

Relaxation techniques may help your patient regain control. Some can be quickly taught, such as deep breathing. Nurses frequently find the use of humor to be helpful. Humor can also be used as a means of reducing tension.

To paraphrase a famous advice columnist, two of the most important words in a relationship are "I apologize." And this columnist recommended making amends immediately when you have made a mistake, because "it is easier to eat crow while it is still warm." Is this advice easier to take (we will not say *swallow*) because it comes with a chuckle? Humor serves as an immediate tension reliever.

Containment

A priority is to maintain a safe environment for yourself and all agency patients. Isolation in a locked room is standard in many psychiatric facilities, as is the use of restraints and pharmaceutical tranquilizers. Sometimes maintaining safety necessitates summoning agency resources, such as a critical incident response team, security, the community police.

Evaluation: Immediate Debriefing

The final strategy is to do an evaluation of the effectiveness of responses. What was the trigger? Sometimes it was something simple, such as having had to wait too long to get information or hearing an insensitive or even hostile comment from a staff person. Your goal is to apply insight toward preventing future occurrences. It is not the responsibility of any nurse to help a patient resolve all conflict. Long-standing conflicts require more expertise to resolve. In such cases, refer them to the appropriate resource.

Each step in the process may need to be taken more than once and refined or revised as circumstances dictate.

Conflict Communication Skills
Be Assertive

Assertive communication means you convey objectives with directness but not with anger or frustration.

Demonstrate Respect

Responsible, assertive statements are made in ways that do not violate the rights of others or diminish their standing. They are conveyed by a relaxed, attentive posture and a calm, friendly tone of voice. Statements should be accompanied by the use of appropriate eye contact.

Use "I" Statements

Statements that begin with "you" sound accusatory and always represent an assumption because it is impossible to know exactly, without validation, why someone acts in a certain way. Because such statements usually point a finger and imply a judgment, most people respond defensively to them.

"We" statements should be used only when you actually mean to look at an issue collaboratively. Thus the statement

"Perhaps we both need to look at this issue a little closer" may be appropriate in certain situations. However, the statement, "Perhaps we shouldn't get so angry when things don't work out the way we think they should" is a condescending statement thinly disguised as a collaborative statement. What is actually being expressed is the expectation that both parties should handle the conflict in one way—the nurse's way.

The use of "I" statements is one of the most effective conflict-management strategies. Assertive statements that begin with "I" suggest that the person making the statement accepts full responsibility for his or her feelings and position in relation to the presence of conflict. It is not necessary to justify your position unless the added message clarifies or adds essential information. "I" statements seem a little clumsy at first and take some practice. The traditional format is this:

"I feel _____ (use a name to claim the emotion you feel) when _____; (describe the behavior nonjudgmentally) because _____; (describe the tangible effects of the behavior)."

Example: *"I feel uncomfortable when a patient's personal problems are discussed in the cafeteria because someone might overhear confidential information."*

Make Clear Statements

Statements, rather than questions, set the stage for assertive responses to conflict. When questions are used, "how" questions are best because they are neutral in nature, they seek more information, and they imply a collaborative effort. "Why" questions ask for an explanation or an evaluation of behavior and often put the other person on the defensive. It is always important to state the situation clearly; describe events or expectations objectively; and maintain a strong, firm, yet tactful manner. The case of Mr. Dixon, presented earlier, shows how a nurse can use the three levels of assertive behavior to meet the patient's needs in a hospital situation without compromising the nurse's own needs for respect and dignity. In this interaction, the nurse's position is defined several times using successively stronger statements before the shift can be made to refocus on underlying patient needs. Notice that even in the final encounter, the nurse labels the behavior, not the patient, as unacceptable. Persistence is an essential feature when first attempts at assertiveness appear too limited. After careful analysis, if you find that a patient's behavior is infringing on your rights, it is essential that the issues be addressed directly in a tactful manner. If they are not, it is quite likely that the undesirable behavior will continue until you are no longer able to tolerate it.

Use Proper Pitch and Tone

The amount of force used in delivery of an assertive statement depends on the nature of the conflict situation as well as on the amount of confrontation needed to resolve the conflict. Starting with the least amount of assertiveness required to meet the demands of the situation conserves energy and does not place the nurse into the bind of overkill. It is not necessary to use all of your resources at one time or to express ideas strongly when this type of response is not needed. You can sometimes lose your effectiveness by becoming long-winded in your explanation when only a simple statement of rights or intentions is needed. Getting to the main point quickly and saying what is necessary in the simplest, most concrete way cuts down on the possibility of misinterpretation. This approach increases the probability that the communication will be received constructively.

Pitch and tone of voice contribute to another person's interpretation of the meaning of your assertive message. A firm but moderate presentation is often as effective as content in conveying the message.

Clinical Encounters With Demanding, Difficult Patients

Every nurse encounters patients who seem overly demanding of the nurse's limited time and resources. Although this may reflect a personality characteristic, most often it is a sign of the patient's anxiety. Box 13.1 describes behaviors that increase anger in others. Reflect on how to avoid these triggers. Conversely, ignoring inappropriate behavior does not make it go away. For example in the case of Mr. Gow, discussed earlier, he is making inappropriate sexual suggestions. The nurse could have ineffectively responded by ignoring his verbal comments or by avoiding him. Instead, she responded assertively in a "no nonsense" professional manner. How would you handle such a situation? Try out some of the more therapeutic approaches outlined in Box 13.3 and Table 13.1. Usually we tend to label people as "difficult to deal with" when our normal way of dealing with them has failed. So remember, we cannot change another's personality, but we can change the way we react to him or her.

Clinical Encounters With Angry Patients
Recognize Signs of Anger

You can expect to encounter patients who express anger. This may take the form of refusal to comply with the treatment plan, withdrawal from any positive interaction with you, or the exhibition of hostile behaviors. Hostility may be verbalized, as when a patient curses at you or even becomes physically violent. When you are dealing with a difficult patient, ask yourself what he or she is gaining from the violent behavior. Some people have not learned how to communicate successfully, so they revert to behavior that has gained them something in the past. For example, as children they may have gotten needed attention only when they acted out in a negative way or when they pouted or sulked. Ask yourself whether a patient who is behaving in a difficult way is being rewarded by becoming the focus of staff attention. Does such an individual only need to learn a more effective way of communicating? Remind yourself that usually a patient's feelings center on their disease or treatment and are not a reflection of their feeling about you. Do not take a patient's frustration or anger personally!

Nonverbal clues to anger include grimacing, clenching one's jaws or fists, turning away, and refusing to maintain eye contact. Verbal cues may, of course, include the use of an angry tone of voice, but they may also be disguised as witty sarcasm or as condescending or insulting remarks. To become comfortable in dealing with anger, the nurse must first become aware of his or her own reactions and learn not to feel threatened or respond in anger. Interventions include those listed in Table 13.1.

Help the Patient Express Anger in an Acceptable Manner

Help patients own their angry feelings by getting them to verbalize things that make them angry. Acknowledging their anger may prevent an expression of abusive ranting. It is essential that you use empathetic statements or active listening to acknowledge their anger and maintain a nonthreatening demeanor *before* moving on to try to discuss an issue. Remember, your goal is to maintain *safety* while helping your patient.

Defuse Hostility

Avoid responding to a patient's anger by getting angry yourself. Verbal attacks follow certain rules, that is, the abusive person expects you to react in specific ways. Usually people will respond by becoming aggressive and attacking back or by becoming defensive and intimidated. Keep your cool, using the strategies discussed earlier. Take a deep breath! Remember, if you lose control, you lose! If you become defensive, you lose! Abusive people want to provoke confrontations as a means of controlling you.

- Use empathy in your communication. An angry person needs to have you acknowledge both the issue and his or her feelings about that issue. Only then can they begin to interact in a meaningful way. Deliberately begin to lower your voice and speak more slowly. When we get upset, we tend to speak quickly and use a higher tone of voice. If you do the opposite, the person may begin to mimic you and thus calm down.

Realistically Analyze the Current Situation That Is Disturbing the Patient

- Be assertive in setting limits. If the behavior persists, you need to assert limits, saying, for example, "Jim, I want to help you sort this out, but if you continue to curse at me and raise your voice, I'm going to have to leave. Which do you want?" Another response might be, "Yelling at me isn't going to get this worked out. I will not argue with you. Come back when you can talk calmly and I will try to help you."
- Help your patients to develop a plan to deal with the situation (e.g., use techniques such as role-playing to help them express anger appropriately, using "I" statements such as, "I feel angry" rather than "You make me angry"). Bringing behavior up to a verbal level should help alleviate the need for acting out and other destructive behaviors.

Prevent Escalation of Conflict

In nurse-patient confrontations, the recognition of "trigger" factors, which often lead to escalation, may help in prevention. Do assess whether the person is intoxicated, disoriented, or whether there may be substance abuse. Using respectful patient-centered care approaches can help to prevent any escalation in interpersonal conflict. Hurt feelings or misunderstandings can quickly grow into a conflict. Keep the focus on the individual's *behavior* rather than on the person. If eye contact seems confrontational, then break eye contact. If the person is acting out by throwing or hitting, set limits: "No ___(hitting) (spitting) (cussing)___ behavior is allowed here. Such behavior is unacceptable." If you set limits, be sure to follow through. Ask the person to verbalize the anger (e.g., "Talk about how you feel instead of throwing things"). Use the strategies described in Table 13.1 for defusing conflict situations.

Strategies Useful in Clinical Encounters With Violent Patients

Your only goal is to lower the individual's level of rage and to protect them and yourself. Always leave yourself a clear exit.

- *Approach.* In an acute situation you **de-escalate** and **contain.** If you are in danger of mortal harm, leave! Using "calming interventions" is recommended if there is no weapon.
- *Actions.* Table 13.1 lists some useful strategies for coping with angry, potentially violent individuals. Remember, your goal is to defuse the threat of violence if possible

and to protect yourself and others from harm. Do not try for a rational discussion, just focus on calming interactions.

- *Reporting.* It has been estimated that a significant number of incidents go unreported; some say up to 80%. This is an international problem for nurses, and ICN urges you to report all incidents of abuse or violence.
- *Analysis.* Postincident analysis may offer insight into how to prevent the next situation. Some patients have mental problems, are truly confused, or have dementia. The AHRQ (2014) recommends that clinicians assess their patients' level of cognitive functioning using the Mini-Mental State Examination (MMSE). It helps you to respond more positively if you perceive that their behavior is not "evil" but a result of their illness. *Be aware that escalating conflict can be a threat not only to your patient but also to you. In no case is violence acceptable.* Limits must be set. Failing this, *you must remove yourself from a potentially harmful situation.* Starcher (1999) describes the behavior of Sam, an emotionally disturbed patient who was admitted to a geriatric unit. Sam's behavior ranged from bullying or pushing other clients to noncompliance with his treatment. Staff tried setting clear limits and identifying specific negative outcomes, including restraints and medication, without success. Eventual successful interventions included a consistent response by all staff members and using written patient contracts for each of his unacceptable behaviors. Outcomes were specifically stated for both negative behaviors (restrictions) and positive acceptable behaviors (rewards with his favorite activities).

An additional strategy for helping nurse-patient problem interactions is the **staff-focused consultation.** Consider the following situation. Students are particularly prone to feeling rebuffed when they first encounter negative feedback from a patient. Support from staff, instructors, and peers, coupled with efforts to understand the underlying reasons for the patient's feelings, can help you to resist the trap of avoiding the relationship. To develop these ideas further, practice.

Defusing Potential Conflicts When You Are Providing Home Health Care

Recognizing potential situations lending themselves to conflict is, of course, an important initial step. Caregivers have been shown to experience conflict through incompatible pressures suffered between caregiver demands and demands from their other roles, such as parenting their children or maintaining employment. In addition to this inter-role conflict, caregivers suffer pressures when a nurse comes into the home to participate in the care of an ill relative. A Canadian study of home health nurses and family caregivers of elderly relatives identified four evolving stages in the nurse-caregiver relationship. The initial stage is "worker-helper," with the nurse providing care to the ill patient and the family helping. Next comes "worker-worker," when the nurse begins teaching the needed care skills to family members. Third is "nurse as manager; family as worker," as the family members learn needed care skills. The final stage, "nurse as nurse for family caregiver," occurs as the family member becomes exhausted (Butt, 2000). A source of conflict for nurses was the dual expectation of the family that the nurse would provide not only care for the identified patient but also relief for the exhausted primary caregiver. When the nurse operated as manager and treated the caregiver as worker, the discrepancy in expectations and values resulted in increased tension in the relationship. Discussion of role expectations is essential. Because of the high cost of providing direct care to the chronically ill, home health nurses may be expected to quickly shift to teaching the necessary skills to the family members. Although this shift in responsibility may result in a reduction of expensive professional time it should not compromise your commitment to the family.

SUMMARY

Conflict represents a struggle between two opposing thoughts, feelings, or needs. It can be intrapersonal in nature, deriving from within a particular individual, or interpersonal, when it represents a clash between two or more people. This chapter focused on conflict between nurse and patient or family.

All conflicts have certain things in common: a concrete content problem issue and relationship issues arising from the process of expressing the conflict. Generally intrapersonal conflicts stimulate feelings of emotional discomfort. Strategies to defuse strong emotion were highlighted. Most interpersonal conflicts involve some threat, either to one's sense of power to control an interpersonal situation or to ways of thinking about the self. Giving up ineffective behavior patterns in conflict situations is difficult, because such patterns are generally perceived to be safer because they are familiar.

Behavioral responses to conflict situations fall into five styles. In the past, nurses most commonly choose avoidance. However, this chapter describes other strategies (e.g., assertion) that have been more successfully used by nurses to manage patient-nurse conflicts. Assertive behaviors range from making a simple statement, directly and honestly, about one's beliefs, to taking a very strong, confrontational stand about what will and will not be tolerated.

The principles of conflict management were described. To apply conflict management principles, you need to identify your own conflictive feelings or reactions. For internal conflict, feelings usually have to be put into words and related to the issue at hand before the meaning of the conflict becomes understandable. In conflict between nurse and patient, you need to think through the possible causes of the conflict as well as your own feelings before making a response. To resolve these kinds of conflict, you need to use "I" statements and respond assertively. This chapter also discussed workplace violence and strategies to maintain or restore a safe environment.

ETHICAL DILEMMA: What Would You Do?

You are caring for Kim, born at the gestational age of 24 weeks in a rural hospital and transferred this morning to your neonatal intensive care unit. Today her father arrives on the unit. Seeing you taking a blood sample from one of the many intravenous lines attached to Kim, he yells at you to "Stop poking at her! What are you trying to prove by keeping her alive? Turn off those machines." This is both a communication problem and an ethics problem. How do you respond to his anger?

DISCUSSION QUESTIONS

1. Select a tone and pitch listed in Simulation Exercise 13.2. Describe how the tone and pitch effect a conflict situation.

2. Using the knowledge gained in the chapter and the behaviors listed in Box 13.1, design a response where you de-escalate a conflict.

REFERENCES

Agency for Healthcare Research and Quality (AHRQ). (n.d.). Retrieved from: www.ahrq.gov. Accessed 10.03.18.

Agency for Healthcare Research and Quality (AHRQ). (2014). *Guide to clinical preventive services, 2014: Recommendations of the U.S. Preventive Services Task Force.* Retrieved from: http://www.ahrq.gov/professionals/clinicians-providers/guidelines-recommendations/guide/index.html. Accessed 10.04.18.

Agency for Healthcare Research and Quality (AHRQ). (2016). *TeamSTEPPS webinar.* Rockville, MD: Agency for Healthcare Research and Quality.

American Association of Critical Care Nurses (AACN). (2004). *Position statement: Workplace violence prevention.* Retrieved from: www.aacn.org/policy-and-advocacy/aacn_advocacy-and-health-policy. [search workplace violence]. Accessed 10.04.18.

American Nurses Association (ANA). (2002). *Preventing workplace violence.* Washington, DC: Author.

American Nurses Association (ANA). (2012). *House of delegates resolution of workplace violence.* Retrieved from: www.nursingworld.org.

Avander, K., Heikki, A., Bjersa, K., & Ergstrom, M. (2016). Trauma nurses' experience of workplace violence and threats: Short and long term consequences in a Swedish setting. *Journal of Trauma Nursing, 23*(2), 51–57.

Brann, M., & Hartley, D. (2016). Nursing student evaluation of NIOSH workplace violence prevention for nurses online course. *Journal of Safety Research,* 1–7. Retrieved from: https://doi.org/10.1016/jsr2016.12.003.

Butt, G. (2000). Nurses and family caregivers of elderly relatives engaged in 4 evolving types of relationships. *Evidence-Based Nursing, 3,* 134.

Campbell, C. L., & Burg, M. A. (2015). Gammonley D: Measures for incident reporting of patient violence and aggression towards healthcare providers: A systematic review. *Aggression and Violent Behavior, 25,* 314–322.

Cheng, F. K. (2016). Mediation skills for conflict resolution in nursing education. *Nurse Education in Practice, 15,* 310–313.

CPI. (2017). *Ten crisis prevention tips.* Retrieved from: www.crisisprevention.com/media/CPI/resources/CPI-s-Top-10-De-Escalation-Tips-US/CPI-Top-10-De-Escalation-Tip. [search crisis]. Accessed 10.04.18.

Dwarswaard, J., & van de Bovenkamp, H. (2015). Self-management support: A qualitative study of ethical dilemmas experienced by nurses. *Patient Education and Counseling, 98,* 1131–1136.

Hahn, S., Muller, M., Hantikainen, V., Dassen, T. W. N., Kok, G., & Halfens, R. J. G. (2013). Risk factors associated with patient and visitor violence in general hospitals: Results of a multiple regression analysis. *International Journal of Nursing Studies, 50,* 374–385.

Haugvaldstad, M. J., & Husum, T. L. (2016). Influence of staff emotional reactions on the escalation of patient aggression in mental health care. *International Journal of Law and Psychiatry, 49,* 130–137.

Hersch, R. K., Cook, R. F., Deitz, D. K., Kaplan, S., Hughes, D., Friesen, M. A., et al. (2016). Reducing nurses' stress: A randomized controlled trial of a web-based stress management program for nurses. *Applied Nursing Research, 32,* 18–25.

International Council of Nurses (ICN). (2006). *Violence: A worldwide epidemic*. Retrieved from: www.icn.ch/nursing-policy/position-statements. Accessed 10.04.18.

Llor-Esteban, B., Sanchez-Munoz, M., Ruiz-Hernandes, J. A., & Jimenez-Barbero, J. A. (2016). User violence towards nursing professionals in mental health services and emergency units. *The European J of Psychology Applied to Legal Context*, 1e–8e, [in press]. https://doi.org/10.1016/j.ejpal.2016.06.002.

Longo, J., Cassidy, L., & Sherman, R. (2016). Charge nurses' experience with horizontal violence: Implications for leadership development. *The Journal of Continuing Education in Nursing*, 47(11), 493–499.

McElhaney, R. (1996). Conflict management in nursing administration. *Nursing Management*, 27(3), 49–50.

NICE Guideline #10. (2015). *Violence and aggression*. London: British Psychological Society.

Nowrouzi, B., & Huyuh, V. (2016). Citation analysis of workplace violence: A review of the top 50 annual and lifetime cited articles. *Aggression & Violent Behavior*, 28, 21–28.

Phillips, J. P. (2016). Workplace violence. *New England Journal of Medicine*, 374, 1661–1669.

Quality and Safety Education for Nurses (QSEN). (n.d.). Retrieved from: www.qsen.org. Accessed 10.02.18.

Riley, J. B. (2017). *Communication in nursing* (8th ed.). St. Louis, MO: Mosby/Elsevier Inc.

Sayer, M. M., McNeese-Smith, D., Leach, L. S., & Phillips, L. R. (2012). An educational intervention to increase 'speaking-up' behaviors in nurses and improve patient safety. *Journal of Nursing Care Quality*, 27(2), 154–160.

Starcher, S. (1999). Sam was an emotional terrorist. *Nursing*, 99(2), 40–41.

The Joint Commission (TJC). (2010). *Preventing violence in the health care setting* Sentinel Event Alert, (45). Retrieved from: www.jointcommission.org/sentinel_event_alert_issue_45_preventing_violence_in_the_healthcaresetting/ http://www.jointcommission.org/assets/1/18/SEA_45.PDF. [SEARC setinel event issue 45]. Accessed 10.04.18.

US Department of Health and Human Services. (2014). *Healthy people 2020: Injury and violence prevention*. Retrieved from: www.healthypeople.gov/2020/topicsobjectives2020/overview.aspx?topicid=24.

US Department of Labor Occupational Safety and Health Administration (OSHA). (2004). *Guidelines for preventing workplace violence for health care and social service workers* OSHA 3148-01R. Retrieved 11 July 2014, from: https://www.osha.gov/OshDoc/data_General_Facts/factsheet-workplace-violence.pdf/. Accessed 10.04.18.

Waschgler, K., Ruiz-Hernandez, J. A., Llor-Esteban, B., & Garcia-Izquierdo, M. (2013). Patients' aggressive behaviours towards nurses: Development and psychometric properties of the hospital aggressive behaviour scale-users. *Journal of Advanced Nursing*, 69(6), 1418–1427.

Watkins, L. E., Sippel, L. M., Pietrzak, R. H., Hoff, R., Harpaz-Rotem, I., Watkins, L. E., et al. (2017). Co-occuring aggression and suicide attempt among veterans entering residential treatment for PTSD: The role of PTSD symptom clusters and alcohol misuse. *Journal of Psychiatric Research*, 87, 8–14.

Wei, C., Chiou, S., Chien, L., & Huang, N. (2016). Workplace violence against nurses: Prevalence and association with hospital organizational characteristics and health-promotion efforts: Cross-sectional study. *International Journal of Nursing Studies*, 56, 63–70.

World Health Organization (WHO). (2012). *Workplace violence*. Geneva: Author. Retrieved from: http://who.int/violence.injury.prevention/injury/work9/en/print.html.

14

Communication Strategies for Health Promotion and Disease Prevention

Elizabeth C. Arnold

OBJECTIVES

At the end of the chapter, the reader will be able to:

1. Define concepts related to health promotion and disease prevention.
2. Identify national agendas for health promotion and disease prevention.
3. Specify relevant conceptual frameworks for health promotion actions.
4. Apply health promotion and disease prevention strategies for individuals.
5. Apply health promotion and disease prevention strategies at the community level.
6. Explain the role of health literacy in health promotion and disease prevention strategies.

INTRODUCTION

An overarching goal of *Healthy People 2020* is to "promote quality of life, healthy development, and healthy behaviors across all life stages" (US Health & Human Services, 2013, p. 3). This chapter focuses on the role of communication as a key nursing strategy in achieving specific health promotion and disease prevention goals. The chapter considers adverse psychosocial determinants of health as underlying challenges to achieving consistent high-quality health promotion and disease prevention outcomes. Applications of communication strategies are designed to help individuals and targeted populations achieve a better health quality of life through education, and lifestyle changes are presented.

BASIC CONCEPTS

Health care reform initiatives have created profound changes in how care is delivered, to whom it is delivered, and where it is delivered. Overall, the United States is undergoing a major paradigm shift that "is about changing the culture of health systems from a curative/reactive to a preventive/responsive orientation" (Litchfield & Jonsdottir, 2008, p. 81).

Health promotion and disease prevention, with special attention to the underlying causes of a health problem, is increasingly recognized as a reimbursable, essential component of comprehensive health care. Evidence of the nation's commitment to health promotion and disease prevention includes new Medicare reimbursement for preventive physicals and action plan generation for older adults. Assisting patients to practice positive health behaviors helps individuals prevent and/or delay chronic disease, functional decline, and related disability.

Definitions

Health is considered a fundamental human right, intimately tied to a nation's social and economic development (*Jakarta Declaration*; World Health Organization [WHO], 1997). **Health promotion** emphasizes "being able to function normally, experiencing well-being, and having a healthy lifestyle" (Fagerlind et al., 2010, p. 104). Factors such as genetics, environment, economics, and social circumstances influence health status. Some population groups are at higher risk for developing chronic health problems because of financial, personal, family, or environmental circumstances. Other factors include the availability of health services and new research findings—even opportunity and luck can enhance a person's ability to achieve optimal health status and well-being. Well-developed social skills, strong family bonds, consistent parenting skills, and active involvement in social institutions such as school, church, and the community provide more opportunities for health promotion/disease prevention strategies.

Health promotion is defined as "the process of enabling individuals to take control over their health" (WHO, 1986). Health promoting activities can include
- Health education
- Preventive health services
- Advocacy and development of public policies
- Safeguarding environmental health
- Community-based education in schools and workplaces
- Population-based targeted strategies for vulnerable populations
- Media outreach in the form of ads and blogs.

DISEASE PREVENTION

Disease prevention is the term used to describe actions designed to reduce or eliminate the onset, progression, complications, or recurrence of chronic disease. The goal of disease prevention is to help individuals "avoid the occurrence of a disease, disorder, or injury, to slow the progression of detectable disease and/or reduce its consequences" (WHO, 1997).

Relevant terminology includes risk, and protective factors. *Risk, and protective factors* are defined as personal and environmental characteristics that increase the probability of having a health problem *(risk factor)* or decrease the probability of its occurrence or progression *(protective factor)*. If a person is obese, eats too many carbohydrates, and leads a sedentary life, the combined risk factors can increase the probability of having a heart attack. Causal risk factors and social determinants of health play a major role in the onset and progression of emergent chronic disorders (Zubialde, Mold, & Eubank, 2009).

Some risk factors are modifiable. Pre-diabetic patients can minimize progression to full symptoms through diet, regular exercise, and leading a balanced life. Smoking, overeating, and excessive alcohol consumption are associated with a range of chronic disorders, including cancer. It has been shown that aggressive reduction of potential threats to full health and well-being is effective. Regular health screenings can identify emerging treatable health problems such as osteoporosis, high blood pressure, and glaucoma. Individuals with a genetic predisposition to chronic diseases—such as obesity, heart disease, arthritis, or diabetes—can reduce the impact of inherited risk factors by actively embracing habits of healthy eating, adequate sleep, regular exercise, and an active lifestyle. The promotion of healthy behaviors involves more than just buzzwords. Many evidence-based studies attest to the effectiveness of promoting health and well-being.

Protective factors are defined as circumstances, resources, and personal characteristics that delay the emergence of chronic disease or lessen its impact. Although protective factors do not guarantee a life free of serious illness or early death, they play a significant role in helping patients improve their health and quality of life. Examples of protective factors include developing a healthy lifestyle, getting daily exercise, eating a healthy diet, having annual medical checkups, increasing the number of available support systems, obtaining health insurance, and so on. Health education, social marketing, and screening services help people to become aware of health risk factors.

Lifestyle

Milio (1976) defines **lifestyle** as "patterns of choices made from the alternatives that are available to people according to their socioeconomic circumstances, and the ease with which they are able to choose certain ones over others" (quoted in Cody, 2006, p. 186). Components of a healthy lifestyle include eating healthy meals, staying active with adequate exercise, getting adequate sleep, managing stress, building supportive relationships, and nurturing one's spirit. Ideally, building a healthy lifestyle begins in childhood. As Frederick Douglass (n.d.) noted years ago, "It is easier to build strong children than to repair broken men." Nurses serve as role models. You will have more credibility in advocating for healthy lifestyles if you practice what you preach.

Social Determinants of Health

Social determinants of health define a wide range of contextual factors influencing the health and well-being of individuals and communities. These social, economic, religious, and political factors are embedded at the level of the community as well as the larger society. They have a significant effect on health and well-being (US Department of Health and Human Services [DHHS], 2010).

Although each person enters the world with a distinct set of constitutional factors (size, gender, intellect, and personality), each grows up within social and community networks and, over time, incorporates the social values of those networks. One's environment interacts with personal factors to influence, enhance, or limit one's health behaviors. Larger social community systems create roles and expectations that further shape and modify the individual's health behaviors (Grey, 2017).

Health Disparities

Health disparities describes fundamental differences in adverse health outcomes and lost opportunities to achieve optimal health and well-being as it relates to demographics, income, education, and access. Nationally, disparities account for significant variations in life expectancy, positive health outcomes, and the incidence of chronic disease and disability. DeWalt et al. (2011) assert that "people with limited health literacy are less likely to engage in disease prevention behaviors, to know about their illness and medicines, and to manage and control a chronic disease" (p. 2).

Social determinants associated with health disparities include lack of adequate health insurance, social isolation, cultural factors, access and availability of services, finances, lack of knowledge or education, food or job security, language barriers, health literacy, and poverty. Social determinants critically affect health, morbidity, and mortality, such that "treatment alone is unlikely to have marked effects on health inequities or health status" (Frankish, Moulton, Rootman, Cole, & Gray, 2006, p. 176). *Healthy People 2020* and the Centers for Disease Control and Prevention (CDC) (2009) identify health disparities as a fundamental health concern, requiring immediate, concentrated attention. The elimination of health disparities is a primary objective of our nation's public health agenda and a central focus of the National Center for Minority Health and Health Disparities within the National Institutes of Health.

Well-Being

Health promotion activities incorporate the WHO concept of a close connection between health and well-being. *Well-being* is defined as an individual's personal life satisfaction in terms of six dimensions: intellectual, physical, emotional, social, occupational, and spiritual (Edlin & Golanty, 2009). People can experience well-being as being at peace with themselves and others even with a serious health problem or terminal diagnosis if they feel peaceful within themselves and receive appropriate support (Saylor, 2004). Fundamental changes in health habits and modifications in lifestyle typically improve health and well-being. Fig. 14.1 displays critical elements for maintaining health and well-being. A healthy lifestyle, a sense of purpose and supportive resources lead to health and well being.

GLOBAL AND NATIONAL HEALTH PROMOTION AGENDAS

Improving the quality of health promotion and disease prevention is a national and global health care reform initiative (Hogg et al., 2009). As you read through this section, note the similar themes in virtually all national and global agenda goals. Strong recommendations appear about the need to explore the close interaction between personal, environmental, and social determinants of health and well-being and the provision of equal opportunity for high-quality health care.

In 1986 the WHO's *Ottawa Charter for Health Promotion* documented the essential prerequisites and resources needed for health promotion as "peace, shelter, education,

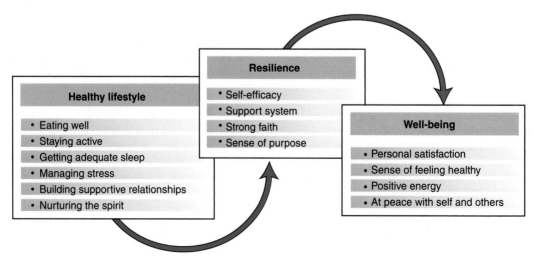

Fig. 14.1 Critical Elements for Maintaining Health and Well-Being.

food, income, a stable ecosystem, sustainable resources, social justice, and equity" (WHO, 1986). The charter identified the prerequisites for improving health as follows:

1. Advocacy for health
2. Enabling equal opportunities and resources for people to achieve health
3. Mediation and coordinated action shared by community groups, health service agencies, and governments targeted toward the pursuit of health

Each decade, the DHHS publishes an updated health promotion and disease prevention agenda for the nation with specific goals and objectives. The latest document of its kind, *Healthy People 2020*, emphasizes the social determinants and environmental factors contributing to the health status of individuals and populations. Its vision is to have "a society in which all people live long, healthy lives" (DHHS, 2010). Proposed goals include the following:

- Eliminate preventable disease, disability, injury, and premature death
- Achieve health equity, eliminate disparities, and improve the health of all groups
- Create social and physical environments that promote good health for all
- Promote healthy development and healthy behaviors across every stage of life

Topic areas proposed to achieve these goals (Box 14.1) identify the population focus of attention. Objectives are organized in three categories—interventions, determinants, and outcomes. *Healthy People 2020* reinforces the importance of social determinants as critical antecedents that influence health and well-being. There is a specific goal related to "ideas of health equity that address social determinants of health and promote health across all stages of life." More information about specific recommendations is available at www.healthypeople.gov/HP2020.

The Jakarta Declaration on Health Promotion is a global initiative that recommends the following to enhance health and well-being (WHO, 1997):

- Building healthy public policy
- Creating supportive environments for health
- Strengthening community action for health
- Developing personal skills
- Reorienting health services

Kushner and Sorensen (2013) suggest that "lifestyle medicine" may represent a new disciplinary approach for the management of chronic illness and disease prevention.

THEORY-BASED FRAMEWORKS

Theory frameworks for health promotion examine how people make choices and decisions about their health.

BOX 14.1 *Healthy People 2020:* Topic Areas With Health Indicators

- Access to Care: Proportion of people with access to health care services
- Healthy Behavior: Proportion of people engaged in healthy behaviors
- Chronic Disease: Prevalence and mortality of chronic disease
- Environmental Determinants: Proportion of people with a healthy physical environment
- Social Determinants: Proportion of people with a healthy social environment
- Injury: Proportion of people that experiences injury
- Mental Health: Proportion of people experiencing positive mental health
- Maternal and Infant Health: Proportion of healthy births
- Responsible Sexual Behavior: Proportion of people engaged in responsible sexual behavior
- Substance Abuse: Proportion of people engaged in substance abuse
- Tobacco: Proportion of people using tobacco
- Quality of Care: Proportion of people receiving quality health care services

Adapted from US Department of Health and Human Services. (2011). Leading health indicators for Healthy People 2020: Letter report. Retrieved from http://iom.edu/Reports/2011/Leading-Health-Indicators-for-Healthy-People-2020.aspx.

Pender's health promotion model, Prochaska's transtheoretical model, and Bandura's social learning theory are useful frameworks to guide health promotion strategies.

Pender's Health Promotion Model

A person's capacity to absorb and use health promotion information depends to a large degree on what people believe about their health, the seriousness of their health conditions, and the extent to which their personal actions can produce positive outcomes. Health promotion interventions target behavioral change. Nurses use Pender's revised health belief model to understand what motivates people to engage in personal health behaviors (Pender, Murdaugh, & Parsons, 2011). The model expands on an earlier health belief model developed by Rosenstock and associates in the 1950s. This model (Fig. 14.2) proposes that a person's willingness to engage in health promotion behaviors is best understood by examining his or her personal beliefs about the nature and seriousness of a health condition and the person's capacity to influence its outcome.

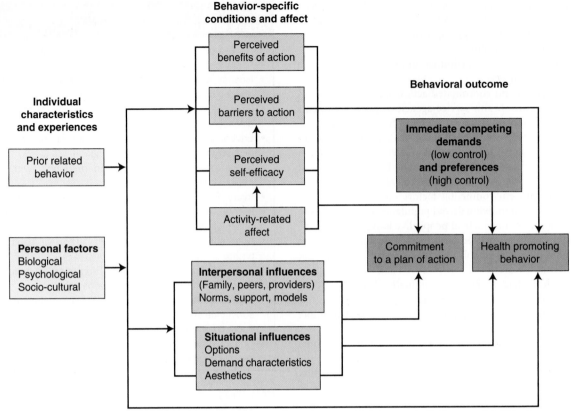

Fig. 14.2 Revised Health Promotion Model. (From Pender, N, Murdaugh C, Parsons M. (2011). *Health promotion in nursing practice* (6th ed., p. 45). Upper Saddle River, NJ: Prentice Hall.)

Pender's model identifies perceived benefits, barriers, and ability to take action related to health and well-being as important components of people's health decision making. These dynamics act as internal or external "cues to action," which influence a person's decision to engage in health promoting activities. **Cues to action** include required school immunizations, interpersonal reminders, past experiences with the health care system, the mass media, and ethnic approval (Fig. 14.3) .

Case Example
Mary Nolan knows that walking will help diminish her risk for developing osteoporosis, but the threat of potentially having this problem in her 60s is not sufficient to motivate her to take action in her 40s. Mary does not feel any signs or symptoms of the disorder, and it is easier to maintain a sedentary lifestyle. To create the most appropriate learning conditions and types of teaching strategies, the nurse will have to understand Mary's value system and other factors that influence Mary's readiness to learn. To remain healthy, Mary will have to effect positive change in her health habits.

Simulation Exercise 14.1 provides practice in applying Pender's model to common health problems.

Transtheoretical Model of Change
Prochaska's transtheoretical model is an evidence-based model used to explore a person's motivational readiness to intentionally change his or her health habits (Prochaska & Norcross, 2013). The model identifies stages of readiness ranging from lack of acknowledgment of a problem to taking and maintaining constructive actions to correct

unhealthy behaviors. Table 14.1 presents Prochaska's model with suggested approaches for each stage and corresponding sample statements.

In the *precontemplation* stage, a person either does not see a health problem (even though it may be obvious to others) or does not have any intention of modifying it in the foreseeable future. The *contemplation* stage is characterized by awareness of a problem. The person is thinking of change but is still ambivalent and lacks a strong commitment to take action. Prochaska and Norcross (2013) refer to contemplation as "knowing where you want to go but not being quite ready to go there" (p. 460). In this *preparation* stage, a person begins to take small tentative steps toward changing poor health habits but is not fully committed to consistent action. An important component in the preparation stage is the setting of goals and priorities. A strong commitment to change and taking consistent definitive actions to make behavioral changes a reality identifies the *action* stage.

A *maintenance* stage, in which patients stabilize and consolidate gains achieved during the action stage, follows. Patients can easily relapse and may need to recycle through previous stages several times before a new health behavior is firmly established. Relapses are treated as temporary setbacks that provide information about triggers and high-risk situations patients need to avoid.

Simulation Exercise 14.2 provides an opportunity to work with the Prochaska's transtheoretical model.

Social Learning Theory

Bandura's (1997) contribution to the study of health promotion is the concept of self-efficacy. *Self-efficacy* is defined as a personal belief in one's ability to execute the actions required to achieve a goal. It represents a powerful mediator of behavior and behavioral change.

Self-efficacy and motivation are reciprocal processes. Increased self-efficacy strengthens motivation, which, in turn, increases an individual's capacity to complete the learning task.

Bandura considers learning to be a social process. He identifies three sets of motivating factors that promote the learning necessary to achieve a predetermined goal: physical motivators, social incentives, and cognitive motivators. *Physical motivators* can be internal, such as memory of previous discomfort or a symptom that the patient cannot ignore. *Social incentives*, such as praise and encouragement, increase self-esteem and give the patient reason to continue learning. Bandura refers to a third set of motivators as *cognitive motivators*, describing them as thought processes associated with change.

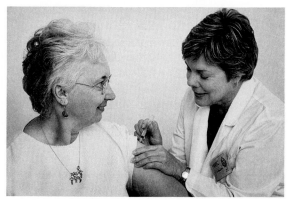

Fig. 14.3 Immunizations are an Important Component of Disease Prevention. (From James Gathany, Centers for Disease Control and Prevention [CDC], 2009.)

SIMULATION EXERCISE 14.1
Motivational Interviewing Using Pender's Model

Purpose
To help students understand the value of the health promotion model in assessing and promoting healthy lifestyles (Fig. 14.4).

Procedure
1. Using the health promotion model as a guide, interview a person in the community about his or her perception of a common health problem (e.g., heart disease, high cholesterol, osteoporosis, breast or prostate cancer, obesity, or diabetes).
2. Record the person's answers in written diagram form following Pender's model of health promotion. Identify the behavior-specific cognitions and affect action that would best fit the person's situation.

3. Share your findings with your classmates, either in a small group of four to six students with a scribe to share common themes with the larger class or in the general class.

Discussion
1. Were you surprised by anything the patient said, his or her perception of the problem, or interpretation of its meaning?
2. As you compare your findings with other classmates, do common themes emerge?
3. How could you use the information you obtained from this exercise in future health care situations?

TABLE 14.1   Prochaska's Stages of Change With Suggested Approaches and Sample Statements Applied to Alcoholism

Stage	Characteristic Behaviors	Suggested Approach	Sample Statement
Precontemplation	Patient does not think there is a problem; is not considering the possibility of change.	Raise doubt; give informational feedback to raise awareness of a problem and health risks.	"Your lab tests show liver damage. These tests can be predictive of serious health problems and premature death."
Contemplation	Patient thinks there may be a problem; is thinking about change; goes back and forth between concern and unconcern.	Tip the balance; allow open discussion of pros and cons of changing behavior; build motivation for change; help patient justify a positive commitment.	"It sounds as though you think you may have a drinking problem but are not sure you are an alcoholic. What would your life be like without alcohol?"
Preparation	Patient decides there is a problem and is willing to make a change: "I guess I do need to stop drinking."	Help the patient choose the best course of action for resolving the problem.	"What kinds of changes will you need to make to stop drinking? Most people find Alcoholics Anonymous (AA) helpful as a support. Have you heard of them?"
Action	Patient engages in concrete actions to effect needed change.	Help the patient take active steps to resolve health problem; review progress; give feedback.	"I am impressed that you went to two AA meetings this week and have not had a drink either. What has this been like for you?"
Maintenance	Patient perseveres with positive behavioral change.	Help the patient identify and use strategies to sustain progress; point out positive changes; accept temporary setbacks and use steps in preparation phase if needed.	"It's hard to let go of old habits, but you have been abstinent for 3 months now, and your liver tests are significantly improved."

SIMULATION EXERCISE 14.2
Assessing Readiness Using Prochaska's Model

Purpose
To identify elements in teaching that can promote readiness, using Prochaska's model.

Procedure
Identify as many specific answers as possible to the following questions:

1. Patrick drinks four to six beers every evening. Last year he lost his job. He has a troubled marriage and few friends. Patrick does not consider himself an alcoholic and blames his chaotic marriage for his need to drink. There is a strong family history of alcoholism. What kinds of information might help Patrick want to learn more about his condition?

2. Lily has just learned she has breast cancer. Although there is a good chance that surgery and chemotherapy will help her, she is scared to commit to the process and has even talked about taking her life. What kinds of health teaching strategies and information might help Lily become ready to learn about her condition?

3. Shawn has just been diagnosed as having epilepsy. He is ashamed to tell his friends and teachers about his condition. Shawn is considering breaking up with his girlfriend because of his newly diagnosed illness. How would you use health teaching to help Shawn cope more effectively with his illness?

In the following case example, the nurse combines the concept of a physical motivator with a social incentive related to something the patient values (his grandson), and relates the process to the desired outcome. The intervention is designed to help Francis recognize how changes in his health behavior can not only improve his health and well-being but also give him a social outlet that could be important to him.

Case Example

Nurse: "I'm worried that you are continuing to smoke, because it affects your breathing. There is nothing you can do about the damage to your lungs that is already there, but if you stop smoking it can help preserve the healthy tissue you still have (physical motivator) and you won't have as much trouble breathing. I bet your grandson would appreciate it if you could breathe better and be able to play with him (social incentive)." As Francis notices that he is coughing less when he gives up smoking, this new perceptual knowledge will act as an internal cognitive motivator to remain abstinent.

DISEASE PREVENTION

Disease prevention frameworks are concerned with identifying modifiable risk and protective factors associated with specific diseases and mental disorders. Nurses use case-finding strategies to identify risk factors in individuals, families, and communities. The goals of prevention emphasize "managing and or preventing the risk of future disease, disability and premature death" (Zubialde et al., 2009, p. 194). Three tiers of prevention—primary, secondary, and tertiary—represent a continuum of disease prevention focus.

- **Primary disease prevention** strategies target modifiable risk factors with suggestions for health promoting activities to facilitate a healthy lifestyle—for example, promoting exercise and a healthy diet in order to prevent obesity and diabetes. Other examples include immunizations; low-cost flu shots; safe-sex counseling; smoking cessation; the use of car seats, seat belts, and motorcycle helmets; and bans on texting while driving. Advocacy for these health protections is easily incorporated into ordinary nursing care.

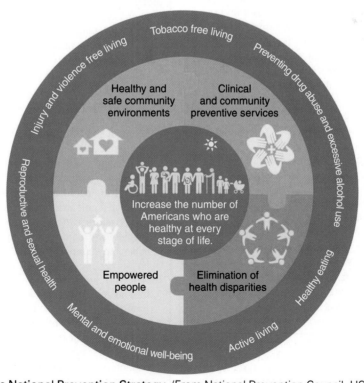

Fig. 14.4 The National Prevention Strategy. (From National Prevention Council, US Department of Health and Human Services, Office of the Surgeon General (2011). *National prevention strategy.* Washington, DC: US Department of Health and Human Services, Office of the Surgeon General.)

- *Secondary prevention* strategies focus on early disease detection through regular health screenings for conditions such as prostate cancer, osteoporosis, and diabetes; regular mammograms and pap smears for women; periodic colonoscopies; and blood pressure screenings. Individuals with known risk factors such as family history, high cholesterol, elevated blood sugar, high blood pressure, and advanced age should be screened periodically. With early case finding, the emergence or course of a chronic disease can be modified to allow a better quality of life. Screening for mental health problems during the course of primary care visits can detect undiagnosed depression, anxiety, and substance abuse.

- *Tertiary prevention* strategies focus on minimizing the damaging effects of a disease or injury once it has occurred. The goal is to help patients achieve a good quality of life regardless of their health circumstances.

Simulation Exercise 14.3 provides an opportunity to look at the role of potential risk factors in your personal health profile.

DEVELOPING AN EVIDENCE-BASED PRACTICE

Background: This meta-analysis and review study was designed to assess the effectiveness of motivational interviewing in improving outcomes for a variety of behavioral problems and chronic diseases as compared with traditional approaches.

Method: Searches using the appropriate search terms were conducted across a variety of evidence-based data bases. Also included were proceedings from the conferences of four diabetes-related associations. The authors of included studies and reviews were contacted for additional information when indicated, and randomized controlled trials were eligible for inclusion. The median duration of follow-up was 12 months, with a range of 2 months to 4 years. Patient participants presented with the following chronic conditions: alcohol abuse, psychiatric issues/addiction, overweight/inactivity, diabetes, asthma, and smoking. The methodology used individual interviews conducted by psychologists, physicians, nurses, and dieticians employing the theoretical counseling approaches developed by Miller and Rollnick (2013). The study identified outcome effects, with stronger results for interviews lasting 60 minutes rather than shorter time frames.

Findings: A total of 72 randomized controlled trials were included and 74% of the research studies demonstrated a positive effect with motivational interviewing.

Application to Your Clinical Practice: Nurses need to be intimately involved in the development of relevant creative public health approaches. Meta-analysis and review demonstrates that motivational interviewing outperforms advice-giving protocols in a range of health care situations.

Modified from Rubak, S., Sandbaek, A., Lauritzen, T., Christensen, B. Motivational interviewing: A systematic review and meta-analysis. University of York, Centre for Reviews and Dissemination. Also published in *British Journal of General Practice;* 55, 305–312 (2005).

SIMULATION EXERCISE 14.3
Developing a Health Profile

Purpose
To help students understand the relationship between lifestyle health assessment factors and related health goals from a personal perspective.

Procedure
Out-of-class assignment: Develop a personal health profile in which you

1. Assess your own personal risk factors related to each of the following:
   a. Family risk factors (diabetes, cardiac, cancer, osteoporosis)
   b. Diet and nutrition
   c. Exercise habits
   d. Weight
   e. Alcohol and drug use
   f. Safe sex practices
   g. Perceived level of stress
   h. Health screening tests: cholesterol, blood pressure, blood sugar
2. Identify unhealthy behaviors or risk factors
3. Develop a personalized action plan to identify strategies to address areas that need strengthening
4. Identify any barriers that might prevent you from achieving your personal goals

Discussion
1. In small groups, discuss findings that you feel comfortable sharing with others.
2. Get input from others about ways to achieve health-related goals.
3. In the larger group, discuss how doing this exercise can inform your practice related to lifestyle changes and health promotion.

APPLICATIONS

The American Association of Colleges of Nursing (AACN, 2008) has declared that "Health promotion, disease, and injury prevention across the lifespan are essential elements of baccalaureate nursing practice at the individual and population levels" (p. 23).

Health promotion strategies should be a part of everyday nursing care. Education and coaching can be introduced informally as you provide care. Community based interventions can be formally presented through patient education, screening programs, and social media.

Nurses need to be public advocates of health promotion actions as well as care agents. They are perceived as trustworthy informants about health matters because of their extensive knowledge base and close caregiving associations with patients and families.

Nurses can be influential in helping communities to create supportive health environments. For example, nurses can serve on health-related community advisory committees and provide relevant discussions regarding care and funding (Hawranik & Strain, 2007). The provision of health fairs for area schools or community groups is another avenue nurses can use to support health promotion and disease prevention at the community level.

Health Education for Health Promotion

Health education is an essential component of effective health promotion and disease prevention strategies (Hoving, Visser, Mullen, & van den Borne, 2010). Clinical approaches to promote healthy behaviors with individuals include motivational interviewing (MI), empowerment, social support, and self-management coaching.

Mol, Moser, and Pols (2010) note that good care involves "persistent tinkering in a world full of complex ambivalence and shifting tensions" (p. 14). Patients requiring the same educational information can demonstrate a wide range of learning, cognitive, experiential, and communication diversity. They differ in intellectual curiosity, learning preferences, motivation for learning, learning styles, and rate of learning, each of which will require adaptations to maximize learning. This is where the art of nursing comes in. It is important to select strategies that hold meaning for patients.

Common examples of general health promotion include developing a healthy lifestyle, good nutrition, regular physical activity, adequate sleep patterns, and stress reduction. But in addition to these desired outcomes, engaging in meaningful health promotion activities supports the development of patient autonomy, personal competence, and social relatedness.

Choosing disease prevention topics of potential interest to higher-risk patient populations offers the best return on investment. For example tuberculosis, hepatitis, and stomach cancer screenings would be of particular interest to Asian immigrant populations. Likewise, screenings for diabetes, hypertension, and prostate cancer would better fit the needs of Latinos and African Americans because of the greater prevalence of these disorders in these populations.

Formal and informal instruction can focus on condition-specific topics. A wide variety of topics lend themselves to a health promotion focus. A sampling includes

- Alcohol, nicotine, and other types of drug abuse prevention
- Anger management
- Prevention, screening, and early detection of common chronic diseases such as human immunodeficiency virus (HIV), diabetes, cancer, heart disease, osteoporosis, and associated disorders
- The fall prevention strategies
- Stress reduction for informal caregivers and organizational work sites
- Healthy dietary practices
- Regular exercise habits
- Developing effective support systems

Health promotion interventions must be responsive to each patient's personal situation, as universal applications may not be appropriately sensitive to the social or economic factors that may be important to an individual or a target population (Carter et al., 2011). For example, attempts to help patients modify food choices or engage in physical activity may mean different things to various cultural and socioeconomic groups.

Motivational Interviewing

Treatment for many chronic diseases such as cancer, heart disease, asthma, diabetes, and arthritis often requires significant ongoing lifestyle changes. Patients are charged with taking a much more active role in designing and implementing the sometimes significant lifestyle changes that are required to live a purpose-filled life while coping with chronic illness. MI is a useful strategy in dealing with ambivalent patients who must make significant lifestyle changes (Brobeck, Bergh, Odencrants, & Hildingh, 2011).

MI is an evidence-based clinical framework designed to help patients incorporate the functional abilities and skills they will need to fully engage in health promotion and disease prevention activities. An overarching goal of individuals who need to improve their health is to develop a better health-related quality of life. To achieve this goal, people must want to change behaviors that compromise their health.

The incorporation of patient preferences and cultural understandings is an essential component of an effective health promotion strategy. Miller and Rollnick (2013) assert that "When you understand what people value, you have a key to what motivates them" (p. 75). People put energy into actions that they believe are essential to their well-being. If they do not understand the link between their actions and their well-being, they are unlikely to sustain their efforts.

MI is "theoretically congruent" with the transtheoretical model of behavior change (Goodwin, Bar, Reid, & Ashford, 2009, p. 204). A motivational intervention encompasses a patient's values, beliefs, and preferences incorporated into relevant functional abilities and learned skills. Motivation is seen as a state of readiness rather than a personality trait (Dart, 2011). The MI framework is based on a person's values, beliefs, and preferences. It fits well with concepts of patient-centered care (Sandelowski, DeVellis, & Campbell, 2008). The MI framework is used with a growing range of chronic health conditions, such as diabetes or obesity exacerbated by unhealthy lifestyle behaviors (Carels et al., 2007; Kirk, Mutrie, Macintyre, & Fisher, 2004).

Since making positive changes in health behaviors is basically the patient's responsibility, it requires a strong commitment of self to engage in such behaviors. MI emphasizes an individual's capacity to take charge of his or her personal health and to control lifestyle factors that interfere with optimal health and well-being. Although initially an MI approach takes longer, it is likely to be more effective because the patient chooses actions having personal meaning and will be more committed to them.

The underlying premise of motivational learning is that learning takes root from within a person. It occurs when the learner is ready and "wants" to learn because she or he believes that it will make a positive difference. The person must also believe that success is 'achievable' with his/her personal efforts and/or resources. The decision to change, the choice of goals, and the commitment to developing new behaviors is always under the patient's control.

Readiness to change can be influenced. Nurses can better understand and influence a patient's deeper perception of a problem through Socratic questioning. This type of questioning allows nurses to point to discrepancies between a patient's goals or values and his or her current behaviors without argument or direct confrontation. MI helps patients address resistance and ambivalence about making health-related lifestyle changes in a nonjudgmental environment (Hall, Gibbie, & Lubman, 2012). Therapeutic strategies center on resolving problem behaviors, increasing committed collaboration, and joint decision-making (Miller & Rollnick, 2013).

Case Example

Patient: "I'm ready to go home now. I know once I get home, that I'll be able to get along without help. I've lived there all my life and I know my way around."

Nurse: "I know that you think you can manage yourself at home. But most people need some rehabilitation after a stroke to help them regain their strength. If you go home now without the rehabilitation, you may be shortchanging yourself by not taking the time to develop the skills you need to be independent at home. Is that something important to you?"

MI is an intervention in which the nurse uses empathetic exploration to help a patient become aware of discrepancies in their behavior that are hurting their health and well-being. This exploration is coupled with teaching them new skills to achieve mpre healthy life goals (Baumann, 2012).

1. What does the patient need to know?

Negotiating behavior change is conceptualized as a shared endeavor in which both patient and provider examine the patient's potential and willingness to change destructive health behaviors (Martin & McNeil, 2009, p. 284). When motivational strategies match an individual's readiness to change, this match increases the likelihood of positive intentional behavioral lifestyle changes.

Miller and Rollnick (2013) describe two phases of MI. The first phase focuses on mutually exploring and resolving ambivalence to change as a collaborative endeavor. This is accomplished through weighing the pros and cons of the current situations and the actions one would have to take to make change possible. With the patient in charge of determining change activities, the second phase emphasizes strengthening and supporting the patient's commitment to change based on the patient's choice and capacity for change.

A good starting point is a simple introductory question, such as, "I wonder if you could tell me what you do to keep yourself healthy? This type of question helps you to see what the patient values or even if he or she thinks about taking a personal role in achieving and maintaining healthy behaviors. It also provides an opportunity to assess for possible issues that actually may be counterproductive.

Case Example

Janet is a 77-year-old woman with osteoporosis. She is health-conscious and walks regularly to build bone strength. She wears a weighted vest to increase her workout strength and recently upped this weight to 15 pounds without consulting her physician. This change caused pain, and Janet was advised to decrease the weight. In this case, the concept of bone strengthening was appropriate, but its application had become inappropriate.

When a patient begins to tell you about his or her personal health habits, you can reflect on the relevant details and ask for clarification. The purpose of the dialogue is to deepen the patient's understanding. Use empathy in your responses. For example, "It sounds like you have been having a tough time and not getting a lot of support."

Open-ended questions allow patients the greatest freedom to respond. Asking a patient if he regularly exercises may yield a one-sentence answer. Inviting the same patient to describe his activity and exercise during a typical day and what makes it easier or harder for him to exercise can provide stronger data. Potential concerns and inconsistency with values, preferences, or goals are more readily identified.

Patient and family perspectives on disease and treatment are not necessarily the same as those of their health care providers. For example, you may think that an emaciated or an obese woman would be worried about her weight and would want to modify it because she values the way she looks. On the other hand, her culture or family values and traditions may be in conflict with making significant behavioral changes. Until the patient can understand a health-related value for making a change, she will not put serious effort into doing so. This level of data allows nurses to tailor interventions based on the patient's readiness to change and the availability of a support system.

As patients progress to the contemplative stage, nurses provide coaching guidance, information, and practical support to help them consider different choices and potential solutions. The pros and cons of each possible choice are explored. Empathy for the challenges faced by the patient and affirming the patient's reflection process encourages patients to consider alternative options and to choose the most viable among them (Levensky, Forcehimes, O'Donohue, & Beitz, 2007). A critical component of MI is acceptance of the patient's right to make the final decision and the need for the clinician to honor the patient's right to do so.

In the preparation stage, your role is to help patients establish realistic goals and develop a plan for achieving them. Goals should be realistic, patient-centered, and achievable. For example, the goal of losing 10 pounds in 3 months sounds more doable than a goal to simply losing weight (too vague) or losing 75 pounds (potentially overwhelming). Incremental goals build a sense of confidence as the patient sequentially meets them.

Personalizing goals and treatment plans for your patients is critical. Each patient has a unique life situation, support system, and way of coping with problems. Unhealthy habits are cumulative and hard to break. Work with patients to monitor their progress, offering suggestions, revising goals or plans when needed, and reminding patients of progress made. It is useful to help patients proactively identify potential obstacles and to anticipate the next steps. You can offer additional suggestions, empathize or commend patient efforts, and revisit actions from the preparation stage if goals need revision. For example, you could say, "You have really worked hard to master your exercises" or "I'm really impressed that you were able to avoid eating sweets this week." Availability to help patients solve problems or rethink plans, if needed, is also key.

Empowerment Strategies

Tengland (2008) distinguishes between empowerment as a *goal* in having control over the determinants of one's quality of life and as a *process* in which one has control over problem formulation, decision making, and the actions one takes to achieve relevant health goals. Patient empowerment takes place through clinician-initiated patient-centered care approaches *and* through actions patients take on their own initiative (Holmstrom & Roing, 2010).

As a process strategy, empowering people to take the initiative with their own health and well-being supports a person's ability to maintain his or her role as a functioning adult and facilitates the self-management of chronic disorders (Zubialde et al., 2009).

Case Example

Mrs. Hixon, who had had a stroke, soon began learning how to dress herself. At first she took an hour to complete this task, but with guidance and practice, she eventually dressed herself in 25 min. Even so, I practically had to sit on my hands as I watched her struggle. I could have done it so much faster for her, but she had to learn and I had to let her (Collier, 1992, p. 63).

Other enabling strategies include a focus on knowledge and skills, tailored education and training, previous successes in solving problems, social supports the patient can lean on, and reviewing the existing supportive assets (Green, 2008). It is empowering to learn as much as possible about healthy lifestyles and how they support the self-management of chronic conditions (Coward, 2006).

Using the Internet as a Resource

The Internet is a powerful resource for knowledge. Patients and families can find specific information on the web regardless of the stage of their illness. Helping people use technology to find information and access related health resources is a form of enabling patients to take charge of their health. Online support groups, chat rooms, and sharing blog experiences provide additional support for people who live in areas that are not geographically convenient to person-to-person contact. Patients can connect with others coping with issues such as weight control and exercise and can share practical strategies through the Internet.

Nurses can help patients and families select, and critically evaluate relevant web data. Not all data are completely accurate or relevant to a particular patient situation. If the patient or family does not use technology, then flyers, fact sheets, and direct dialogue with opportunity for questions and follow-up can be used to reinforce information.

A participatory learning format that encourages different ways of thinking and opportunities to try out new behaviors is more effective than giving simple instructions to a patient or family or offering patients a demonstration without enabling feedback (Willison, Mitmaker, & Andrews, 2005). When time is short, focus on topics that address the most pressing lifestyle changes. Literacy involves more than a person's capacity to read (Cornett, 2009). People need to be able to turn information into meaningful actions needed to meet life and health goals. Teaching strategies presented in Chapter 15 can be used or modified for health promotion teaching.

Empowerment Through Social Support

Andam (2011) suggests that "Empowerment implies a gathering of power, in a dynamic way, over a period of time" (p. 50). Social support from friends and family is an important empowerment resource in health promotion activities. *Social support* describes a person's "integration within a social network," and "the perceived availability of support" when it is needed (MacGeorge, Feng, & Burleson, 2011, p. 320). The interested support of significant others can strengthen a person's resolve, provide input for innovative solutions, and nurture the development of self-efficacy.

Health-related support groups in the community are available for a wide variety of diagnoses, providing relevant information, direct assistance, referral to appropriate resources, and the opportunity to simply interact with others experiencing similar challenges. For example, the Alzheimer's Association (for Alzheimer disease and related disorders) holds regularly scheduled support groups in most major locations to assist family members. Community-based cancer support groups provide valuable information and support for many common cancer diagnoses. Educational and referral supports enable patients and families to learn the skills they need to effectively manage chronic conditions and to live healthy lives.

Health Promotion as a Population Concept

Community is defined as "any group of citizens that have either a geographic, population-based, or self-defined relationship and whose health may be improved by a health promotion approach" (Frankish et al., 2006, p. 174). The community offers a natural social system with special significance for facilitating health promotion activities, particularly for people who are economically or socially disadvantaged. It is difficult to change attitudes and lifestyles to promote health when a patient's social or economic environment does not support prevention efforts.

Successful community-based health promotion activities start with a community analysis of health issues identified by the community. Consciousness raising is critical, as engagement and buy-in of the community in which the activity is to take place is essential. The WHO notes that health promotion activities should be "carried out by and with people, not on or to people" (WHO, 1997). The active participation of individuals, communities, and systems means a stronger and more authentic commitment to the establishment of the realistic regulatory, organizational, and sociopolitical supports that will be needed to achieve targeted health outcomes (Kline & Huff, 2008).

Health Disparities and Empowerment

Major advances in health promotion and prevention have not benefited all segments of nation's population equally (Kline & Huff, 2008). *Health disparities* is the term used to describe cohort differences in health status across ethnic groups, gender, education, or income. The term is also associated with inequalities in access, service use, and health outcomes. People with the greatest health burdens often have inadequate financial resources and the least access to information, communication technologies, health care, and supporting social services. Individuals living in extreme poverty do not have access to preventive care, adequate nutrition, or the opportunity to live in a healthy environment. When they are at the survival level, most people are not in a position to think about health promotion techniques to acquire a better quality of life. Being mindful of the patient's environment helps nurses proactively tailor interventions to engage and meet their health promotion and disease prevention needs.

Equity and empowerment related to health care are the expected outcome of health promotion activities at the community level. Equity corresponds to the WHO directive that all people should have an equal opportunity to enjoy good health and well-being. Key health issues in economically disadvantaged communities are often those with social roots such as violence or abuse, substance abuse, teen pregnancies, and acquired immunodeficiency syndrome (AIDS) (Blumenthal, 2009).

Community empowerment "seeks to enhance a community's ability to identify, mobilize, and address the issues that it faces to improve the overall health of the community"

(Yoo et al., 2004, p. 256). This type of empowerment is fueled by *both* public policy and targeted education. Successful health promotion programs require individuals, groups, and organizations to act as active agents in shaping health practices and policies that have meaning to a target population. Specific interventions are designed to engage those people who are most involved as active participants in a common environmental concern related to health. Proactive social and political action to enhance health services can augment educational efforts to ensure program viability.

Health promotion activists recognize the community as their principal voice in promoting health and well-being. Health promotion represents a multidisciplinary approach, also inclusive of health education, public health, and environmental health (Corcoran, 2013). Health promotion strategies are relevant in clinics, schools, communities, and parishes; they can be introduced during many aspects of routine care in hospitals.

PRECEDE-PROCEED Model

The PRECEDE-PROCEED model is a community education structural framework for designing, implementing, and evaluating community-based health promotion. Developed by Green and Kreuter (2005), this model consists of two components. The PRECEDE dimension refers to the assessment and planning components of program. The acronym PRECEDE stands for the predisposing, reinforcing and enabling factors contributing to the educational/organizational diagnosis, which are directly addressed in the proceed component. Factors that can affect the success of the program are presented in Table 14.2.

TABLE 14.2 **PRECEDE-PROCEED Model: Examples of PRECEDE Diagnostic Behavioral Factors**	
Factors	**Examples**
Predisposing factors	Previous experience, knowledge, beliefs, and values that can affect the teaching process (e.g., culture and prior learning)
Enabling factors	Environmental factors that facilitate or present obstacles to change (e.g., transportation, scheduling, and availability of follow-up)
Reinforcing factors	Perceived positive or negative effects of adopting the new learned behaviors, including social support (e.g., family support, risk for recurrence, and avoidance of a health risk)

Nurses also determine population needs and establish evaluation methods in the PRECEDE phase. Evaluation is a continuous process that begins when the program is implemented and is exercised throughout the educational experience. Sufficient resources, knowledge about target populations, and leadership training are part of an essential infrastructure needed to support health promotion approaches in the community.

A sustainable educational model needs political, managerial, and administrative supports for full implementation of a community-based approach to health promotion and disease prevention. Green later added the PROCEED component (policy, regulatory, organizational constructs in educational and environmental development). This component considers critical environmental and cost variables such as budget, personnel, and critical organizational relationships as part of the implementation phase. Having resources in place and assessing their sustainability is important in successful health promotion programs, although it is not always thought through in the planning phase.

Components of The PRECEDE-PROCEED model are presented in Table 14.3.

As with all types of education and counseling, learners need to be actively engaged in goal setting and developing action plans that have meaning to them. The health care system is complex and requires a new level of patient decision making. Simulation Exercise 14.4 and 14.5 provides an opportunity to reflect on the complex factors inherent in community health problems.

Choosing the right strategies requires special attention to the learner's readiness, capabilities, and skills. Box 14.2 presents health promotion educational strategies. Evaluation of health promotion activities is essential. In addition to evaluating immediate program effects, longitudinal evaluation of the impact of health promotion activities on morbidity, mortality, and quality of life is desirable. Keep in mind that what constitutes quality of life is a subjective reality for each patient and may differ from person to person (Fagerlind et al., 2010).

Health Promotion Models for Community Empowerment

Community empowerment strategies are used to help identify and address environmental and social issues needed to improve the overall health of the community. This strategy is sometimes referred to as "capacity building." Community-focused empowerment strategies build on the personal strengths, community resources, and problem-solving capabilities already existing among individuals and within communities that can be used to

TABLE 14.3 PRECEDE-PROCEED Model Definitions

Phase	Definition
PRECEDE Components	
1. Social diagnosis	People's perceptions of their own health needs and quality of life
2. Epidemiological diagnosis	Determination of the extent, distribution, and causes of a health problem in the target population
3. Behavioral and environmental diagnosis	Determination of specific health-related actions likely to affect a (behavioral) problem; systematic assessment of factors in the environment likely to influence health and quality-of-life (environmental) outcomes
4. Educational and organizational diagnosis	Assessment of all factors that must be changed to initiate or sustain desired behavioral changes and outcomes
5. Administrative and policy diagnosis	Analysis of organizational policies, resources, and circumstances relevant to the development of the health program
PROCEED Components	
6. Implementation	Conversion of program objectives into actions taken at the organizational level
7. Process evaluation	Assessment of materials, personnel performance, quality of practice or services offered, and activity experiences
8. Impact evaluation	Assessment of program effects of intermediate objectives inclusive of all changes as a result of the training
9. Outcome evaluation	Assessment of the teaching program on the ultimate objectives related to changes in health, well-being, and quality of life

Adapted from Green, L., Kreuter, M. (2005). *Health program planning: An educational and ecological approach* (4th ed.). New York: McGraw-Hill.

SIMULATION EXERCISE 14.4
Analyzing Community Health Problems for Health Promotion Interventions

Purpose
To develop an appreciation for the multidimensional elements of a community health problem.

Procedure
In small groups of three to five students, brainstorm about health problems you believe exist in your community and develop a consensus about one public health problem that your group would prioritize as being most important.

Use the following questions to direct your thinking about developing health promotion activities for a health-related problem in your community.

- What are the most pressing health problems in your community?
- What are the underlying causes or contributing factors to this problem?
- In what ways does the selected problem affect the health and well-being of the larger community?
- What is the population of interest you want to target for intervention?
- What additional information would you need to have to propose a solution?
- Who are the stakeholders, and how should they be involved?
- What step would you recommend as an initial response to this health problem?
- What is one step the nurse could take to increase awareness of this problem as a health promotion issue?

Discussion
How hard was it for your group to arrive at a consensus about the most pressing problem? Were you surprised with any of the discussion that took place about this health problem? How could you use what you learned in doing this exercise in your nursing practice?

address potential and actual health problems. Capacity building requires the inclusion of informal and formal community leaders as valued stakeholders. Networking, partnering, and creating joint ventures with indigenous and local religious organizations is a powerful consensus-building strategy that communities can use for effective health education planning and implementation. Box 14.3 outlines a process for engaging the community in health promotion activities.

SIMULATION EXERCISE 14.5
Developing Relevant Teaching Aids

Purpose

To develop skill in adapting learning materials for patients with limited literacy.

Procedure

1. Develop a one-paragraph case study, preferably from a patient experience.
2. Choose a related health promotion topic such as exercise, diet, stress reduction, or medication adherence.
3. Use the topic to develop a simple poster or teaching aid for a patient with limited literacy skills.
4. Use clear plain language consistent with a fifth- to sixth-grade reading level to develop your project.
5. Check your content for accuracy.
6. Use your teaching aid with your patient and ask for feedback about the patient understanding of your message, and reaction to the teaching aid.

Discussion

How difficult was it to develop the teaching aid? What factors did you have to take into consideration to make it interesting and informative for your patient? Were you surprised at any of the feedback you received from the patient? Would you do anything differently as a result of the feedback?

BOX 14.2   Strategies in Health Education and Counseling: Recommendations of the US Preventive Services Task Force

- Frame the teaching to match the patient's perceptions. Consider and incorporate the patient's preferences, beliefs, and concerns.
- Fully inform patients of the purposes and expected outcomes of interventions and when to expect these effects.
- Suggest small changes and baby steps rather than large ones.
- Be specific.
- Add new behaviors rather than eliminating established behaviors whenever possible.
- Link new behaviors to old behaviors.
- Obtain explicit commitments from the patient; ask patients to state exactly how they plan to achieve goals (what, when, and how often—start with "How will you begin?"
- Refer patients to appropriate community resources that are accessible and convenient.
- Use a combination of strategies to achieve outcomes tailored to individual needs.
- Monitor progress through follow-up contact.

Adapted from Agency for Healthcare Research and Quality (AHRQ). (2002). *Guide to clinical preventive services: report of the U.S. Preventive Services Task Force* (2nd ed., p. lxxvii–lxxx). New York: International Medical Publishing.

Health Literacy in Health Promotion and Disease Prevention

The AACN, and the Institute of Medicine have specified that health literacy be incorporated as an essential component in undergraduate nursing curricula (Mosley & Taylor, 2017). Health literacy differs from overall literacy and IQ. People with inadequate health literacy may be highly intelligent but functionally unable to fully grasp medical terminology due to the lack of education or language differences. Many of the words and meanings associated with medical terminology are complex and not easily understood by the lay public.

Health Literacy Is Central to Achieving Good Health and Well-Being

Health literacy "is defined as the degree to which an individual has the capacity to obtain, communicate, process, and understand health information and services in order to make appropriate health decisions" (Coleman, Hudson, & Maine, 2013, p. 82), consent forms and fully negotiating directions in the health system (Davis, Michiellutte, Askov,

Williams, & Weiss, 1998). This has disastrous implications for self-management, as indicated in the following case example.

Case Example

Jonathan is a 14-year-old adolescent recently discharged from a mental health unit. This was his fourth admission over an 18-month period. His mother assumed responsibility for seeing that he took his medications as directed. His mother knew the names of his medications and faithfully monitored his taking of them. But Jonathan's behavior began to deteriorate again. At one of Jonathan's follow-up visits, the nurse asked him to show her the meds he was on, and how he was taking them. It turned out that Jonathan's mother could not read, got the meds mixed up, and was administering the daily med three times a day and the thrice daily medication once daily.

BOX 14.3   Guiding Principles for Community Engagement

Before starting a community engagement effort,
- Be clear about the purposes or goals of the engagement effort and the populations and/or communities you want to engage.
- Become knowledgeable about the community's culture, economic conditions, political and power structures, norms and values, demographic trends, history, and experience with the efforts by outside groups to engage it in various programs. Learn about the community's perceptions of those initiating the engagement activities.

For ***engagement to occur***, it is necessary to
- Go to the community, establish relationships, build trust, work with the formal and informal leadership, and seek commitment from community organizations and leaders to create processes for mobilizing the community.
- Remember and accept that collective self-determination is the responsibility and right of all people who are in a community. No external entity should assume it can bestow to a community the power to act in its own self-interest.

For engagement to succeed,
- Partnering with the community is necessary to create change and improve health.
- All aspects of community engagement must recognize and respect the diversity of the community. Awareness of the various cultures of a community and other factors of diversity must be paramount in designing and implementing community engagement approaches.
- Community engagement can be sustained only by identifying and mobilizing community assets and strengths and by developing the community's capacity and resources to make decisions and take action.
- Organizations that wish to engage a community as well as individuals seeking to effect change must be prepared to release control of actions or interventions to the community and be flexible enough to meet the changing needs of the community.
- Community collaboration requires long-term commitment by the engaging organization and its partners.

From (2011). *Clinical and Translational Science Awards (CTSA) Consortium and Community Engagement Key Function Committee Task Force on the Principles of Community Engagement: Principles of community engagement* (2nd ed., pp. 46–52). NIH Publication No. 11-7782. Washington, DC: National Academies Press. Retrieved from http://www.atsdr.cdc.gov/communityengagement/pdf/PCE_Report_508_FINAL.pdf

Responsibility for health literacy is a collaborative initiative that lies with both providers and patients. Special attention needs to be given to patients disadvantaged by social determinants that limit their understanding of health-related materials. A more proactive approach needs to be extended to lower socioeconomic groups and minority populations, as health illiteracy disproportionately affects these population groups. Patients need to be encouraged to ask questions about anything they do not understand. You can reinforce the expectation that people need to ask questions for complete understanding, by saying something such as, "many people find it difficult to fully understand what is going on with them. They ask a lot of questions and I am hoping you will too." "Teach-back" (see Chapter 15), in addition to written instructions, also helps patients to grasp complex clinical instructions.

Literacy is not just about reading and writing. It is also about speaking, listening for understanding, asking questions for clarification, and checking in with patients to see that the messages sent are the same as those received. Simply providing information to low-literacy patients using "plain language" is *not* sufficient in and of itself to encourage behavioral changes. Even when patients seem to understand information at the time, they may have trouble keeping complex information straight once they leave. It can be difficult to comprehend and retain new and complex information.

Health literacy can be compromised by background noise, individual visual or auditory impairment, diminished mental alertness, fatigue, and acute illness. For example, a hard-of-hearing patient may not hear the words correctly and assign meanings that are incorrect. A patient with poor vision can misread a medication label or misinterpret individual words on a consent form. It is important to ask relevant questions or to use teach-back strategies (see Chapter 15) to ensure understanding.

The American Medical Association (AMA, 1999) defines **functional health literacy** as "the ability to read and comprehend prescription bottles, appointment slips, and other essential health-related materials to successfully function as a patient" (p. 552) Health illiteracy can include inability to understand the complexity and implications of medical treatments or essential system navigation skills (Dewalt & Pignone, 2005). A few well-placed questions can reveal this problem. People with inadequate health literacy skills often do not know what to do about their health or how to manage a chronic condition. They may not understand why their medical management is important, especially if they have not previously been exposed to medical settings. Even when patients can comprehend the words, their level of understanding may be too limited to weigh possible alternative meanings or to know what questions to ask for a better interpretation or to effectively make appropriate choices. Table 14.4 presents examples of the core constructs of health literacy.

TABLE 14.4 Core Constructs of Health Literacy With Application Examples

Core Construct	Application Examples
I. Basic literacy or comprehension	Reading various texts, such as appointment cards
	Interpreting medical tests, dosages and instructions, side effects, contraindications
	Understanding what is read, including brochures, medication labels, informed consent, insurance documents
II. Interactive and participatory literacy (able to engage in two-way interactions)	Provision of appropriate and usable information
	Comprehension and ability to act on information
	Mutual decision making
	Remembering and acting on information
III. Critical literacy	Ability to weigh critical scientific facts; capacity to assess competing treatment options

Adapted from Marks, R. (2009). Ethics and patient education: Health literacy and cultural dilemmas. *Health Promotion Practice, 10*(3), 328–332.

A less common but related literacy skill is numeracy. *Numeracy* is defined as "the ability to understand and use numbers in daily life" (Rothman, Montori, & Pignone, 2008, p. 583). Lack of numeracy can affect a patient's ability to understand expiration dates and timing related to medications as well as to comprehend the dosing of oral medications, the importance of time intervals between medications, and so forth. Inadequate numeracy is particularly relevant for patients who rely on prescribed medications given at different times and as-needed meds to cope with their illness (Rothman et al., 2008).

Partial understanding or a lack of full step-by-step instructions can result in unintentional noncompliance. Some patients try to hide the fact that they have trouble understanding the meaning of complex words or making sense of numbers. They may fake an ability to understand by appearing to agree with the nurse, by saying they will read the instructions later, or by not asking questions. Here are some issues patients and significant caregivers present related to poor health literacy:

- Inability to adequately describe symptoms or health problems
- Taking instructions too literally
- Having a limited ability to generalize information to new situations

- Decoding one word at a time rather than reading a passage as a whole
- Skipping over uncommon or hard words
- Thinking in individual rather than categorical terms (Doak, Doak, & Root, 1996)

Case Example

A 2-year-old is diagnosed with an inner ear infection and prescribed an antibiotic. Her mother understands that her daughter should take the prescribed medication twice a day. After carefully studying the label on the bottle and deciding that it does not tell how to take the medicine, she fills a teaspoon and pours the antibiotic into her daughter's painful ear.

Parker, Ratzan, and Lurie., 2003, p. 150

Educationally disadvantaged or functionally health illiterate people are interested in learning, but nurses need to adapt teaching situations to accommodate literacy learning differences. Marks (2009) suggests having materials written at sixth- to eighth-grade reading levels and providing lists of key instructions for use after visits. Using symbols and images with which the patient is familiar makes the material easier to comprehend. Taking the time to understand a patient's use of words and phrases provides the nurse with concrete words and ideas that may be more familiar to the patient and family. If you have any concerns about a patient's ability to interpret or understand health-related instructions, it is important to check with the patient or caregiver about the availability of additional supports needed for self-management strategies. Do not assume that the patient understands the implications of a clinical recommendation without some form of back-and-forth dialogue.

It is important to check with the patient or family about any circumstances that might get in the way of understanding any other special directions. Health literacy is both content and context specific (Nutbeam, 2009)

Case Example #1

Michelle is a nurse practitioner in an inner-city pediatric clinic. After examining a child with strep throat, she prescribed an antibiotic for her. She instructed the mother to give her child the medication two times a day and to store it in the refrigerator between doses. She asked the mother if she had any questions or concerns. Mom indicated she did not have any. But as the mother and child were leaving the exam room, the mother turned to the nurse practitioner and said, "We don't have a refrigerator. Will anything happen if I don't refrigerate the medication?"

If you were the nurse in this situation, how would you respond to this patient?

Case Example #2

Jose is filling out a routine clinical information form that asks questions about his health, use of medications, past surgeries, and family history of illnesses. Jose fills out his personal identifying information because he understands this section. There is a lot of reading involved in filling out the rest of form, and he is puzzled by some of the other medical history questions. He leaves these questions blank because he is not sure what they mean. He signs his name and returns the form. Working on filling out a clinical form as a joint exercise between nurse and patient may make difference between understanding and unintentional noncompliance.

The following are guidelines for improving communication with patients and caregivers who may have a low level of health literacy:

1. Use common concrete words rather than abstractions or medical terminology; for example, "Call the doctor on Monday if you still have pain or swelling in your knee."
2. Use the same words to describe the same thing. Name the medication or procedure and use the same words to describe it each time. Otherwise there can be slippage as a patient struggles to understand whether the different words mean the same thing. The same instructions, written exactly as they were spoken, act as a reminder once the person leaves the actual teaching situation.
3. Sequence the content logically beginning with the most important core concept.
4. Remember that the patient with low health literacy may not be able to read or interpret the label instructions on the bottle. Go over the instructions verbally with the patient holding the bottle.
5. Medications for children often have dosing charts, which identify age and weight recommendations for dose requirements. This can be confusing when the correct age or weight on the medication bottle does not match the reality of the child's presentation.
6. *Guide the patient to think about the following sequence when taking a new medication*:
   What do I take?
   How much do I take?
   When do I take it?
   What will it do for me?
   What do I do if I experience a problem or a side effect?
7. If there are multiple oral medications, describe each medication's appearance and let the patient actually see the med.
8. *Apply common simple concrete words,* such as "You should take your medicine apart from your meals" instead of "take this medication on an empty stomach." Sophisticated terminology, while accurate, may not be understood.
9. Whenever possible, *link new information and tasks with what the patient already knows.* This strategy builds on previous knowledge and reinforces self-efficacy in mastering new concepts.
10. Keep sentences short and precise (no more than 15–20 words).
11. The use of active verbs helps patients better understand what is being taught. When technical words are necessary for patients to communicate about their condition with health professionals, patients may need additional instruction or coaching about the appropriate words to use.
12. When the complexity resides in the concept rather than the words, you may need to guide the patient through the explanation. For example, you may have to explain the meaning and clinical implications of certain lab tests, offer help with filling out insurance forms, and so on.

Developmental Level

Developmental level affects both teaching strategies and the delivery of content. You will have patients at all levels of the learning spectrum with regard to their social, emotional, and cognitive development.

Developmental learning capability is not necessarily age-related; it is easily influenced by culture and stress. Social and emotional development does not always parallel cognitive maturity or literacy. Mirroring the patient's communication style and framing messages to reflect cultural characteristics helps improve comprehension and understanding. Parents and other family members can provide information about their child's immediate life experiences and suggest commonly used words to be incorporated into the nurse's health teaching.

Avoid information overload and giving vague or conflicting health information to older adults, particularly if there is any evidence of cognitive processing issues (Baur, 2011). For example, it is better to say, 'Take the white pill when you get up and before you eat your breakfast" than it is to say, "You need to take this medication on an empty stomach." Written plus oral instructions reinforce messages. Another issue for older adults is that they often have multiple medications, some of which may look alike.

Incorporating Cultural Understandings

Cultural understandings add to the complexity of health promotion strategies in health care (Lie, Carter-Pokras, Braun, & Coleman, 2012). Values, norms, and beliefs are an integral part of a person's self; they influence individual and community lifestyles and health perceptions (see Chapter 7).

Respecting a patient's cultural values increases a patient's trust of individual care providers. Eliciting and integrating explanatory information regarding health and illness into health teaching promotes better understanding *and* greater acceptance of health promotion and disease prevention recommendations. Cultural sensitivity includes knowledge of the preferred communication styles of different cultural groups. For example, Native Americans are known for learning through stories. The tradition of oral storytelling is a primary means of teaching that nurses can use for health promotion purposes. Patient motivation and participation can also be promoted through the use of indigenous teachers and counselors. If health literacy is related to language, qualified interpreters should be used for the translation and preparation of written materials.

Nurses participate routinely in community health promotion and disease prevention activities. They have an ethical and legal responsibility to maintain the expertise and interpersonal sensitivity required to promote effective patient learning.

SUMMARY

This chapter focuses on communication strategies nurses can use, to help people increase understanding of personal health care across clinical settings. National and global agendas over the last decade reinforce the importance of developing public health policies to create supportive health environments. Specific attention to reducing health disparities, negative social determinants through strengthened community action for health, and increased access for all is advocated. Optimal health and well-being are considered the desired outcomes of health promotion activities.

Three individual health promotion frameworks are presented. Pender's health belief model identifies perceptions of benefits, barriers, and ability to take action related to health and well-being as components of the individual's willingness to engage in health promotion activities.

Prochaska's transtheoretical model is used to explore a person's readiness to intentionally change his or her health habits. This theory serves as foundation for MI, developed by Miller and Rollnick.

Bandura's social learning theory explores the role of self-efficacy in empowering patients to use health promotion and disease prevention recommendations to take better care of their health.

Community-based interventions are critical in addressing broader causal influences on health, referred to as social determinants. The PRECEDE-PROCEED model is used to plan, implement, and evaluate community-based health promotion interventions. Chapter 14 also describes the important role of health literacy. Lack of health literacy, culture, and developmental status are described as factors that can compromise a patient's ability to fully engage in healthy lifestyle behaviors.

ETHICAL DILEMMA: What Would You Do?

Jack Marks is a 16-year-old adolescent who comes to the clinic complaining of symptoms of a sexually transmitted disease (STD). He receives antibiotics and you give him information about safe sex and preventing STDs. Two months later he returns to the clinic with similar symptoms. It is clear that Jack has not followed instructions and has no intention of doing so. He tells you he's a regular jock and just can't get used to the idea of condoms. He says he cannot tell you the names of his partners—there are just too many of them. What are your ethical responsibilities as his nurse in caring for Jack? What are the implications of your potential decisions?

DISCUSSION QUESTIONS

1. In what ways are the concepts of health literacy and functional health literacy different and alike and why is this important?
2. Why are health promotion and disease prevention strategies receiving so much emphasis in contemporary health care?
3. How would you implement Pender's model to enhance personal responsibility for health promotion and disease prevention practices?
4. Discuss how you could use MI as a tool for helping patients to learn self-management strategies.

REFERENCES

American Association of Colleges of Nursing (AACN). (2008). *The essentials of Baccalaureate Education for Professional Nursing Practice*. Washington, DC: Author.

American Medical Association Ad Hoc Committee on Health Literacy for the Council on Scientific Affairs (AMA). (1999). Health literacy: Report of the council on scientific affairs. *Journal of the American Medical Association, 281*, 552–557.

Andam, R. (2011). *Planning in Health Promotion Work*. Routledge, NY: An Empowerment Model.

Bandura, A. (1997). *Self-Efficacy: The Exercise of Control*. New York: W. H. Freeman.

Baumann, S. (2012). Motivational interviewing for emergency nurses. *Journal of Emergency Nursing, 38*, 254–257.

Baur, C. (2011). Calling the nation to act: Implementing the national action plan to improve health literacy. *Nursing Outlook, 59*, 63–69.

Blumenthal, D. S. (2009). Clinical community health: revisiting "the community as patient. *Education for Health, 22*(2), 1–8. Retrieved from: http://www.educationforhealth.net.

Brobeck, E., Bergh, H., Odencrants, S., & Hildingh, C. (2011). Primary health care nurses' experiences with motivation interviewing in health promotion practice. *Journal of Clinical Nursing, 20*, 33322–33330.

Carels, R., Darby, L., Cacciapaglia, H., Konrad, K., Coit, C., Harper, J., et al. (2007). Using motivational interviewing as a supplement to obesity treatment: A stepped-care approach. *Health Psychology, 26*(3), 369–374.

Centers for Disease Control and Prevention. (2009). *Improving health literacy for older adults: expert panel report 2009*. Atlanta: U.S. Department of Health and Human Services.

Cody, W. (2006). *Philosophical and Theoretical Perspectives for Advanced Practice Nursing* (4th ed.). Sudbury, MA: Jones and Bartlett.

Coleman, C. A., Hudson, S., & Maine, L. L. (2013). Health literacy practices and educational competencies for health professionals: A consensus study. *Journal of Health Communication, 18*, 82–102.

Collier, S. (1992). Mrs. Hixon was more than the "CVA" in 251. *Nursing, 22*(5) 62–62.

Corcoran, N. (2013). *Communicating Health: Strategies for Health Promotion* (2nd ed.). Thousand Oaks, CA: Sage Publications.

Cornett, S. (2009). Assessing and addressing health literacy. *Online Journal of Issues in Nursing, 14*(3) Article 2.

Coward, D. (2006). Supporting health promotion in adults with cancer. *Family Community Health, 29*(Suppl. 1), S52–S60.

Dart, M. (2011). *Motivational Interviewing in Nursing Practice*. Salisbury, MA: Jones & Bartlett.

Davis, T., Michiellutte, E., Askov, E., Williams, M. V., & Weiss, B. D. (1998). Practical assessment of adult literacy in health care. *Health Education & Behavior, 22*(5), 613–624.

DeWalt, D. A., Broucksou, K. A., Hawk, V. H., Brach, C., Hink, A., Rudd, R., & Callahan, L. F. (2011). Developing and testing the health literacy universal precautions toolkit. *Nursing Outlook, 59*, 85–94.

Dewalt, D. A., & Pignone, M. (2005). The role of literacy in health and health care. *American Family Physician, 72*(3), 387–388.

Doak, C. C., Doak, L. G., & Root, J. H. (1996). *Teaching Patients With Low Literacy Skills* (2nd ed.). Philadelphia: J. B. Lippincott.

Douglass F. (n.d.): BrainyQuote.com: Frederick Douglass, Retrieved from: http://www.brainy-quote.com/quotes/quotes/f/frederickd201574.html.

Edlin, G., & Golanty, E. (2009). *Health and Wellness* (10 ed.). Sudbury, MA: Jones & Bartlett.

Fagerlind, H., Ring, L., Feltelius, N., Lindblad, A. (2010). Patients' understanding of the concepts of health and quality of life. *Patient Education and Counseling, 78*(1), 104–110.

Frankish, C. J., Moulton, G., Rootman, I., Cole, C., & Gray, D. (2006). Setting a foundation: Underlying values and structures of health promotion in primary health care settings. *Primary Health Care Research & Development, 7*, 172–182.

Goodwin, A., Bar, B., Reid, G., & Ashford, S. (2009). Knowledge of motivational interviewing. *Journal of Holistic Nursing, 27*(3), 203–209.

Green, J. (2008). Health education—the case for rehabilitation. *Critical Public Health, 18*(4), 447–456.

Green, L., & Kreuter, M. W. (2005). *Health Program Planning: An Educational and Ecological Approach* (4th ed.). New York: McGraw-Hill.

Grey, M. (2017). Lifestyle determinants of health. Isn't it all about genetics and environment? *Nursing Outlook, 1–5*.

Hall, K., Gibbie, T., & Lubman, D. (2012). Motivational interviewing techniques: Facilitating behavior change in the general practice setting. *Australian Family Physician, 42*, 660–667.

Hawranik, P., & Strain, S. (2007). Giving voice to informal caregivers of older adults. *Canadian Journal of Nursing Research, 39*(1), 156–172.

Holmstrom, I., & Roing, M. (2010). The relation between patient-centeredness and patient empowerment: A discussion on concepts. *Patient Education and Counseling, 72*(2), 167–172.

Hogg, W., Dahrouge, S., Russell, G., Tuna, M., Geneau, R., Muldoon, L., et al. (2009). Health promotion activity in primary care: performance of models and associated factors. *Open Medicine, 3*(3), e165–e173.

Hoving, C., Visser, A., Mullen, P. D., & van den Borne, B. (2010). A history of patient education by health professionals in Europe and North America. *Patient Education and Counseling, 78*(3), 275–281.

Kirk, A., Mutrie, N., Macintyre, P., & Fisher, M. (2004). Promoting and maintaining physical activity in people with type 2 diabetes. *American Journal of Preventive Medicine, 27*, 289–296.

Kline, M., & Huff, R. (2008). *Health Promotion in Multicultural Populations: A handbook for Practitioners and Students* (2nd ed.). Thousand Oaks, CA: Sage Publications.

Kushner, R. F., & Sorensen, K. W. (2013). Lifestyle medicine: the future of chronic disease management. *Current Opinion in Endocrinology, Diabetes and Obesity, 20*(5), 389–395.

Levensky, E., Forcehimes, A., O'Donohue, W., & Beitz, K. (2007). Motivational interviewing: an evidence-based approach to counseling helps patients follow treatment recommendations. *American Journal of Nursing, 107*(10), 50–58.

Lie, D., Carter-Pokras, O., Braun, B., & Coleman, C. (2012). What do health literacy and cultural competence have in common? Calling for a collaborative health professional pedagogy. *Journal of Health Communication. International Perspectives, 17*(Suppl. 3), 13–22.

Litchfield, M., & Jonsdottir, H. (2008). A practice discipline that is here and now. *Advances in Nursing Science, 31*(1), 79–91.

MacGeorge, E., Feng, B., & Burleson, B. (2011). Chapter 10: Supportive communication. In M. Knapp, & J. Daly (Eds.), *The Sage handbook of interpersonal communication* (pp. 317–354). Thousand Oaks, CA: Sage.

Marks, R. (2009). Ethics and patient education: health literacy and cultural dilemmas. *Health Promotion Practice, 10*(3), 328–332.

Martins, R., & McNeil, D. (2009). Review of motivational interviewing in promoting health behaviors. *Clinical Psychology Review, 29*, 283–293.

Mosley, C., & Taylor, B. (2017). Integration of health literacy content into nursing curriculum utilizing the health literacy expanded model. *Teaching and Learning in Nursing, 12*(2), 109–116.

Milio, N. (1976). A framework for prevention: Changing health-damaging to health-generating life patterns. *American Journal of Public Health, 66*, 435–439.

Miller, W., & Rollnick, S. (2013). *Motivational Interviewing: Preparing People for Change* (3rd ed.). New York: Guilford Press.

Mol, A., Moser, I., & Pols, J. (Eds.). (2010). *Care in practice: On tinkering in clinics, homes and farms.* www.transcript-verlag.de /ts1447/ts1447.php.

Nutbeam, D. (2009). Defining and measuring health literacy: What can we learn from literacy studies? *International Journal of Public Health, 54*, 303–305.

Parker, R., Ratzan, S., Lurie, N., & Health illiteracy (2003). A policy challenge for advancing high-quality health care. *Health Affairs (Millwood), 22*(4), 147–153.

Pender, N., Murdaugh, C., & Parsons, M. (2011). *Health Promotion in Nursing Practice* (6th ed.). Upper Saddle River, NJ: Prentice Hall.

Prochaska, J., & Norcross, J. (2013). *The Transtheoretical Model in Systems of Psychotherapy: A Transtheoretical Analysis* (8th ed.). Stamford, CT: Cengage Learning.

Rothman, R., Montori, V., & Pignone, M. (2008). Perspective: the role of numeracy in health care. *Journal of Health Communication, 13*(6), 583–595.

Sandelowski, M., DeVellis, B., & Campbell, M. (2008). Variations in meanings of the personal core value "health". *Patient Education and Counseling, 73*(2), 347–353.

Saylor, C. (2004). The circle of health: a health definition model. *Journal of Holistic Nursing, 22*(2), 98–115.

Tengland, P.A. (2008). Empowerment: A conceptual discussion. *Health Care Analysis, 16*(2), 77–96.

US Department of Health and Human Services (DHHS). (2013). *Healthy People 2020.* Retrieved from: www.healthypeople.gov/HP2020.

US Department of Health and Human Services (DHHS). (2010). *National action plan to improve health literacy.* Washington, DC: Author.

Willison, K., Mitmaker, L., & Andrews, G. (2005). Integrating complementary and alternative medicine with primary health care through public health to improve chronic disease management. *Journal of Complement Integrative Medicine, 2*(1), 1–24.

World Health Organization (WHO). (1997). *Jakarta Declaration on Leading Health Promotion into the 21st Century.* Retrieved from: www.who.int/hpr/NPH/docs/jakarta_declaration_en.pdf.

World Health Organization (WHO). (1986). *Ottawa Charter for Health Promotion: First International Conference on Health Promotion.* Ottawa, Retrieved from: http://www.who.int/healthpromotion/conferences/previous/ottawa/en/.

Yoo, S., Weed, N., Lempa, M., Mbondo, M., Shada, R. E., & Goodman, R. M. (2004). Collaborative community empowerment: An illustration of a six-step process. *Health Promotion Practice, 5*(3), 256–265.

Zubialde, J., Mold, J., & Eubank, D. (2009). Outcomes that matter in chronic illness: a taxonomy informed by self-determination and adult-learning theory. *Families, Systems and Health, 27*(30), 193–200.

SUGGESTED READING

Dennison-Himmelfarb, C. R., & Hughes, S. (2011). Are you assessing the communication "vital sign"? *Journal of Cardiovascular Nursing, 26*, 177–179.

Dudas, K. (Patient Centered Care: Assessment of Health Literacy. Retrieved from: http://qsen.org/patient-centered-care-assessment-of-health-Literacy. 2011.

Elliot, D. L., Goldberg, L., MacKinnon, D. P., Ranby, K. W., Kuehl, K. S., Fagerlind, H., et al. (2010). Patients' understanding of the concepts of health and quality of life. *Patient Education and Counseling, 78*, 104–110.

Heinrich, C. (2012). Health literacy: the sixth vital sign. *Journal of the American Association of Nurse Practitioners, 24*(4), 218–223.

Institute of Medicine (IOM). (2001). *Crossing the Quality Chasm: A New Health System for the 21st Century.* Washington, DC: National Academies Press.

Institute of Medicine (IOM). (2003). *The Future of the Public's Health in the 21st Century.* Washington, DC: National Academies Press.

Institute of Medicine (IOM). (2011). *Health Literacy Implications for Health Care Reform.* Washington, DC: National Academies Press.

Institute of Medicine (IOM). (2012). *Primary Care and Public Health: Exploring Integration to Improve Population Health.* Washington, DC: National Academies Press.

Jager, A. J., & Wynia, M. K. (2012). Who gets a teach-back? Patient-reported incidence experiencing a teach-back. *Journal of Health Communication, 17*(Suppl. 3), 294–302.

Lorig, K., & Halsted, R. H. (2017). Self-management education, outcomes and mechanisms. *Annals of Behavioral Medicine, 26*(1), 1–7.

Miller, W. R., & Rollnick, S. (2014). The effectiveness and ineffectiveness of complex behavioral interventions: Impact of treatment fidelity. *Contemporary Clinical Trials, 37*, 234–241.

Owens, L., & Walden, D. (2007). Health literacy: The new essential in nursing education. *Nurse Educator, 32*(6), 238–239.

Saint Onge, J. M., & Krueger, P. M. (2017). Health lifestyle behaviors among US adults. *Society for Social Medicine & Population Health, 3*, 89–98.

Sentell, T. L., & Halpin, H. A. (2006). Importance of adult literacy in understanding health disparities. *Journal of General Internal Medicine, 21*, 862–866.

Sheridan, S. L., Halpern, D. J., Viera, A. J., Berkman, N. D., Donahue, K. E., & Crotty, K. (2011). Interventions for individuals with low health literacy: A systematic review. *Journal of Health Communication, 16*(Suppl. 3), 30–54.

Sørensen, K., Van den Broucke, S., Fullam, J., Doyle, G., Pelikan, J., Slonska, Z., & Brand, H. (2012). Health literacy and public health: A systematic review and integration of definitions and models. *BioMed Central Public Health, 12* Article 80.

Speros, C. I. (2005). Health literacy: Concept analysis. *Journal of Advanced Nursing, 50*, 633–640. https://doi.org/10.1111/j.1365-2648.2005.03448.x.

Speros, C. I. (2009). More than words: promoting health literacy in older adults. *Online Journal of Issues in Nursing, 14*(3) Article.

Volandes, A. E., & Paasche-Orlow, M. K. (2007). Health literacy, health inequality and a just healthcare system. *American Journal of Bioethics, 7*(11), 5–10.

Yip, M. (2012). A health literacy model for limited English speaking populations: sources, context, process, and outcomes. *Contemporary Nurse, 40*(2), 160–168.

Zoorob, R., & Morelli, V. (2008). Disease prevention and wellness in the 21st century. *Primary Care, 35*(4), 663–667.

WEB RESOURCES

Harvard School of Public Health. (Health Literacy Studies. www.hsph.harvard.edu/healthliteracy.

Health, & Literacy Special Collection. http://healthliteracy.worlded.org/.

Joint Commission Report. What Did the Doctor Say?: Improving Health Literacy to Protect Patient Safety. www.jointcommission.org/NR/rdonlyres/D5248B2E-E7E6-4121-8874-99C7B4888301/0/improving_health_literacy.pdf.

National Institute for Literacy. Health Literacy Discussion List. www.nifl.gov/mailman/listinfo/Healthliteracy.

Office of Disease Prevention and Health Promotion. Health Literacy Outline. http://www.health.gov/healthliteracyonline/.

15

Communication in Health Teaching and Coaching

Elizabeth C. Arnold

OBJECTIVES

At the end of the chapter, the reader will be able to:
1. Describe patient-centered health education.
2. Identify the domains of learning.
3. Discuss theoretical frameworks used in patient-centered health teaching.
4. Discuss health teaching applications in different settings.
5. Describe coaching strategies for the self-management of chronic conditions.
6. Apply the teach-back strategy.

INTRODUCTION

This chapter examines evidence-based patient education communication strategies in health care. Health teaching is a defined professional standard for professional nurses. Nurses are legally and ethically charged with providing relevant health-related education to patients, family, caregivers, and the community across clinical settings (Baur, 2011). The chapter identifies selected theories of teaching and learning as an evidence-based foundation for effective health teaching and coaching of patients needed to self-manage their chronic illness, and work effectively with community resources to maximize their health, and well-being (Deek et al., 2016).

BASIC CONCEPTS

Patient Education represents a focused form of instructional communication. Its purpose and design is to provide patients and families with the specific knowledge, life skills, and practical and emotional support needed to
- Cope with diagnosed health disruptions
- Self-manage and minimize the effects of chronic disorders
- Make effective health-related decisions
- Slow or prevent disease progression
- Promote patient's attainment of a high quality of life

The Complexity of Patient Education

Chronic illness usually requires long-term consistent self-management. Patient education is complex, particularly for the long-term treatment of patients with chronic illnesses. The overarching goals of patient education are to assist patients and caregivers to:
- Understand the nature of their chronic conditions
- Develop personally relevant lifestyle changes to cope with chronic health problems and to maximize health and well-being

The "learner" can be a patient, a family member or caregiver, a school group, or a community group. Each learning experience is unique. The same medical diagnosis each learning experience is uniquely human and individual creates different realities for people related to diverse cultural beliefs, life experiences, personal perception of impact, and financial or social resources. Learning characteristics of patients and families from different socioeconomic, educational, cultural, and life experience backgrounds vary across the spectrum and are further complicated by degrees of interest.

The goals of patient education are presented in Fig. 15.1.

Health teaching related to chronic conditions extends beyond simple medical and clinical data. Each teaching situation requires an individualized teaching approach and "learner buy-in" to ensure successful outcomes. Assessment of a patient's readiness to learn and learning

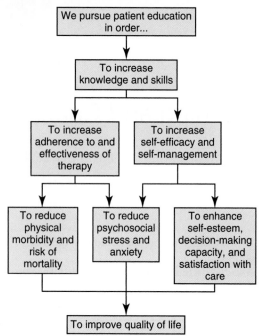

Fig. 15.1 Goals of Patient Education. (From Feudtner, C. [2001]. What are the goals of patient education? *Western Journal of Medicine, 174*(3), 174.)

style are important details in developing tailored nursing approaches with patients and families. Self-management skills require patients and families to

- Develop personalized problem-solving strategies related to the patient's particular health care and related needs
- Identify, access, and use resources across clinical settings (Lorig & Holman, 2003)
- Demonstrate mastery of skill, reflecting an understanding of underlying skill dynamics

Professional standards specify health teaching and health promotion as required components of professional nursing practice (Standard 5B) (American Nurses Association [ANA], 2004). Medicare also identifies health teaching as a skilled nursing intervention for reimbursement purposes. Documentation of patient-specific education provided to patients about treatment options in a language the patient can fully understand is required for informed consent. Although the informed consent document is the physician's responsibility, nurses play an important role in providing appropriate pre- and follow-up health teaching, particularly with patients having limited mental or literacy capacity and with surrogate decision makers (Menendez, 2013).

BASIC CONCEPTS

Theoretical Frameworks

Carl Rogers

Carl Rogers' (1983) learner-centered approach engages learners as active partners in all aspects of the learning process. In health care, nurses act as health guides for patients, families, and ancillary personnel. Rogers advises that the "teacher" must start where the learner is. For example, some patients initially are disinterested and others have a natural desire to learn. Relationship conditions of unconditional positive regard, empathy, and authenticity in interpersonal relationships are conceptual threads in health teaching environments.

Participatory strategies build on personal strengths. They support a patient's effectiveness in learning new behaviors because they incorporate skills that a patient is already practicing. When information is provided in a meaningful context, it has greater impact (Benner, Sutphen, Leonard, & Day, 2010; Su, Herron, & Osisek, 2011). The learner is in charge of processing and acting on personally relevant information in partnership with the health care providers. In health teaching situations, nurses should offer sufficient background information, specific instructions, coaching, and emotional support about the topic under discussion but no more than is required to reinforce forward movement. Each patient should be encouraged to take responsibility for personal self-management. Health teaching related to self management strategies must be a participatory sport. It has to be a shared endeavor, with both patient and professional working together to achieve specified goals. Without this alliance, optimal outcomes may be compromised.

Science of Teaching

Andragogy refers to the "art and science of helping adults learn" (Knowles, Holton, & Swanson, 2011). Adult learners tend to be self-directed, action-oriented, and practical. They want to see the usefulness of what they are learning. Generally adults favor a problem-focused approach to learning. They want to be directly engaged in developing the skills needed to master immediate life problems. The adult learner expects the nurse to inquire about previous life experience and to incorporate this knowledge into a jointly agreed upon teaching plan. Fig. 15.2 presents Knowles' model of adult learning principles.

Pedagogy describes the processes used to help children learn. Children need direct health education, but they come to the learning experience with far less life experience that can be tapped as resources for learning. They pass through cognitive and psychosocial stages, which dictate different teaching formats for successful participation (see Chapter 18).

A key difference between pedagogy and andragogy is the need to provide the child learner with additional direct guidance and structure in learning content. Parent

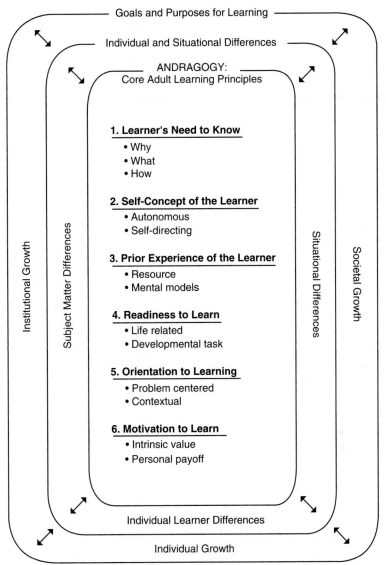

Fig. 15.2 Andragogy Model: A Core Set of Adult Learning Principles. (From Knowles M, Holton E, Swanson R: *The adult learner: the definitive classic on adult education and training,* Terre Haute, IL, 1998, Butterworth-Heinemann, p. 182.)

participation is critical to successful education with school-aged children. It provides both oversight management guidance and essential emotional support (Kelo, Eriksson, and Eriksson, 2013).

Bastable (2017) describes learning approaches in older adulthood as *gerogogy*. In normal aging a person's knowledge changes, and asking about the particular life experiences of older adults is essential for successful health teaching. It can be much harder for an older adult to adapt

to new ways of managing his or her health. Others may have significant mobility or sensory deficits that interfere with ease in learning formats. These impairments can make performing self-management skills challenging.

Older patients may need a slower pace, as many are likely to be cautious about trying new self-management strategies. Simple accommodations such as cueing, brighter lighting, and enlarged print can facilitate learning. Encouragement and positive reinforcement also improve motivation, self-efficacy, and performance. More commu-nities are making community-based efforts to provide free or low-cost exercise and stress-management programs for older adults. Specfic targeted classes on fall prevention, and bone strengthening are available in many communities.

Bandura's Social Cognitive Model

Bandura's social cognitive model links successful behav-ioral changes to a person's perception that he or she has the capability to carry out the actions (self-efficacy) required to meet identified goals (outcome expectancy) within his or her unique social context. If people think they have the skills or can easily learn them, they tend to be more confi-dent and are more likely to succeed.

Health teaching is a dynamic interactive process. A patient's knowledge about the reasons for using the skill and the steps involved provides a stronger foun-dation in the cognitive domain. For example, health teaching for a person a person with a recent diagnosis of diabetes might include knowledge of the disease; the roles of diet, exercise, and insulin in diabetic control, and guidance about how to identify trouble signs requiring immediate attention. Concrete information—provided through ver-bal discussions, images and line drawings, written instruc-tions, and Web data—can help to explain the steps needed to achieve negotiated health goals. Paying attention to the emotional impact of a diabetes diagnosis allows patients to work through emotional issues that potentially could com-promise compliance with essential treatment. Emotions are a powerful backdrop for self efficacy and motivation.

The Bloom Taxonomy: Classifying Behavioral Objectives

Objectives are essentially guides to action related to achiev-ing goals. Nurses use the Bloom taxonomy as a guide to writing behavioral objectives in health care. The utility of the taxonomy, originally described by Bloom and associ-ates, is that it provides "a common language about learning goals to facilitate communication across persons and sub-ject matter" (Krau, 2011, p. 305).

The Bloom taxonomy identifies a hierarchy of learn-ing objectives ranging from simple to the most complex. Fig. 15.3 shows leveled objectives using it. These objectives were revised in the 21st century to represent verbs rather than nouns (Su, Osisek, & Starnes, 2004). The revised Bloom taxonomy consists of

- **Remembering**: recognizing, recalling information and facts
- **Understanding**: interpreting, explaining, or construct-ing meaning
- **Applying**: carrying out or executing a procedure, using information in a new way

- **Analyzing**: considering individual components of the whole and how they relate to each other and the whole
- **Evaluating**: making judgments, critiquing, prioritizing, selecting, verifying
- **Creating**: putting material together into a coherent whole, reorganizing material into a new pattern, creat-ing something new (Anderson et al., 2000)

Behavioral objectives begin with the phrase "the patient will," followed by step-by-step achievable, measurable patient behaviors toward treatment goals. Ideally, there should be an objective for each significant component of the teaching session. An example of leveled objectives, applied to patient teaching for diabetes is presented in Fig. 15.3.

Simulation Exercise 15.1 provides practice with devel-oping behavioral objectives.

Learning in the **affective domain** focuses on emotional attitudes related to acceptance, compliance, valuing, and taking personal responsibility. It is more complex because of its association with values and beliefs. Objectives focusing on affective understanding are useful when patients demon-strate compliance issues or seem stalled in moving forward.

DOMAINS OF LEARNING

The psychomotor domain focuses on hands-on practice (performance learning). Performance learning promotes greater understanding than reading or hearing about a skill. Think of the first time you rode a bike. Chances are it was not until you made the bike move through your personal efforts that you really "owned" the skill of bike riding. Coaching a patient through a psychomotor skill step by step is a helpful strategy to achieving competence. Encouragement and teach-back in which the patient ver-bally goes through the steps can reinforce psychomotor task performance. Developing proficiency in performing the required psychomotor skill also involves building per-sonal confidence and the coping skills needed to adjust when challenged with unexpected circumstances. Learning in the affective domain helps to keep the patient on track when challenges arise, and to maintain the emotional com-mitment needed to achieve success.

Case Example

Jack "knows" that following his diabetic diet is essen-tial to control his diabetes. He can tell you everything there is to know about the relationship of diet to dia-betic control. Although he follows his diet at home, he eats snack foods at work and insists on extra helpings at dinner, especially when he is stressed. He says he does not mind taking extra insulin and that it is his choice to do so. Jack's problem with compliance lies

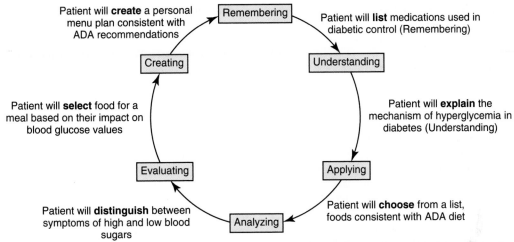

Fig. 15.3 Leveled Objectives Using Bloom's Revised Taxonomy. (Text adapted from Krau S: Creating educational objectives for patient education using the new Bloom's taxonomy, Nurs Clin North Am 46(3):302, 2011.)

in the affective domain; he resents having a lifelong condition that limits his food selections. Motivational interviewing might be useful in working with this patient to look at his health picture from a broader perspective. This strategy would allow him to explore his ambivalence and frustration at dietary restrictions imposed by his health condition. Without such a discussion, his behavior is unlikely to change. The cognitive domain consists of the knowledge base for the self management skill and an understanding of the nature and dimensions of the underlying medical and psychological issues associated with the patient's diagnosis.

CORE DIMENSIONS OF CONTEMPORARY PATIENT EDUCATION

Contemporary health education embraces a broad spectrum of related activities (Farin, Gramm, & Schmidt, 2013). Taking personal actions to achieve health goals helps people connect the dots related to physical, social, and lifestyle modifications needed for self-managed health promotion, and treatment compliance, as presented in the following paragraphs.

Patient's Perspective

Patient-centered education should start with and incorporate the patient's perspective across all activities. Health teaching and coaching approaches should be built on give-and-take relationships between health care professionals and patients, which in turn are based on "mutual trust, understanding and

sharing of collective knowledge" (McCormack & McCance, 2006, p. 473). Patient-centered education is a joint endeavor.

The teaching-learning process is designed to *empower* patients with the conceptual understandings and skills they need to self-manage their health and quality of life. Rather than a stand-alone nursing intervention, health teaching represents an element of quality care that should be integrated with other aspects of care interactions. Freda (2004) notes that "the goal of patient education has changed from telling the patient the best actions to take, to now assisting patients in learning about their health care to improve their own health" (p. 203). As with other aspects of patient-centered care, effective health teaching tailors interventions to be compatible with patient values, goals, and resources. Nurses also provide coaching cues and behavioral counseling and promote the concept of social support as an essential component of chronic disease self-management. Patients expect health care providers to be familiar with community resources and to facilitate access.

Self-Management

Self-management strategies are designed to optimize chronic disease management for patients and families in the home and community. The focus is on skill enhancement, with full patient engagement in clinical decision making and consistent self-management activities.

New models related to self-management skill development are *competency-based*. Teaching strategies include coaching, shared decision making and personal self-management of the individual's health condition(s). Strategies start with

SIMULATION EXERCISE 15.1
Developing Behavioral Goals

Purpose
To provide practical experience with developing teaching goals.

Procedure
Establish a nursing diagnosis related to health teaching and a teaching goal that supports the diagnosis in each of the following situations:

1. Jimmy is a 15-year-old adolescent who has been admitted to a mental health unit with disorders associated with impulse control and conduct. He wants to lie on his bed and read Stephen King novels. He refuses to attend unit therapy activities.
2. Maria, a 19-year-old single woman, is in the clinic for the first time because of cramping. She is 7 months pregnant and has had no prenatal care.
3. Jennifer is overweight and desperately wants to lose weight. However, she cannot walk past the refrigerator without stopping, and she finds it difficult to resist the snack machines at work. She wants a plan to help her lose weight and resist her impulses to eat.

Discussion
1. What factors did you have to consider in developing the most appropriate diagnosis and teaching goals for each patient?
2. In considering the diagnosis and teaching goals for each situation, what common themes did you find?
3. What differences in each situation contributed to variations in diagnosis and teaching goals? What contributed to these differences?
4. In what ways can you use the information in this exercise in your future nursing practice?

obtaining an active provider/patient collaborative commitment to setting realistic, achievable health goals.

The next step is to mutually identify specific learning outcomes with the patient and incorporate the support of essential others in the coaching process. This is followed by developing specific action plans to meet learning outcomes and evaluating their effectiveness (Su et al., 2011).

What is taught and how it is taught are critical elements of competency-based health teaching. Applications are grounded in evidence-based and nursing practice guidelines tailored to each patient's presenting needs, preferences, and available resources. The linkage between assessment needs and tailored actions should be transparent to everyone involved with the patient's care.

Tailoring interventions begin with listening for hidden emotional cues. Accommodating individual differences into teaching plans whenever possible shows respect for patient preferences. For example, a patient with normal cognitive functioning might respond well to a suggestion to shower, while a patient with mental issues or mild dementia might respond poorly. Accommodations for some flexibility in timing, built into the teaching process, can make a major difference. When self-management health related tactics fit within a patient's daily routine, they are more likely to be followed with cooperation. Scheduled times for exercising and taking medications also help new habits assume a regular place in the patient's life.

Patients are expected to be active participants and to take responsibility for their health care with collaborative support from their health care team. Contemporary patient education involves multilevel interventions linked to a common purpose of maximizing a patient's health and well-being. Nurses should use evidence-based knowledge and guidelines to facilitate and support individualized patient and family decision making (Inott & Kennedy, 2011). Meaningful patient-centered teaching does more than supply a basis for action; this process can improve patient self-esteem and reduce health anxiety (Feudtner, 2001).

Opportunities for Health Teaching

Patient-centered education should be evidenced as a continuous thread, extending across health care settings and community systems. Opportunities for health teaching occur in the community, school, parish, home, hospital, and clinic (Dreeben, 2010). Teaching formats range from informal one-to-one health sessions, to formal structured group sessions, family conferences, and scheduled presentations in the care setting or community. Even emergency departments provide opportunities for "teachable moments" for patients (Szpiro, Harrison, Van Den Kerkhof, & Lougheed, 2008). Health teaching can occur spontaneously during home visits as the nurse observes patients having specific difficulties with aspects of health care. Referred to as *guided care*, this type of on-the-spot health teaching is targeted to respond to specific health issues as they appear (Doherty, 2009). The media provides health-related patient information related to primary prevention (e.g., safe sex and drug abuse prevention commercials) to targeted community groups. Health fairs for children and preventive screenings for adults provide natural health teaching spot opportunities in the community.

Using Plain Language

Plain language is defined as a major instructional strategy for making written and oral information easier to understand, especially for individuals with lower literacy

capabilities, English as a second language, and older adults. Key elements of plain language include
- Organizing information so that the most important points come first
- Breaking complex information into easily understandable chunks
- Using simple language and defining technical terms
- Using the active voice
- Reading level is at the eighth grade or lower
- Using less than 15 words in each sentence
- Using phrasing that is easy to understand

Technology Integration

Technological advances have expanded the depth and breadth of health information available to the health consumer. In addition to basic tailored health information, decision support systems can assist patients in making better health care decisions (Lewis, 2003). The Internet provides instant health information, with a wide range of learning resources to accommodate different levels of knowledge and learning styles. For example, MedlinePlus from the National Library of Medicine provides accurate current information about the most common health conditions, palliative care, and drug information (Smith, 2013). Patients can type in a layperson's description of a problem and quickly receive links to tutorials and appropriate web sites. Web-based information on the Internet is searchable, up to date, inexpensive to obtain, and accessible at any time of day. Search engines such as Google and Bing allow patients to type in a few key words, which grant immediate access with immediate access to web sites related to their diagnosis (Gordon, 2011). National organizations, such as the American Diabetes Association and the American Cancer Society, have online tools to help patients understand their disease and treatment options. These and other web sites offer specific ideas for self-management with a wide range of in information and learning tools. Patients have free access to computers in public libraries and selected community centers (Bastable, 2017).

Although it is a powerful learning resource, the Internet has human and resource limitations. Many patients do not have easy access to computers or know how to use them. In most well populated areas, people have free access to the web in public libraries. Not all health information is equally relevant or directly applicable. Nurses can educate patients on how to begin searches and how to access information and also to evaluate its quality (Gordon, 2011). Patients and families find online sharing with others coping with similar health conditions helpful.

Holt, Flint, and Bowers (2011) describe using cell phone technology as a health teaching aid for patients. They

---

DEVELOPING AN EVIDENCE-BASED PRACTICE

Purpose:
The goal of this scoping review study was to provide a comprehensive review of the different beneficial and challenging aspects of patient participation in self-management education programs for people living and coping with chronic illness.

This scoping review of the literature searched eight evidence-based literature databases. The Arksey and O'Malley framework was used to guide the review process, and thematic analysis was used to synthesize the extracted data.

Results:
Forty-seven articles met the criteria for inclusion in this literature review. Positive benefits of participation in the education programs included less symptom distress, improved execution of self-management strategies, peer support, hope, and better learning.

Application to Your Clinical Practice:
The results of this review study can assist health care professionals in developing and carrying out effective education programs related to self-management strategies.

Stenberg, U., Haaland-Overby, M., Fredriksen, K., Westerman, K., & Kvisvik, T. (2016). A scoping review of the literature on benefits and challenges of participating in patient education program aimed at promoting self-management for people living with chronic illness. *Patient Education and Counseling, 99*(11), 1759–1771.

created an app consisting of personalized step-by-step photos beginning with essential equipment and accompanied by voice memo directions for complicated self-management of wound care.

APPLICATIONS

Professional, Legal, and Ethical Mandates for Patient Education

Within the last decade, the Joint Commission established standards requiring health care agencies to provide systematic health education and training for patients and families. These include the following:
- Information sufficient for patients to make informed decisions, and to take responsibility for self-management activities related to their needs

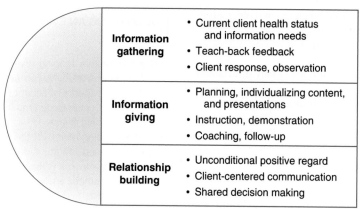

Fig. 15.4 Health Teaching Categories.

- Information provided to patients and families in a manner understandable to them and designed to accommodate various learning styles
- Information including documentation that patients and families have received appropriate health information and their response to this medical information (The Joint Commission, 2014).

DEVELOPING INDIVIDUALIZED TEACHING PLANS

Preparation

Health Teaching Responsibilities

Individualized teaching plans follow the nursing process, beginning with an assessment of patient learning needs, strengths, and limitations and ending with an evaluation of clinical outcomes. Common categories of health teaching responsibilities are featured in Fig. 15.4.

Health teaching is a complex nursing intervention consisting of many interlocking parts. Research demonstrates that structured patient-specific teaching is more effective than generalized approaches (Friedman, Cosby, Boyko, Hatton-Bauer, & Turnbull, 2011). As a health professional, you are responsible for the quality of health teaching, even though only the patient can assure the outcome. Prior to beginning the teaching process, you should review evidence-based care guidelines for the patient's condition (Bonaldi-Moore, 2009). Taking time to look over *key concepts and verifiable bottom-line information* needed to achieve designated patient health goals facilitates later content discussion. Effective teaching plans provide patients and families with new or reorganized knowledge, skills, and attitudes based on scientific evidence and personally tailored to patient needs, resources, preferences, and values.

Case Example

There was Nadine, who was an excellent preoperative teacher. She was the first person who clearly explained what a bladder augmentation entailed. She described different tubes I'd have and the purpose of each. When I returned from surgery, she helped me cope with my body image by teaching me how to use my bladder and by being a compassionate listener (Manning, 1992, p. 47)

Coaching

As patients assume stronger collaborative responsibility for the self-management of their conditions, coaching becomes a major nursing strategy in health education. The nurse acts not only as an information provider but also as a guide, resource, and knowledgeable emotional support. As *guides,* nurses coach patients on actions they can take to improve their health. They offer suggestions on modifications as their condition changes. As *information providers,* they help patients become more aware of why, what, and how they can learn to take better care of themselves. As *resource supports,* nurses help patients connect with appropriate community social and health supports to promote health and well-being while preventing the emergence of chronic disorders and disability.

Nurses act as a knowledge source and emotional support, encouraging positive learning efforts by helping patients minimize the impact of temporary setbacks and never giving up on them. For example, helping patients to anticipate actual and potential effects of a medication or treatment reduces anxiety and the incidence of errors.

Self-Awareness

It is easier to remain engaged with self-directed, motivated patient learners. It takes energy and imagination to stimulate interest in learning when a patient sees little reason to participate in making essential lifestyle changes.

Health teaching is a two-way process. This means rising above personal stereotypes to fully understand and appreciate each patient's unique worldview. Incorporating a discovery approach to health teaching means encouraging questions and using the patient's life experiences whenever possible to help him or her apply new knowledge. Try to imagine yourself in the patient's or patient's family's health situation. Empathy and understanding of motivational commitment broaden health-teaching perspectives and convey respect for the patient and family.

Assessment Data for Health Teaching and Coaching

Each learning situation has a past and a present reality. Patient education and coaching begins with a comprehensive assessment of each patient's needs, issues, strengths, and concerns. Start with what patients already know about their health condition and treatment. When what a patient "already knows" is inaccurate, a different set of evidence-based data should be shared with the patient. Sometimes such data has meaning for patients. If not, new data can be presented as another source of information.

Past experience and beliefs about illness, medications and treatments, cultural values, and the reactions of others produce assumptions that directly affect motivation and the acceptance of health teaching. Finding out what the patient feels is his or her primary health concern is important, as this may differ from the reason that the patient is seeking treatment.

Apart from a patient's symptom history, contextual factors such as impact on work or social relationships are often of considerable concern to patients. Asking open-ended questions can help nurses understand the unique learning needs of individual patients and families in a practical way. Box 15.1 provides examples of questions nurses can use to assess patient learning needs; for example, "Can you tell me what this illness has been like for you so far?"

Assessing Personal Learning Characteristics

Personal learning characteristics have a significant influence on achieving positive clinical outcomes. Preferred learning style, developmental stage, learning readiness and motivation, and low health literacy affect successful learning (Bastable, 2017).

BOX 15.1 Characteristics of Different Learning Styles

Visual
- Learns best by seeing
- Likes to watch demonstrations
- Organizes thoughts by writing them down
- Needs detail
- Looks around; examines situation

Auditory
- Learns best with verbal instructions
- Likes to talk things through
- Detail is not as important
- Talks about situation and pros and cons

Kinetic
- Learns best by doing
- Hands-on involvement
- Needs action and likes to touch, feel
- Loses interest with detailed instructions
- Tries things out

BOX 15.2 Questions to Assess Learning Needs

- What does the patient already know about his or her condition and treatment?
- In what ways is the patient affected by it?
- In what ways are those persons intimately involved with the patient affected by the patient's condition or treatment?
- What does the patient identify as his or her most important learning need?
- To what extent is the patient willing to take personal responsibility for seeking solutions?
- What goals would the patient like to achieve?
- What will the patient need to do to achieve those goals?
- What resources are available to the patient and family that might affect the learning process?
- What barriers to learning exist?

Preferred Learning Style

There are three major types of learning styles: visual, auditory, and kinesthetic. A visual learner learns best by reading or viewing web-based material and graphic images rather than listening to explanations. Auditory learners need to hear the information and appreciate discussion rather than strictly depending on visual material. Kinesthetic learners learn best with demonstration and hands-on practice. Beagley (2011) notes that although most patients can learn using any of these learning styles, each person has a preference and responds best when his or her preference is incorporated in the teaching plan. Box 15.2 presents the characteristics of different learning styles.

Learning Readiness

Learning readiness refers to a person's mind set and openness to engaging in a learning or counseling process for the purpose of adopting new behaviors. Motivational interviewing is a widely used strategy designed to assess and enhance the potential for patient learning readiness when internal motivation seems to be lacking. Nurses use empathy, acceptance, and respect for the patient's autonomy to help patients choose and commit to positive health behavior changes. Rather than challenging a patient's resistance directly, nurses should guide patients from wherever they are in the continuum of assuming responsibility for health promotion. Four stages of change applicable to current behaviors and patient investment in making positive behavioral change (precontemplation, contemplation, action, maintenance) direct the teaching learning process.

Emotional issues can increase learning readiness as well as interfere with it. Crisis anxiety (if it is not extreme) can create an immediate need to learn (Mezirow, 1990). Uninsured and medically underserved patients, who may lack the resources or inclination to engage in health care otherwise, also seek crisis intervention services (Gravely, Hensley, & Hagood-Thompson, 2011). Health teaching for these patients should be practical and carefully orchestrated to meet their immediate needs. If patients experience professional support as a helpful relationship, they may be more receptive to less crisis-oriented teaching interventions related to chronic conditions.

Ability to Learn

Some patients are ready to learn but are unable to do so with traditional learning formats. Assessing the patient's ability to learn and adapting the learning format to the learner's unique characteristics makes a difference. For example, a patient's physical condition or emotional state can temporarily preclude teaching. Patients in pain can focus on little else. Nausea or weakness makes it difficult for patients to sustain attention. Medications, or a temporary period of disorientation after a diagnostic test or surgical procedure can inhibit concentration.

Accurately assessing and managing a patient's level of anxiety before health teaching is essential, as is choosing a time when the patient energy wise is most likely to be receptive (Stephenson, 2006). The shock of a difficult diagnosis may require teaching in small segments or postponement of serious teaching sessions until the patient has understood the diagnosis. Patients with significant thought disorders have difficulty processing information. They may need simple, concrete instructions and frequent prompts to perform adequately. Comorbid health problems, if not recognized, can interfere with the goals of patient education. For example, an exercise program might be useful for an overweight person, but if the patient also has asthma or another activity-limiting issue, the intervention might require modification. Elevated stress and anxiety affect a patient's ability to focus attention and process material.

Health Literacy

If the patient cannot understand what is being taught, learning does not take place.

Patients, especially when they are in crisis mode, do not always ask questions. Anxiety limits cognitive skills even in the best of us and medical vocabulary can be daunting. The World Health Organization (WHO, 2009) defines health literacy as "the cognitive and social skills, which determine the motivation and ability of individuals to gain access to, understand, and use information in ways that promote and maintain good health." This broader definition heightens awareness of the social aspects of health literacy, which are sometimes overlooked in immediate hectic teaching situations. Low literacy is related to but not the same as low health literacy; medical vocabulary can be daunting for many people (Schwartzberg, Cowett, Vangeest, & Wolf, 2007).

Case Example

"Everything was happening so fast and everybody was so busy," and that is why Mitch Winston, 66 years old and suffering from atrial fibrillation, did not ask his doctor to clarify the complex and potentially dangerous medication regimen that had been prescribed for him on leaving the hospital emergency department. When he returned to the emergency department via ambulance, bleeding internally from an overdose of warfarin (Coumadin), his doctor was surprised to learn that Mitch had not understood the verbal instructions he had received and that he had ignored the written instructions and orders for follow-up visits that the doctor had provided. In fact, Mitch had never retrieved these from his wallet. Despite their importance, they were useless pieces of paper, as Mitch cannot read (The Joint Commission, 2007, p. 5).

In addition to being able to read and understand words and numbers, literacy includes being able to "orally express oneself, understand and recall spoken instructions, make inferences, utilize technology, critically weigh options and make decisions, and sustain often complex behaviors" (Wolf, Curtis, &

Baker, 2012, p. 1302). Since nurses are identified as key providers of patient education across clinical settings, it is especially important for us to incorporate health literacy strategies in all aspects of care. Baker et al. (2011) suggest using a limited set of essential learning goals related to

- Explaining the outcome behavior
- Essential background information to understand the recommended behavior
- Explanation of how the behavior change will help the patient feel better
- What barriers exist and how they can be overcome to produce the desired result (p. 11)

Patients with limited literacy struggle harder to understand and usually need more time to process information. They tend to decode messages one word at a time and may not grasp the whole message. To facilitate understanding, use fewer rather than more words to explain a concept and allow extra time to practice psychomotor skills with ongoing feedback. Learning goals should be simple and stated in words familiar to the learner. Provide only essential basic information in a sequential format and avoid information overload. Using open-ended questions and other listening responses can help you clarify your information for the patient.

Some patients have adequate literacy skills but a limited background or lack of interest in medical matters. This makes it difficult for a patient to understand medical terminology and complex medical explanations. The advice to keep information simple and straightforward applies to all health education situations.

Developmental Factors

The patient's developmental learning factors significantly influence his or her ability to learn (Bastable, 2017). Children at different levels of cognitive development need health teaching that is specifically tailored to their developmental level. For example, children who cannot think abstractly will not understand a conceptual explanation of what is happening to them. Instead, they need simple, concrete explanations and examples. Recommended teaching strategies for patient learners at different developmental levels are presented in Table 15.1.

Social Determinants

Socioenvironmental factors can undermine the effectiveness of health teaching and even produce dangerous outcomes. Commonly overlooked potential barriers, because of poverty, include preauthorizations for medical care, limited health insurance, transportation difficulties, lack of follow-up facilities, lack of access to food markets and health facilities, cultural considerations, and choice of priorities.

TABLE 15.1   Recommended Teaching Strategies at Different Development Levels

Developmental Level	Recommended Teaching Strategies
Preschool	Allow child to touch and play with safe equipment. Relate teaching to child's immediate experience. Use child's vocabulary whenever possible. Involve parents in teaching.
School age	Give factual information in simple, concrete terms. Focus teaching on developing competency. Use simple drawings and models to emphasize points. Answer questions honestly and factually.
Adolescent	Use metaphors and analogies in teaching. Give choices and multiple perspectives. Incorporate the patient's norm group values and personal identity issues in teaching strategies.
Adult	Involve patient as an active partner in learning process. Encourage self-directed learning. Keep content and strategies relevant and practical. Incorporate previous life experience into teaching.
Older adult	Explain why the information should be important to the patient. Incorporate previous life experience into teaching. Accommodate for sensory and dexterity deficits. Use short, frequent learning sessions (<30 minutes).

Patients may not have the money for medication. A visit to the pediatrician for an ear infection may have a copay that the mother cannot afford. Health illiteracy can be a product of poverty as well as culture (Lowenstein, Foord-May, & Romano, 2009). Nurses need to explore the level and types of situational support available to patients and families as part of any teaching plan.

Planning

Family Involvement

Constructive family involvement is an essential component of successful self-management. The Joint Commission's standards (2014) require evidence of direct education provided to the family as well as the patient. Health teaching similar to that provided to fully functional patients is required of anyone actively involved in the patient's care as a primary caregiver or reliable supportive influence. Information and anticipatory guidance about what to expect when the patient goes home, and early warning signs of complications or potential problem, should also be given to family members. Knowing when to seek professional assistance and resource support is critical. Examples of appropriate goals for family teaching relate to empowerment of family members in using equipment, understanding what is happening to their loved one, and promoting direct involvement in therapeutic care.

Note changes in the level of support from primary caregivers, as this circumstance can affect a patient's willingness or ability to learn. When these supports are no longer available through death, incapacity, or for other reasons, the patient may lack not only motivation but also the skills to cope with complex health problems.

Case Example

Edward Flanigan, an 82-year-old recently widowed man, has severe diabetes. There is no evidence of memory problems, but there are significant emotional components to his current health care needs. All his life, his wife pampered him and did everything for him, from meal preparation to monitoring his diabetes. Since her death, Edward has taken no interest in controlling his diabetes. He does not follow his prescribed diabetic diet and is not consistent in taking his medication. Predictably, his diabetes has become increasingly unstable. His family worries about him, but he is unwilling to consider leaving his home of 42 years. To enhance Edward's learning readiness, how could Edward's teaching plan related to diabetic self-care management skills be individualized?

Considering Special Learning Needs

Cultural Diversity

Patients interpret health care messages within the context of their culturally bound traditions, beliefs, and values. Tailoring teaching interventions to meet the specific cultural needs and resources of patients is key to improving outcomes through patient education (Peek et al., 2012). Explanatory models for why symptoms develop and personalized cultural attitudes toward common treatment protocols are important to know, primarily because they may be wrong or harmful. Inquire about home remedies and applicable spiritual influences. The use of folk medicine and recommendations from indigenous health informants and providers is critically important to know about. Differences should be treated with the utmost respect. When you are working with culturally diverse patients, it is important to put information in a culturally familiar context. Doing so can be a collaborative venture in which you ask the patient to tell you how the health problem would be treated in his or her culture and negotiate for an acceptable treatment option. Culturally unique perspectives and preferences for treatment can be incorporated in many situations if they are not harmful. When this is not the case, negotiating an acceptable compromise respects a patient's cultural values and, most important, the person exhibiting them.

There are several reasons for including cultural values. Culturally diverse patients are more likely to trust traditional health care solutions than modern medical approaches. Patients prefer a teaching plan that integrates cultural practices with mainstream biomedical approaches because the traditional sounds familiar. They are more likely to follow suggestions that correspond with their preferences and to use the provider relationship as a valued resource.

Focusing on accurate information without destroying the credibility of influential cultural health advisors is part of the art of health teaching. Nothing is gained by injuring the reputation of the person who gave the patient information, and only those findings with potentially adverse health consequences should be addressed. To stimulate further discussion, you could say: "There have been some new findings that I think you might be interested in… or, current thinking suggests that (and give a relevant example) works well in situations like this." With this type of statement you can expand the patient's thinking without challenging the status of the person a patient considers as expert. (See Chapters 7 and 14 for more ideas tailoring communication and teaching strategies to use in teaching culturally diverse patients.)

Sometimes there is a tendency for people to speak louder when instructing someone from a different culture. Instead, speak *slowly* in a normal conversational tone. When teaching a patient for whom English is a second language, keep in mind that words from one language do not necessarily translate with the same meaning in another. Certain concepts may not exist or the phrases used for expressing and describing them may differ significantly. It is best to use simple, concrete words and images in explaining options and to ask frequently for validation of understanding. Lorig (2001) suggests that when you are preparing teaching materials for translation, the following are important:

- Use nouns rather than pronouns and simple unambiguous language.
- Use short, simple sentences of less than 16 words each.
- Avoid the use of metaphors and informal slang.
- Avoid verb forms that have more than one meaning or include *would* or *could* (p. 181).

If a patient still is unable to understand important concepts with accommodations, enlisting the services of a trained medical interpreter becomes an essential intervention.

Adaptations for Cognitive Processing Deficits

Learners with memory deficits, lack of insight, poor judgment, and limited problem-solving abilities require accommodations. Special needs learners respond best when the content is presented in a consistent, concrete, and patient manner, with clear and frequent cues to action. Patience and the repetition of key ideas are essential. Illustrated materials can result in greater comprehension and recall, but they should be simple, without distracting details (Friedman et al., 2011). If the deficit is more than minimal, it may be helpful to include significant others in the teaching session, as this may increase the chance of follow through with instructions.

Creating a Successful Teaching Plan

Teaching plans provide a guide for choosing and sequencing content and for identifying the best approach. Box 15.3 provides a sample format for developing a relevant teaching plan.

- What **essential** *information* does the patient **need** to have for self-management of his or her disease process?
- What *attitudes* does the patient hold that could **enable** or **hinder** the learning process?
- What specific *skills* does this patient **need** for self-management?
- What does the patient **want** from this health experience to improve his or her quality of life?
- What *cultural* or *socioenvironmental* factors could **facilitate** or **sabotage** the learning process?

Periodically asking the patient and primary caregivers, "Do you have any questions for me?" gives nurses a sense of what is most important to the patient or what may not be fully understood. Suggest that if things come up that the patient has questions about later, the patient should ask for

---

BOX 15.3 Suggested Format for Teaching Care Plans

- Briefly identify patient's needs and preferences.
- Write summary statement of what is to be taught (three to four main points).
- Identify realistic goal(s) or outcome(s) you want the patient to achieve with your teaching in one or two sentences.
- State two to three specific measurable behavioral objectives related to goal achievement.
- Specify content (relate to objectives) in bulleted outline form.
- Describe teaching methodology (e.g., discussion, demonstration, diagrams).
- Identify materials, handouts, and resources needed to achieve patient success.
- Stipulate specific evaluation measures such as teach-back or return demonstration.

---

further clarification. Often hours or days after health teaching takes place, patients have questions or concerns about received information. You can offer additional opportunities for discussion after the patient has had time to absorb the initial information and/or ask questions to determine comprehension.

Health Teaching Goals

Setting realistic collaborative goals with patients with periodic reviews not only helps motivate patients but also serves as a benchmark for evaluating changes. Establish goals *with* your patient rather than *for* your patient. Clear step-by-step learning goals that the patient agrees to are more likely to be met.

Identify outcome goals with a general statement of what the patient needs to achieve as a result of the teaching (e.g., "After health teaching, the patient will maintain dietary control of her diabetes"; an interim goal might be, "After health teaching, the patient will develop an appropriate diet plan for 1 week"). Setting realistic goals prevents disappointment.

Developing Measurable Objectives

Objectives help organize content and identify logical action steps. Box 15.4 provides guidelines for developing effective health teaching goals and objectives.

Collaboratively developed objectives should describe an immediate action step-by-step plan for goal achievement based on the patient's most pressing clinical issues (Edwards, 2013). Each action step should build on the

BOX 15.4   Guidelines for Developing Effective Goals and Objectives

- Link goals to the nursing diagnosis.
- Make goals action-oriented.
- Make goals specific and measurable.
- Define objectives as behavioral outcomes.
- Design objectives with a specific time frame for achievement.
- Show a logical progression with established priorities.
- Review periodically and modify goals as needed.

previous one for maximum effectiveness. Objectives should be achievable within the allotted time frame. To determine whether an objective is achievable, consider the patient's level of experience, educational level, resources, skills, and motivation. This information helps ensure that the objectives are defined in specific measurable behavioral terms. Objectives also should directly relate to medical and nursing diagnoses and support the overall health outcome.

Timing

Health teaching is an essential nursing intervention; it is not an add-on. Teaching interventions should never be eliminated because the nurse lacks time. Even in the most limited situation, schedule a block of time for health teaching. Because time is a precious commodity in health care, choosing the most effective and efficient ways to achieve identified clinical goals is vital (Stephenson, 2006). You need to consider how much time is required to learn a particular skill or body of knowledge and build this into the learning situation. Complicated skill development may need blocks of time for repeated practice with feedback. Pick times for teaching when energy levels are high, other things do not distract the patient, it is not visiting time, and the patient is alert and not in pain. Careful observation of the patient helps determine the most appropriate times for health teaching.

Even under the best of circumstances, people can absorb only so many details and fine points at a time (Suter & Suter, 2008). Keep the teaching session short, interesting, and to the point. Ideally teaching sessions should last no longer than about 20 minutes, including time for questions. Otherwise the patient may tire or lose interest. By scheduling shorter sessions with time in between to process information, you can help to prevent sensory overload and reinforce teaching points.

Nurses also have opportunities for informal teaching during the course of providing care. Simple, spontaneous health teaching takes minutes, but can have immeasurable effects. The following case example, taken from *Heartsounds* (Lear, 1980), illustrates this point.

Implementation

Each teaching session should be a collaborative process with a reciprocal exchange of information, feedback, and opportunities to ask questions.

Building a Logical Information Teaching Flow

No one teaching strategy can meet the needs of all patients (Su et al., 2011). Introductory content should build on the patient's experiences, abilities, interests, motivation, and skills. Most patients learn best when there is a logical flow and a building of information from simple to complex. Begin by presenting a simple overview of what will be taught and why the information is important to learn. Include only essential information in your overview; for example, give a brief explanation of the health care problem, risk factors, treatment, and self-care skills the patient will need to manage at home. Incorporate or ask about previous related experience.

Concrete application of knowledge in a meaningful context increases learning (Benner et al., 2010). Ideally you should solicit input frequently and offer opportunities for patient feedback and questioning. Complex information can be delivered in smaller stepwise learning segments. For example, diabetic teaching could include the following segments:

- Introduction, including what the patient does know
- Basic pathophysiology of diabetes (keep description simple and short)
- Diet and exercise
- Demonstration of insulin injection with return demonstration
- Recognizing signs and symptoms of hyperglycemia and hypoglycemia
- Care of skin and feet
- How to talk to the doctor

A strong closing statement summarizing major points reinforces the learning process. Simulation Exercise 15.2 provides practice with developing a mini teaching plan.

Using Clear Concrete Language

Use simple familiar words and limit the number of ideas in each learning segment. General or vague language leaves the learner wondering what the nurse actually meant. For example, "Call the doctor if you have any problems" has more than one meaning. "Problems" can refer to side effects of the medication, a return of symptoms, problems with family acceptance, changed

SIMULATION EXERCISE 15.2
Developing Teaching Plans

Purpose

To provide practice with developing teaching plans.

Procedure

1. Using the teaching plan format, develop a mini teaching plan for one of your patients. Alternative: Develop a "mini" teaching plan for one of the following patient situations:
   a. Jim Dolan feels stressed about returning to work after his accident. He is requesting health teaching on stress management and relaxation techniques.
   b. Adrienne Parker is a newly diagnosed diabetic. Her grandfather had diabetes.
   c. Marion Hill just gave birth to her first child. She wants to breastfeed her infant but she is afraid that she does not have enough milk.
   d. Barbara Scott weighs 210 pounds and wants to lose weight.
2. Include the following data: a brief statement of patient learning needs and a list of related nursing diagnoses in order of priority.
3. For one nursing diagnosis, develop a mini teaching plan outlining objectives, topical content, planned teaching strategies, time frame for planned activities, and evaluation criteria.

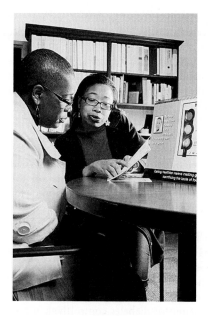

relationships, and even alterations in self-concept. You could say, "If you should develop a headache or feel dizzy in the next 24 hours, call the emergency department doctor right away." Providing the physician's name and phone number.

Checking with patients to confirm a common understanding of words and concepts is critical to knowledge transfer in health teaching. Doak, Doak, Gordon, and Lorig (2001) suggest asking the patient, "What does this material tell you about _____ [subject]? What does it tell you to do?" (p. 188). Concrete examples help patients understand abstract material. You also can ask the patient for relevant examples to make a point.

Written directions should demonstrate similar language clarity. From a study of patient input about written care instructions, Buckley et al. (2013) suggest highlighting key words, for example: "After cleaning, you can **apply antibiotic ointment** 'Neosporin or bacitracin' to the wound and then put on a clean bandage" (p. 556).

Incorporating Visual Aids

Line drawings and simple diagrams of body parts or physiology related to a procedure help to increase comprehension. Simple images and plain language work better than complicated visual aids and technical terms. For example, an illustrated chart showing how the heart pumps blood might help a patient understand the anatomy and physiology of a cardiac problem better than words. Perdue, Degazon, and Lunny (1999) suggest that DVDs are useful in teaching patients with limited reading skills. They have the advantage of allowing patients to watch them again at their convenience. Related discussions help to correct misinterpretations and emphasize pertinent points.

Preparing Written Handouts

Written materials reinforce learning. Attention to the patient's reading level and health care literacy helps ensure that the pamphlets will be read (CDC, 2009). Most reading materials should be geared to a sixth-grade reading level. Even people with adequate health literacy comprehend written information better when the language is simple and clear using layperson's language. Large-print pamphlets and audiotapes are helpful learning aids for those with sight problems and auditory learners.

Guidelines for preparing effective written materials include the following:

- Present the most important information first.
- Use clear illustrations and diagrams designed to enhance clarity and appeal.

- Make sure that the content is current, accurate, objective, *and* consistent with information provided by other team members.
- Use simple language at a literacy level that the reader can understand easily.
- Use a 12-point font and avoid using all capital letters for reading ease.
- Define technical terms in lay language (plain language); avoid medical jargon.
- Bold important points.
- Check for spelling errors and avoid complicated sentences.
- Include resources with contact information that the patient can refer to for further information or for help with problems.

Advance Organizers

Advance organizers, called *mnemonics*, consist of cue words, phrases, or letters related to more complex data. They are memory aids to help patients remember difficult concepts. For example, each letter in the word *diabetes* can represent an action for diabetes control. Taken together, mnemonics give the patient a useful tool for remembering related concepts. For example, in the case of diabetes, the following mnemonic can be useful:

D = diet
I = infections
A = administering medications
B = basic pathophysiology
E = eating schedules
T = treatment for hyperglycemia or hypoglycemia
E = exercise
S = symptom recognition

Evaluation and Documentation

Teach-Three and Teach-Back

Teach-back is a simple, effective means of checking patient comprehension of care concepts, and execute self-management skills post discharge. Patients are initially taught up to three key actions, knowledge concepts, and care skills related to self-management of the patient's condition. This information should be delivered in small chunks of data or skill demonstrations using terminology that the patient can easily understand.

The first step in the process is to determine what the patient knows about his or her medical condition. Listen to questions, explain the patient's condition in terms that he or she can understand, and teach-back or "show me" is a participatory evaluation method used to confirm a patient's understanding of and/or ability to execute self-management skills through demonstration or explanation of major points. It involves having the patient explain

relevant information and treatment instructions in his or her own words (Lorenzen, Melby, & Earles, 2008). Teach-back offers nurses valuable data about areas of skill learning needing additional attention.

Start with a statement such as, "I just want to be sure that I have explained everything you need to know. Can you tell me, in your own words, how you will determine that your blood sugar is low, and what you will do if it is?" Encourage the patient to ask questions. If the content is complex, consider using teach-back after each segment, before moving on to the next concept. Redo instruction if needed. Document your use of teach-back and the patient's response (Simulation Exercise 15.3).

Documenting Health Teaching

The Joint Commission (2014) requires written documentation of all patient health teaching. Notes about the initial assessment should be succinct but comprehensive and objective. Teaching content should be linked to assessment data, including patient preferences, previous knowledge, and values. Included in the documentation are the teaching actions, the patient response, and any clinical issues or barriers to compliance. If family members are involved, you

---

SIMULATION EXERCISE 15.3
Teach-Back

Purpose
To help students understand the teach-back process.

Procedure
Review what you learned in class about the teach-back method. Break into class groups of three students: nurse, patient, and observer. Each student will take a turn being the nurse, the patient, and the observer. Using one medication that your patient is on, role-play the teach-back process with one person taking the role of nurse, another the patient receiving the medication for the first time, and the third person an observer. Rotate roles so each student has the opportunity to role-play the part of the nurse.

Discussion
After *each* teach-back role-play:
1. The nurse should reflect on what he or she did well or would have changed.
2. The observer should provide feedback on what the nurse did well and what he or she could have done better.
3. The patient should add his or her perspective and anything that was not addressed by the other two participants.

should identify their role, content provided, and teaching outcomes in your documentation. Accurate documentation promotes continuity of care and prevents duplication of teaching efforts. The record informs other health care providers of completed teaching and what areas need further work.

Self-Management Strategies

People are living much longer than in years past, and the contemporary focus on helping patients and families develop self-management strategies in contemporary health care reflects the expanded extent of chronic illness reform. Examples of chronic illnesses requiring self-management include cancer, dementias, asthma, osteoporosis, diabetes, multiple sclerosis, arthritis, hypertension, macular degeneration, cardiovascular disorders, chronic obstructive pulmonary disease, stroke, and chronic mental illness. Cystic fibrosis, developmental delays and abnormalities, juvenile diabetes, sickle cell anemia, and childhood cancer are significant chronic disorders seen particularly in younger patients. Participatory self-management from patients related to chronic disorders represents a logical way of reducing health costs while still providing quality care (Peeters, Wiegers, & Friele, 2013).

Skill support for patients and families requires more than basic informative education about a person's medical information and treatment. Holman and Lorig's (2004) research findings indicate that patients desire data about further access to information and continuity of care as part of learning about their condition and how to self-manage their symptoms.

COMPONENTS OF SELF-MANAGEMENT PATIENT EDUCATION

The Center for the Advancement of Health (2002) identifies problem solving, decision-making structures, goal setting, utilization of resources, development of patient/provider partnerships, and taking action as essential self-management skills.

Simple, direct pieces of information help patients and families understand and effectively support their management of chronic disorders. You can reinforce relevant information with a guidebook or check list. Collaborative development of a self-management plan helps patients feel more committed to a self-management plan in line with their values, health and life needs, and resources.

Learning self-management strategies takes time and social support. Approaches must be tailored to each patient's unique life situation, values, opportunities, and skills. Care plans and self-management plans can be useful in facilitating patients' discussion of self-care actions

and lifestyle management. Organizational factors affect opportunities for professionals to support patient self-care management. These include time, resources, the opportunity for open access to appointments, and early referral to other professional groups. Correlational design studies indicated that individual psychological factors, such as attachment style and autonomy support given to a patient during a patient-practitioner encounter, have a relationship to self-care behaviors and outcomes. Correlational design studies indicated that both general communication and diabetic specific communication used during a patient-practitioner encounter have a positive effect on patient self-care management and outcomes for patients with diabetes.

SELF-MANAGEMENT SKILL DEVELOPMENT

Mickley, Burkhart, and Sigler (2013) define self-management as "the skills and activities necessary to control symptoms of a chronic condition" (p. 323). Development of self-management skills requires a problem-based teaching approach. Key skills involve "monitoring, interpreting, making decisions, taking actions, making adjustments, accessing resources, providing hands-on care, working together with the ill person, and navigating the health care system" (Schumacher & Marren, 2004, p. 460). In addition to acquiring specific knowledge and skills, patients and families need to learn how to cope effectively with a chronic illness. This usually involves special attention to the social consequences and lifestyle changes occurring as a result of the chronic condition.

A multistrategy approach is useful, including the activation of essential resources such as social services, joining support groups, choosing different activities, and so forth (Barlow, Wright, Sheasby, Turner, & Hainsworth, 2002). Children usually require consistent parental support and encouragement to follow through with care tasks and reinforcement for small successes. Because of their developmental needs, children may require special adaptations to lead normal healthy lives. It is critically important to be aware of the school and community supports available for children with chronic disabilities.

Active patient participation with support of the patient's family is essential in the daily management of chronic medical conditions (Udlis, 2011). Participatory decision making is a vital component of meaningful action planning and tailoring of teaching strategies for individual patients and families is a critical dimension. *Repetition is important*, as is careful inquiry with open-ended questions about new issues. Patients must understand why an action is important, what can be expected with a medication or treatment protocol, what are the risks and benefits of treatment options, and what are the warning signs of adverse reactions. A specific plan about what to do when something goes wrong is essential content. Unforeseen factors affecting the self-management process such as changes in the environmental context, interactions with health professionals, and changes imposed by the chronic illness make this information essential content. Incomplete patient education, resulting in patients not knowing how to self-monitor symptoms and recognize side effects, is not only unsafe but also ethically indefensible (Redman, 2011). Patients need support as they take the first steps toward autonomously assuming responsibility for self-care and whenever a health situation changes. Living with chronic illness produces unexpected transitions in care requirements associated with exacerbations. Self-monitoring should focus on changes in symptoms and achieving treatment goals. Patient and family input, combined with professional contributions, are essential for the development of personalized self-care applications. They help to incorporate specific self-management actions into a patient's daily routine.

COACHING

Coaching provides tailored support for people learning self-management and problem-solving skills when patients and families are learning to deal with unfamiliar tasks and procedures (Huffman, 2007). For example, you can help patients and families choose the most appropriate questions to ask their provider. A coaching intervention can be as simple as helping people seek information from several sources rather than calling only one and waiting for a response (Lorig & Holman, 2003).

Coaching "builds on the patient's strengths rather than attempting to fix weaknesses" (Dossey & Hess, 2013, p. 10). A coaching process emphasizes the patient's autonomy in acquiring self-management skills because the patient is always in charge of the pace and direction of the learning.

Coaching involves a number of skills presented in Fig. 15.5. Start an assessment with an examination of patient's current health issue followed by an exploration of its meaning in the patient's life. This dual dialogue provides a basis for looking at current options through the lens of personal values and beliefs. The next step is to encourage patients to critically think about the elements of a situation. Only then is it possible to consider multiple options, and new perspectives. The final step is to evaluate the appropriateness of choosing one option over another and to choose a course of action.

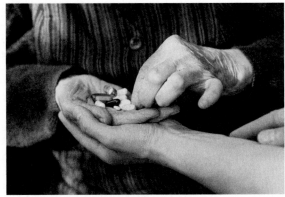

Fig. 15.5 "Teach-back" helps patients anchor their knowledge about Important aspects of self-management. (Copyright © Ocskaymark/iStock/Thinkstock.)

The coaching process involves taking the patient step by step through a procedure or activities with the patient taking the lead in choice of actions. The secret of successful coaching is to provide enough information and/or support to help the patient take the next step without taking over (Fig. 15.6).

Coaching strategies can include supervised skill practice and role-playing. For example, role-playing a potentially difficult conversation can inform the patient about timing of actions, and potential outcomes. The exercise highlights areas that need special attention, and related issues that might not otherwise emerge in a teaching situation. Simulation Exercise 15.4 provides practice with coaching as a teaching strategy.

Providing Transitional Cues

Patients sometimes have difficulty learning essential information because they do not see how information fits together as applied to their particular circumstances. Transitional cues should do the following:

- Link purpose with action, for example, follow the purpose of taking a medication or doing an exercise, with the actions you want the patient to take. This dual approach helps fix the process in a person's mind and makes it easier for patients to remember related instructions.
- Specify what is important, and why. When you tell a patient that a medication should be taken with meals, be specific about what this means and why it is important.
- Ask the patient (teach-back) how he or she will implement essential health management skills, such as using an inhaler or adhering to a therapeutic diet. Ask the patient if he or she has any issues or concerns that you

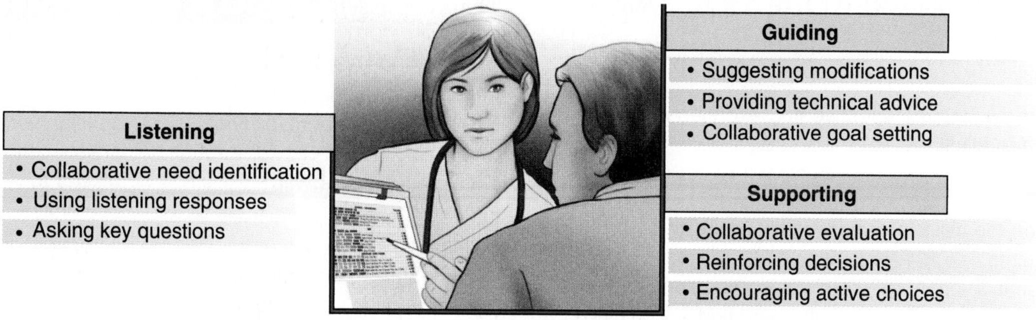

Fig. 15.6 The Nurse's Role in Coaching Patients.

SIMULATION EXERCISE 15.4
Coaching

Purpose
To help students understand the process of coaching.

Procedure
Identify the steps you would use to coach a current patient or a patient with one of the chronic health conditions listed. Use Fig. 15.1 as a guide to develop your plan.
1. A patient returning from hip replacement surgery
2. A patient recovering from a myocardial infarction
3. A patient with newly diagnosed type II diabetes
4. A child with partially controlled asthma
   Share your suggestions with your classmates.

Discussion
1. What were the different coaching strategies you used with the patient?
2. In what ways were your coaching strategies similar to or unlike those of your classmates?
3. How could you use the information you gained from this exercise to improve the quality of your coaching?

have not addressed. Visual cues such as a sticky note to remember to take medication or to keep an appointment are helpful too. Ask patients to keep a self-report log and share it with you as needed.

Giving Feedback
Feedback is of central importance in successful health coaching. Giving immediate feedback is important with learning psychomotor tasks. To appreciate its significance in learning new skills, consider the effect on your performance if you never received feedback from your instructor. For maximum effectiveness, give feedback as soon as possible after the learning event or observation. Consider the impact on the patient. Encourage patient reflection by asking open-ended questions such as, "How did you feel about doing your treatment by yourself?" "Is there anything you would do differently next time?"

Indirect feedback—provided through nodding, smiling, and sharing information about the process and experiences of others—also reinforces learning. When providing feedback, keep it *participatory and simple*. Focus only on behaviors that can be changed. Include strengths as well as areas needing improvement. Simulation Exercise 15.5 provides practice with giving feedback.

BEHAVIORAL APPROACHES

Behavioral approaches are based on the work of B. F. Skinner (1971). Behaviorists believe that reinforcement strengthens learner responses. Premack principle: Reward must have meaning to the learner in order to be effective. This is critical because what is reinforcing to one person may not be so for another. Rewarded behaviors (positive reinforcement) tend to be repeated. Negative reinforcement (reward withdrawal) and ignoring behaviors tend to diminish their occurrence. Different types of reinforcement with examples are found in Table 15.2. Reinforcement schedules describe the timing of rewards. Schedules start with continuous reinforcement for each completed attempt. Once a new behavior is in place, interval schedules in which reinforcement is given after a certain number of successful attempts (fixed interval), or after a random number of responses (variable ratio) are introduced. Tangible rewards are gradually replaced with social reinforcement such as praise. Over time, improved health outcomes become a source of reinforcement to patients. For example, significant weight loss and the way it makes a person feel about his or her personal appearance is a strong motivator to continue with a healthy diet.

SIMULATION EXERCISE 15.5 Usable Feedback

Purpose
To give students perspective and experience in giving usable feedback.

Procedure
1. Divide the class into working groups of three or four students.
2. Present a 3-minute sketch of some aspect of your current learning situation that you find difficult (e.g., writing a paper, speaking in class, coordinating study schedules, or studying certain material).
3. Each person, in turn, offers one piece of usable informative feedback to the presenter. In making suggestions, use the guidelines on feedback given in this chapter.
4. Place feedback suggestions on a flip chart or chalkboard.

Discussion
1. What were your thoughts and feelings about the feedback you heard in relation to resolving the problem you presented to the group?
2. What were your thoughts and feelings in giving feedback to each presenter?
3. Was it harder to give feedback in some cases than in others? In what ways?
4. What common themes emerged in your group?
5. In what ways can you use the self-exploration about feedback in this exercise in teaching conversations with patients?

TABLE 15.2 Types of Reinforcement

Concept	Purpose	Example
Positive reinforcer	Increases probability of behavior through reward	Stars on a board, smiling, verbal praise, candy, tokens to "purchase" items
Negative reinforcer	Increases probability of behavior by removing aversive consequence	Restoring privileges when patient performs desired behavior
Punishment	Decreases behavior by presenting a negative consequence or removing a positive one	Time-outs, denial of privileges
Ignoring	Decreases behavior by not reinforcing it	Not paying attention to whining, tantrums, or provocative behaviors

A behavioral approach starts with a careful description of a concrete behavior requiring change. Describe each action as a single behavioral unit (e.g., failing to take a medication, cheating on a diet, or not participating in unit activities). It is important to start small so that the patient will experience success.

A behavioral approach requires the cooperation of the patient and a shared understanding of the problem. Count the number of times the patient engages in a behavior as a baseline before implementing the behavioral approach. This allows the nurse and the patient to monitor progress as the process progresses.

Behavioral objectives should be action oriented. They reframe the problem in a solution statement (e.g., "The patient will lose 2 pounds"). Begin with the simplest and most likely behavior to stimulate patient interest. Identify the tasks in sequential order; define specific consequences, positive and negative, for behavioral responses; and solicit the patient's cooperation.

Behavioral Strategies

Modeling describes learning a behavior by observing another person who is performing it. Nurses model behaviors in their normal conduct of nursing activities and teaching situations. Bathing an infant, feeding an older person, and talking to a scared child in front of significant caregivers provides informal modeling.

Shaping refers to the reinforcement of successive approximations of the target behavior. The long-term goal is broken down into smaller steps. The person is reinforced for any behavior (successive approximations) that gets him or her closer to accomplishing the desired behavior.

Learning Contracts

A learning contract with the patient serves as a formal commitment to a behavioral learning process. Contracts spell out the responsibilities of each party, expected behaviors, and reinforcements. Contracts are especially useful as part of learning self-management strategies for school-aged children (Burkhart, Oakley, & Mickley, 2012). The contract should include

- Behavioral changes that are to occur
- Conditions under which they are to occur
- A reinforcement schedule
- A time frame

Initially, each instance of expected behavior should be rewarded. If the patient is noncompliant or needs to pay more attention to a particular aspect of behavior, the nurse can say, "This (name the behavior or skill) needs a little more work." One advantage of a behavioral approach is that it never considers the patient as bad or unworthy.

Group Presentations

Group presentations offer the advantage of being able to teach a number of people at one time. Group formats allow people to hear the questions of others and to learn from their experiences and approaches (Tucker, 2013). Health teaching topics that lend themselves to a group format include care of the newborn, diabetes, oncology, and prenatal and postnatal care (Redman, 2007).

Formal group teaching should occur in a space large enough to accommodate all participants. The learner should be able to hear and see the instructor and visual aids without strain. Technical equipment (if used) should be available and in working order. Should the equipment not work, it is better to eliminate the planned teaching aid completely than to spend a portion of the teaching session trying to fix it. Preparation and practice can ensure that your presentation will be clear, concise, and well spoken.

Establish rapport with your audience. Extension of eye contact to all participants communicates acceptance and inclusion. Make eye contact immediately and continue to do so throughout the presentation. An initial quote capturing the meaning of the presentation or a humorous opening grabs the audience's attention. Logical organization of the material is essential. Strengthen content statements with careful use of specific examples. Citing a specific problem and the ways another person dealt with it offers a broader perspective. Repeating key points and summarizing them again at the conclusion of the session helps reinforce learning.

Use slides to identify key points. Slides help you stay on track and move through the agenda. The font should be large enough to be seen from a distance (32 point is recommended). Include no more than four or five items per slide. Face the audience, not the slides. Practice your presentation to ensure that you keep within the time

frame and allot time for short discussion points. It is up to you as the presenter to set the pace. No matter how interesting the presentation and the dialogue that it stimulates, running out of time is frustrating for the audience.

Anticipate questions and be on the alert for blank looks. No matter how good a nurse educator you are, from time to time you will experience the blank look. When this occurs, it is appropriate to ask, "Do you have any questions about anything I have said so far." Give reinforcement for comments, such as "I'm so glad you brought that up," or "That's a really interesting question (or comment)." Smiling and nodding your head are nonverbal reinforcers. If a participant has a question that you cannot answer, do not bluff. Instead, say, "That is a good question. I don't have an answer at this moment, but I will get back to you with it." This should not be the end point. Sometimes another person will have the required information and will share it. Handouts provide reinforcement. Make sure that the information is accurate, complete, easy to understand, logical, and very important, and that you have enough for all participants. Simulation Exercise 15.6 provides an opportunity to practice health teaching in a group setting.

Health Teaching in the Home

Health teaching in the home includes assessment of the home environment, family supports, and resources, as well as patient needs and family needs. In many ways the home offers a teaching laboratory unparalleled in the hospital. The nurse can "see" improvisations in equipment and technique that are possible in the home environment. Family members may have ideas that the nurse would not

---

SIMULATION EXERCISE 15.6 Group Health Teaching

Purpose

To provide practice with presenting a health topic in a group setting.

Procedure

1. Plan a 15- to 20-minute health presentation on a health topic of interest to you, including teaching aids and methods for evaluation. Suggested topics:

Nutrition	Weight control
Drinking and driving	Mammograms
High blood pressure	Safe sex

2. Present your topic to your class group.

have thought of and the nurse can see obstacles the family face. Nurses should review the basic pathophysiology and course of the patient's health condition with the patient and family. Everyone should understand the nature of chronic illness, the potential for exacerbation episodes. Teach-back evaluation helps reinforce learning.

The nurse is a guest in the patient's home. Always call before going to the patient's home. This is common courtesy; it also protects the nurse's time if the patient is going to be out. Teaching in home care settings is rewarding. Often the nurse is the patient's only visitor. Family members often display a curiosity and willingness to be a part of the learning group, particularly if the nurse actively uses knowledge of the home environment to make suggestions about needed modifications.

Teaching in home settings should center on self-management essentials. Encourage patients or caregivers to write down their questions between visits, so critical issues can be addressed during the home visit. Start each session with an open-ended question as to how are things going. Ask if there are any new or unresolved concerns.

You need to review medications with the patient or caregiver on every visit. Tips for teaching patients and caregivers about medications are presented in Box 15.5. Other content should reflect specific information the patient and family need to support self-care management.

An understanding of Medicare, Medicaid, and other insurance regulations, required documentation, and

> **BOX 15.5   Medication Teaching Tips**
>
> - Provide patients with written drug information, particularly for metered-dose inhalants and high-alert medications such as insulin.
> - Include family or caregivers in the teaching sessions for patients who need extra support or reminders.
> - Do not wait until discharge to begin education about complex drug regimens.
> - Clearly explain directions for using each medication.
> - Always require repeat demonstrations or explanations about medications to be taken at home, particularly for those requiring special drug administration techniques.
> - Use the time you already spend with patients during assessments and daily care to evaluate their level of understanding about their medications.
> - Keep medication administration schedule as simple and easy to follow as possible.
>
> Modified from Institute for Safe Medication Practices. (2006). *Patient medication teaching tips*. Huntingdon Valley, PAthor.

reimbursement schedules is important, as is knowledge of community resources *and* helping patients access them. Expert nurses know that patients often can be a source of information about resources they may not know about.

SUMMARY

This chapter describes the nurse's role in health teaching. Theoretical frameworks, patient-centered teaching, as well as developmental and behavioral approaches guide the nurse in implementing health teaching. Teaching is designed to access one or more of the three domains of learning: cognitive, affective, and psychomotor. Box 15.1 provides characteristics associated with each of these domains.

Constructing the Teaching Plan

Health teaching consists of three interrrelated components: Health teaching consists of three categories: information gathering, information sharing, and relationship building as shown in Fig. 5.4.

Essential content in all teaching plans includes information about the health care problem, risk factors, and self-care skills needed to manage at home. Patient learning needs help define relevant teaching strategies. Assessment for purposes of constructing a teaching plan centers on three areas: What does the patient already know? What is important for the patient to know? What is the patient ready to learn?

Several teaching strategies, such as coaching, use of mnemonics, and visual aids, are described. Repetition of key concepts and frequent feedback make the difference between simple instruction and teaching that informs. Nurses use teach-back methods to confirm understanding.

The Joint Commission (2014) requires documentation of patient education. The patient's record becomes a permanent communication tool, informing other health care workers what has been taught and what areas need to be addressed in future teaching sessions.

DISCUSSION QUESTIONS

1. How can you best integrate chronic disease–related personal self-management skills with lifestyle and other aspects of the patient's life?
2. Discuss what is meant by the following statement: "Patient education is essential to safe, ethical clinical practice."
3. What *specific* strategies would you use to help low-literacy patients learn essential health information?

ETHICAL DILEMMA: What Would You Do?

Louisa is a low-literacy patient at the mental health clinic who wants a refill of her medication. She states that she has reduced her medication to every other day rather than every day because she thinks it "works better for her." She does not want to lower her dose. She also tells the nurse that she gave several of her extra pills to her brother because he ran out of his pills. Although she listens politely to the nurse's concerns, Louisa tells her that she thinks her current regimen is appropriate for her. She sees nothing wrong with sharing her meds with her brother as he is on the same medication. If you were the nurse, how would you respond to this patient?

REFERENCES

American Nurses Association (ANA). (2004). *Scope and standards of practice.* Washington DC: Author.

Anderson, L. W., Krathwohl, D. R., Airasian, P. W., Cruikshank, K. A., Mayer, R. E., Pintrich, P. R., et al. (2000). *A taxonomy for learning, teaching, and assessing: A revision of Bloom's taxonomy of educational objectives.* New York: Pearson, Allyn & Bacon.

Baker, D., DeWalt, D., Schillinger, D., Hawk, V., Ruo, B., Bibbins-Domingo, K., et al. (2011). Teach to goal: Theory and design principles of an intervention to improve heart failure self-management skills of patients with low literacy. *Journal of Health Communication,* 16(Suppl. 3) 7, 3–88.

Barlow, J., Wright, C., Sheasby, J., Turner, A., & Hainsworth, J. (2002). Self-management approaches for people with chronic conditions a review. *Patient Education and Counseling,* 48(2), 177–187.

Bastable, S. (2017). *Nurse as educator: principles of teaching and learning for nursing practice* (5th ed.). Sudbury: MA: Jones & Bartlett.

Baur, C. (2011). Calling the nation to act: Implementing the national action. *Nursing Outlook,* 59(2), 63–69.

Beagley, L. (2011). Educating patients: Understanding barriers, learning styles, and teaching techniques. *Journal of Perianesthesia Nursing,* 26(5), 331–337.

Benner, P., Sutphen, M., Leonard, V., & Day, L. (2010). *Educating nurses: a call for radical transformation.* Standford, CA: Jossey-Bass.

Bonaldi-Moore, L. (2009). The nurse's role in educating post-mastectomy breast cancer patients. *Plastic Surgical Nursing,* 29(4), 212–219.

Buckley, B. A., McCarthy, D. M., Forth, V. E., Tanabe, P., Schmidt, M. J., Adams, J. G., et al. (2013). Patient input into the development and enhancement of ED discharge instructions: a focus group study. *Journal of Emergency Nursing,* 39(6), 553–561. https://doi.org/10.1016/j.jen.2011.12.018.

CDC. (2009). *Simply put: A guide for creating easy-to-understand materials* (3rd ed.). www.cdc.gov/healthliteracy/pdf/simply_put.pdf.

Center for the Advancement of Health. (2002). *Essential elements of self-management interventions.* Washington, DC: Author.

Deek, H., Hamilton, S., Brown, N., Inglis, S., Digiacom, M., Newton, P., et al. (2016). Family-centered approaches to healthcare interventions in chronic diseases in adults: A quantitative systemic review. *Journal of Advanced Nursing,* 72, 968–979.

Doak, C., Doak, L., Gordon, L., & Lorig, K. (2001). Selecting, preparing and using materials. In K. Lorig (Ed.), *Patient education: a practical approach* (3rd ed.) (pp. 183–197). Thousand Oaks, CA: SAGE.

Doherty, D. (2009). Guided care nurses help chronically ill patients. *Patient education management,* 16(12), 139–141.

Dossey, B., & Hess, D. (2013). Professional nurse coaching: advances in global healthcare transformation. *Global Advances in Health and Medicine,* 40(2), 10–16.

Dreeben, O. (2010). *Patient education in rehabilitation.* Sudbury MA: Jones & Bartlett Publishers.

Edwards, A. (2013). Asthma action plans and self-management: Beyond the traffic light. *Nursing Clinics of North America,* 48, 47–51.

Farin, E., Gramm, L., & Schmidt, E. (2013). Predictors of communication preferences in patients with chronic low pain. *Patient Prefer Adherence,* 7, 1117–1127.

Feudtner, C. (2001). What are the goals of patient education? *Western Journal of Medicine,* 174(3), 173–174.

Freda, M. (2004). Issues in patient education. *Journal of Midwifery & Women's Health,* 39(3), 203–209.

Friedman, A. J., Cosby, R., Boyko, S., Hatton-Bauer, J., & Turnbull, G. (2011). Effective teaching strategies and methods of delivering for patient education: A systemic review and practice guideline recommendations. *Journal of Cancer Education,* 26, 12–21.

Gordon, J. (2011). Educating the patient: Challenges and opportunities with current technology. *Nursing Clinics of North America, 46*, 341–350.

Gravely, S., Hensley, B., & Hagood-Thompson, C. (2011). Comparison of three types of diabetic foot ulcer education plans to determine patient recall of education. *Journal of Vascular Nursing, 29*, 113–119.

Holman, H., & Lorig, K. (2004). Patient self-management: a key to effectiveness and efficacy in care of chronic disease. *Public Health Reports, 119*, 239–243.

Holt, J. E., Flint, E. P., & Bowers, M. T. (2011). Got the picture? Using mobile phone technology to reinforce discharge instructions. *American Journal of Nursing, 111*(8), 47–51.

Huffman, M., & Health coaching. (2007). A new and exciting technique to enhance patient self-management and improve outcomes. *Home Health Nurse, 25*(4), 271–274.

Inott, T., & Kennedy, B. (2011). Assessing learning styles: Practical tips for patient education. *Nursing Clinics of North America, 46*(3), 313–320.

Kelo, M., Eriksson, E., & Eriksson, I. (2013). Pilot educational program to enhance empowering patient education of school-age children with diabetes. *Journal of Diabetes & Metabolic Disorders, 12*, 18.

Knowles, M., Holton, E., & Swanson, R. (2011). *The adult learner: the definitive classic on adult education and training* (7th ed.). Oxford UK: Elsevier.

Krau, S. (2011). Creating educational objectives for patient education using the new Bloom's taxonomy. *Nursing Clinics of North America, 46*, 299–321.

Lear, M. W. (1980). *Heartsounds pocket books.* New York: Simon & Schuster.

Lewis, D. (2003). Computers in patient education. *Computers, Informatics, Nursing, 21*(2), 88–96.

Lorenzen, B., Melby, C., & Earles, B. (2008). Using principles of health literacy to enhance the informed consent process. *Association of Operative Registered Nurses Journal, 88*(1), 23–29.

Lorig, K. (2001). *Patient education: a practical approach* (3rd ed.). Thousand Oaks, CA: SAGE.

Lorig, K., & Holman, H. (2003). Self-management education: History, definition, outcomes and mechanisms. *Annals of Behavioral Medicine, 26*(1), 1–7.

Lowenstein, A. A., Foord-May, L. L., & Romano, J. J. (2009). *Teaching strategies for health education and health promotion.* Sudbury, MA: Jones & Bartlett.

Manning, S. (1992). The nurses I'll never forget. *Nursing, 22*(8), 47.

McCormack, B., & McCance, T. (2006). Development of a framework for person-centered nursing. *Journal of Advanced Nursing, 56*(5), 472–479.

Menendez, J. (2013). Informed consent: Essential legal and ethical principles for nurses. *JONAS Healthcare Law, Ethics, and Regulation, 15*(4), 140–144.

Mezirow, J. (1990). *fostering critical reflection in adulthood: a guide to transformative and emancipatory learning.* San Francisco, CA: Jossey-Bass.

Mickley, K., Burkhart, P., & Sigler, A. (2013). Promoting normal development and self-efficacy in school age children managing chronic conditions. *Nursing Clinics of North America, 48*(2), 319–328.

Peek, M., Harmon, S., Scott, J., Eder, M., Roberson, T. S., Tang, H., et al. (2012). Culturally tailoring patient education and communication skills training to empower African Americans with diabetes. *Translational Behavioral Medicine, 2*(3), 296–308.

Peeters, J., Wiegers, T., & Friele, R. (2013). How technology in care at home affects patient self-care and self-management: A scoping review. *International Journal of Environmental Research and Public Health, 10*(11), 5541–5564.

Perdue, B., Degazon, C., & Lunny, M. (1999). Diagnoses and interventions with low literacy. *Nursing Diagnosis, 10*(1), 36–39.

Redman, B. K. (2007). *The practice of patient education: a case study approach* (10th ed.). St. Louis, MO: Mosby.

Redman, B. K. (2011). Ethics of patient education and how do we make it everyone's ethics. *Nursing Clinics of North America, 46*, 283–289.

Rogers, C. (1983). *Freedom to learn for the '80s.* Columbus, OH: Merrill.

Skinner, B. F. (1971). *Beyond freedom and dignity.* New York: Knopf.

Schumacher, K., & Marren, J. (2004). Home care nursing for older adults: State of the science. *Nursing Clinics of North America, 39*, 443–471.

Schwartzberg, J., Cowett, A., Vangeest, J., & Wolf, M. (2007). Communication techniques for patients with low literacy: a survey of physicians, nurses, and pharmacists. *American Journal of Health Behavior, 31*(9), S96–S104.

Smith, L. (2013). Help your patients access government health information. *Nursing, 2013*, 32–34.

Stephenson, P. (2006). Before the teaching begins: Managing patient anxiety prior to providing education. *Clinical Journal of Oncology Nursing, 10*(2), 241–245.

Su, W. M., Herron, B., & Osisek, P. (2011). Using a competency based approach to patient education: achieving congruence among learning, teaching and evaluation. *Nursing Clinics of North America, 46*(3), 291–298.

Su, W. M., Osisek, P., & Starnes, B. (2004). Applying the revised Bloom's taxonomy to a medical–surgical nursing lesson. *Nurse Education, 29*(3), 116–120.

Suter, P. M., & Suter, W. N. (2008). Timeless principles of learning: a solid foundation for enhancing chronic disease self-management. *Home Health Nurse, 26*(2), 83–88.

Szpiro, K., Harrison, M., Van Den Kerkhof, E. G., & Lougheed, M. M. D. (2008). Patient education in the emergency department. *Advanced Emergency Nursing Journal, 30*(1), 34–49.

Tucker, M. (2013). Older Diabetes patients benefit from group education. *Medscape.*

Udlis, K. (2011). Self-management in chronic illness: Concept and dimensional analysis. *Journal of Nursing and Health Care in Chronic Illness, 3*(2), 130–139.

Wolf, M., Curtis, L., & Baker, D. (2012). Literacy, cognitive function, and health: Results of the LigCog study. *Journal of General Internal Medicine, 27*(100), 1300–1307.

World Health Organization (WHO). (2009). Health promotion. Track 2: health literacy and health behaviour 7th global conference on health promotion. *Track themes.* http://www.who.int/healthpromotion/conferences/7gchp/track2/en/index.html Accessed February 11, 2014.

SUGGESTED READING

Ajzen, I. (1991). The theory of planned behavior. *Organizational Behavior and Human Decision Processes, 50,* 179–211.

Bennett, H., Coleman, E., Parry, C., Bodenheimer, T., & Chen, E. (2010). Health coaching for patients with chronic illness. *Family Practice Management, 17*(5), 24–29.

de Boer, D., Delnoij, D., & Rademakers, J. (2013). The importance of patient-centered care for various patient groups. *Patient Education and Counseling, 90*(3), 405–410.

Durham, B. (2015). The nurse's role in medication safety. *Nursing, 45*(4), 1–4.

Dykes, P., & Collins, S. (2013). *Building linkages between nursing care and improved patient outcomes: the role of health information technology.* http://www.nursingworld.org/MainMenu-Categories/ANAMarketplace/ANAPerio dical.

Hudon, C., Tribble, D., Bravo, G., Hogg, W., Lambert, M., & Poitras, M. E. (2013). Family physician enabling attitudes: a study of patient perceptions. *BMC Family Practice, 14,* 8–16.

Koh, H., Brach, C., Harris, M., & Parchman, M. (2013). A proposed 'Health Literate Care Model' would constitute a systems approach to improving patients' engagement in care. *Health Affairs, 32*(2), 357–367.

Masters, K. (2017). *Role development in professional nursing.* Sudbury MA: Jones & Bartlett.

Speros, C. L. (2011). Promoting health literacy: a nursing imperative. *Nursing Clinics of North America, 46*(3), 321–333.

The Joint Commission. (2014). *Comprehensive accreditation manual for hospitals (CAMH),* Oakbrook Terrace, IL: Author

The Joint Commission. (2007). *What did the doctor say? Improving health literacy to promote patient safety. Health Care at the Crossroads Reports.* Oakbrook Terrace, IL: Author

The Joint Commission. (2009). *"What did the doctor say?: improving health literacy to protect patient safety.* Oakbrook Terrace: The Joint Commission.

Ward, B. W. (2014). Multiple chronic conditions among US adults: a 2012 update. *Preventing Chronic Diseas, 11,* E62.

WEB RESOURCES

MedlinePlus (n.d.). Health topics. U.S. *National Library of Medicine and National Institutes of Health.* www.nlm.nih.gov/medlineplus/healthtopics.html; www.cdc.gov/healthliteracy/pdf/Simply_Put.pdf.

16

Communication in Stressful Situations

Elizabeth C. Arnold

OBJECTIVES

At the end of the chapter, the reader will be able to:
1. Define stress and associated concepts.
2. Describe biological and psychosocial models of stress.
3. Identify concepts related to coping with stress.
4. Discuss stress assessment strategies.

5. Describe stress reduction strategies nurses can use in stressful situations.
6. Identify stress management therapies.
7. Address burnout in nurses.

INTRODUCTION

Stress is both a cause and a consequence of illness and injury; it stems from functional disruptions and unrealistic self-expectations. Stress has been linked to the six leading causes of death, including heart disease, cancer, lung ailments, accidents, cirrhosis of the liver, and suicide (American Psychological Association [APA], 2007).

When a person is admitted to the hospital, that person enters a new and usually unfamiliar world. This circumstance, in itself, represents a stressful situation. Chapter 16 focuses on understanding the role of stress, and helping patients develop coping strategies to reduce the impact of stress reactions in health care relationships. Included in this chapter are descriptions of biological and psychosocial models of stress reactions and the types of coping mechanisms used to deal with stress. Nurses and other primary providers of care, especially those working in highly acute nursing situations, are especially vulnerable to stress and burnout. This chapter identifies communication strategies nurses can use to help patients and families reduce stress levels in health care situations.

BASIC CONCEPTS

Definition

Hans Selye (1950) defined stress as a nonspecific response of the body to any demand made upon it, regardless of whether it is caused by a pleasant or unpleasant situation. McEwen (2012) describes stress as a state of mind, "involving both brain and body as well as their interactions" (p. 17180). A stress response is a common reaction to serious illness that affects quality of life for all family members as well as the patient's ability to function (Haugland, Veenstra, Vatn, & Wahl, 2013).

Stress represents a natural physiological, psychological, and spiritual response to the presence of a stressor. A stress reaction differs from a crisis situation. Unlike crisis, stress responses usually are less dramatic and may not lessen over time. Strengthening a patient's capacity to cope effectively with stress has important implications for clinical outcomes as well as the patient's motivation and capacity to perform self-management (Jaser et al., 2012). A stress assessment should be incorporated as part of the complex data needed to support a person's ability to adapt to chronic illness.

A *stressor* is defined as any demand, situation, internal stimulus, or circumstance that threatens an individual's personal security or integrity. Internal stressors such as pregnancy, fever, menopause, or emotions originate within the body. External stressors—such as social or work stressors, accidents, debt, and exams—start outside the self. *Crisis* (detailed in Chapter 20) represents an extreme acute stressor situation for which coping mechanisms fail and the person is unable to function normally. By definition a crisis situation will resolve within 6 weeks.

Sources of Stress

Stress is a common part of life. For each individual, stress represents a personal experience. What is stressful for one person may not be for another. Stress can develop over time or can strike without warning. Stressors can affect many people at the same time—for example, war, hurricane, earthquake or severe flood damage, community mass murders in schools, or the Twin Towers destruction. They can be cumulative, continuous, or just minor hassles. Personal stress can be related to a major life change (marriage, divorce, death, moving to a new area, becoming a parent, graduating from college, starting a new job) or an illness or injury. A new diagnosis, loss of social ties, premature death, and potential damage from adjuvant therapy are common health-related stressors (Antoni, 2013). Some of the more common personal sources of stress are identified in Box 16.1.

In health care situations, sources of emotional stress include watching a loved one steadily decline physically or mentally, concern about finances, uncertainty about the future, balancing other family responsibilities with patient care, and coping with personal frustration. Stressors likely to stimulate an intense stress response are those where a person has limited control over the situation, the situation is ambiguous, or aspects of the current situation resemble past unresolved stressful events for.

The intensity and duration of stress varies according to the circumstances, level of social support, and the person's emotional state. Significant or prolonged stress can increase the impact of a current stressful situation. (Meyers, 2011). Mentally ill patients have a double set of chronic stressors. Some stem from their mental disorder, which lowers a patient's threshold for stress and diminishes a person's capacity to act effectively to reduce the stress (Lavoie, 2013). Daily hassles (traffic jam, child misbehavior, too many competing tasks, computer crashes) are mild stressors that can turn into chronic stress, especially when they are cumulative. The stress response is commonly present in most health care situations.

Levels of Stress

Selye used the term *eustress* to describe a mild level of stress, which is a positive response with protective and adaptive functions. Mild stress heightens awareness and can motivate people to master challenges and develop new skills. Coping skills learned in mastering a stressful situation help people cope better with other life circumstances as well (Aldwin & Levenson, 2004).

Distress, defined as a negative stress level, creates a level of anxiety exceeding a person's normal coping abilities. Distress diminishes performance and quality of life. High stress levels interfere with a person's ability to function. Severe, chronic stress weakens the immune system, thereby contributing to the development of stress-related illnesses (Martin, Lae, & Reece, 2007).

- *Chronic stress* is implicated in the development and exacerbation of cardiac conditions, migraine, and digestive disorders. Stress and coping are said to account for up to 50% of the variation in psychological symptoms (Sinha & Watson, 2007).
- *Acute stress* requires immediate attention. It creates a very intense form of anxiety, which is disabling for the person experiencing it. Once the situation is resolved, homeostasis is reestablished. Untreated, severe mental stress reactions associated with traumatic events can develop into posttraumatic stress disorder, a clinical syndrome requiring psychiatric intervention.

Variation in Stress Responses

Although stress is a universal occurrence, it is a subjective personal experience. People have different tolerance levels for stress. Some people are extremely sensitive to any stressor. Others are laid back and appear less disturbed by unexpected stressful circumstances.

More than mild stress reduces the efficiency of cognitive functions and clouds perceptual acuity. Secondary stressors, such as insomnia caused by worry and financial issues, can heighten the impact of primary stressors on

---

BOX 16.1 Personal Sources of Stress

Physical Stressors
- Acute or chronic illness
- Trauma or injury
- Pain
- Insomnia
- Mental disorder

Psychological Stressors
- Loss of job or job security
- Loss of a significant person or pet
- Significant change in residence, relationship, work
- Personal finances
- Work relationships
- High-stress work environment
- Caretaking (frail elderly, children)
- Significant change or loss of role

Spiritual Stressors
- Loss of purpose
- Loss of hope
- Questioning of values or meaning

a person's personal life and routines (Wittenberg-Lyles, 2012). The level of social and resource support that a person receives when stressed can reduce the impact of a stressor.

Current research suggests that men and women respond to stress differently. Men respond with patterns of "fight or flight," whereas women use a "tend and befriend" approach (Taylor, 2006). Women use nurturing activities to reduce stress and promote safety for self and others as priority interventions. They seek social support from others, particularly from other women. Children express stress through behavior, usually corresponding with their developmental stage and family patterns. Acting out behaviors and psychosomatic illness can mask a child's distress.

STRESS MODELS

Systemic Physiological Response

Walter Cannon (1932) described stress as a systemic physiological response to a perceived threat. It occurs in a similar way regardless of the stressor. Cannon believed that when people feel physically well, emotionally centered, and personally secure, they are in a state of dynamic equilibrium, or **homeostasis**. Stress disturbs homeostasis. Physiologically, the sympathetic nervous system sets in motion an immediate hormonal cascade designed to mobilize the body's energy resources to cope with acute stress.

Cannon proposed that people attempt to adapt to stress using either a "fight or flight" response. The "fight" response refers to a person's inclination to take action against a threat. This response is used if the threat appears to be resolvable. People use a flight response if they perceive that the threat cannot be overcome through personal effort.

General Adaptation Syndrome

Hans Selye (1950) described stress as a physiological whole body response to stress, evidenced primarily through the endocrine and autonomic nervous systems. Referred to as the ***general adaptation syndrome***, this set of symptoms "was so general that it was like a single burglar alarm that sounds, no matter what intrudes" (Meyers, 2011, p. 275). The same physiological response occurs regardless of whether a stressor is psychological, or physical.

Selye described a three-stage progressive pattern of nonspecific physiological responses: alarm, resistance, and exhaustion. The "***alarm*** stage" is similar to Cannon's acute stress response. If the stressor is not resolved in the initial alarm stage, a second level adaptive phase, ***"resistance stage"*** occurs as the body tries to accommodate for the stressor. In the resistance stage, overt alarm symptoms subside as the immune system helps the body to adapt to the demands of the stressor. If the body fails to adapt or is unable to resist the continued stress, it leads to an ***"exhaustion stage."*** At this point, the person becomes higher risk for a stress-related illness, or mental disorder. The longer the physiological stress response remains elevated, the greater is the negative impact on the person.

Allostasis

Allostasis, a recent theory of stress response, describes how the human organism "maintains physiological homeostasis through changing circumstances" (Huber et al., 2011). The brain serves as a "primary mediator" between the "current exposure, internal regulation of bodily processes, and health outcomes" (Gaelan, Morris, & Wethingon, 2010, p. 134).

Allostatic accommodation is the physiological process through which the brain tries to find a new homeostasis, using a range of adaptive functioning. McEwen (2000) refers to this phenomenon as "stability through change" (p. 1219). The interaction between stressors and physical responses is ongoing, such that individuals become more or less susceptible to the negative consequences of stress over time. Inclusion of genetic risk factors, early life events, and adaptive lifestyle behaviors offers a way to understand the interaction between stressful events and physiological adaptation processes (McEwen, 2012). Fig. 16.1 identifies the relationships in the model.

Stress hormones protect the body against short-term acute stress (allostasis). Stress mediators, such as social support, can provide protective effects. When slight or moderate levels of stressor exposure are encountered and social support is available, coping with stress can actually work to strengthen well-being and quality of life.

Complex or prolonged stress levels are more problematic. According to McEwen (2007), early life experiences with stress can have implications for later biological stress experiences, and a "cumulative wear and tear of the physical and social environment on the brain and body". If a stressor presents continued challenges or coping responses are ineffective, there is "wear and tear" on the body, which can have a damaging effect. McEwen terms this phenomenon ***allostatic load***. The allostatic load can be negligible, severe, or protracted enough to result in significant illness or death if untreated.

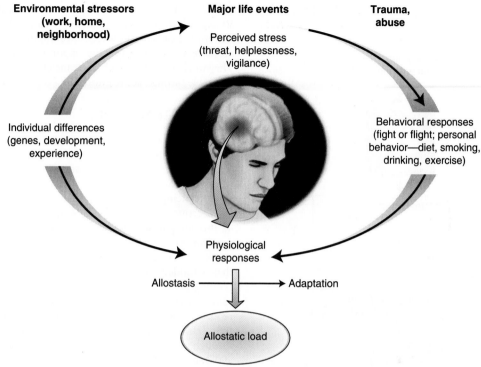

Fig. 16.1 Allostasis Model of Stress.

Psychosocial Frameworks

Critical Life Events

Holmes and Rahe (1967) consider stressful life events—such as marriage, divorce, death, and losing a job—as stimuli sufficient to disrupt homeostasis and thus create stress. The Holmes and Rahe scale assigns each life event a weighted numeric score reflecting its potential impact. Stressors requiring a significant change in the person's lifestyle have greater impact, as do the number of cumulative stresses on the scale. A higher score reflects a person's potential for the later development of physical illness (Pearlin, 1989).

Transactional Model of Stress

Lazarus and Folkman's (1984, 1991) transactional appraisal model of stress is widely used in health care. Basically this is a psychological model; it considers stress as a two way interactive process involving both the stressor, and the individual's interpretive response to the stressor. According to the transactional model of stress and coping, when stress occurs, the stressor creates a significant adaptive demand requiring a response from the individual Dolbier, Smith, & Steinhardt, 2007. It is not the objective stressor that accounts for how a person responds to a stressor. Rather, primary response

mediators are (1) Primary appraisal refers to a person's interpretation of the severity of a stressor. (2) Secondary appraisal describes a person's perception of his or her personal ability to resolve the stressful situation (Fig. 16.2). The transactional model is as applicable to daily "hassles as it is to major events" (Maybery, Neale, Arentz, & Jones-Ellis, 2007).

Lazarus's (1984) transactional model helps explain individual differences in personal responses to stressors that objectively could be thought of as having the same stress value. There are two forms of appraisal. A primary appraisal examines the strength of a person's belief about the potential harm that a stressor holds for a person. The stronger the perceived threat to self-integrity, the greater the stress response. The secondary appraisal considers a person's perception of personal coping skills, and availability of appropriate social environmental resources to reduce a stressor's impact. Both appraisals are required to determine whether a stressor will be considered to be a harmful threat or challenge (Folkman, 2008). People experience stress if they appraise the stressor to be threatening and/or feel incapable of meeting the stressor's demands with available resources.

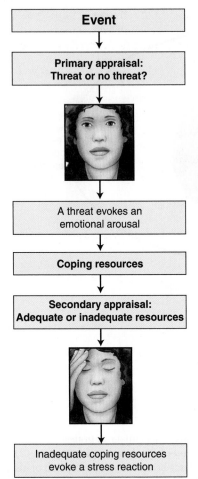

Fig. 16.2 Primary and Secondary Appraisal in Stress Reactions.

COPING

Coping is "defined as the constantly changing cognitive and behavioural efforts to manage specific external or internal demands that are appraised as taxing or exceeding the resources of the person (Bayuo & Agbenorku, 2018, p. 47). In a classic work, Pearlin and Schooler (1978) define coping as "any response to external life strains that serves to prevent, avoid, or control emotional distress" (p. 2). They identify three purposes of coping strategies:

- To change the stressful situation (problem-focused)
- To change the meaning of the stressor (meaning-focused)
- To help the person relax enough to take the stress in stride (emotion-focused)

In general, using problem-focused coping strategies to actively reduce the impact of a stressful situation and make it less stressful is more effective in controllable situations

(Thoits, 2010). By contrast, emotion or meaning-focused strategies have a stronger impact when less controllable situations are causing the stress. Meaning-focused strategies are designed to diminish the importance of the stressor. They work best when work or financial issues are not easily reducible through active efforts.

COPING STRATEGIES

Culture plays a role in determining a person's stress and coping behaviors by

1. Shaping the types of stressors a person is likely to experience
2. Influencing the patient's appraisal of stress
3. Affecting the choice of coping strategies
4. Providing different resources and institutional mechanism as coping options (Aldwin, 2010, p. 564)

Skinner, Edge, Altman, and Sherwood (2003) suggest that a fundamental problem in defining coping is that "coping is not a specific behavior that can be unequivocally observed or a particular belief that can be reliably reported" (p. 217). For example, in certain collective cultures (Hispanic and Asian), *distress* is commonly expressed through somatic symptoms (Lehrer, Woolfolk, & Sime, 2007). In addition to cultural differences, previous stressful experiences, financial assets, and social/self-management support influence a patient's and family's ability to solve problems and cope effectively with their health conditions.

People learn coping strategies from their parents, peers, and life experiences. Those with varied life opportunities and supportive people in their lives have an advantage over those who lack opportunity, and/or support systems. People who have been overprotected or were repeatedly exposed to danger without support generally lack adequate coping skills. Simulation Exercise 16.1 is intended to help identify common personal coping strategies.

Types of Coping

Appraisal theory describes coping as "a process by which a person makes cognitive and behavioral efforts to manage psychological stress" (Bippus & Young, 2012, p. 177). Two types of coping: an approach problem focused style, and an emotion focused style are the most commonly used coping strategies (Wagland, Fenlon, Tarrant, Howard-Jones, & Richardson, 2015). **Problem-focused coping strategies** are purposeful active, task-oriented methods to reduce stress. Examples include confronting a problem directly, negotiating for a different solution, seeking social support, constructive problem solving, and taking action. In general, problem-focused coping strategies have been found to be the most effective in reducing stress. For example, Jaser et al. (2012) found that adolescents who used problem-solving strategies to control their diabetes

SIMULATION EXERCISE 16.1 Examining Personal Coping Strategies

Purpose
To help students identify the wide range of adaptive and maladaptive coping strategies.

Procedure
1. Identify all of the ways in which you handle stressful situations.
2. List three personal strategies that you have used successfully in coping with stress.
3. List one personal coping strategy that did not work and identify your perceptions of the reasons it was inadequate or insufficient to reduce your stress level.
4. List on a chalkboard or flip chart the different coping strategies identified by students.

Discussion
1. What common themes did you find in the ways people handle stress?
2. Were you surprised at the number and variety of ways in which people handle stress?
3. What new coping strategy might you use to reduce your stress level?
4. Are there any circumstances that increase or decrease your automatic reactions to stress?

demonstrated better diabetic control, and experienced a higher quality of life than those who did not.

Emotion-focused coping strategies act in a different way to minimize the influence of stress in the patient's mind. These strategies can be effective when the stressor is perceived as an overwhelming irreversible situation or a person needs respite from overthinking about a stressful situation. Emotion-focused coping strategies—such as meditation, yoga, or spirituality—are constructive when a person deliberately chooses to "let go" of negative feelings associated with an unmanageable stressor and employ other strategies.

Most people use both types of coping strategies, with the choice of strategy dependent on the nature of the stressor and a person's typical coping style. Awareness of personal and external resources adds options. Individuals who believe that they have options are generally better able to cope with stress. Common personal coping assets, referred to as "resource options," include health, energy, problem-solving skills, the amount and availability of social supports, and other material resources to cope effectively with the stressor.

Meaning-focused coping strategies help to reframe the meaning or significance of the stressor so that it loses its power as an overwhelming challenge and becomes a challenge in need of a change in focus level. The stressor may still exist, but the greater calmness that the behavioral focused coping strategies provides a realignment of its impact. Simulation Exercise 16.1 provides an opportunity to examine your personal use of coping strategies.

Defensive Coping Strategies

Although some forms of coping yield positive results to reduce stress, others are negative influences. Rumination, denial, anger, excessive anxiety, use of drugs, or alcohol can increase the effects of stressors and further add to distress. **Ego defense mechanisms** are defined as a coping style that people use to protect the self from full awareness of challenging conflict situations. They are designed to protect the ego from anxiety and loss of self-esteem by denying, avoiding, or projecting responsibility for a challenging conflict to an external source.

Ego defense mechanisms can be temporarily adaptive by minimizing the threat of a potentially overwhelming stressor (Richards & Steele, 2007). Persistent use of the **ego defense mechanisms** presented in Table 16.1 is considered pathological. As a primary stress reducer, defense mechanisms are ineffective because avoidant behavior typically delays action and compromises trust in relationships. Some defense mechanisms—humor, anticipation, affiliation (asking for help), and sublimation—can be adaptive if not used exclusively as coping strategies (Reich, Zautra, & Hall, 2010).

Case Example
Lynn was diagnosed as having high cholesterol and was advised to lose weight. She sees no purpose in going on a diet because "it's all in the genes." Both her parents had high cholesterol and died of heart problems. Lynn claims that there is nothing she can do about it, even though her physician advised her differently. Her defensive interpretation prevents her from taking actions needed to reduce her risk for cardiovascular disease. Motivational interviewing (see Chapter 14) offers guidelines for gently casting doubt, providing new information, and introducing problem solving to resistant patients. Her nurse inquires about Lynn's personal health goals and provides her with information about the link between diet, exercise, and heart disease. Linking information to Lynn's stated life goals provides her with a different frame of reference.

Resilience

Resilience is a concept linked to well-being and burnout prevention (Arrogante & Aparicio-Zaldivar, 2017). It is defined as the ability of individuals who are exposed

TABLE 16.1   Ego Defense Mechanisms

Ego Defense Mechanism	Clinical Example
Regression: returning to an earlier, more primitive form of behavior in the face of a threat to self-esteem	Julie was completely toilet trained by 2 years of age. When her younger brother was born, she began wetting her pants and wanting a pacifier at night.
Repression: unconscious forgetting of parts or all of an experience	Elizabeth has just lost her job. Her friends would not know from her behavior that she has any anxiety about it. She continues to spend money as if she were still getting a paycheck.
Denial: unconscious refusal to allow painful facts, feelings, or perceptions into awareness	Bill Marshall has had a massive heart attack. His physician advises him to exercise in moderation with caution. Bill continues to jog 6 miles a day.
Rationalization: offering a plausible excuse or explanation for unacceptable behavior	Ann Marie tells her friends she is not an alcoholic, even though she has blackouts, because she drinks only on weekends and when she is not working.
Projection: attributing unacceptable feelings, facts, behaviors, or attitudes to others; usually expressed as blame	Ruby just received a critical performance evaluation from her supervisor. She tells her friends that her supervisor does not like her.
Displacement: redirecting feelings onto an object or person considered less of a threat than the original object or person	Mrs. Jones took Mary to the doctor for bronchitis. She is not satisfied with the doctor's explanation and feels he was condescending, but she says nothing. When she gets to the receptionist's desk to make the next appointment, she yells at her for not having the prescription ready and taking too much time to set the appointment.
Intellectualization: unconscious focusing on only the intellectual and not the emotional aspects of a situation or circumstance	Johnnie has been badly hurt in a car accident. There is reason to believe he will not survive surgery. His father, waiting for his son to return to the intensive care unit, asks the nurse many questions about the equipment, and philosophizes about the meaning of life and death.
Reaction formation: unconscious assumption of traits that are the opposite of undesirable behaviors	John has a strong family history of alcoholism on both sides. He abstains from liquor and is known in the community as an advocate of prohibition.
Sublimation: redirecting socially unacceptable unconscious thoughts and feelings into socially approved outlets	Bob has a lot of aggressive tendencies. He decided to become a butcher and thoroughly enjoys his work.
Undoing: verbal expression or actions representing one feeling, followed by expression of the direct opposite	Barbara criticizes her subordinate, Carol, before a large group of people. Later, she sees Carol on the street and tells her how important she is to the organization.

to highly disruptive stressors to remain relatively stable and functional despite the stress (Garcia-Dia, DiNapoli, Garcia-Ona, Jakuboski, & O'Flaherty, 2013). Resilience explains why some people seem to weather stress and adversity more easily than others and are able to grow from the experience. Through development of a strong internal sense of control and a positive attitude, patients can develop the skills needed to override their stress and move forward despite stressful life events (Marsiglia, Kulis, Garcia Perez, & Bermudez-Parsai, 2011).

Characteristics of resilience include empowerment and creativity (Lin, Rong, & Lee, 2013). Resilient people develop coping mechanisms that allow them to see a situation as it is, to focus on what can be changed, and to accept what cannot be altered (Schieveld, 2009). Helping patients develop clear goals, shape relevant problem-solving skills, and take baby steps toward identified goals is a means of improving personal resilience. A person develops resiliency through practice, social support, and learning self-efficacy strategies. Examples of relevant strategies include developing an organized way of coping with challenges and cultivating a meaningful support system. A strong faith and sense of purpose are other factors associated with resilience (Freedman, 2008).

Hardiness. Hardiness is considered as a protective factor that can minimize the effects of stress. The concept of *hardiness* consists of three basic elements:

- *Challenge* (looking at stressors and characterizing the need for change as an opportunity for personal growth)
- *Commitment* (developing a sense of purpose and a strong involvement in directing one's life)
- *Taking control* (the belief that one can help to influence one's life's outcomes, Dolbier et al. 2007)

Resilience and hardiness act as protective factors that influence a person's ability to view global stress events as ultimately being manageable.

DEVELOPING AN EVIDENCE-BASED PRACTICE

The purpose of this qualitative exploratory study was to describe occupational stressors and ways they could be reduced from the nurse's perspective. Thirty-eight registered nurses (RNs) participated in six focus groups to discuss sources of occupational stress and possible ways to reduce the stress.

Results

This sample group of nurses identified high workloads, shift work, unsupportive management, unavailability of physicians, poor parking facilities and other human resource issues, and issues regarding patients and their relatives. Suggestions for modification included workload and shift hour changes, organizational development, better work conditions, and acknowledgment from management.

Application to Your Clinical Practice

All nurses have a responsibility to participate in making health care environments better and less stressful. Nurse managers should make opportunities available to discuss occupational stressors and encourage nurses to engage in stress reduction activities.

From Happell, B., Dwyer, T., Reid-Searl, K., Burke, K. J., Caperchione, C. M., & Gaskin, C. J. (2013). Nurses and stress: Recognizing causes and seeking solutions. *Journal of Nursing Management, 21*(4), 638–647.

APPLICATIONS

Stress Assessment

Stress is an unwelcome part of most illnesses and injury. It is rarely a personal choice. People experience and cope with stress in different and sometimes unexpected ways. Nurses can be instrumental in helping patients cope with

---

BOX 16.2   Factors That Influence the Impact of Stress

- Magnitude and demands of the stressor on self and others
- Multiple stressors occurring at the same time
- Suddenness or unpredictability of a stressful situation
- Accumulation of stressors and duration of the stress demand
- Level of social support available to the patient and family
- Previous trauma, which can activate unresolved fears
- Presence of an associated mental disorder
- Developmental level of the patient
- Normal attitude and outlook
- Knowledge, expectations, and realistic picture

---

stress effectively so that their anxiety does not dominate their health experience and they are able to function effectively. Factors that influence the impact of stress are identified in Box 16.2.

Addressing stress issues and teaching patients related coping strategies enhances clinical outcomes and recovery potential. An initial assessment should include the patient's

- Perception of current stressors
- Perception of the stressor causing the greatest stress
- Insight about the value or meaning attached to the stressor
- Identification of usual coping strategies used to manage stressful situations
- Assessment of linked issues such as developmental stage, culture, family ways of coping, and level of support
- Religious and spiritual beliefs and activities

Understanding how a stressful event relates to other life issues, including stressors from the past and current financial or family concerns, is helpful. Ask open-ended questions about changes in daily routines, new roles and responsibilities. Explore the patient's and family's current understanding of diagnosis and treatment options. Pay close attention to cultural values. What is a small stressor in one culture can be huge in another, and normal coping strategies can be quite different.

Sources of Stress in Health Care

All health disruptions create a sense of vulnerability. Health-related stressors for patients and families include fear of death, uncertainty about diagnosis, clinical outcomes, changes in roles, disruption of family life, and financial concerns. Hospital-related sources of stress include

---

BOX 16.3   Assessment and Intervention Tool

Assessment

A. Perception of stressors
   1. Major stress area or health concern
   2. Present circumstances related to usual pattern
   3. Experienced similar problem? How was it handled?
   4. Anticipation of future consequences
   5. Expectations of self
   6. Expectations of caregivers
B. Intrapersonal factors
   1. Physical (mobility, body function)
   2. Psychosociocultural (attitudes, values, coping patterns)
   3. Developmental (age, factors related to present situation)
   4. Spiritual belief system (hope and sustaining factors)
C. Interpersonal factors
   1. Resources and relationship of family or significant others as they relate to or influence interpersonal factors
D. Environmental factors
   1. Resources and relationships of community as they relate to or influence interpersonal factors

Prevention as Intervention

A. Primary
   1. Classify stressor
   2. Provide information to maintain or strengthen strengths
   3. Support positive coping mechanisms
   4. Educate patient and family
B. Secondary
   1. Mobilize resources
   2. Motivate, educate, involve patient in health care goals
   3. Facilitate appropriate interventions; refer to external resources as needed
   4. Provide information on primary prevention or intervention as needed
C. Tertiary
   1. Attain/maintain wellness
   2. Educate or reeducate as needed
   3. Coordinate resources
   4. Provide information about primary and secondary interventions

Unpublished, Developed by Conrad, J. (1993). Baltimore, MD: University of Maryland School of Nursing.

---

physical discomfort, strange noises and lights, unfamiliar people asking personal questions, and strange equipment. Patients and their families experience stress with a patient transfer to the intensive care unit, again when the patient is transferred to a step-down or regular unit, and still again when patients are transitioning to home (Chaboyer et al., 2005) . Providing immediate practical and emotional support during such transitions helps reduce excessive stress.

A patient-centered approach pays attention to the *type* of stress a patient is experiencing. When stress presents as anxiety, the nurse might suggest problem-solving techniques. However, if the stress is related to a significant loss, the nurse would want to focus on the loss and work with the patient from a grief perspective. Box 16.3, developed by a nursing student, provides an assessment and intervention tool that you can use to organize assessment data and plan interventions.

Behavioral Observations

Stress behaviors are sometimes hard to understand or accept. Distress often presents through behavior rather than through words. For example, anxiety can present in the form of heart palpations, shortness of breath, sweating, and muscle tension (Grillon, 2005). Other physical and mental symptoms of stress include

- Significant changes in eating or sleeping habits
- Headaches, gastric problems, muscular tension, aches and pains, tightness in the throat
- Restlessness and irritability
- Inability to cope with normal everyday concerns and obligations
- Inability to concentrate

Anger and Hostility

Anger and hostility are common stress responses associated with feeling helpless or psychologically threatened. Patients (and/or families) become hostile when they feel threatened about what is happening or feel they have little control in a situation. Anxiety usually exists as the underpinning of anger. What hostile patients or families need most, despite their hostile behavior, is understanding, comfort, and human caring.

Blame is a frequent form of hostility. Family members blame each other for undesired outcomes, or the physician for operating (or not operating) on a loved one. They criticize the nurse for not responding quickly enough. Recognizing hostility as a cry for help in coping with escalating stress makes it easier to respond empathetically. Nurses can help a patient stabilize an out-of-control situation by providing a calming supportive presence, and working with the patient to find a viable resolution to personal anxiety.

SIMULATION EXERCISE 16.2
Relationships Between Anger and Anxiety

Purpose

To help students appreciate the links between anger and anxiety and understand how anger is triggered.

Procedure

1. Think of a time when you were really angry. It need not be a significant event, or one that would necessarily make anyone else angry.
2. Identify your thoughts, feelings, and behavior in separate columns of a table you construct. For example, what were the thoughts that went through your head when you were feeling this anger? What were your physical and emotional responses to this experience? Write down words or phrases to express what you were feeling at the time. How did you respond when you were angry?
3. Identify what was going on with you before experiencing the anger. Sometimes it is not the event itself but your feelings before the incident that make the event the straw that breaks the camel's back.
4. Identify underlying threats to your self-concept in the situation (e.g., you were not treated with respect, your opinion was discounted, you lost status, you were rejected, you feared the unknown).

Reflective Analysis Discussion

1. In what ways were your answers similar to and different from those of your classmates?
2. What role did anxiety and threat to your self-concept play in the development of the anger response? What percentage of your anger related to the actual event and to your self-concept?
3. In what ways did you see anger as a multidetermined behavioral response to threats to your self-concept?
4. Did this exercise change any of your ideas about how you might handle your feelings and behavior in a similar situation?
5. What are the common threads in the events that made people in your group angry?
6. In what ways could experiential knowledge of the close association between anger and anxiety be helpful in your nursing practice?

Carefully listening to a patient's concerns goes a long way toward neutralizing anger and hostility. The patient feels heard, even if the issues cannot be fully resolved to the patient's satisfaction. In the course of the conversation, both nurse and patient can sort out how the patient experiences a stressor. This data can serve as a basis for choosing productive solutions. Set limits if necessary, but do so with a calm attitude and empathetic matter of fact manner. If patient and/or family expectations are unrealistic, or cannot be met in the current situation, alternative explanations and suggestions can be introduced. Simulation Exercise 16.2 is designed to address the relationship between anger and anxiety.

Social Withdrawal

Stress does not always look like a "stressor response" to observers. Some people internalize stress. Culture and circumstance play a role. People may withdraw or seem disengaged from an obvious stressor when they are feeling stressed. Unexpressed emotions of anxiety and anger are toxic and debilitating. Nurses can help patients externalize their stress. Putting their observations into words helps patients link emotional states to specific stress reactions using words rather than behavior to express them. Words put limits on the stress experience and make it more manageable. For example, you might say, "This (name stressor) must be very upsetting," or "It seems like you are pretty anxious about…" Offering your presence, together with a simple statement such as "when people put their stress into words they usually experience less anxiety," can help to normalize the feelings.

Assessment of Coping Skills

Assessment of a patient's coping behaviors and social support network is critical to understanding stress from a holistic perspective. Ask about coping strategies a patient has used in the past and what he or she is currently doing to resolve stress. Relevant issues include culturally sanctioned coping approaches and typical family coping strategies. Sample questions might include

- What do you do to relieve your stress?
- Who can you rely on when you are feeling stressed?

Discussing stress can be difficult in part because it is so uncomfortable. Patients feel more comfortable when their nurse presents an open, nonthreatening stance and a calm attitude. Use an informal conversational format. Being patient and willing to listen is important. Your patient's reactions will serve as a guide as to how much and how quickly the information can be gathered.

Social Support

Social support is an essential buffer against stress. Families can be a major support for patients in managing health-related distress (Antoni, 2013). To be sure that everyone is on the same page, nurses should inquire about the following as part of the initial assessment:

- What are the family's expectations of care?
- In what ways, if any, are family, patient, and provider expectations different?

- What does the family or patient need from you as the nurse? From each other?
- Is there a family spokesperson?
- What are the family's cultural, religious, and values concerning the meaning of the stressor?
- What does the family identify as sources of strength and hope? Are these similar or different from the patient's list?

Community resources include support groups, social services, and other public health agencies that provide practical support, as well as social contacts. Nurses need to be aware of community support services. Simulation Exercise 16.3 is designed to help you become better acquainted with resources in your community.

Belief in a personal god or higher power provides interested patients with an incomparable personal resource. Multiple studies reveal that spiritual interventions can help prevent and improve physical illnesses, and have helped patient cope with chronic pain and death (Moeini, Taleghani, Mehrabi, & Musarzale, 2014). Some people rely on faith to facilitate their acceptance of a reality that cannot be changed. Assessing and providing spiritual comfort to patients is an important consideration in caring for patients

experiencing stress. For example, African Americans tend to use spirituality and religious activities as preferred coping strategies (Samuel-Hodge, Watkins, Rowell, & Hooten, 2008).

Assessing Impact on Family Relationships
Stress Issues for Children

Health disruptions create special stress for children; they lack the words and life experience to sort out the meaning of illness, either their own, or that of a significant family member (Compas et al., 2001). Children express their stress through behavior. Signs of distress, such as academic decline, gastric distress, and headaches, can alert the nurse to unvoiced stress. In the hospital, children withdraw, demonstrate clinging behaviors, or have frequent meltdowns. Uncertainty creates stress for both parents and children (Stewart & Mishel, 2000). Parents may need help with communicating information about serious illness to children, with anticipating their child's reactions, or with setting realistic limits with an ill child.

Children need to have their questions answered simply and honestly, consistent with their developmental stage. Hearing information from someone they trust is important in modifying the uncertainty of a serious illness. Small children can be encouraged to express their stress feelings through drawings and manipulating puppets.

STRESS ISSUES FOR OLDER ADULTS

Stress issues for older adults often relate to multiple health challenges, and an increased potential for loss of important interpersonal supports during this phase of life. Worry about finances and fears of not being able to live independently are common. Older adults living alone often feel vulnerable about their safety or ability to reach help, should they experience a fall or sudden physical change. The loss of significant supportive people, isolation, and loneliness can complicate treatment issues.

Stress management strategies for older adults from a health promotion perspective include maintaining an active social life, and a healthy lifestyle to keep mind and body actively engaged with life. Developing leisure or volunteer interests helps older adults build a well-balanced lifestyle that not only reduces stress but also improves quality of life. Sometimes all it takes are simple suggestions and well-timed questions about recreational activities or hobbies that the older adult has not considered. Many communities have low-impact exercise programs, senior centers, continuing education, and social programs for older adults. The activity provides a venue for socialization that may not be available otherwise. Caregivers of patients with dementia can benefit from some of the suggestions in Chapter 19 to reduce stress as they care for a family member with dementia.

STRESS REDUCTION STRATEGIES

In stressful situations, normal feelings are overlaid by anxiety. Your initial goal is to help patients and families feel secure. A calm empathetic approach helps establish a safe holding environment. It creates the space patients need to express fears, anger, and negative feelings. Slowing the pace is essential to allow feelings to emerge. Name the feelings: "You seem to be really struggling right now." This can be followed by a simple question, "How can I best help you?"

Providing Information

Information is an essential stress reducer. Relevant information can range from providing basic data about visiting hours, the timing of tests and procedures, plans for discharge, or contact phone numbers, to complex facts about the patient's condition or treatment. Information sharing should begin with orienting patients and families to the health care situation or unit. Types of information patients and families find helpful during a hospital stay include the following:

- What will happen during tests or surgery
- Who is likely to interview the patient, and why
- How the patient can best cooperate or assist in his or her treatment process

In stressful situations, the perceptual field narrows. Information and directions given in the first 48 hours of an admission should be repeated, usually more than once, because this is the time of high stress. The same is true when there is a change in treatment plans, or prognosis. A calm approach and repetition help patients in stressful situations relax enough to hear new information. Providing simple written instructions, particularly about medications, that can be discussed at the time and then left with the patient or family enhances understanding. Allow time to answer questions and provide the patient's family with the health provider's contact numbers to call if other issues arise.

Processing Strong Feelings

When strong stress feelings get bottled up in the patient, constructive problem-solving ceases. Often nurses can tell that patients are stressed from their body language, even when they deny strong feelings. Helpful statements include, "This must be very difficult for you to absorb" or "Can you tell me what you are experiencing?" Your immediate goal is to help patients step back, and take a second look at their situation from a broader perspective.

A calm accepting presence and willingness to listen to the patient's story allows nurses and patients to develop a shared understanding of a stressful event. You can help a patient normalize stressful feelings such as, "I think I'm losing my mind," with a statement such as, "What you are feeling is not unusual; although it feels that way, you are having a normal response to a sudden, overwhelming situation. Can you tell me what worries you the most?" Notice in both probes, the nurse acknowledges the legitimacy of feelings as a normal response to an abnormal situation. Once the patient begins to calm down, it becomes possible to look at the situation more realistically.

Simulation Exercise 16.4 provides practice with helping patients handle stressful situations.

SIMULATION EXERCISE 16.4
Role-Play: Handling Stressful Situations

Purpose

To give students experience in responding to stressful situations.

Procedure

Use the following case study as the basis for this exercise.

Dave is a 66-year-old man with colon cancer. In the past he had a colostomy. Recently he was readmitted to your unit and had an exploratory laparotomy for small-bowel obstruction. Very little can be done for him because the cancer has spread. He is in pain, and he has to have a feeding tube. His family has many questions for the nurse: "Why is he vomiting?" "How come the pain medication isn't working?" "Why isn't he feeling any better than he did before the surgery?" You have just entered the patient's room; his family is sitting near him, and they want answers now.

1. Have different members of your group role-play the patient, the nurse, the son, the daughter-in-law, and the wife. One person should act as observer.
2. Identify the factors that will need to be clarified in this situation to help the nurse provide the most appropriate intervention.
3. Using the strategies suggested in this chapter, intervene to help the patient and family reduce their anxiety.
4. Role-play the situation for 10 to 15 minutes.

Reflective Analysis Discussion

1. Have each player identify the interventions that were most helpful.
2. From the nurse's perspective, which parts of the patient and family stress were hardest to handle?
3. How could you use what you learned from doing this exercise in your clinical practice?

Reappraisal of either the stress event itself (primary appraisal) or secondary appraisal of coping and personal resources can help a patient change the meaning of a stress event from being a failure to viewing it as a challenge or opportunity for personal growth. Jamieson, Nock, and Mendes (2011) propose that when people believe they have the resources to cope with stressors, they begin to perceive a stressful situation as a challenge rather than a threat. Pointing out personal or community resources the patient has not considered can reduce the impact of the stressor and make strengthen coping efforts. Group formats provide social support and practical education. It is important to help patients choose supports that are convenient and compatible with their stage of life, other commitments and health issues (Arnold, 1997). Concrete assistance with negotiating appropriate referral resources may be needed.

Developing Realistic Goals

Without command over controllable parts of life, most people feel helpless and stressed. Relevant goals for stress reduction should relate to assessment data, for example, patient-identified needs, strengths, resources, barriers, and goal achievement priorities. Treatment goals and objectives should build on past successful coping efforts and preferences. Choosing personal responses to stress is empowering and has a ripple effect on patient self-efficacy around other health issues.

Coping mechanisms such as negotiation, specific actions, seeking advice, and rearranging priorities can significantly diminish stress through direct action. Once stressors are named, nurses can use health teaching formats and coaching that help patients to

- Develop a realistic plan to offset stress.
- Deal directly with obstacles as they emerge.
- Evaluate action steps.
- Make needed modifications in the plan and essential lifestyle adjustments.

Case Example

Sam Hamilton received a diagnosis of prostate cancer on a routine physical examination. His way of coping (problem-focused) included obtaining as much information on the disease as possible. He researched treatment options and sought advice from physician friends as to which surgeons had the most experience with this type of surgery. As he shared his diagnosis with friends and colleagues, he found several men who had successfully survived without a cancer recurrence. Sam used the time between diagnosis and surgery to finish projects and delegate work responsibilities. He attended a

support group with his wife and was able to obtain valuable advice on handling his emotional responses to what would happen. When the time came for his surgery, Sam's actions before surgery reduced his stress.

Priority Setting

Patients do not always know where to start. Priority setting helps reduce hesitation and offers a stepwise framework for resolving stress. You can help patients determine which task elements are critical and achievable, and which can be addressed later. Break objective tasks into smaller manageable progressive segments. The most important tasks should be scheduled during times when the patient or family has the most energy, and freedom from interruption.

The next step is to help patients identify the concrete tasks needed to achieve treatment goals, including the people involved, necessary contacts, amount of time each task will take, and specific hours or days for each task.

Some tasks are more important than others in reducing stressful situations and not everything can be handled at once. A helpful suggestion might be, "Let's see what you need to do right now and what can wait a little while." Tasks that someone else can do and those that are not essential to the achievement of goals should be delegated or ignored for the moment.

Anticipatory Guidance

Fear of the unknown intensifies the impact of a stressor. Anticipatory guidance is a proactive strategy to help patients cope effectively with stressful situations. The term refers to the process of sharing information about a circumstance, concern, or situation before it occurs. Knowing what lies ahead often prevents the development of a crisis (Hoff, Hallisey, & Hoff, 2009). In framing a response, you might reflect on the following:

- What type of information would be most helpful to this patient at this particular time, given what the patient has told me?
- How would I feel if I was in this person's position?
- What would I want to know that might bring me comfort in this situation?

Providing anticipatory guidance can put needless worry to rest. You can prepare your patients for a procedure, beginning with a simple statement, "You've never had this procedure before. Let me explain how it works" (Keller & Baker, 2000). When you are providing anticipatory guidance, do not offer more than what the situation dictates. Encourage the patient to expand on suggestions rather than outlining a full plan. The growth in patient ability to set priorities, develop a plan with personal meaning, and establish benchmarks to measure progress stimulates self-confidence and decreases stress.

Anticipatory guidance should relate only to behaviors that can be changed. Stress-related questions about uncertainties do not qualify, for example, "If I take this chemotherapy, will I be cured, or am I going to die anyway?" The reality is that there may be no single answer. It helps to ask the patient what prompted the question and to have a good idea of the patient's level of knowledge before answering. Honest communication is essential, but sensitivity to the patient's experience also is critical.

Social Support

Social support is defined as the emotional comfort, advice, and instrumental assistance that a person receives from other people in their social network (Taylor, Welch, Kim, & Sherman, 2007). The concept has three distinct functions in helping patients reduce stress levels: validation, emotional support, and correction of distorted thinking. *Social support* refers to both the "perceived availability of help, or support actually received" (Schwarzer & Knoll, 2007, p. 244). A person's social networks are drawn from family, friends, church, work, social groups, or school. Being able to contact family and friends when you need an emergency babysitter or an extra hand in a stressful situation immediately lessens stress. Not only does sharing with others reduce stress by "externalizing" negative emotions, but family, friends and support groups can provide a sounding board, practical assistance, and tangible encouragement. Seeking help can empower both seeker and provider of emotional support. Sharing a laugh, eating a meal with others, and being in good company helps people feel more relaxed, which, in turn, reduces stress levels.

Social support does not have the same meaning for all cultures in terms of self-disclosure. Taylor et al. (2007) report that Asian American patients may be more comfortable with an implicit form of social support that does not require the sharing of thoughts. Examples of implicit social support include showing kindness, caring, acceptance, and positive regard for a patient.

Helping Families Reduce Health-Related Stress

Contemporary health care environments with advanced technology, shorter stays, and multiple caregivers are complex and anxiety producing. Sources of stress for families can include "fear of death, uncertain outcome, emotional turmoil, financial concerns, role changes, disruption of routines, and unfamiliar hospital environments" (Leske, 2002, p. 61). Families look to nurses for support and direction.

Regular communication and providing updated information about a family member's condition is a key component of stress reduction. Listen carefully to the family. Statements such as "Most people would feel anxious in this situation," or "It would be hard for anyone to have all the answers in a situation like this" can normalize difficult situations.

Ongoing direct family contact can sometimes provide additional information about patient preferences, health care needs, and resources. This strategy is particularly helpful when the patient is unable to provide information (Davidson et al., 2007). It also helps family members feel more connected.

Nurses play an important role in helping families reduce their stress levels to a workable level in health care. You can explore the presence of stress by linking the immediate health situation with expected feelings: "Seeing your husband like this must be a terrible shock. I suspect you might be wondering how you are going to cope with his care at home." This type of statement normalizes feelings and introduces subjects that are difficult but necessary to talk about. Nurses can help families process complex information and address specific concerns. Topics should focus on what will happen next, how to explain the illness to others, or what the patient or family is experiencing related to the stressor. Table 16.2 identifies interventions to decrease family stress.

In critical care situations, families have a strong need to remain physically close to the patient; there is a strong correlation between proximity to the patient and satisfaction with care (Davidson et al., 2007). It is important to support the presence of key family members in "every area of the hospital, including the emergency department and the intensive care unit" (Leape et al., 2009, p. 426).

Family members often want to provide support and comfort to critically ill patients. They want to be full "partners in care." Being able to "do something" for the patient helps them feel less helpless and defuses stress. Allowing family members to provide comfort measures and participate in the patient's care to whatever extent is possible for the patient and comfortable for the family can be a meaningful experience for both.

Even the most dedicated family members, however, need respite periods. A helpful strategy is suggesting that family members take short breaks. Family members may need "permission" to go to a movie or eat in a restaurant outside the hospital. Sometimes they will do so with an assurance that they will be called should there be any change in the patient's condition.

Promoting a Healthy Lifestyle

Encouraging a healthy lifestyle is an essential but sometimes overlooked component of stress-management strategies. Good health habits improve stress resistance. Eating a healthy diet and avoiding emotional eating gives people

TABLE 16.2	**Nursing Interventions to Decrease Family Anxiety**
Recommendation	**Specific Actions**
Identify a family spokesperson and support persons involved in decision making	Choose a person the family and patient trusts; establish mechanisms for contact.
Identify a primary nursing contact for the family	If possible, choose the nurse most in contact with the patient. Meet with the family within 24 hours of admission to explain roles of each health care team member. Provide contact number to family spokesperson.
Discuss family access to the patient	Arrange for visitation based on unit protocols, patient condition and needs, family preferences. Educate the family about visiting hours, how to reach the hospitalist, when rounds occur. Involve family in patient care whenever possible and desired.
Call the family about any changes in patient condition or treatment	Inform family of changes as they occur. Provide frequent status reports. Allow time for questions.
Provide complete data in easily understandable terms	Ask questions about what the patient and family understand about the patient's condition, how they are coping, what they fear. Check for misunderstandings, incomplete information. Provide information based on family needs. Respect cultural and personal desire for level of information disclosure.
Actively involve the patient and family in all clinical decisions	Hold formal care conferences for important care decisions. Take into account and respect patient preferences as well as spiritual and cultural attitudes. Allow time for questions. Strive for consensus in decisions.
Connect family with support services	Provide information about support groups, hospital-based social, spiritual, Medicare, hospice, home care, and other care services as needed.
Ensure collaborative rapport and support among health care team members	Maintain clear communication among health care team members. Avoid conflicting messages to the family. Provide opportunities for staff to decompress and discuss difficult situations and feelings.

Data from Davidson, J., Powers, K., Hedayat, K., Tieszen, M., Kon, A. A., Shepard, E., et al. (2007). Clinical practice guidelines for support of the family in the patient-centered intensive care unit: American College of Critical Care Medicine Task Force 2004–2005. *Critical Care Medicine, 35*(2), 605–622; Leske, J. (2002). Interventions to decrease family anxiety. *Critical Care Nursing, 22*(6), 61–65.

a sense of control and well-being. Too much caffeine and alcohol can exacerbate stress. Laughter dissolves it, and reduces stress levels.

Quality sleep is restorative. Healthy nighttime habits, such as establishing a scheduled bedtime and having a small snack before bedtime, encourages sleep. Regular exercise helps the body release tension, as well as contributes to fitness. Exercise can be accomplished in a social setting, for example, hiking or biking. Certain exercise programs such as yoga or tai chi meditation, deep breathing, and muscle stretching are well known stress reducers. Organizing time and deliberately choosing activities that energize rather than stress, balancing work with leisure activities, and eliminating unnecessary obligations reduce stress.

Therapeutic Approaches for Chronic Stress Management

Cognitive Behavioral Approaches

Cognitive-behavioral approaches have proven useful in addressing stressful negative attributions about oneself, and modifying negative core beliefs. The cognitive behavioral therapy (CBT) model (Beck & Beck, 2011) uses a person-centered approach aimed at helping individuals troubled by faulty thinking reframe the meaning of difficult situations. According to Beck, the relationship between a person's thoughts and feelings influences behaviors. Optimistic or neutral thoughts can lead to positive emotions and tend to create cooperative constructive actions. Negative thinking does the opposite. Faulty thinking causes a person to interpret neutral situations in unrealistic, exaggerated, or negative ways. Helping people become aware of and modify negative or dysfunctional thoughts, beliefs, and perceptions (cognitive distortions) makes it possible for them to change behavior patterns. Awareness can result in a more constructive approach to a problem situation.

Stress symptoms look similar on the surface, but the cognitive beliefs supporting the stress reaction can be quite different. *Cognitive restructuring* is a strategy, which "involves teaching patients to question the automatic beliefs, assumptions and predictions that often lead to negative emotions and to replace negative thinking with more realistic and positive beliefs" (Schacter, Gilbert, & Wegner, 2010, p. 599). The focus of CBT is not on the behavior itself but on the inner perceptions and thoughts that create and perpetuate negative self-evaluations and self-defeating behaviors.

Automatic negative thoughts are classified as **cognitive distortions**. Examples include magnifying or minimizing the impact of a single behavior as a commentary on the person. Failing a test is experienced as "I am stupid," instead of "I messed up on a test—what can I do so this doesn't happen again?"

Mind reading or having rigid rules about what a person "should" do is another example. Over time a person develops a set of related automatic distortions referred to as a *schema*. The person uses core schemas to filter incoming information and determine its meaning related to self, others, and the world. Schemas become a template for understanding the meaning of incoming information and appraising its value to the self. They are pervasive and hard to dislodge. Although distortions seem to be legitimate assessments, they are not valid.

Nurses can help patients challenge distortions through Socratic questioning. By gathering and weighing evidence to support a different position, people are able to distinguish between a distorted perception and a realistic appraisal of its validity. Ridding oneself of unrealistic expectations and negative self-thoughts allows cognitive space for thinking about possible options and broader choices. Once a problem is appropriately categorized, solutions become more apparent. You can help patients understand that they have choices and that no matter what feeling they have, it is not permanent. Initially people have to force themselves to challenge negative thoughts and replace them with more balanced thoughts. Over time this becomes easier.

> ### BOX 16.4 Meditation Techniques
>
> 1. Choose a quiet, calm environment with as few distractions as possible.
> 2. Get in a comfortable position, preferably a sitting position.
> 3. To shift the mind from logical, externally oriented thought, use a constant stimulus: a sound, word, phrase, or object. The eyes are closed if a repetitive sound or word is used.
> 4. Pay attention to the rhythm of your breathing.
> 5. When distracting thoughts occur, discard the thought(s) and redirect your attention to the repetition of the word or gazing at the object. Distracting thoughts will occur and do not mean you are performing the techniques incorrectly. Do not worry about how you are doing. Redirect your focus to the constant stimulus and assume a passive attitude.

Modified from Benson, H. (1975). *The relaxation response.* New York: Morrow.

Nurses can use open-ended questions such as
- What is the worst thing that can happen?
- If *(worst thing)* did happen, what could you do?

Mind-Body Therapies and Meditation

Using mind/body exercises to lessen the intensity of a stressor on a person, helps. Examples include meditation, relaxation techniques, yoga, and cognitive restructuring.

Meditation is a stress-reduction strategy that people use to develop a sense of inner peace and tranquility. Meditation clears the mind of disturbing thoughts and neutralizes toxic feelings. This activity helps to reduce the concentration of stress hormones attached to stressful thinking. A guide to meditation is provided in Box 16.4.

Mindfulness meditation uses a nonjudgmental personal conscious awareness related to the present moment, and what is happening in the here and now. Mindfulness is a stress management tool that can be used at any point. It can be as simple as focusing on deep breathing. Focusing completely on your breathing, music, or what is happening in the current moment forces a person to at least momentarily let go of stressful thoughts. It is an easy way of quieting the mind and decreasing the intensity of stressful feelings.

Progressive Relaxation

Progressive relaxation is a technique that focuses the patient's attention on conscious control of voluntary skeletal muscles. Originally developed by Edmund Jacobson (1938), the technique consists of alternately tensing and relaxing muscle groups. Davis, Eshelman, and McKay

(2008) provide an excellent step-by-step description of the basic procedure for progressive relaxation.

A variant of progressive relaxation is deep breathing. This can be accomplished anywhere and at any time a person experiences stress. Try doing it as follows:

- Deeply inhale to the count of 10 and hold your breath.
- Exhale slowly, again to the count of 10.
- Concentrate as you do this exercise only on your breathing.
- Feel the tension leave your body.

Focusing your mind on the continuous rhythm of inhaling and exhaling turns the mind away from thinking about specific stressors. To experience the progressive relaxation technique, use Simulation Exercise 16.5.

Yoga and Tai Chi

Yoga is a mind-body exercise practice rooted in ancient India. The practice of yoga has proven useful as a treatment for depression, and for promotion of physical and mental health (Rao, Varambally, & Gangadhar, 2013). Yoga emphasizes correct alignment, controlled postures or poses, and regulated breathing to help people relax and reduce stress. Controlling breathing helps to quiet the

---

SIMULATION EXERCISE 16.5   Progressive Relaxation

Purpose

To help students experience the beneficial effects of progressive relaxation in reducing tension.

Procedure

This exercise consists of alternately tensing and relaxing skeletal muscles.

1. Sit in a comfortable chair with arm supports. Place the arms on the arm supports, and sit in a comfortable upright position with legs uncrossed and feet flat on the floor.
2. Close your eyes and take 10 deep breaths, concentrating on inhaling and exhaling.
3. Your faculty or a student member of the group should give the following instructions, and you should follow them exactly:
   - I want you to focus on your feet and to tense the muscles in your feet. Feel the tension in your feet. Hold it, and now let go. Feel the tension leaving your feet.
   - I would like you to tense the muscles in your calves. Feel the tension in your calves and hold it. Now let go and feel the tension leaving your calves. Experience how that feels.
   - Tense the muscles in your thighs. Most people do this by pressing their thighs against the chair. Feel the tension in your muscles and experience how that feels. Now release the tension and experience how that feels.
   - I would like you to feel the tension in your abdomen. Tense the muscles in your abdomen and hold it. Hold it for a few more seconds. Now release those muscles and experience how that feels.
   - Tense the muscles in your chest. The only way you can really do this is to take a very deep breath and hold it. (The guide counts to 10.) Concentrate on feeling how that feels. Now let it go and experience how that feels.

- I would like you to tense your muscles in your hands. Clench your fist and hold it as hard as you can. Harder, harder. Now release it and concentrate on how that feels.
- Tense the muscles in your arms. You can do this by pressing down as hard as you can on the arm supports. Feel the tension in your arms and continue pressing. Now let go and experience how that feels.
- I would like to you to feel the tension in your shoulders. Tense your shoulders as hard as you can and hold it. Concentrate on how that feels. Now release your shoulder muscles and experience the feeling.
- Feel the tension in your jaw. Clench your jaw and teeth as hard as you can. Feel the tension in your jaw and hold it. Now let it go and feel the tension leave your jaw.
- Now that you are in this relaxed state, keep your eyes closed and think of a time when you were really happy. Let the images and sounds surround you. Imagine yourself back in that situation. What were you thinking? What are you feeling?
- Open your eyes. Students who feel comfortable in doing so may share the images that emerged in the relaxed state.

Reflective Analysis Discussion

1. What are your impressions in doing this exercise?
2. Do you feel more relaxed after doing this exercise?
3. If applicable, after doing the exercise, in what ways did you feel differently?
4. Were you surprised at the images that emerged in your relaxed state?
5. In what ways do you think you could use this exercise in your nursing practice?

mind. Some forms of yoga involve meditation and developing self-awareness.

Tai chi is an exercise system consisting of stretching and rhythmic movements coordinated with controlled breathing. The postures and movements are practiced in a slow, graceful manner. The concentration required for both yoga and tai chi requires a person to relax and forget distressing thoughts.

Guided Imagery

Guided imagery is a technique often used in combination with relaxation strategies for cancer pain and stress (Kwekkeboom, 2008). Imagery techniques use the patient's imagination to stimulate healing mental images designed to promote stress relief. The process involves asking a patient to imagine a scene, previously experienced as safe, peaceful, or beautiful. Supportive prompts to engage all of senses deepen the imagery experience. This scene can be used each time that the patient begins to experience stress. Inspirational tapes and music are also used in connection with guided imagery.

Support Groups

Support groups for patients or families struggling with the same health situation or crisis can be extremely helpful in helping them defuse stress and learn coping strategies to self-manage difficult health issues. Examples include bereavement groups, cancer support groups, dementia family groups, and specialized groups for abuse or alcoholism. Psychoeducational groups with supportive interventions include the National Alliance on Mental Illness (NAMI), cardiac rehabilitation, and health promotion groups for targeted populations.

Stress Issues for Nurses: Burnout

Nurses face many adverse situations and high-risk conditions that people in other professions do not experience or witness on as regular a basis (Cross, 2015). Over time, prolonged work-related stress takes its toll. Khamisa and Peltzer Oldenburg (2013) notes that nurses experience a greater vulnerability to burnout because they work in high-stress service environments, helping people cope with serious life and death situations every day.

Freudenberger (1980) defines **burnout** as "a state of fatigue or frustration brought about by devotion to a cause, way of life, or relationship that failed to produce an expected reward" (p. 13). He refers to burnout as the "overachievement syndrome." Burnout is characterized by emotional exhaustion, depersonalization, and a sense of diminished professional accomplishment. Although burnout shares some characteristics with depression and

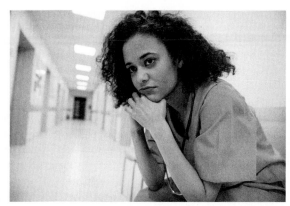

Fig. 16.3 Burnout is a form of occupational stress, which compromises performance and professional commitment. (Copyright © gpointstudio/iStock/Thinkstock.)

anxiety, it is a different syndrome, clearly linked to work environments, and personal expectations of self and others within that setting.

Burnout develops from combined factors in work related environments, and within the person. Unchecked, it is a progressive syndrome associated with emotional exhaustion and loss of meaning. High achievers and committed nurses, who are passionate about their work, are more at risk. Burnout begins insidiously, particularly in nurses who strive for perfection. Sources of work-related burnout for nurses include working too many hours or at an accelerated pace with no respite, feeling unappreciated, giving too much to needy patients, trying to meet multiple demands of administrators, unrealistic commitment to work demands, and loss of balance with other life interests, lack of community with coworkers, and feeling resentment, in place of the meaning that work once held. Fig. 16.3 displays the symptoms of burnout.

Symptoms of Burnout

Khamisa and Peltzer Oldenburg (2013) note typical characteristics of burnout as emotional exhaustion, depersonalization, and a reduced sense of competence. Nurses experiencing burnout usually feel disillusioned and lack zest for their work. Other signs include loss of motivation and ideals, boredom or dissatisfaction at work, irritability and cynicism, resentment of expectations, and avoidance of meaningful encounters with patients and families. Headaches, gastric disturbances, skipping meals or eating compulsively on the run, feeling irritated by the intrusion of others, and a lack of balance between a nurse's work and personal life can signal the onset of burnout. In a study of coworkers' perceptions of colleagues suffering from

TABLE 16.3   ABCs of Burnout Prevention

Suggested Strategy	
Awareness	Use self-reflection and conversations with others to sort out priorities and identify parts of life out of balance. Recognize and allow feelings.
Balance	Maintain a healthy lifestyle. Balance care of others with self-care and self-renewal needs.
Choice	Differentiate between things you can change and those you cannot. Deliberately make choices that are purpose driven and meaningful.
Detachment	Detach from excessive ego involvement and personal ambition. Share responsibility and credit for care. Use meditation to center self.
Altruistic egoism	Take scheduled time for self, learn to say no, practice meditation, and develop outside interests that enrich the spirit.
Faith	Burnout is a malaise of the spirit. Trust in a higher power or purpose to center yourself when you do not know what will happen next.
Goals	Identify and develop realistic goals in line with your personal strengths. Seek feedback and support.
Hope	Hope is nurtured through conversations with others that lighten the burden and a belief in one's possibilities and personal worth in the greater scheme of things.
Integrity	Recognize that each of us is the only person who can determine the design and application of meaning in our lives.

Data from Arnold, E. (2008). Spirituality in educational and work environments. In V. Carson & H. Koenig (Eds.), *Spiritual dimensions of nursing practice* (revised ed., pp. 386–399). Conshohocken, PA: Templeton Foundation Press.

burnout, signs observed included a struggle to achieve unobtainable goals, wanting to manage alone, and becoming isolated from others (Ericson-Lidman & Strandberg, 2007).

Burnout Prevention Strategies

The ABCs of burnout prevention (Arnold, 2008) are presented in Table 16.3.

Reflecting on the sources of stress in your life puts boundaries on it. Think about your goals, and what is important to you. Seek opportunities to talk with trusted coworkers who can offer you the support and sensitivity you need to become aware of what is going on in your life—and *what steps you need to recharge of your life* so it is more fulfilling and meaningful. Then take the steps to make the changes needed. Self-care is one of the most effective mechanisms for coping with workplace stress (Cross, 2015).

A useful exercise is to imagine yourself a year from now, and ask yourself what do you need to do to be happy, a year from now? Identify the first step you need to take that will move you toward this goal. Then do it!

Identifying realistic, achievable goals in line with your personal values is an excellent burnout prevention strategy. Goals should be aligned with purpose and values.

Focusing on one thing at a time and finishing one project before starting another has several benefits. Achieving small related goals promotes self-efficacy and offers hope that more complex goals are achievable.

Give yourself a break! Maintaining a healthy balance between work, family, leisure, and lifelong learning activities enhances personal judgments, satisfaction, and productivity in all three spheres. Actively schedule a time for each of these activities and stick to it. You actually will be a better nurse if you choose a balanced life.

Remember, you always have choices, even it is to change your attitudes to allow "caring for yourself" as an essential part of providing excellent nursing care. People experiencing burnout lose sight of this fact. Life is a series of choices and negotiations. The choices we make help to create the fabric of our lives. Refusing to delegate work because someone else cannot do it as well or not going out to dinner with friends because you have too much work to do are choices.

Detachment from ego is a critical component of burnout prevention. It means that you do not allow emotional involvement in a task, or relationship undermine your own quality of life, values, and needs. Someone once asked Mother Teresa how she was able to remain so energetic and hopeful in the midst of the unrelenting suffering she encountered in

SIMULATION EXERCISE 16.6 Burnout Assessment

Purpose

To help students understand the symptoms of burnout.

Procedure

Consider your life over the past year. Complete the questionnaire by answering with a 5 if the situation is a constant occurrence, 4 if it occurs most of the time, 3 if it occurs occasionally, 2 if it has occurred once or twice during the last 6 months, and 1 if it is not a problem at all. Scores ranging from 60 to 75 indicate burnout. Scores ranging from 45 to 60 indicate you are stressed and in danger of developing burnout. Scores ranging from 20 to 44 indicate a normal stress level, and scores of less than 20 suggest that you are not a candidate for burnout.

1. Do you find yourself taking on or being overwhelmed by other people's problems?
2. Do you feel resentful about the amount or nature of claims on your time?
3. Do you find you have less time for social activities?
4. Have you lost your sense of humor?
5. Are you having trouble sleeping?
6. Do you find you are more impatient and less tolerant of others?
7. Is it difficult for you to say no?
8. Are the things that used to be important to you slipping away from you because you do not have time?
9. Do you feel a sense of urgency and not enough time to complete tasks?
10. Are you forgetting appointments, friends' birthdays?
11. Do you feel overwhelmed and unable to pace yourself?
12. Have you lost interest in intimacy?
13. Are you overeating or have you begun to skip meals?
14. Is it difficult to feel enthusiastic about your work?
15. Do you feel it is difficult to connect on a meaningful level with others?

Creating an Antidote to Burnout

Tally up your scores. Nursing school is a strong breeding ground for the development of burnout (demands exceed resources). To offset the possibility of developing burnout symptoms, do the following:

1. Think about the last time you took time for yourself. If you cannot think of a time, you really need to do this exercise.
2. Identify a leisure activity that you can do during the next week to break the cycle of burnout.
3. Describe the steps you will need to take to implement the activity.
4. Identify the time required for this activity and what other activities will need rearrangement to make it possible.
5. Describe any obstacles to implementing your activity and how you might resolve them.

Reflective Analysis Discussion

1. Was it difficult for you to come up with an activity? If so, why?
2. Were you able to develop a logical way to implement your activity?
3. Were the activities chosen by others or helpful to you in any way?
4. How might you be able to use this exercise in your future practice?

Calcutta. She replied that it was because she did the best she could and did not worry about the outcome because she could not control it. The same is true for the work that all nurses do. We can control our professional contribution to the care process, but not patient outcomes. It is important to pay as much attention to your own personal needs as you do to the needs of others. Although it seems obvious to do so, nurses sometimes consider attention to their own needs as being selfish, especially when the patient needs are worrying. However, one cannot give from an empty cupboard. Replenishing the self actually improves the quality of care a nurse can give to others.

Simulation Exercise 16.6 provides an opportunity to think about your personal burnout potential and ways to achieve better balance in your life.

Burnout challenges personal integrity when important values are ignored or devalued. When you begin to forget who you are and try to become what everyone else expects of you, you are in trouble. Reclaim yourself! Taking responsibility for you as a person *and* as a professional means that you respect yourself *and* your patient. Take the risk to be all that you are, as well as all that you can be, without worrying about what others think. Seek professional supports such as training, staff retreats, staff support networks, and job rotation to stimulate new ideas and insights. Professional support groups are effective as a means of providing encouragement to nurses in acute settings. Schedule times for fun and self-replenishment!

SUMMARY

This chapter focuses on the stress response in health care and supporting patient and family coping with stress through nurse-patient relationships. Stress can negatively impact patient outcomes, level of satisfaction with care, and compliance with treatment. A fundamental goal in the nurse-patient relationship is to empower patients and families with the knowledge, support, and resources they need to cope effectively with stress.

Stress is a part of everyone's life. Mild stress can be beneficial, but greater stress levels can be unhealthy. Concurrent and cumulative stresses increase the response level. Theoretical models address stress as a physiological response, as a stimulus, and as a transaction between person and environment. Factors that influence the development of a stress reaction include the nature of the stressor, personal interpretation of its meaning, number of previous and concurrent stressors, previous experiences with similar stressors, and availability of support systems and personal coping abilities.

People use problem- and emotion-focused coping strategies to minimize stress. Social support is key to effectively coping with stress. Assessment should focus on stress factors the person is experiencing, the context in which they occur, and identification of coping strategies. Supportive interventions include giving information, opportunities to express their feelings, thoughts, and worries, and anticipatory guidance.

Nurses are at the forefront of health care delivery to patients and families experiencing complex health and life issues. They too can experience stress and need support to do their job effectively. Burnout prevention requires recognition and resolution of organizational and personal factors contributing to job-related stress in professional nurses.

ETHICAL DILEMMA: What Would You Do?

The mother of a patient with acquired immunodeficiency syndrome (AIDS) does not know her son's diagnosis because her son does not want to worry her and fears her disapproval if she knew that he is gay. The mother asks the nurse if the family should have an oncology consult because she does not understand why, if her son has leukemia as he says he does, an oncologist is not seeing him. What should the nurse do?

DISCUSSION QUESTIONS

- What would you identify as tips for self-care to prevent the development of burnout?
- Stress is characterized by physical and emotional symptoms of tension. In what ways does stress manifest itself in your patient's behaviors?
- In what ways does stress manifest itself in your behavior as a student nurse?
- What are some of the stress management strategies you have tried or observed that seem to work better than others?

REFERENCES

Aldwin, C. M. (2010). Culture, coping and resilience to stress. In *Gross National Happiness and Development—Proceedings of the First International Conference on Operationalization of Gross National Happiness*. Thimphu: Centre for Bhutan Studies.

Aldwin, C. M., & Levenson, M. R. (2004). Posttraumatic growth: a developmental perspective. *Psychological Inquiry, 15*(1), 19–22.

American Psychological Association. (2007). *How does stress affect us?*. Retrieved from: http://psychcentral.com/lib/how-does-stress-affect-us/0001130.

Antoni, M. (2013). Psychosocial intervention effects on adaptation, disease course and biobehavioral processes in cancer. *Brain, Behavior, and Immunity, 30*(Suppl), S88–S98.

Arnold, E. (1997). The stress connection: Women and coronary heart disease. *Critical Care Nursing Clinics of North America, 9*(4), 565–575.

Arnold, E. (2008). Spirituality in educational and work environments. In V. Carson, & H. Koenig (Eds.), *Spiritual dimensions of nursing practice (revised ed* (pp. 368–399). Conshohocken, PA: Templeton Foundation Press.

Arrogante, O., & Aparicio-Zaldivar, E. (2017). Burnout and health among critical care professionals: the mediational role of resilience. *Intensive and Critical Care Nursing, 42*, 110–125.

Bayuo, J., & agbenorku, P. (2018). Coping strategies among nurses in the burn intensive unit A qualitative study. *Burns Open, 2*, 47–52.

Beck, J., & Beck, A. T. (2011). *Cognitive Behavior Therapy: Basics and beyond*. New York, NY: The Guilford Press.

Benson, H. (1975). *The relaxation response*. New York: Morrow.

Bippus, A., & Young, S. (2012). Using appraisal theory to predict emotional and coping responses to hurtful messages. *Interpersonal, 6*(2), 176–190.

Cannon, W. B. (1932). *The wisdom of the body*. New York: Norton Pub.

Chaboyer, W., James, H., & Kendall, M. (2005). Transitional care after the intensive care unit: current trends and future directions. *Critical Care Nurse, 25*, 16–28.

Compas, B., Connor-Smith, J., Thomsen, A., Salzman, H., & Wadsworth, M. (2001). Coping with stress during childhood and adolescence: progress, problems and potential in theory and research. *Psychological Bulletin, 127*, 87–127.

Cross, W. (2015). Building resilience in nurses: The need for a multiple pronged approach. *Journal of Nursing and Care, 4*, e124–e135.

Davidson, J., Powers, K., Hedayat, L., Tieszen, M., Kon, A., Shepard, E., et al. (2007). Clinical practice guidelines for support of the family in the patient-centered intensive care unit: American college of critical care medicine task force 2004–2005. *Critical Care Medicine, 35*(2), 605–622.

Davis, M., Eshelman, E., & McKay, M. (2008). *The relaxation and stress reduction workbook*. Oakland CA: New Harbinger Publications, Inc.

Dolbier, C., Smith, S., & Steinhardt, M. A. (2007). Relationships of protective factors to stress and symptoms of illness. *American Journal of Health Behavior, 31*(4), 423–433.

Ericson-Lidman, E., & Strandberg, G. (2007). Burnout: Co-workers' perceptions of signs preceding workmates' burnout. *Journal of Advanced Nursing, 60*(2), 199–208.

Folkman, S. (2008). The case for positive emotions in the stress process. *Anxiety Stress Coping, 21*(1), 3–14.

Freedman, R. (2008). Coping, resilience, and outcome. *American Journal of Psychiatry, 165*(12), 1505–1506.

Freudenberger, H. (1980). *Burn-out: The high cost of high achievement*. Garden City, NY: Doubleday.

Ganzel, B., Morris, P., & Wethington, E. (2010). Allostasis and the human brain: integrating models of stress from the social and life sciences. *Psychological Review, 117*(1), 134–174.

Garcia-Dia, M. J., DiNapoli, J. M., Garcia-Ona, L., Jakuboski, R., & O'Flaherty, D. (2013). Concept analysis: Resilience. *Archives of Psychiatric Nursing, 27*, 264–270.

Grillon, C. (2005). In B. Saddock, & V. Saddock (Eds.), *Anxiety disorders: Psychophysiological aspects* (pp. 1728–1739). Philadelphia, PA: Lippincott, Williams and Wilkins.

Haugland, T., Veenstra, M., Vatn, M., & Wahl, A. (2013). Improvement in stress, general self-efficacy and health related quality of life following patient education for patients with neuroendocrine tumors: a pilot study. *Nursing Research and Practice*. https://doi.org/10.1155/2013/695820. Epub 2013.

Hoff, L., Hallisey, B., & Hoff, M. (2009). *People in crisis: Clinical diversity perspectives* (6th ed.). New York, NY: Routledge.

Holmes, T. H., & Rahe, R. (1967). The social readjustment rating scale. *Journal of Psychosomatic Research, 11*, 213–218.

Huber, M., Knottnerus, J. A., Green, L., Van der Horst, H., Jadad, A. R., Leonard, B., et al. (2011). How should we define health? *British Medical Journal, 343*, d4163. https://doi.org/10.1135/bmj.

Jacobson, E. (1938). *Progressive relaxation*. University of Chicago: Chicago Press.

Jamieson, J., Nock, M., & Mendes, W. (2011). Mind over matter: Reappraising arousal improves cardiovascular and cognitive responses to stress. *The Journal of Experimental Psychology: Genera, 141*, 417–422 2011.

Jaser, S., Faulkner, M., Whittemore, R., Sangchoon, J., Murphy, K., Delamater, A., et al. (2012). Coping, self-management, and adaptation in adolescents with type 1 diabetes. *Annals of Behavioral Medicine, 43*(3), 311–319.

Keller, V., & Baker, L. (2000). Communicate with care. *Registered Nurse, 63*(1), 32–33.

Khamisa, N., & Peltzer Oldenburg, B. (2013). Burnout in relation to specific contributing factors and health outcomes among nurses: a systematic review. *International Journal of Environmental Research and Public Health, 10*(6), 2214–2240.

Kwekkeboom, K. (2008). Patients' perceptions of the effectiveness of guided imagery and progressive muscle relaxation. *Complementary Therapies in Clinical Practice, 14*(3), 185–194.

Lavoie, J. (2013). Eye of the beholder: Perceived stress, coping style, and coping effectiveness of discharged psychiatric patients. *Archives of Psychiatric Nursing, 27*, 185–190.

Lazarus, R. S., & Folkman, S. (1984, 1991). *Stress, appraisal and coping*. New York: Springer.

Leape, L., Bearwick, D., Clancy, C., Conway, J., Gluck, P., Guest, J., et al. (2009). Transforming health care: A safety imperative. *Quality & Safety in Health Care, 18*, 424–428.

Lehrer, P., Woolfolk, R., & Sime, W. (2007). *Principles and practice of stress management*. New York: Guilford Press.

Leske, J. (2002). Interventions to decrease family anxiety. *Critical Care Nursing, 22*(6), 61–65.

Lin, F. Y., Rong, J. R., & Lee, T. Y. (2013). Resilience among caregivers of children with chronic conditions: A concept analysis. *Journal of Multidisciplinary Healthcare, 6*, 324–333.

Marsiglia, F. F., Kulis, S., Garcia Perez, H., & Bermudez-Parsai, M. (2011). Hopelessness, family stress, and depression among Mexican-heritage mothers in the southwest. *Health & Social Work, 36*(1), 7–18.

Maybery, D. J., Neale, D., Arentz, A., & Jones-Ellis, J. (2007). The negative event scale: Measuring frequency and intensity of adult hassles. *Anxiety Stress Coping, 20*(2), 163–176.

McEwen, B. (2000). Allostasis, allostatic load, and the aging nervous system: Role of excitatory amino acids and excito-toxicity. *Neurochemical Research, 9*(10), 1219–1231.

McEwen, B. (2007). Physiology and neurobiology of stress and adaptation: Central role of the brain. *Physiological Reviews*, *87*(3), 873–904.

McEwen, B. (2012). Brain on stress: How the social environment gets under the skin. *Proceedings of the National Academy of Sciences of the United States of America*, *109*(Suppl. 2), 17180–17185.

Meyers, D. (2011). *Psychology in everyday life*. New York, NY: Worth Publications.

Moeini, M., Taleghani, F., Mehrabi, T., & Musarzale, A. (2014). Effects of a spiritual care program on levels of anxiety in patients with leukemia. *Iranian Journal of Nursing and Midwifery Research*, *19*(1), 88–93.

Pearlin, L., & Schooler, C. (1978). The structure of coping. *Journal of Health and Social Behavior*, *19*, 2–21.

Pearlin, L.I. (1989). The sociological study of stress. *Journal of Health and Social Behavior*, *30*(3), 241–256.

Rao, N., Varambally, S., & Gangadhar, B. (2013). Yoga school of thought and psychiatry: Therapeutic potential. *Indian Journal of Psychiatry*, *55*(Suppl. 2), S145–S149.

Reich, J., Zautra, A., & Hall, J. (2010). *Handbook of adult resilience*. New York, NY: Guilford.

Richards, M., & Steele, R. (2007). Children's self-reported coping strategies: the role of defensiveness and repressive adaptation. *Anxiety Stress Coping*, *20*(2), 209–222.

Samuel-Hodge, C., Watkins, D., Rowell, K., & Hooten, E. G. (2008). Coping styles, well-being and self-care behaviors among African Americans with type 2 diabetes. *Diabetes Education*, *34*(3), 501–510.

Schacter, D., Gilbert, D., & Wegner, D. (2010). *Psychology* (2nd ed.). New York: Worth.

Schieveld, J. (2009). On grief and despair versus resilience and personal growth in critical illness. *Intensive Care Medicine*, *35*, 779–780.

Schwarzer, R., & Knoll, N. (2007). Functional roles of social support within the stress and coping process. *International Journal of Psychology*, *42*(4), 243–252.

Selye, H. (1950). Stress and the general adaptation syndrome. *British Medical Journal*, *4667*, 1383–1392.

Sinha, B., & Watson, D. (2007). Stress, coping and psychological illness: a cross-cultural study. *International Journal of Stress Management*, *14*(4), 386–397.

Skinner, E., Edge, K., Altman, J., & Sherwood, H. (2003). Searching for the structure of coping: A review and critique of category systems for classifying ways of coping. *Psychological Bulletin*, *129*(2), 216–269.

Taylor, S. E., Welch, W., Kim, H. S., & Sherman, D. K. (2007). Cultural differences in the impact of social support on psychological and biological stress responses. *Psychological Science*, *18*, 831–837.

Thoits, P. (2010). In W. Avison, et al. *Compensatory Coping With Stressors*, 23–34.

Wagland, R., Fenlon, D., Tarrant, R., Howard-Jones, G., & Richardson, A. (2015). Rebuilding self-confidence after cancer: a feasibility study of life-coaching. *Support Care Cancer*, *23*(3), e651–e659.

Wittenberg-Lyles, E. (2012). *Communication in Palliative Nursing*. New York: Oxford University Press.

SUGGESTED READING

American Psychological Association. (2012). *Stress in America: Missing the health care connection*. Retrieved from: https://www.apa.org/news/press/releases/stress/2012/full- report.pdf.

American Psychological Association. (2013). *Stress in America: Are teens adopting adults' stress habits?*. Retrieved from: http://www.apa.org/news/press/releases/stress/2013/stress-report.pdf.

Berry, J. W. (2005). Acculturation: Living successfully in two cultures. *International Journal of Intercultural Relations*, *29*(6), 697–712. https://doi.org/10.1016/j.ijintrel.2005.07.013.

Boss, P. (2011). *Loving someone who has dementia: How to find hope while coping with stress and grief*. San Francisco, CA: Jossey-Bass.

Bourne, E. J. (2010). *The anxiety and phobia workbook*. Oakland, CA: New Harbinger.

Brown, K. W., Ryan, R. M., & Creswell, J. D. (2007). Mindfulness: Theoretical foundations and evidence for its salutary effects. *Psychological Inquiry*, *18*(4), 211–237.

Carmody, J., & Baer, R. A. (2008). Relationships between mindfulness practice and levels of mindfulness, medical and psychological symptoms and well-being in a mindfulness-based stress reduction program. *Journal of Behavioral Medicine*, *31*(1), 23–33.

Earvolino-Ramirea, M. (2007). Resilience: A concept analysis. *Nursing Forum*, *42*, 73–82.

Fink, G. (2017). Stress: Concepts, definition and history. In *Reference Module in Neuroscience and Biobehavioral Psychology*. St Louis, MO: Elsevier.

Gessler, R., & Ferron, L. (2012). When caregiving ignites burnout—New ways to douse the flames. *American Nurse Today*, 7.

Grazzi, L., & Andrasik, F. (2010). Non-pharmacological approaches in migraine prophylaxis: Behavioral medicine. *Neurological Sciences*, *31*(Suppl. 1), S133–S135.

Hart, P. L., Brannan, J., & De Chesnay, M. (2014). Resilience in nurses: an integrative review. *Journal of Nursing Management*, *22*, 720–734.

Jackson, D., Firtko, A., & Edenborough, M. (2007). Personal resilience as a strategy for surviving and thriving in the face of workplace adversity: A literature review. *Journal of Advanced Nursing*, *60*, 1–9.

Miller, G., & Wrosch, C. (2007). You've gotta know when to fold them. *Psychological Science*, *18*, 773–777.

Park, E. R., Traeger, L., Vranceanu, A. M., Scult, M., Lerner, J. A., Benson, H., et al. (2013). The development of a patient-centered program based on the relaxation response: The relaxation response resiliency program (3RP). *Psychosomatics*, *54*, 165–174.

Posadzki, P., & Jacques, S. (2014). Tai chi and meditation: A conceptual (re)synthesis. *Journal of Holistic Nursing*, *27*(2), 103–114.

Strachan, P., Currie, K., Harkness, K., Spaling, M., & Clark, M. (2014). Context matters in heart failure self-care: A qualitative systematic review. *Journal of Cardiac Failure*, *20*(6), 448–455.

Tay, L., Tan, K., Diener, E., & Gonzalez, E. (2013). Social relations, health behaviors, and health outcomes: A survey and synthesis. *Applied Psychology: Health and Well Being*, *5*(1), 28–78.

Communicating With Patients Experiencing Communication Deficits

Kathleen Underman Boggs

OBJECTIVES

At the end of the chapter, the reader will be able to:

1. Describe nursing strategies for communicating with patients experiencing communication deficits secondary to visual, auditory, cognitive, or stimuli-related disabilities or that are treatment related.
2. Describe a specific communication deficit advocacy issue for nurses.
3. Access evidence-based databases for communication deficits and discuss application of these evidence-based practices and research findings to your clinical practice.

Communication is necessary for safe health care, but this can be problematic for patients with communication impairments (Sharpe & Hemsley, 2016). An inability to communicate leaves patients at risk for unsafe situations and preventable adverse events (Rodriguez et al., 2016; Yuksel & Unver, 2016). Access to appropriate health care providers occurs less often, because people with communication deficits are more likely to forego needed care (Barnett et al., 2017). For some, the underlying problem is related to physiological impairments making it difficult to communicate their needs. This chapter presents an overview of communication difficulties commonly encountered when caring for patients with communication deficits. Most nurses will be challenged with caring for patients with specialized communication problems. Consider the following case of Private Tim Dakota.

Case Example: Private Tim Dakota

Private Tim Dakota, age 22 years, is 3 weeks post-traumatic brain injury and has been a patient in your neurological intensive care unit for 2 weeks.

Nurse: Good morning, Tim Dakota. I am Sue Nance, your nurse for this fine Sunday morning. I am going to give you your bath now. The water will feel a little warm to you. After your bath, your wife will be in to see you. She stayed in the waiting room last night because she wanted to be with you. (No answer is necessary if the patient is unable to talk, but the sound of a human voice and attention to his unspoken concerns can be very healing.)

Summary of the strategies this nurse used:

- Called Tim by name
- Introduced self
- Established time (date, time, place would be better)
- Explained procedure before beginning
- Changed his position frequently

Changing the patient's position frequently benefits the person physiologically and offers us something to talk about. Recovered patients have reported that our efforts to create a more stimulating environment, to offer reassurance and support, have later been reported to have been meaningful to the patient.

The United Nations has affirmed the rights of those with communication problems, among all disabled (n.d. [no date]). As we strive to meet our Quality and Safety Education for Nurses (QSEN) competency of coordinating patient-centered care, we are also charged with using our skills to communicate their needs to the other members of the health care team. In this chapter, we describe strategies for enhancing communication for this population.

BASIC CONCEPTS

A communication deficit is an impairment in the ability to receive, send, process, and comprehend concepts or verbal, nonverbal, and graphic symbol systems, as defined by the American Speech-Language-Hearing Association (ASHA, 1993). These include deficits such as compromised hearing, vision, speech, or language or problems with cognitive processing. They may be congenital or acquired; they range from mild to severe. Severe cognitive and sensory deficits interfere with communication, decrease access to health care, and lead to feelings of frustration. Globally health conditions related to communication deficits are much more prevalent in developing countries. Many of the physical conditions are preventable or treatable, if only health care were accessible. Worldwide, more than a billion people, or 15% of the population, have some form of disability (World Health Organization [WHO], 2017). Nearly one in six Americans, nearly 50 million people (US Department of Health and Human Services, n.d.), has a sensory or communication deficit. Improving access to care for these people is one of the goals of *Healthy People 2020*. Many of these individuals report delays or difficulties obtaining health care.

In 2001 the WHO's International Classification of Functioning, Disability, and Health shifted away from a medical diagnosis model to a functional model (i.e., how people with a sensory impairment function in their daily lives). Under this model, a communication disability definition includes any person who has any impairment in body structure or function that interferes with communication. Specifically, the patient has a communication difficulty because of impaired functioning of one or more of the five senses or has impaired cognitive processing functioning. Communication deficits can also arise from the kind of sensory deprivation that occurs in some agencies and units, such as intensive care units (ICUs). The degree of difficulty in communicating is an interaction between the patient's type of functional impairment, personal adaptability, and the health care environment (i.e., body factors, personal factors, and environmental factors as stated in WHO's model).

Any impairment of patients' abilities to send and/or receive information from health care providers may compromise their health, safety, health care, and rights to make decisions. When working with patients having communication disabilities, you may need to modify communication strategies presented earlier in this textbook. Assess *every* patient's communication abilities. Two individuals can have the same sensory impairment but not be equally communication disabled. Each person compensates for his or her impairment in different ways.

Goal

Our primary nursing goal is to maximize our patient's ability to successfully communicate and to interact with the health care system to ensure optimal health and quality of life. Evidence shows us that when nurses are unable to understand them, patients with communication disabilities become frustrated, angry, anxious, depressed, or uncertain. Some become so frustrated that they exhibit behavioral problems or even omit needed care. Even when care is accessed, communication deficits interfere with the therapeutic relationship and delivery of optimum care. The patient's deficit is one barrier, but other barriers may include staff's negative attitude or inability to adapt communication.

LEGAL MANDATES

In the legal system, the standard of "effective communication" is based on statutes. Many countries have laws against discrimination similar to the Americans with Disabilities Act (ADA) which prohibit discrimination on the basis of a disability.

HOME-BASED HEALTH CARE

Visiting patients with communication deficits in their home allows nurses the time to engage in collaborative negotiations for which there may not have been time during acute care management. Home health nurses can build the infrastructure needed to prevent worsening of disability, as demonstrated in a study of elders by Liebel (2012).

TYPES OF DEFICITS

Hearing Loss

Hearing loss is a common problem, with approximately 15% of the world's population reporting trouble hearing (NIDCD, 2016). Globally, approximately 360 million, or 5%, have disabling hearing loss, defined as loss greater than 40 decibels (WHO, 2017). More than half of hearing loss is preventable.

More than 28 million Americans have some problem hearing. Loss can be conductive, sensorineural, or functional. Causes can be genetic, congenital, or acquired, such as due to infections, medication toxicity, or even to exposure to excessive noise, such as occurs in combat. Hearing

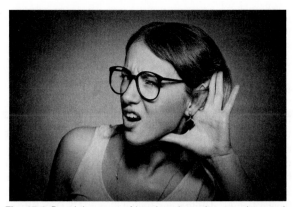

Fig. 17.1 People's sense of hearing alerts them to changes in the environment so they can respond effectively. (Copyright © Slphotography/iStock/Thinkstock.)

losses, especially in higher ranges, are most often found in older-aged patients, with approximately 50% of those older than 75 years and 80% of those older than 85 years affected (Blazer, Domnitz, & Liverman, 2013; NIDCD, 2016; also see Chapter 19). Nurses have both a legal and ethical obligation to provide appropriate care. People who have hearing loss from birth learn American Sign Language (ASL) as their first language. Think of them as folks for whom English is a second language. They may be unable to read health handouts written in English. Title III of the ADA delineates rights of the deaf and applies to communication between deaf clients and medical services.

People's sense of hearing alerts them to changes in the environment so they can respond effectively (Fig. 17.1). The listener hears sounds and words and also a speaker's vocal pitch, loudness, and intricate inflections accompanying the verbalization. Subtle variations can completely change the sense of the communication. Combined with the sound and intensity, the organization of the verbal symbols allows individuals to perceive and interpret the meaning of the sender's message. The extent of your patient's loss is not always appreciated because they often look and act in a normal fashion. Even mild to moderate hearing losses can lead to significant functional impairments (George, Farrell, & Griswold, 2012). Deprived of a primary means of receiving signals from the environment, patients with hearing loss may try to hide deficits, withdraw from relationships, become depressed, or be less likely to seek information from health care providers. Millions could benefit from hearing aids yet have never used them (NIDCD, 2016).

Children

Nearly 3 of every 1000 newborns are deaf or have hearing loss (US Department of Health and Human Services, n.d.). Fortunately, many of these deficits are diagnosed at birth.

Newborn hearing is tested in the nursery via auditory brainstem response tests (see the National Institute on Deafness and Other Communication Disorders website at www.nidcd.nih.gov).

Older Adults

As we age, we have an increased likelihood for *presbycusis*, or degeneration of ear structures, which is a sensorineural dysfunction that normally occurs with aging.

Vision Loss

Humans rely more heavily on vision than do most species. Globally, vision problems occur in approximately 285 million people; 180 million are visually disabled. The majority of these would be treatable if care were accessible (WHO, 2001). The WHO has mounted a call for global action to promote eye care, "Vision 2020."

Nearly 5 million Americans are blind or have uncorrectable visual impairments (National Eye Institute, n.d.). In addition to total loss, visual impairment is defined as at least 3/60 or having less than a 20-degree visual field (McGrath, Rudman, Polgar, & Spafford, 2016). The majority of these are older than 50 years of age. People who lack vision lose a primary method to decode the meaning of messages. All of the nonverbal cues that accompany speech communication (e.g., facial expression, nodding, and leaning toward the patient) are lost to those who are blind. Even with partial loss, it is important for you to assess whether your patient can read directions, medication labels, and so forth.

Children

Children with visual impairments lack access to visual cues, such as the facial expressions that encourage them to develop communication skills. The United States Preventive Services Task Force (USPSTF) recommends testing children younger than 5 years for amblyopia, strabismus, and acuity, but traditional vision screening requires a verbal child and cannot be done reliably until age 3 years.

Older Adults

As we age, the lens of the eye becomes less flexible, making it difficult to accommodate shifts from far to near vision; this is a condition known as *presbyopia*. Macular degeneration has also become a major cause of vision loss in older adults.

Impaired Verbal Communication Secondary to Speech and Language Deficits

A speech disorder involves impaired articulation, whereas a language disorder is impaired comprehension or use of spoken sounds (ASLHA, 2013). Patients who have speech and language deficits resulting from neurological trauma present a different type of communication problem. Normal communication allows people to perceive and interact with the world in an organized and systematic manner. People use language to express self-need and to control environmental events. Language is the system people rely on to represent what they know about the world. Early identification of children with at-risk prelinguistic skills may allow intervention to improve communication competencies. Patients unable to speak, even temporarily because of intubation or ventilator dependency, incur feelings of frustration, anxiety, fear, or even panic.

When the ability to process and express language is disrupted, many areas of functioning are assaulted simultaneously. *Aphasia* is a neurological linguistic deficit, such as occurs after a stroke. Aphasia can present as primarily an expressive or receptive disorder. The person with *expressive aphasia* can understand what is being said but cannot express thoughts or feelings in words.

Receptive aphasia creates difficulties in receiving and processing written and oral messages. With *global aphasia*, the patient has difficulty with both expressive language and reception of messages. Your patient may have feelings of loss and social isolation imposed by the communication impairment. Although there may be no cognitive impairment, they may need more "think time" for cognitive processing during a conversation.

Impaired Cognitive Processing

Impaired cognitive processing ability can interfere with the communication process and leads to anxiety and confusion. Understanding involves receiving new information and integrating it meaningfully with prior knowledge. Individuals with impaired processing ability have to work harder and require more time for conceptual integration. The responsibility for assessing ability to understand, to give consent, and to overcome communication difficulties rests with both social services and health care workers. You need to continually determine the extent of your patients' understanding and even their ability to understand self-care activities. Assess their use of alternative communication aids.

Children

Because there is a significant increase in the prevalence of children with developmental disabilities, more nurses will be caring for them both in clinical agencies and in the community (Betz, 2012). Atypical communication is often the first behavioral clue to cognitive impairment in young children, associated with conditions such as mental retardation, autism, and affective disorders. As these children grow, subtle distortions in communication may exist.

Older Adults

Cognitively impaired older clients may have altered communication pathways. Although most older adults retain

their mental acuity, we need to assess risks. For example, memory loss can interfere with ability to correctly take prescribed medications.

Communication Deficits Associated With Some Mental Disorders

Patients with serious mental disorders may have a different type of communication deficit resulting from a malfunctioning of the neurotransmitters that normally transmit and make sense out of messages in the brain. Global incidence is unknown but is estimated as affecting 400 million by the WHO, which has made mental health a part of their 2030 goals (WHO, 2017). Thirteen million Americans have a serious, debilitating mental illness (US Department of Health and Human Services, n.d.), as do 20% of children and adolescents (Agency for Healthcare and Quality [AHRQ], 2016). Some of these have communication difficulties. In addition to illness-related communication problems, social isolation and impaired coping may accompany your patient's inability to receive or express language signals.

Mental Illness

Communication problems occur with different mental disorders. As an example, some patients with mental disorders can perhaps have intact sensory channels, but they cannot process and respond appropriately to what they hear, see, smell, or touch. In some forms of *schizophrenia* there are alterations in the biochemical neurotransmitters in the brain, which normally conduct messages between nerve cells and help to orchestrate the person's response to the external environment. Messages have distorted meanings. It is beyond the scope of this text to discuss psychosis. Some patients with mental disorders present with a poverty of speech and limited content. Speech appears blocked, reflecting disturbed patterns of perception, thought, emotions, and motivation. You may notice a lack of vocal inflection and an unchanging facial expression. A "flat affect" makes it difficult for you to truly understand. Illogical thinking processes may manifest in the form of illusions, hallucinations, and delusions. Common words assume new meanings known only to the person experiencing them.

Dementia

An increasing percentage of people, especially older adults, develop dementia, including Alzheimer disease, affecting their ability to communicate. Communication skill training is recommended especially for family members (Mamo et al., 2017; Memory Matters, interview, March 7, 2017), and for all staff employed in extended care facilities (Fig. 17.2). Some communication strategies are listed in Table 17.1.

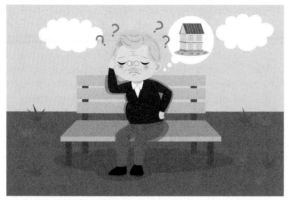

Fig. 17.2 Patients with dementia may need assistance with cognitive processing. (Copyright © Lin Shao-hua/iStock/Thinkstock.)

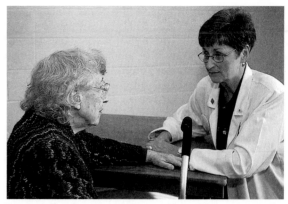

Fig. 17.3 Touch, eye movement and sounds can be used to communicate with patients experiencing aphasia.

TABLE 17.1 **Tips for Communicating With Patients Who Have Dementia**
The literature lacks agreement on definitions of dementia and little empirical backing for communication interventions, rather these suggestions are based on expert opinion (Machiels, Metzelthin, Hamers, & Zwakhalen, 2017)
• Gain your patient's attention before speaking (face the patient)
• Use your active listening skills, especially eye contact
• Use brief sentences (fewer words)
• Speak clearly and slightly slowly
• Use more nonverbal cues
• Observe your patient for his or her nonverbal cues
• Use positive reinforcement (keep messages short and sweet)
• Use familiar objects to give cues, such as holding up a hairbrush when you want to groom the head
• Use "memory books" or family photos, especially when patient keeps asking about someone
• Verify patient's understanding by having him or her restate (summarize not just repeat).

Environmental Deprivation as Related to Illness

Communication is particularly important in nursing situations characterized by sensory deprivation, physical immobility, limited environmental stimuli, or excessive, constant stimuli (Fig. 17.3). Nurses show sensitivity for patients in bewildering situations, such as emergency departments or ICUs. Patients may be frightened, in pain, and unable to communicate easily with others because of intubation or other complications.

Fig. 17.4 The following are situational factors that affect *patient* responses to critical care hospital situations:
- Anxiety and fear
- Pain
- Altered stimuli—too much or too little, including unusual noises and isolation
- Sleep deprivation
- Unmet physiological needs such as thirst
- Losing track of time
- Multiple life changes
- Multiple care providers
- Immobility
- Frequent diagnostic procedures
- Lack of easily understood information

Absent Stimulation

Patients who are immobile, isolated, or intubated, such as in ICUs, often experience absence of stimulation resulting in gradual decline of cognitive abilities. Patients with normal intellectual capacity can appear dull, uninterested, and lacking in problem-solving abilities if they do not have frequent interpersonal stimulation (Fig. 17.4).

Pain. When assessing pain in patients with communication disabilities, it is difficult to be exact with "yes/no" nodding. Critical care nurses have validated use of a number of pain assessment graphic assessment scales such as FACES (Rahu et al., 2015). Never assume a nonverbal patient is cognitively impaired (Booker & Haedtke, 2016).

Applications

Communication deficits may be developmental or acquired. The emphasis on patient-centered care embodies a need for those with communication deficits to become active participants in their care.

Developing an Evidence-Based Practice

Access some of the many databases that summarize research to compile "best practice" guidelines for adapting communication, especially pertinent for those who have communication deficits. Most sites rank the strength of the research evidence from strong to poor. Access www.guideline.gov/content.aspx?id=34160&search=best+evidence+statement+multiple+means for the "best evidence statement" (BESt). They offer suggestions such as using active verbs and short sentences with all patients having communication deficits. Another suggestion is to supplement your oral information with visual aids such as picture, PowerPoint presentations, or videos.

For another Evidence Based Practice (EBP) scenario, consider that thousands of babies born each year have totally preventable birth defects. Some are the result of the pregnant mother taking medications (teratogenic side effects, category D medication). According to Schwarz (2013), it is estimated that 12 million American women are prescribed medications annually that increase risk for birth defects. A common example is prescription of fluconazole [Diflucan] for vaginal yeast infection. Several studies found many prescribers did not counsel women who were pregnant or who wanted to become pregnant to use contraceptives while on this medication, despite alerts from their clinical decision support system warning of potential harm (Howley et al., 2016; Schwarz, 2013). Compounding the problem, women, especially teens, often have unplanned pregnancies. Therefore they do not have a prenatal health plan, such as taking folic acid to decrease likelihood of neurotube defects in their babies. Pediatricians are the primary providers for adolescents, yet the study by Kaskowitz et al. (2017) found many do not view prescribing contraception as their responsibility.

APPLICATION TO YOUR CLINICAL PRACTICE

How can nurses help prevent birth defects? Make a list of possible interventions you could apply in practice such as compiling each patient's medication list and assessing them for possible teratogenic side effects, then determining whether your patient is acting to prevent conception. If they are teens, consider using more effective methods for teaching contraception such as using a multimedia, developmental counseling strategy.

In a hospital, all staff need to be aware of the patient's communication disability, perhaps by posting a sign or symbol on the door. Mutual goals involve fostering effective communication with all members of the health team. Nurses with heavy workloads do not always choose to take the time to find alternative communication strategies, sometimes opting just to avoid direct communication, leading to high patient frustration levels. Even when we are aware of a patient's communication deficit, we sometimes lack the ability to communicate effectively. Applying communication accommodation theory, nurses can choose to use strategies in boxes in this chapter. A variety of communication devices are available to assist in communication. Always let your patients know when you cannot understand their communication.

EARLY RECOGNITION OF COMMUNICATION DEFICITS

Identification of communication deficit is one aspect of your role. For example, if a 4-year-old child fails to speak at all or uses a noticeably limited vocabulary for his or her age and cannot name objects or follow your directions, would you recognize the need for further assessment? Given this history, you could urge the health team to make a referral for speech and language evaluation.

ASSESSMENT OF CURRENT COMMUNICATION ABILITIES

Are you assessing each patient for communication problems? Do you tailor you plan of care to help meet identified communication needs? Provision of alternative communication methods is a legal requirement.

COMMUNICATION STRATEGIES

Specific strategies are contained in the accompanying boxes. In general, evidence-based practice suggests you create a quiet environment, allocate more of your time to facilitate communication, take time to listen, ask yes/no questions, observe nonverbal cues, repeat back comments, effectively use communication equipment, assign same staff for care continuity, and encourage family members to be present to assist in communications (access www.AHRQ.gov).

Mobile App use to communicate. Handheld devices such as smartphones have downloadable applications (apps) which provide picture-to-speech or text-to-speech options. An Australian study reported mixed attitudes from nurses regarding this. Nurses expressed concern about their time constraints, device security, and patient conditions/ability to use. On the other hand, they acknowledged mobile Apps could aid in more complex communication than picture boards and could improve communication (Sharpe & Hemsley, 2016). Rodriguez et al. (2016), in a study of American critical care units, tested customized recorded messages and words on tablets. All but two subjects reported higher satisfaction with communication and less frustration than those in the control group. Chapter 26 will discuss use of mobile technology for communication.

Patients With Hearing Loss

Assessment of functional hearing ability is recommended for all your patients. Assessment of auditory sensory losses can provide an opportunity for referral. Your assessment should include the age of onset and the severity of the deficit. Hearing loss that occurs after the development of speech means that the patient has access to word symbols and language skills. Deafness in children can cause developmental delays, which may need to be taken into account in planning the most appropriate communication strategies. Clues to hearing loss occur when people appear unresponsive to sound or respond only when the speaker is directly facing them. Ask patients whether they use a hearing aid and whether it is working properly.

Strategies for communicating with patients who have a hearing loss depend on the severity of the deafness. Covering your face with a mask or speaking with an accent may make it impossible for a lip reader to understand you. Communication-assisting equipment should be available. We need to know how to operate auditory amplifiers such as assisted listening devices, hearing aids, and telephone attachments. Often, patients have hearing aids but fail to use them unless family or nurses assists them. Simulation Exercises 17.1 and 17.2 will help you to understand what it is like to have a sensory deficit. Refer to Box 17.1 to adapt

---

SIMULATION EXERCISE 17.1   Loss of Sensory Function in Geriatric Populations

Purpose:
To assist students in getting in touch with the feelings often experienced by older adults as they lose sensory function. If the younger individual is able to "walk in the older person's shoes," he or she will be more sensitive to the losses and needs created by those losses in the older person.

Procedure:
1. The class separates into three groups.
2. Group A: Place cotton balls in your ears. Group B: Cover your eyes with drugstore glasses covered in Vaseline. Group C: Place kernels of hard corn in your shoes to simulate walking with arthritis. A student from group B should be approached by a student from group A. The student from group B is to talk to the student from group A using a whispered voice. The group A student is to verify the message heard with the student who spoke. The student from group B is then to identify the student from group A.
3. The students in group C are expected to make a statement to the others and have that individual retell what they were told.

Reflective Analysis:
1. Explain how the loss you experienced during the activity made you feel. Be sure to describe your comfort level while performing the functions expected of you with your limitation.
2. Evaluate this experience to determine what you think could have been done to make you feel less disabled?
3. Critique and justify how you would feel if "normal" level of functioning was restored, and how you would feel if it was permanent.
4. Construct a response that explains how the knowledge gained from this chapter impacts your future interactions with individuals who have sensory loss.

---

your communication techniques. Consider the case of Timmy.

Case Example: Timmy

Two student nurses were assigned to care for 9-year-old Timmy, who is deaf and mute. When they went into his room for assessment, he was alone and appeared anxious. No information was available as to his ability to read lips, the nurses were not sure what reading skills he had, and they did not know sign language. So, instead of using a pad and paper for communication, they decided to role-play taking vital signs by using some funny facial expressions and demonstrating on a doll.

Patients With Vision Loss

Vision assessment for impairment is recommended for all patients routinely. Nurses caring for anyone with vision limitations should perform some evaluation and ensure that glasses and other equipment are available to hospitalized patients. Refer to Box 17.1 for strategies of use in caring for those with vision impairments. Use of vocal cues (e.g., speaking as you approach) helps prevent startling. Because the visually impaired cannot see our faces or observe our nonverbal signals, we need to use words to express what they cannot see in the message. It also is helpful to mention your name as you enter the patent's presence. Even people who are partially blind appreciate hearing the name of the person to whom they are speaking. Communication-enhancing equipment for the vision impaired includes electronic magnifier machines, auditory teaching materials, and computer screen readers with voice synthesizers, Braille keypads or cards, and video magnifying machines.

When caring for patients with macular degeneration, remember to stand to their side, an exception to the "face them directly" rule applied with patients with hearing loss. Macular degeneration patients often still have some peripheral vision. Enhanced lighting and use of light filters to reduce glare may help you to communicate with those who have reduced vision.

With blind patients, the use of touch acts as a social reinforcer and can orient them to your presence. However, use of verbal greetings may better alert your patients. Voice tones and pauses that reinforce the verbal content are helpful. They need to be informed when you are leaving the room. Consider the following case of Ms. Shu.

SIMULATION EXERCISE 17.2 Sensory Loss: Hearing or Vision

Purpose:
To help raise consciousness regarding loss of a sensory function.

Procedure:
- Pair up with another student. One student should be blindfolded. The other student should guide the "blind" student on a walk around the campus.
- During a 5- to 10-minute walk, the student guide should converse with the "blind" student about the route they are taking.
  or
- Watch the first 2 minutes of a television show with the sound turned off. All students should watch the same show (e.g., the news report or a rerun of a situation comedy).
- In class, students share observations and answer the following questions.

Discussion:
1. Determine perceptual differences experienced during this exercise. Describe any frustrations experienced and how this made you feel.
2. Evaluate the implications these differences have in working with blind or deaf patients.
3. Appraise what you have learned about yourself from this exercise, and share how you would apply this knowledge to your nursing practice.

Case Example: Ms. Shu

You can use words to supply additional information to counterbalance the missing visual cues. Ms. Sue Shu is a blind, elderly patient who commented to the student nurse Ruth that she felt Ruth was uncomfortable talking with her and perhaps did not like her. Not being able to see Ruth, Ms. Shu interpreted the hesitant uneasiness in Ruth's voice as evidence that Ruth did not wish to be with her. Ruth agreed with Ms. Shu that she was quite uncomfortable but did not explain further. Had Ms. Shu been able to see Ruth's apprehensive body posture, she would have realized that Ruth was quite shy and ill at ease with *any* interpersonal relationship. To avoid this serious error in communication, Ruth might have clarified the reasons for her discomfort, and the relationship could have moved forward.

Orientation to Environmental Hazards

When a blind person is being introduced to a new environmental setting, you should orient them by describing the size of the room and the position of the furniture and equipment. When placing your patient's food tray, describe the position of items, perhaps using a clock face analogy (e.g., "Carrots are at 2 o'clock, potatoes at 11 o'clock"). If other people are present, you could name each person. A good communication strategy is to ask the other people in

BOX 17.1 Suggestions for Helping the Patient With Sensory Loss

- Assess psychological readiness to communicate.
- Introduce yourself and convey respect, an understanding of patient frustrations, and your willingness to communicate.
- Be concise.
- Always maximize the use of sensory aids, such as communication boards, pictures, sign language, and electronic aids.
- Pick the means of available communication best suited to your patient. Multiple pathways using both audio and visual are standard recommendations.
- Always help patients to use their assistive equipment (adjust hearing aids, glasses, smartphones for texting, etc.).
- Assess the patient's understanding of what was said by having them signal or repeat the message.

For Hearing-Impaired Patients

- Tap on the floor or table to get the patient's attention via the vibration.
- Communicate in a well-lighted room and face the patient, so they focus their attention, see your facial expression, and watch your lips move.
- Choose a quiet, private place; close doors and turn off TVs or radios to decrease environmental noise.
- Use facial expressions, hand signals, and gestures that reinforce verbal content, or request a sign language interpreter, perhaps a family member.
- Speak distinctly without exaggerating words or shouting. Partially deaf patients respond best to well-articulated words spoken in a moderate, even tone. Speak only as loudly as you need to.

- Write important ideas and allow the patient the same option to increase the chances of communication. Always have a writing pad or smartphone available.
- Arrange for a TTY or an amplified telephone handset for those with partial hearing loss, if they do not text.
- If the patient is unable to hear, rely primarily on visual materials.
- Arrange for closed-captioned television.
- Use text messaging, e-mail, and Apps on patient's phone.
- Encourage the patient with hearing loss to verbalize speech, even if the person uses only a few words or the words are difficult to understand at first.
- Use an intermediary, such as a family member who knows sign language, to facilitate communication with deaf patients who sign.

For Vision-Impaired Patients

- Let the person know when you approach by identifying yourself, use a simple touch, and always indicate when you are leaving.
- Adapt communication to compensate for lack of nonverbal messaging.
- Adapt teaching for low vision by using large print, audio information, or Braille.
- Do not lead or hold the patient's arm when walking; instead, allow the person to take your arm.
- Use touch and close physical proximity while you are with the client; give the person something substantial to touch in your absence.
- Develop and use signals to indicate changes in pace or direction while walking.

TTY, Teletypewriter.

the room to introduce themselves. In this way, he or she gains an appreciation for their voice configurations. You should avoid any tendency to speak with a blind patient in a louder voice than usual or to enunciate words in an exaggerated manner. This may be perceived by some as insensitive to the nature of the handicap. Voice tones should be kept natural.

A blind patient may need guidance in moving around in unfamiliar surroundings. For example, surveyed blind people said they needed assistance getting to and from their bathroom. One way of preserving autonomy is to offer your arm to them instead of taking their arm. Mention steps and changes in movement as they are about to occur to help them go new places with differences in terrain. Some blind people use wearable navigation systems.

Impaired Verbal Communication Secondary to Speech and Language Deficits

Assessment of speech and language is part of the initial evaluation. Difficulties arise when people are unable to speak (**aphasia**). For these, an assessment of the type of disorder experienced will aid in selecting the most appropriate intervention. Expressive language problems are evidenced in an inability to find words or to associate ideas with accurate word symbols. Some with **expressive aphasia** can find the correct word if given enough time and support. Others have difficulty organizing their words into meaningful sentences or describing a sequence of events. Individuals with receptive communication deficits have trouble following directions, reading information, writing, or relating data to previous knowledge. Even when your patient appears not to understand, you should explain in simple terms what is happening. Using touch, gestures, eye movements, and squeezing of the hand should be attempted. Patients appreciate nurses who take the time to respond to communication attempts.

Refer to Box 17.2 for strategies to use with those having speech deficits. People who lose both expressive and receptive communication abilities have **global aphasia**. Individuals with these deficits can become frustrated when they are not understood. Struggling to speak causes fatigue. Short, positive sessions are used to communicate. Otherwise, they may become nonverbal as a way of regaining energy and composure. Changes in self-image occasioned by physical changes, the uncertain recovery course and outcome of strokes, shifts in family roles, and the disruption of free-flowing verbal interaction among family members all make the loss of functional communication particularly agonizing. Any language skills that are preserved should be exploited.

Alternative means of communication, such as pointing, gesturing, or using pictures, can be used, as well as speech-generating electronic devices. Augmentative and alternative communication (AAC) methods have been found to help nurses better communicate with patients who are unable to speak. AAC options include communication boards, picture cards, and use of picture pain rating scales, but the preferred AAC method for many is use of **speech-generating devices**. There are several **smartphone Apps** available that allow the patient to touch a picture on-screen causing a mechanical voice to speak, conveying the intended message.

Communication With Patients Who Have Mental Processing Deficits

Cognitive understanding involves recognition of words and integrating them into schemata of acquired knowledge. Some have difficulty ignoring irrelevant information or have difficulty organizing input meaningfully.

Learning Delays

As a nurse providing care to learning delay (LD) patients, you need to adapt your messages to an understandable level. This is crucial in all communication but especially when you are seeking to gain informed consent for treatment. To what extent should you involve your cognitively impaired patient in decision making? In communicating about general health care, adaptations include simple explanations, touch, and use of familiar objects.

Communication Deficits Associated With Some Mental Disorders

When working with some patients with mental disorders, you will face a formidable challenge in trying to establish a relationship. Those with altered reality discrimination

---

> ### BOX 17.2 Strategies to Assist the Patient With Cognitive Processing Deficits or Speech and Language Difficulties
>
> - Speak slowly, using simple sentences; ask yes or no questions.
> - Talk about one thing at a time, or ask one question at a time; do not rush.
> - Give extra time to process and formulate a response; do not interrupt.
> - Avoid prolonged, continuous conversations; instead, use frequent, short talks. Present small amounts of information at a time.
> - When your patient falters in written or oral expression, supply needed compensatory support.
> - Praise efforts to communicate.
> - Provide regular mental stimulation in a nontaxing way.
> - Help patients to focus on the faculties still available to them for communication.
> - Use visual cues; for print materials, use short, bulleted lists.
> - Make referrals so patients can obtain and use AAC devices.

AAC, Augmentative and alternative communication.

---

have both verbal and nonverbal communication deficits. Rarely will this person approach you directly. They generally respond to questions, but their answers are likely to be brief, and they do not elaborate without further probes. Although the patient appears to rebuff any social interaction, it is important to keep trying to connect. People with mental disorders such as schizophrenia are easily overwhelmed by the external environment. It has been demonstrated that schizophrenic patients have the same expressive deficits as do those with depression. Keeping in mind that their unresponsiveness to words, failure to make eye contact, unchanging facial expression, and monotonic voice are parts of the disorder and not a commentary on your communication skills helps you to continue to engage.

If your patient is hallucinating or using delusions as a primary form of communication, you should neither challenge their validity directly nor enter into a prolonged discussion of illogical thinking. Often you can identify the underlying theme they are trying to convey with the delusional statement. For example, when they say, "Voices are telling me to do…," you might reply, "It sounds as though you feel powerless and afraid at this moment." Listening carefully, using alert posture, nodding to demonstrate active listening, and trying to make sense out of their underlying feelings model effective communication and help you to decode nonsensical messages. Simulation Exercise 17.3 may help you to gain some understanding of communication problems experienced by the person with schizophrenia (Fig. 17.5).

Patients Experiencing Treatment-Related Communication Disabilities

Communication disabilities can stem from sedative medications, mechanical ventilation, isolation in an ICU, or isolation such as occurs when older adults are in long-term care facilities. A number of studies of communication in intensive care show that patients are very dependent on their nurse to institute communication. Specific recommended skills are listed in Box 17.3. Many items such as mobile devices with text-to-speech apps, computers with gaze-controlled programs, or communication boards are useful with ventilator-dependent patients temporarily unable to speak. Better communication leads to psychological improvements such as decreased anxiety and depression.

Lack of Communication Due to Lowered Level of Consciousness

When a patient is not fully alert, it is not uncommon for nurses to speak in his or her presence in ways they would not if they thought the patient could fully understand what is being said, forgetting that hearing can remain acute. It is not possible to be certain about what level of awareness remains. Good practice suggests you never say anything you would not want them to hear. Always calling them by name; orienting to time, place, and location; explaining all procedures; and using touch are considered best practice. Consider the following case of Mr. Lopez.

Case Example: Mr. Lopez

Mr. Lopez is totally paralyzed and seems unresponsive immediately after a rupture of a blood vessel in his brain. Mrs. Lopez thinks he can still blink his eyes. You say: "Mr. Lopez, you are in the emergency department of General Hospital. I am your nurse, Kathleen. I need to draw a sample of your blood. Can you feel this? Blink once for yes and twice for no."

For all communication-impaired patients, convey a caring, compassionate attitude, use alternative communication strategies, and give frequent orienting cues, linking events to routines (e.g., saying, "The x-ray technician will take your chest x-ray right after lunch."). When they are unable or unwilling to engage in a dialogue, you should continue to initiate communication in a one-way mode.

SIMULATION EXERCISE 17.3
Schizophrenia Communication Simulation

Purpose:
To gain insight into communication deficits encountered by clients with schizophrenia.

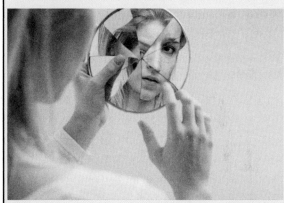

Fig. 17.5 Nurse tries to understand patient's underlying feelings. (Copyright © KatarzynaBialasiewicz/iStock/Thinkstock.)

Procedure:
1. Break class into groups of three (triads) by counting off 1, 2, 3.
2. Person 1 (the nurse) reads a paragraph of rules to the patient and then quizzes him or her afterward about the content.
3. Person 2 (the patient with schizophrenia) listens to everything and tries to answer the nurse's questions correctly to get 100% on the test.
4. Person 3 (representing the mental illness) speaks loudly and continuously in the patient's ear while the nurse is communicating, saying things like "You are so stupid," "You have done bad things," and "It is coming to get you," over and over.

Reflective Analysis and Discussion:
Determine if any patient has 100% recall after this activity. Critique the simulation. Describe difficulties communicating when the patient is "hearing voices."

Courtesy Ann Newman, PhD, University of North Carolina, Charlotte, NC.

BOX 17.3 Strategies for Communicating With Patients With Treatment-Related Communication Deficits Such as Occur in the Intensive Care Unit

- Encourage your patient to display pictures or a simple object from home.
- Orient them to the environment, time, and place.
- Ask many questions, especially questions the patient can answer with a yes or no.
- Frequently provide information about condition and progress.
- Reassure your patient that cognitive and psychological disturbances are common.
- Give explanations before procedures by providing information about the sounds, sights, and feelings the patient is experiencing.
- Make communication assistive devices available, ranging from paper and pencil or communication cards to computerized communication.
- Always assess whether your communication was successful by having the patient signal back.

Referrals

There are a host of communication specialists available to help patients with communication deficits. As the health team member having the most daily contact with a patient, you may be best positioned to know when they are ready for a referral.

PATIENT ADVOCACY

Our nurse role also includes acting as an advocate for our patients who have communication disabilities. Too often they are discounted. Medical treatment decisions may be made without seeking input from them. Appropriate communication aids may be withheld while they are hospitalized. In the larger community, we need to advocate for community services designed to foster communication, including referrals to speech and language therapists.

SUMMARY

This chapter discusses the specialized communication needs of patients with communication deficits. Adapting our communication skills and projecting a caring, positive attitude are important in overcoming barriers. Basic issues and applications for communicating with those experiencing sensory loss of hearing and sight are outlined. Sensory stimulation and compensatory channels of communication are needed for patients with sensory deprivation. All workers who come in contact with them need to be aware of their communication impairments. We need to learn how to operate and fit equipment such as hearing aids, because hospitalized patients often need help with devices. The mentally ill patient has intact senses, but information processing and language are affected by the disorder. It is important for you to develop a proactive communication approach with the learning impaired or those who suffer from mental disorders. Patients can experience communication isolation and temporary distortion of reality. They need frequent cues that orient them to time and place, as well as providing sensory stimulation and alternative methods of communication. Evidence shows that we need to be careful not to associate communication disability with intellectual dysfunction. Our skill in adapting communication is important to the patient.

ETHICAL DILEMMA: What Would You Do?

Working in a health department clinic, the nurse—through a Spanish-speaking translator—interviews a 46-year-old married woman about the missing results of her recent breast biopsy for suspected cancer. Because the translator is of the same culture as the patient and holds the same cultural belief that suicide is shameful, he chooses to withhold from the nurse information he obtained about a recent suicide attempt. If this information remains hidden from the nurse and doctor, could this adversely affect the patient? What ethical principle is being violated?

REVIEW QUESTIONS

As part of our QSEN patient-centered care expected competencies, evaluate answers for the following situations.

1. You notice your patients on the medical wing at Shangri-La Long-Term Care Facility are rarely out of their rooms and seem withdrawn. Determine what patient-centered interventions might be used to ameliorate stimuli-related communication disabilities.
2. Evaluate opportunities for patient advocacy. Describe one way in which you can advocate for a deficit issue affecting communication
3. Create a scenario of your first meeting with your confused patient as you begin the 3 to 11 p.m. shift in General Medical Centers ICU. (Hint: check Box 17.3)

REFERENCES

Agency for Healthcare and Quality (AHRQ). (2016). Strategies to improve mental health care for children and adolescents. Executive Summary. www.effectivehealthcare.ahrq.gov/ Accessed 10.4.18.

American Speech-Language-Hearing Association (ASLHA). (1993). Definitions of communication disorders and variations [Relevant Paper]. Accessed 10.4.18. www.asha.org/policy.

Barnett, S. L., Mathews, K. A., Sutter, E. J., DeWindt, L. A., Pransky, J. A., O'Hearn, A. M., et al. (2017). Collaboration with deaf communities to conduct accessible health surveillance. *American Journal of Preventive Medicine, 52*(353), s250–s254.

Betz, C. (2012). Opportunities to create nurse-directed, evidence-based services and programs for children and youth with special health care needs and developmental disabilities. *Journal of Pediatric Nursing, 27*(6), 1–2.

Blazer, D. G., Domnitz, S., & Liverman, C. T. (Eds.). (2013). *Hearing health care for adults: Priorities for improving access & affordability.* Washington, DC: National Academy Press.

Booker, S, Q., Haedtke, C. (2016). Assessing pain in nonverbal older adults. *Nursing, 46*(5), 66–69.

George, P., Farrell, T. W., & Griswold, M. F. (2012). Hearing loss: Help for the young and old. *The Journal of Family Practice, 61*(5), 268–270.

Howley, M. M., Carter, T. C., Browne, M. L., Romitti, P. A., Cunniff, C. M., Druschel, C. M., et al. (2016). Fluconazole use and birth defects in the National Birth Defects Prevention study. *American Journal of Obstetrics & Gynecology, 214*(5), 657e1–657e9. Retrieved from: http://www.nap.edn/23446.

Kaskowitz, A., Quint, E., Zochowski, M., Caldwell, A., Vinekar, K., & Dalton, V. K. (2017). Contraception delivery in pediatric and specialist pediatric practices. *Journal of Pediatric Adolesc Gynecology, 30*, e184–e187.

Liebel, D. V., Powers, B. A., Friedman, B., Watson, N. M. (2012). Barriers and facilitators to optimize function and prevent disability worsening: a content analysis of a nurse home visit intervention. Journal of Advanced Nursing, *68*(1),80-93.

Machiels, M., Metzelthin, S. F., Hamers, J., & Zwakhalen, S. (2017). Interventions to improve communication between people with dementia and nursing staff during daily nursing care: a systematic review. *International Journal of Nursing Studies, 66*, 37–46.

Mamo, S. K., Nirmalasari, O., Nieman, C. L., McNabney, M. K., Simpson, A., Oh, E. S., et al. (2017). Hearing care intervention for persons with dementia: A pilot study. *American Journal of Geriatric Psychiatry, 25*(1), 91–101.

McGrath, C., Rudman, D. L., Polgar, J., Spafford, M. M., & Trentham, B. (2016). Negotiating 'positive' aging in the presence of age-related vision loss (ARVL): The shaping and perpetuation of disability. *Journal of Aging Studies, 39*, 1–10.

National Eye Institute. (n.d.) Available online at: www.nei.nih.gov/. Eye Data Statistics Accessed 10.4.18.

NIDCD. (2016). United States national institute of deafness and communication disorders. https://www.nidcd.nih.gov- /health/statistics/quick-statistics-hearing Accessed 10.4.18.

Rahu, M. A., Grap, M. J., Ferguson, P., Joseph, P., Sherman, S., & Elswick, R. K., Jr. (2015). Validity and sensitivity of 6 pain scales in critically ill intubated adults. *American Journal of Critical Care, 24*(6), 514–524.

Rodriguez, C. S., Rowe, M., Thomas, L., Schuster, J., Koeppel, B., & Cairns, P. (2016). Enhancing the communication of suddenly speechless Critical Care patients. *American Journal of Critical Care, 25*(3), e40–e47.

Schwarz, E. B., Parisi, S. M., Handler, S. M., Koren, G., Shevchik, G., & Fischer, G. S. (2013). Counseling about medication-induced birth defects with clinical depression support in primary care. *Journal of Women's Health, 22*(10), 817–824.

Sharpe, B., & Hemsley, B. (2016). Improving nurse-patient communication with patients with communication impairments: hospital nurses' view on feasibility of using mobile communication technologies. *Applied Nursing Research, 30*, 228–236.

US Department of Health and Human Services (n.d.). *Healthy people 2020: topics and objectives. Hearing and other sensory or communication disorders.* www.healthypeople.gov/2020/topic-sobjectives2020/overview.aspx?topicid=20 Accessed 10.4.18.

World Health Organization (WHO). (2001). *International classification of functioning, disability, and health.* Switzerland: Geneva: World Health Organization: Author.

World Health Organization (WHO). (2017). Fact sheets.[disability, hearing, vision, mental illness]. Available online at: www.who/int/mediacentre/factsheets/.

Yuksel, C., & Unver, V. (2016). Use of simulated patient method to teach communication with deaf patients in the Emergency Department. *Clinical Simulation Nursing, 12*, 281–289.

SUGGESTED READING

Agency for Healthcare Research and Quality (AHRQ). (2012). Guide to clinical preventive services: recommendations of the U.S. preventive services task force. http://www.ahrq. gov/professionals/clinicians-providers/guidelines-recommendations/guide/index.html Accessed 10.4.18.

Agency for Healthcare Research and Quality (AHRQ). www.ahrq.gov/topicsobjectives2020/ Refer to Goal DH-8 and sections on hearing and other sensory or communication disorders Accessed 10.4.18.

18

Communicating With Children

Kathleen Underman Boggs

OBJECTIVES

At the end of the chapter, the reader will be able to:

1. Identify how developmental levels impact the child's ability to communicate within interpersonal relationships with caregivers.
2. Discuss evidenced-based practice applications for communicating with a child in clinical practice.
3. Describe modifications in communication strategies to meet the specialized needs of children.
4. Describe interpersonal techniques needed to interact with concerned parents of ill children.
5. Use a pediatric website to access data for evidence-based pediatric practice.

This chapter is designed to help you recognize and apply communication concepts related to the nurse-child-family relationship in pediatric clinical situations. Quality patient-family–centered care has been associated with improved child health outcomes regardless of income or ethnicity (Bleser, Young, & Mirand, 2017). In mastering the Quality and Safety Education for Nurses (QSEN) competency of patient-centered care, effective tools need be cognitively, attitudinally, and developmentally appropriate. For each of these domains, the child's and family's socioeconomic status and cultural background must be considered.

Communicating with children at different age levels requires modifications of the skills learned in previous chapters. By understanding the child's cognitive and functional level, you are able to select the most appropriate communication strategies. Children undergo significant age-related changes in the ability to process cognitive information and in the capacity to interact effectively with the environment. To have an effective therapeutic relationship with a child, you need to understand the feelings and thought processes from the child's perspective and convey honesty, respect, and acceptance of feelings.

Communicating with parents of seriously ill children requires a deliberate effort. Parents need explanations they can understand, need to have established trust with the nurse, and need to feel they have some control over what

is happening to their child. This chapter identifies strategies to enhance communication with parents, as well as children.

BASIC CONCEPTS

LOCATION

Just as there is a nationwide emphasis on outpatient procedures and home care for adults, the same is true for children. More than 70% of pediatric illness care occurs in ambulatory settings. Inpatient care continues to decline significantly.

ATTITUDE

Quality of care studies indicate that, in all settings, children may receive less than half of "best evidence" interventions. Could this be due to overreliance on health care providers' own experience or lack of time to access the latest data and protocols? Major changes in society are mirrored in changing health care for children. Involving children in their own health care decision making is a part of QSEN's "patient-centered care." Making the child a (limited) partner might lead to better health outcomes than treating the child as a target for our delivery of care. Do you see this as desirable?

COGNITIVE DEVELOPMENT

Childhood is very different from adulthood. A child has fewer life experiences from which to draw and is still in the process of developing skills needed for reasoning and communicating. Every child's concept of health and illness must be considered within a developmental framework. Erikson's (1963) concepts of ego development and Piaget's (1972) description of the progressive development of the child's cognitive thought processes together form the theoretical basis for the child-centered nursing interventions described in this chapter. Both theorists say that the child's thought processes, ways of perceiving the world, judgments, and emotional responses to life situations are different from those of the adult. Cognitive and psychosocial developments unfold according to an ordered hierarchical scheme, increasing in depth and complexity as the child matures.

Developmentally Appropriate

Piaget's descriptions of stages of cognitive development provide a valuable contribution toward understanding a child's perceptions and communication abilities. Cognitive development and early language development are integrally related. Although current developmental theorists expand on Piaget's theoretical model by recognizing the

effects of the parent-child relationship and a stimulating environment on developing communication abilities, his work forms the foundation for the understanding of childhood cognitive development. Piaget observed cognitive development occurring in sequential stages (Table 18.1). The ages are only approximated because Piaget himself was not specific.

Wide individual differences exist in the intellectual functioning of same-age children. Variations also occur across situations, so that the child under stress or in a different environment may process information at a lower level than under normal conditions. Because two children of the same choronological age may have quite different skills as information processors, we need to assess level of functioning. Language alternatives familiar to one child because of certain life experiences may not be useful in providing health care and teaching with another. Integrating cognitive and psychosocial developmental approaches into communication with children at different ages enhances effectiveness.

Speech Development

Children progress through stages of communication abilities. When an infant uses gestures or cries to get attention to meet a need, this is termed *intentional communication*. This stage continues through age 7

TABLE 18.1	Stages of Cognitive Development		
Age	**Piaget's Stage**	**Characteristics**	**Language Development**
Birth to 2 years	**Sensorimotor**	Infant learns by manipulating objects. At birth, reflexive communication, then moves through six stages to reach actual thinking.	**Presymbolic** Communication largely nonverbal. Vocabulary of more than 4 words by 12 months, increases to >200 words and use of short sentences before age 2 years.
2–6 years	**Preoperational**	Beginning use of symbolic thinking. Imaginative play. Masters reversibility.	**Symbolic** Actual use of structured grammar and language to communicate. Uses pronouns. Average vocabulary >10,000 words by age 6 years.
7–11 years	**Concrete operations**	Logical thinking. Masters use of numbers and other concrete ideas such as classification and conservation.	Mastery of passive tense by age 7 years and complex grammatical skills by age 10 years.
12+ years	**Formal operations**	Abstract thinking. Futuristic; takes a broader, more theoretical perspective.	Near adultlike skills.

Adapted from Piaget, J. (1972). *The child's conception of the world.* Savage, MD: Littlefield, Adams.

months or so and includes making babbling noises. By 16 months, in the next stage of *symbolic communication,* the child uses single words perhaps combined with gestures in interactions to get what is wanted. With further development the child enters the *linguistic communication* phase using two words, then increasing until approximately at age 5 when full sentences are used (Brown & Elder, 2015).

INTERPERSONAL

Gender Differences in Communication

Some studies show school-age children are more satisfied if their health care provider is the same sex. Past studies showed that communication by female providers was more social and more encouraging. Use of good age-appropriate communication strategies probably outweighs gender as a factor in successful communication with a child, but gender cannot be excluded as a factor affecting communication.

Understanding the Ill Child's Needs

Difficulties arise in adult-child communication, in part because of the child's limited experience in interpreting subtle nuances of facial expression, inflection, and word meanings. When illness and physical or developmental disabilities occur during formative years, situational stressors are added that affect the way children perceive themselves and the environment. Illness may lead to significant alterations in role relationships with family and peers. You need to assess not only the physical care needs of the child but the impact of the illness on the child's self-esteem and on relationships with family and friends. Responses to hospitalization vary with the individual according to age. Negative responses may include separation anxiety, night terrors, feeding disturbances, or regression to earlier developmental stage behavior. Things that affect a child's response may include the chronicity of illness, its impact on lifestyle, the child's cognitive understanding of the disease process, and the family's ability to cope with care demands.

Children With Special Health Care Needs

Some children have chronic physical, developmental, behavioral, or emotional conditions that require health services. In developed countries, one in every five child-rearing households has a child with a chronic health condition (US Department of Health and Human Services [DHHS], n.d.). Many of these children previously would have died but were saved by current technology, leaving some with chronic problems.

Family-Centered Care

In pediatric situations, patient-centered care is really family centered with attention to family diversity and family processes. Evidence documents relationships between such processes and child health outcomes. If the child needs to be hospitalized, this is a *situational crisis* for the child and the entire family. Hospitalization is always stressful. *Prehospitalization preparation* can be done to decrease the child's anxiety. Before elective procedures, many hospitals now offer orientation education tours to youngsters. There are many good books, available in most public libraries, designed to prepare children for their hospitalization.

Child Coping Strategies: Ill children have been shown to successfully develop their own coping strategies (Sposito et al., 2015). For example, they seek cognitive understanding about their disease, employ distractions, and use electronic devices, television, music, and drawing, among other strategies. Hospitalized children have to contend not only with physical changes but with possible separation from family and friends, as well as living in a strange, frightening, and probably painful environment. Usually having a family member stay with them helps.

Parent Coping Strategies: Parents are reported to have a strong desire to create a sense of normalcy for their ill child, even to the point of not revealing or discussing a diagnosis (O'Toole, Lambert, Gallagler, Shahwan, & Austin, 2016). Parenting a seriously ill child has been documented to be very stressful, especially for young parents or those with illness-related perceived financial hardship. Their child's suffering impairs their own coping ability. Nurses are in a position to identify those who are highly stressed. Jones, Taylor, Watson, and Dordic (2015), Kodjebacheva, Sabot, and Xiong (2016), Mullen Reynolds, and Larson (2015) and others suggest we can help parents to cope by:

- Providing emotional support. We need to be accessible and caring and demonstrate continuity of care. Expectations for care and information about treatment need to be clearly communicated with consistent team members.
- Involving parents in care decisions
- Providing needed information. Written literature needs to be used to supplement our teaching.
- Enabling direct care giving by the parent. The extent of responsibility the family assumes for basic care of their hospitalized child needs to be negotiated with staff. Some parents prefer to bathe or feed their child themselves.
- Assisting parents to master procedures needed to care for their child, especially those that will be done in the home.
- Fostering good open communication between parents and health team members.

- Parents repeatedly express a desire to be present during team rounds. Bedside rounds not only improve communication, they also assist a parent in coping.

With chronically ill children, the family needs to learn new interactional patterns and coping strategies that take into consideration the meaning of an illness and disability in family life. Caring for a chronically ill child demands considerable resources.

DEVELOPING AN EVIDENCE-BASED PRACTICE

Much progress has been made in recognizing pediatric pain, although we continue to under-manage children's pain despite published guidelines (Twycross, 2015). According to Young (2017), literature cites a combination of reasons, including the proven falsehood that children do not feel pain or do not have sufficient communication skills to describe pain, while nurses lack adequate methods to assess child pain or fear adverse effects from opioid administration. Finding from LaFond, Vincent, Oosterhouse, and Wilkie's (2016) survey of nurses verifies these reasons, with the addition of a widespread belief that a nurse must verify child pain with observable physiological markers. Limke, Peabody, and Kullgren (2015) describes an mHealth pilot study using electronic tablets' (iPads) application programs (Apps) to enable children to self-manage their pain. For example, they use relaxation techniques such as an App titled "Breathe2Relax." Several biofeedback Apps such as "Inner Balance" are also being used on tablets loaned to hospitalized children older than 5 years. Parents and staff are encouraged to coach each child to practice with the Apps to manage his or her pain.

Results. Anecdotal reporting showed unanimous agreement that App use increased parent satisfaction with treatment and taught children new coping skills. Staff said the Apps enhanced their ability to teach pain management skills and increased child enthusiasm for practicing these skills.

Application to your clinical practice: Although better research is needed to validate effective interventions, this study holds promise. In addition to recognizing that infants and children experience the same or greater pain as do adults with the same disease or undergoing the same procedure, you can provide nonpharmacological interventions that actually help a child to manage his or her pain, such as diaphragmatic breathing. Download a few of the many Apps available, and try them out. There are many evidence-based data websites you can use to aid your pediatric practice. The Cumulative Index to Nursing and Allied Health (CINAHL) website has compiled "Evidence-Based Care Sheets" you can access. For example, they have summarized the best evidence to list strategies for *pediatric pain assessment*. They describe research results showing that three-quarters of the children admitted to emergency departments are in pain but that only half of these children receive analgesics. This may be because emergency department nurses are not all using age-appropriate visual pain scales to assess the child's pain, even though data show self-reporting is the most reliable tool in children older than age 4 years.

Access CINAHL for application to your practice:
1. Which pain assessment scales are available?
2. How much time does it take to use one to assess a child's pain?
3. What reasons do nurses and physicians use to justify not giving pain relief?

APPLICATIONS

Although children historically have not been the subjects of study, research has contributed to our knowledge of child learning and development. Children are more vulnerable and thus are entitled to extra protection as research subjects. Findings are limited because of overreliance on what parents have told us. Agencies tend to see children as similar, without consideration of differences because of age, gender, race, or culture. To give one example, many of the medicines we use to treat children have been tested only on adults by pharmaceutical companies.

Major sources of stress for parents of critically ill children include uncertainty about current condition or prognosis, lack of control, and lack of knowledge about how to best help their hospitalized child or how to deal with their child's response. Although more nursing research is being conducted on effective communication with both parents and their ill children, many of the applications we discuss are based more on experience than on research.

ASSESSMENT

Assessing a child's reaction to illness requires knowing the child's normal patterns of communication. Interactions are observed between parent and child. The child's behavioral responses to the entire interpersonal environment (including nurse and peers) are assessed. Are the child's interactions age appropriate? Are behaviors organized, or is the child unable to complete activities? Does the child act out an entire play sequence, or is such play fragmented and disorganized? Do the child's interactions with others suggest imagination and a broad repertoire of relating behaviors, or is communication devoid of possibilities? Because children cannot communicate fully with us, we have a special responsibility to assess for problems. For example, 25% of the world's adults report being physically abused as children, and 20% of girls are sexually abused (WHO, n.d.). Six million American children are reported victims of neglect, physical abuse, psychological abuse, or even sexual abuse (DHHS, n.d.). Once baseline data have been collected, you can plan specific communication strategies to meet the specialized needs of the child (Fig. 18.1). An overview of nursing adaptations needed to communicate effectively with children is summarized in Box 18.1.

Regression as a form of Childhood Communication

A severe illness can cause a child to show behaviors that are reminiscent of an earlier stage of development. A certain amount of regression is normal. Common behaviors in younger children include whining, demanding undue attention, withdrawal, or having toileting "accidents." These behaviors might stem from the powerlessness the child feels in attempting to cope with an overwhelming, frightening environment. Reassuring the parent that this is a common response to the stress of illness can be helpful (Fig. 18.2).

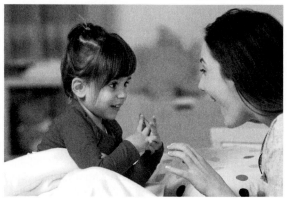

Fig. 18.1 Adapt communication to child's appropriate developmental level. (Copyright © AntonioGuillem/iStock/Thinkstock.)

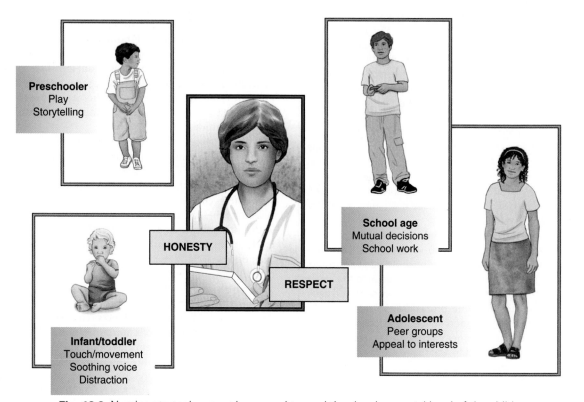

Preschooler
Play
Storytelling

HONESTY

RESPECT

Infant/toddler
Touch/movement
Soothing voice
Distraction

School age
Mutual decisions
School work

Adolescent
Peer groups
Appeal to interests

Fig. 18.2 Nursing strategies must be geared toward the developmental level of the child.

Because children have limited life experience to draw from, they exhibit a narrower range of behaviors in coping with threat. The quiet, overly compliant child who does not complain may be more frightened than the child who screams or cries. This should alert you to the child's emotional distress. You need to obtain detailed information regarding the usual behavioral responses of the family and child. Some behaviors that look regressive may be a typical behavioral response for the child (e.g., the 2-year-old who wants a bedtime bottle). A complete baseline history offers a good counterpoint for assessing the meaning of current behaviors.

Age-Appropriate Communication

An assessment of vocabulary and understanding is essential in fostering communications. Whenever possible, you should communicate using words familiar to the child. Parents are valuable resources in helping to interpret behavioral data. You might assist a child who is having difficulty finding the right words by reframing what he said and repeating it in a slightly different way.

The ill child's peers often have difficulty accepting individual differences created by health deviations. They lack the knowledge and sensitivity to deal with physical changes that they do not understand, as evidenced by "bald" jokes about the child receiving chemotherapy. Children with hidden disorders such as diabetes, some forms of epilepsy, or minimal brain dysfunction seem particularly susceptible to interpersonal distress. For example, it may be difficult for diabetics to regulate their intake of fast foods when all of their friends are able to eat what they want. When peer pressure is at its peak in adolescence, teenagers with newly diagnosed convulsive seizure disorders may find it difficult to tell peers they no longer can ride bicycles or drive cars. Unless the family and nurse provide support, such children have to cope with an indistinct assault to their self-concept alone. A summary of age-appropriate strategies is provided in Box 18.2.

COMMUNICATING WITH CHILDREN WITH PSYCHOLOGICAL BEHAVIORAL PROBLEMS

One out of 10 adolescents and children in our society suffer from a mental illness. These illnesses lead to some level of interactional problems, which may be encountered by nurses in schools, hospitals, clinics, or during home visits to treat physical illnesses. Discussion of nursing interventions with mentally ill children is beyond the scope of this textbook. An excellent source is available via Web links from the Maternal and Child Health Bureau of the US Department of Health and Human Services (2011, www.HRSA.gov).

BOX 18.1

- Nurse-Child Communication Strategies: Adapting Communication to Meet the Needs of the Ill Child Develops an understanding of age-related norms of development.
- Let the child know you are interested in him or her; convey respect and authenticity.
- Let the child know how to summon you (call bell, etc.).
- Develop trust through honesty and consistency in meeting the child's needs.
- Use "transitional objects" such as familiar pictures or toys from home.
- Assess:
  - Level of understandings
  - The child's needs in relation to the immediate situation
  - The child's capacity to cope successfully with change
- Observe for nonverbal cues.
- Use *nonverbal* communication:
  - Tactile (soothing strokes)
  - Kinesthetic (rocking)
  - Get down to the child's height; do not tower over him or her
  - Make eye contact and use reassuring facial expressions
  - Interpret the child's nonverbal cues verbally back to him
  - Instead of conversation, use some indirect age-appropriate communication techniques (e.g., storytelling, picture drawing, music, and creative writing)
- Use *verbal* communication:
  - Use familiar words
  - Use age-appropriate vocabulary
  - Listen without interrupting
  - Humor and active listening to foster the relationship
  - Use open-ended questions
  - Use "I" statements
  - Help child to clarify his or her ideas and feelings ("Tell me more…"; "You got scared when…")
- Respect the child's privacy.
- Accept child's emotions.
- Help child to understand the difference between thoughts and actions.
- Increase coping skills by providing play opportunities; use creative, unstructured play, medical role play, and pantomime.
- Use alternative, supplementary communication devices for children with specialized needs (e.g., sign language and computer-enhanced communication programs).

BOX 18.2   Key Points in Communicating With Children According to Age Group

Updated from material originally supplied by Joyce Ruth, MSN, University of North Carolina Charlotte, College of Health Sciences.

Infants

- Nonverbal communication is a primary mode.
- Infants are biologically "wired" to pay close attention to words. In first year, infants are able to distinguish all conversational sounds.
- Infants are bonded to primary caregivers only. Those older than 8 months may display separation anxiety when separated from parent or when approached by strangers.

Use Kinesthetic Communication

- Use stroking, soft touching, and holding.
- Use motion (e.g., rocking) to reassure. Allow freedom of movement and avoid restraining when possible.
- Learn specifically how the primary caregiver provides care in terms of sleeping, bathing, and feeding, and attempt to mimic these approaches.

Hold Close to Adapt to Limited Vision (20/200 to 20/300 at Birth)

- Encourage the infant's caregivers (parents) to use a lot of intimate space interaction (e.g., 8–18 inches). Mimic the same when trust is established.

Talk with Infants

- Talk with infants in normal conversational tones; soothe them with crooning voice tone.

Establish Trust

- Use parents to give care. Arrange for one or both parents to remain within the child's sight.

Shorten Your Stature

- Sit down on chair, stool, or carpet to decrease posture superiority, so as to look less imposing.

Handle Separation Anxiety When Primary Caregiver Is Absent

- Establish rapport with the caregiver (parent) and encourage the caregiver to be with child and reassure child that staff will be there if caregiver is away. At first, keep at least 2 feet between nurse and infant. Talk to and touch the infant and initially smile often. Provide for kinesthetic approaches; offer self while infant is protesting (e.g., stay with the child; pick the child up and rock or walk; talk to the child about Mommy and Daddy and how much the child cares for them).

1- to 3-Year-Olds

- Child begins to talk around 1 year of age; learns nine new words a day after 18 months.
- By age 2, child begins to use phrases; should be able to respond to "what" and "where" type questions.
- By age 3, child uses and understands sentences.

Adapt to Limited Vocabulary and Verbal Skills

- Make explanations brief and clear. Use the child's own vocabulary words for basic care activities (e.g., use the child's words for defecate [poop, goodies] and urinate [pee-pee, tinkle]). Learn and use self-name of the child.
- Rephrase the child's message in a simple, complete sentence; avoid baby talk. Child should be able to follow two simple directions.

Continue to Use Kinesthetic Communication

- Allow ambulating where possible (e.g., using toddler chairs or walkers). Pull the child in a wagon often if child cannot achieve mobility.

Facilitate Child's Struggle with Issues of Autonomy and Control

- Allow the child some control (e.g., "Do you want a half a glass or a whole glass of milk?").
- Reassure the child if he or she displays some regressive behavior (e.g., if child wets pants, say, "We will get a dry pair of pants and let you find something fun to do.").
- Allow the child to express anger and to protest about his or her care (e.g., "It's okay to cry when you are angry or hurt.").
- Allow the child to sit up or walk as often as possible and as soon as possible after intrusive or hurtful procedures (e.g., "It's all over and we can do something more fun.").
- Use nondirective modes, such as reflecting an aspect of appearance or temperament (e.g., "You smile so often.") or playing with a toy and slowly coming closer to and including the child in play.

Recognize Fear of Bodily Injury

- Show hands (free of hurtful items) and say, "There is nothing to hurt you. I came to play/talk."

Accept Egocentrism and Possible Regression

- Allow child to be self-oriented. Use distraction if another child wants the same item or toy rather than expect the child to share. Some children cope with stress of hospitalization by regressing to an earlier mode of behavior, such as wanting to suck on a bottle, and so forth.

BOX 18.2   Key Points in Communicating With Children According to Age Group—cont'd

Redirect Behavior to a Verbal Level

- Use a nondirective approach. Sit down and join the parallel play of the child. Reflect messages sent by toddler (nonverbally) in a verbal and nonverbal manner (e.g., "Yes, that toy does lots of interesting and fun things.").

Deal with Separation Anxiety

- Accept protesting when parent(s) leave. Hug, rock the child, and say, "You miss Mommy and Daddy! They miss you, too." Play peek-a-boo games with the child. Make a big deal about saying, "Now I am here."
- Show an interest in one of the child's favorite toys. Say, "I wonder what it does" or the like. If the child responds with actions, reflect them back.

3- to 5-Year-Olds

- Most children this age can make themselves understood to strangers.
- They speak in sentences but are unable to comprehend abstract ideas.
- Unable to recognize their own anxiety, at this age some will somaticize (i.e., complain only of stomachache, etc.)
- They begin to understand cause-and-effect relationships; should be able to understand, "If you do…, then we can…"
- Can follow a series of up to four directions unless anxious about being hurt, and so on.

Use Age-Appropriate, Simple Vocabulary

- Use simple vocabulary; avoid lengthy explanations. Focus on the present, not the distant future; use concrete, meaningful references. For example, say, "Mommy will be back after you eat your lunch" (instead of "at 1 o'clock").

Behave in a Culturally Sensitive Manner

- In some cultures, a child is unable to tolerate direct eye-to-eye contact, so use some eye contact and attending posture. Sit or stoop, and use a slow, soft tone of voice.

Attempt to Decrease Anxiety about Being Hurt

- Use brief, concrete, simple explanations. Delays and long explanations before a painful procedure increase anxiety.
- Be quick to complete the procedure; give explanations about its purpose afterward. For example, say, "Jimmy, I'm going to give you a shot," then quickly administer the injection. Then say, "There. All done. It's okay to cry when you hurt. I'd complain too. This medicine will make your tummy feel better." Some experts suggest you create a "safe zone" in the child's bed by doing all painful procedures elsewhere, perhaps in a treatment room.

Use Play Therapy

- Explanations and education can be done using imagination (puppetry, drama with costumes), music, or drawings.
- Allow the child to play with safe equipment used in treatment. Talk about the needed procedure happening to a doll or teddy bear, and state simply how it will occur and be experienced. Use sensory data (e.g., "The teddy bear will hear a buzzing sound.").

Use Distraction and a Sense of Humor

- Tell corny jokes and laugh with the child.

Allow for Child's Continuing Need to Have Control

- Provide for many choices (e.g., "Do you want to get dressed now or after breakfast?").

5- to 10-Year-Olds

- They are developing their ability to comprehend. Can understand sequencing of events if clearly explained: "First this happens…, then…"
- They can use written materials to learn.

Facilitate Child to Assume Increased Responsibility for Own Health Care Practices

- Include the child in concrete explanations about condition, treatment, and protocols.
- Use draw-a-person to identify basic knowledge the child has and build on it.
- Use some of the same words the child uses in giving explanations.
- Use sensory information in giving explanations (e.g., "You will smell alcohol in the cast room.").
- Reinforce basic health self-care activities in teaching.

Respect Increased Need for Privacy

- Knock on the door before entering; tell the client when and for what reasons you will need to return to his or her room.

11-Year-Olds and Older

- Have an increased comprehension about possible negative threats to life or body integrity, yet some difficulty in adhering to long-term goals.

Continued

BOX 18.2   Key Points in Communicating With Children According to Age Group—cont'd

- Continue to use mainly concrete rather than abstract thinking.
- They are struggling to establish identity and be independent.

Verbalize Issues in Age-Appropriate Ways
- Talk about treatment protocols that require giving up immediate gratifications for long-term gain. Explore alternative options (e.g., tell a diabetic adolescent who must give up after-school fries with friends that he or she could save two breads and four fats exchanges to have a milkshake). If you use abstract thinking, look for nonverbal cues (e.g., puzzled face) that may indicate lack of understanding; then clarify in more concrete terms. Use humor or street slang, if appropriate.

Remember That Confidentiality May Be an Issue
- Reassure the adolescent about the confidentiality of your discussion, but clearly state the limits of this

confidentiality. If, for example, the child should talk of killing himself, be clear that this information needs to be shared with parents and staff.

Foster and Allow a Sense of Independence
- Allow participation in decision making, such as wearing own clothes. Avoid an authoritarian or judgmental approach.
- Accept behaviors such as regression, but set limits on injurious behavior.
- Encourage responsibility for keeping own appointments, bedtime poutiness, administration of own medications such as insulin and so forth.

Assess Sexual Awareness and Maturation
- Demonstrate a willingness to listen. Provide value-free, accurate information.

COMMUNICATING WITH PHYSICALLY ILL CHILDREN IN THE HOSPITAL AND AMBULATORY CLINIC

Overestimating a child's understanding of information about illness results in confusion, increased anxiety, anger, or sadness. Beyond physiological care, ill children of all ages need support from every member of the health team—support that they normally would receive from parents. The nurse must provide stimulation to talk, listen, and play. Play is their language, especially because children have major difficulties verbalizing their true feelings about the treatment experience. As nurses, we adapt our communication to meet the ill child's needs. Many agencies have play therapists who serve as excellent resources for staff.

COMMUNICATION WITH INFANTS FROM BIRTH TO 12 MONTHS

Cues to assessment of the preverbal infant include tone of the cry, facial appearance, and body movements. Because the infant uses the senses to receive information, nonverbal communication (e.g., touch) is an important tool for the pediatric nurse. Tone of voice, rocking motion, use of distraction, and a soothing touch can be used in addition to or in conjunction with verbal explanations.

Face-to-face position, bending or moving to the child's eye level, maintaining eye contact, and making a reassuring facial expression further help in interactions with infants.

Anticipate developmental behaviors such as "stranger anxiety" in infants between 9 and 18 months of age. Rather than reaching to pick a child up immediately, you might smile and extend a hand toward the child or stroke the child's arm before attempting to hold the child. If the child is able to talk, asking the child's name and pointing out a notable pleasant physical characteristic conveys the impression that you see the child as a unique person. To a tiny child, this treatment can be synonymous with caring.

COMMUNICATION WITH CHILDREN 1 TO 3 YEARS OF AGE (TODDLERS)

Almost all small children receiving invasive treatment feel some threat to their safety and security, one of Maslow's hierarchies of human needs. This need is exaggerated in toddlers and young children, who cannot articulate their needs or understand why they are ill. To help the child's comprehension, use phrases rather than long sentences and repeat words for emphasis. Because the toddler has a limited vocabulary, you may need to put into words the feelings that the ill child is conveying nonverbally.

Evaluate the Agency Environment

Is it safe? Does it allow for some independence and autonomy? Care in the ambulatory setting is facilitated if a parent or caregiver is present. Agency policies should promote parent-child contact (e.g., unlimited visiting hours, rooming in, or use of CDs, Skype, or podcasts of a parent's voice). Familiar objects make the environment feel safer. Use transitional objects such as a teddy bear, blanket, or favorite toy to remind the alone or frightened child that the security of the parent is still available even when the parent is not physically present. Distraction is a successful strategy with toddlers in ambulatory settings. Use of stuffed animals, windup toys, or "magic" exam lights that blow out "like a birthday candle" can turn fright into delight. The author wears a small toy bear on her stethoscope and asks the child to help listen for a heart sound from the bear, so the child focuses on the toy, making it easier to listen to the child's heart.

COMMUNICATION WITH CHILDREN 3 TO 5 YEARS (PRESCHOOLERS)

Throughout the preoperational period, young children tend to interpret language in a literal way. For example, the child who is told that he will be "put to sleep" during the operation tomorrow may think it means the same as the action recently taken for a pet dog who was too ill to live. Children do not ask for clarification, so messages can be misunderstood quite easily. Preschool children have limited auditory recall and are unable to process auditory information quickly. They have a short attention span. Verbal communication with the preschool child should be clear, succinct, and easy to understand.

Before the age of 7 years, most children cannot make a clear distinction between fantasy and reality. Everything is "real," and anything strange is perceived as potentially harmful. In the hospital, preschool children need frequent concrete reminders to reinforce reality. Assigning the same caregiver reduces insecurity. Visiting the preschooler at the same time each day and posting family pictures are simple strategies to reduce the child's fears of abandonment. You can link information to activities of daily living. For example, saying, "Your mother will come after you take your nap," rather than "at 2 o'clock" is much more understandable to the preschool child.

Children need to be assessed for misconceptions and troubling problems, preferably using free play and fantasy storytelling exercises. Egocentrism can be a normal developmental process that may prevent children from understanding why they cannot have a drink when they are fasting before a scheduled test. Explanations given a long time beforehand may not be remembered. If something is going to hurt, you should be forthright about it, while at the same time reassuring the child. Simple explanations reduce the child's anxiety. No child should ever be left to figure out what is happening without some type of simple explanation. Reinforce the child's communication by praising the willingness to tell you how he or she feels. Avoid judging or censuring the child who yells such things as, "I hate you," or "You are mean for hurting me." Not being able to recognize or communicate anxiety, the child may just complain of a physical symptom, like a headache or stomachache. Box 18.2 can help you to focus on specific communication strategies with the hospitalized preschooler.

Play as a Communication Strategy

The preschooler lacks a suitable vocabulary to express complex thoughts and feelings. Small children cannot picture what they have never experienced. Play is an effective means by which a puzzling and sometimes painful real world can be approached. Play allows the child to create a concrete experience of something unknown and potentially frightening. By constructing a situation in play, the child is able to put together the components of the situation in ways that promote recognition and make it a concrete reality. When the child can deal with things that are small or inanimate, the child masters situations that might otherwise be overwhelming. Cartoons, pictures, or puppets can be used to demonstrate actions and terminology. Dolls with removable cloth organs help children to understand scheduled operations.

Preschoolers tend to think of their illness, their separation from parents, and any painful treatments as punishment. Play can be used to help children express their feelings about an illness and to role-play coping strategies. Allowing the young child to manipulate syringes and give "shots" to a doll or put a bandage or restraint on a teddy bear's arm allows the child to act out feelings. The child masters fear by becoming "the aggressor." Play can be a major channel for communication. Preschool children develop communication themes through their play and work through conflict situations in their own good time; the process cannot be rushed.

Play materials vary with the age and developmental status of the child. Simple, large toys are used with young children; more intricate playthings are used with older preschoolers. Clay, crayons, and paper become modes of expression for important feelings and thoughts about problems. Play can be your primary tool for assessing preschool children's perceptions about their hospital experience, their anxieties, and their fears. Play can increase their coping ability. Preschoolers love jokes, puns, and riddles—the cornier, the better. Using jokes during the physical assessment, such as "Let me hear your lunch," or "Golly, could that be a potato in your ear?" helps to form the bonds needed for a successful relationship with the preschool child.

Storytelling as a Communication Strategy

A communication strategy often used with young children is the use of story plots. As early as 1986, Gardner described a mutual storytelling technique. You ask the child to help make up a story. If the child is a little reluctant, you may begin, as described in Simulation Exercise 18.1. At the end of the story, the child is asked to indicate what lesson might be learned from the story. If the child seems a little reluctant to give a moral to the story, you might suggest that all stories have something that can be learned from them. Analyze the themes presented by the child, which usually reveal important feelings. Is the story fearful? Are the characters scary or pleasing? The child should be praised for telling the story. The next step in the process is to ask yourself what would be a healthier resolution than the one used by the child. Then suggest an alternative ending. In your version of the story, the characters and other details remain the same initially, but the story contains a more positive solution or suggests alternative answers to problems. The object of mutual storytelling is to offer the child an opportunity to explore different alternatives in a neutral communication process with a helping person.

COMMUNICATION WITH CHILDREN 6 TO 11 YEARS (SCHOOL AGE)

As children move into concrete operational thinking, they begin to internalize the reasons for illness: illness is caused by germs, or you have cavities because you ate too much candy or did not brush your teeth. In later childhood, most children become better able to work with you verbally. It still is important to prepare responses carefully and to anticipate problems, but the child is capable of expressing feelings and venting frustration more directly through words. Use Simulation Exercise 18.2 to reformulate medical technology into age-appropriate expressions.

Assessment of the child's cognitive level of understanding continues to be essential. Search for concrete examples to which the child can relate rather than giving abstract examples. If children are to learn from a model, they must see the model performing the skill to be learned. School-age

children thrive on explanations of how their bodies work and enjoy understanding the scientific rationales for their treatment. Ask questions directly to the child, consulting the parent for validation.

SIMULATION EXERCISE 18.1   Using a Mutual Storytelling Technique

Purpose:
To give practical experience with the mutual storytelling technique.

Procedure:
1. Use the mutual storytelling process described in the text with a 5- to 8-year-old child in your neighborhood.
2. Write down the story the child told. Read the story this child told, and suggest alternative endings.
3. Analyze commonalities.

Reflective Analysis:
1. Explain any surprises from the child's story.
2. Describe what you learned about the child when using this technique?
3. Determine any difficulties in engaging the child and explain what techniques you would use next time.
4. After listening to all scenarios, draw conclusions to determine what were the most effective and least effective techniques?

Sample Answer:
Nurse: Once upon a time in a land far away, there lived a...
  Child: Dragon.
  Nurse: A dragon who ate...
  Child: Carrots.
  Nurse: The dragon ate carrots and slept...
  Child: In a cave.
  Nurse: One day he left the cave to go out and find many sweet carrots to eat, but as he walked along he ran into a...
  Child: Bike.
  Nurse: He was afraid of the bike and so he...
  Child: Kicked it and ran away.
  Nurse: After he ran away, is there any more to the story?
  Child (upset): He got hit with a stick.
  Nurse: What is the message to this story? What does it tell us?
  Child: About running away not to be punished.
  Activity

SIMULATION EXERCISE 18.2 Age-Appropriate Medical Terminology

Purpose:
To help students think of terminology appropriate to use with young clients.

Procedure:
This can be fun if the instructor quickly asks students, going around the room.

Reformulate the following expressions using words a child can understand:

Anesthesia	Inflammation	NPO
Cardiac catheterization	Injection	Operating room
Disease	Intake and output	Sedation
Dressings	Isolation	Urine specimen
Enema	IV needle	Vital signs
Infection	Nausea	Hydration

Discussion:
Higher level vocabulary words can be difficult for some children. Try explaining the meaning of the above words.

IV, intravenous; *NPO,* nothing by mouth.

Using Audiovisual AIDS or Hobbies as a Communication Strategy

Audiovisual aids and reading material geared to the child's level of understanding may supplement verbal explanations and diagrams. Details about what the child will hear, see, smell, and feel are important. For the younger school-age child, expressive art can be a useful method to convey feelings and to open up communication. The older school-age child or adolescent might best convey feelings by blogging or posting on social media or writing a poem or story. Written or digital materials such as in Cary's case can assist you in understanding hidden thoughts or emotions.

Case Example: Cary

Ashley, a first-year student nurse, becomes frustrated during the course of her conversation with her assigned child, 11-year-old Cary, admitted 5 days ago to the psychiatric unit. Despite a genuine desire to engage him in a therapeutic alliance, he will not talk. Attempts to get to know him on a verbal level seemed to increase rather than decrease his anxiety. The nurse correctly inferred that despite his age, this adolescent needed a more tangible approach. Knowing that he likes cars, Ashley brought in an automotive magazine.

Together, they looked at the magazine; the publication soon became their special vehicle for communication, bridging the gap between inner reality and his ability to express himself verbally in a meaningful way. Feelings about cars gradually generalized to verbal expressions about other situations, and Cary began describing his attitudes about himself. When Ashley left the unit, he asked to keep the magazine and frequently spoke of her with fondness. This simple recognition of his awkwardness in verbal communication and use of another tool to facilitate the relationship had a positive effect.

Mutuality in Decision Making

Children of this age need to be involved in discussions of their illness and in planning for their care. Explanations giving the rationale for care are useful. Involving the child in decision making may decrease fears about the illness, the treatment, or the effect on family life. Videos and written materials may be useful in involving the child in the management phase of care.

COMMUNICATION WITH CHILDREN OLDER THAN 11 YEARS OF AGE (ADOLESCENTS)

An understanding of adolescent developmental principles is essential in working with teens. Adolescence is the time when we clinicians encourage a shift in responsibility for health-related decisions from parent to the teen. Even teens enjoying good health are forced to deal with new health issues such as acne, menstrual problems, or sexual activity. The adolescent vacillates between childhood and adulthood and is emotionally vulnerable. The ambivalence of the adolescent period may be normally expressed through withdrawal, rebellion, lost motivation, and rapid mood changes. A teen may look adultlike but in illness especially may be unable to communicate easily with care providers. Identity issues become more difficult to resolve when the normal opportunities for physical independence, privacy, and social contacts are compromised by illness or handicap. All adolescents have questions about their developing body and sexuality. Ill teens have the same longings, but problems may be greater because the natural outlets for their expression with peers are curtailed by the disorder or by hospitalization. Use of peer groups, adolescent lounges (separate from the small children's playroom), and smartphones, as well as provisions for wearing one's own clothes, fixing one's hair, or attending hospital school, may help teenagers to adjust to hospitalization. When the developmental identity crisis becomes too uncomfortable, adolescents may project their fury and frustration onto family or staff. Identifying rage as a normal response to a difficult situation can be reassuring.

Assessment of the adolescent should occur in a private setting. Attention to the comfort and space of an adolescent will have a tremendous impact on the quality of the interaction. To the teenager, the nurse represents an authority figure. The need for compassion, concern, and respect is perhaps greater during adolescence than at any other time in the life span. Often lacking the verbal skills of adults, yet wishing to appear in control, adolescents do well with direct questions. Innocuous questions are used first to allow the teenager enough space to check the validity of his or her reactions to the nurse. In caring for a teen in an ambulatory office or clinic, conduct part of the history interview without the parent present. If the parent will not leave the examination room, this can be done while walking the teen down to the laboratory. Questions about substance use or sexual activity demand confidentiality.

To assess a teen's cognitive level, find out about the teen's ability to make long-term plans. An easy way to do this is the "three wishes question." Ask the teen to name three things he or she would expect to have in 5 years. Answers can be analyzed for factors such as concreteness, realism, and goal-directness.

Some teens lack sufficient experience to recognize that life has ups and downs and that things will eventually be better. Suicide is the second leading cause of death in teenagers, and many experts think that the actual rate is greater because many deaths from the number one cause, motor vehicle accidents, may actually be attributed to this cause. Be aware of danger signs such as apathy, persistent depression, or self-destructive behavior. When faced with a tragedy, teens tend to mourn in doses with wide mood swings. Grieving teens may need periods of privacy but also need the opportunity for relief through distracting activities, music, and games. In communicating with an ill adolescent, remember to listen. When teens ask direct questions, they are ready to hear the answer. Answer directly and honestly.

Using Hobbies as a Communication Strategy

Adolescents still rely primarily on feedback from adults and from friends to judge their own competency. A teen may not yet have developed proficiency and comfort in carrying on verbal conversations with adults. The teen may respond best if the nurse uses several modalities to communicate. Using empathy, conveying acceptance, and using open-ended questions are three useful strategies. Sometimes more innovative communication strategies are needed.

Dealing With Care Problems
Pain

The literature reflects major concern that pain in children is underestimated and inadequately relieved. Lack of adequate pain relief may, in part, be due to fears of

---

SIMULATION EXERCISE 18.3 Pediatric Nursing Procedures

Purpose:
To give practice in preparing for painful procedures.

Procedure:
Timmy, age 4, is going to have a bone marrow aspiration. (The insertion of a large needle into the hip is a painful procedure.) Answer the following questions:
1. Create a dialog between nurse and young patient that will help to prepare them for a painful procedure.
2. If this is a frequently repeated procedure, how can you make him feel safe before and after the procedure?
3. How soon in advance should you prepare him?
   Reflective Analysis and Discussion:
   In a group critically examine the responses of others. Try to reach consensus on the best practices for pain intervention.

---

oversedating a child but more likely is due to the child's limited capacity to communicate the nature of their discomfort. We need to adapt our pain assessments to be age appropriate. A major transition in pediatric pain management is the shift from the pharmacological intervention model to a biopsychosocial model, which gives us many more intervention strategies to be used instead of or in conjunction with medication.

Infants indicate pain with physiological changes (e.g., diaphoresis, pallor, increased heart rate, increased respirations, and decreased oxygen saturation). With other children, we use one of the many child-based assessment scales, such as smiley faces or poker chips with toddlers and preschoolers. We also need to instigate protocols for preventing pain associated with treatment. Examples include use of local anesthetics for effective reduction of the pain associated with venipuncture. Effective nonpharmacological interventions for pain include nonnutritive sucking/pacifiers, rocking, physical contact, and swaddling. Use Simulation Exercise 18.3 to develop your own approach to caring for children in pain.

Anxiety

Illness is often an unanticipated event. Uncertainty and even anxiety should be expected when both treatment and outcome are unknown. Young children react to unexpected stimuli, to painful procedures, and even to the presence of strangers with fear. Older children fear separation from parents but also may fear injury, loss of body function, or even a sense of shame for being perceived by friends as different. Many children with chronic health problems

SIMULATION EXERCISE 18.4   Preparing Children for Treatment Procedures

Purpose:
To help students apply developmental concepts to age-appropriate nursing interventions.

Procedure:
Students divide into four small groups and role play interventions in the following situation. As a large group, each small group spokesperson writes the intervention on the board under the label for the age group.

Situation:
Jamie is scheduled to go to the surgical suite later today to have a central infusion catheter inserted for hyperalimentation. This is Jamie's first procedure on the first day of this first hospitalization experience.

Reflective Analysis:
Group focuses on comparing and contrasting interventions across the various age spans to determine age-appropriate nursing interventions.
1. How does each intervention differ according to the age of the child? (Describe age-appropriate interventions for preschooler, school-age child, and adolescent.)
2. What concept themes are common across the age spans? (education components; assessing initial level

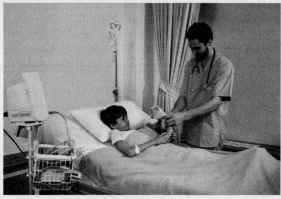

Fig. 18.3 Nurse uses toy bear to explain procedure. (Copyright © Wavebreakmedia/iStock/Thinkstock.)

of knowledge; assessing ability to comprehend information, readiness to receive information; adapting information to cognitive level of child)
3. What formats might be best used for each age group? (Role-play with tools such as dolls, pictures, comic books, educational pamphlets, and peer group sessions.)

---

experience tension between balancing the restrictions of their treatment regime and their own desires for normal activities (Sparapani, Jacob, & Nascimento, 2015). Think of the diabetic teen who goes to a friend's birthday party and is urged to eat cake! Simulation Exercise 18.4 helps to develop age-appropriate explanations that may reduce anxiety.

Acting-Out Behaviors

Behavior problems present a special challenge to the nurse. Clear communication of expectations, treatment protocols, and rules is of value. As much as possible, adolescents should be allowed to act on their own behalf in making choices. At the same time, limits need to be set on acting-out behavior. Limits define the boundaries of acceptable behaviors in a relationship. Initially determined by the parents or the nurse, limits can be developed mutually as an important part of the relationship as the child matures. Determining consequences has a positive value in that it provides the child with a model for handling frustrating situations in a more adult manner.

Once the conflict is resolved and the child has accepted the consequences of his or her behavior, he or she should be given an opportunity to discuss attitudes and feelings that led up to the need for limits, as well as reaction to the limits set. Serious symptoms such as substance abuse require specialist interventions.

Although communication about limits is necessary for the survival of the relationship, it needs to be balanced with time for interaction that is pleasant and positive. Sometimes with children who need limits set on a regular basis, discussion of the restrictions is the only conversation that takes place between nurse and child. When this is noted, nurses might ask themselves what feelings the child might be expressing through their actions. Putting into words the feelings that are being acted out helps children to trust the nurse's competence and concern. Usually it is necessary for the entire staff to share this responsibility. Box 18.3 presents ideas for setting limits.

More Helpful Strategies for Communicating With Children

Adapting communication strategies presented earlier in this book to interactions with children requires some imagination and creativity. Working with children is rewarding, hard work that sometimes must be evaluated indirectly. For example, George was the primary care nurse who had worked very hard with a 13-year-old girl over a 6-month period while the girl was on a bone marrow transplant unit. He felt bad when, at discharge, the girl stated, "I never want to see any of you people again." However, just before

BOX 18.3   Guidelines for Developing Workable Limit-Setting Plan

1. Have the child describe his or her behavior.
2. *Key:* Evaluate realistically.
3. Encourage the child to assess behavior. Is it helpful for others and him or her?
4. *Key:* Evaluate realistically.
5. Encourage the child to develop an alternative plan for governing behavior.
6. *Key:* Set reasonable goals.
7. Have the child sign a statement about his or her plan.
8. *Key:* Commit to goals.
9. Consequences for unacceptable behavior are logical and fit the situation.
10. *Key:* Consequences are known.
11. At the end of the appropriate time period, have the child assess his or her performance.
12. *Key:* Evaluate realistically.
13. Consequences are applied in a matter-of-fact manner, without lengthy discussion.
14. *Key:* Consequences immediately follow the transgression.
15. Provide positive reinforcement for those aspects of performance that were successful.[1]
16. *Key:* Evaluate realistically.
17. Encourage the child to make a positive statement about his or her performance.
18. *Key:* Teach self-praise.

[1]If the child's performance does not meet the criteria set in the plan, return to Step 3 and assist the child in modifying the plan so that success is more possible. If, conversely, the child's performance is successful, help him or her to develop a more ambitious plan (e.g., for a longer period or for a larger set of behaviors).

leaving, the nurse found her sobbing on her bed. No words were spoken, but the child threw her arms around George and clung to him for comfort. For this nurse, the child's expression of grief was an acknowledgment of the meaning of the relationship. Children, even those who can use words, often communicate through behavior rather than verbally when under stress.

Active Listening

The process of active listening takes form initially from watching the behaviors of children as they play and interact with their environments. As a child's vocabulary increases and the capacity to engage with others develops, listening begins to approximate the communication process that occurs between adults, with one important difference: Because the perceptual world of the child is concrete, the nurse's communication should be at the child's developmental level.

Authenticity and Veracity

Sometimes adults ignore children's feelings or else deceive them about procedures, illness, or hospitalization in the mistaken belief that they will be overwhelmed by the truth. Just the opposite is true. Children, like adults, can cope with most stressors as long as they are presented in a manner they can understand and given enough time and support from the environment to cope. Teens rate honesty, attention to pain, and respect as the three most important factors in their quality of care. You should never allow any individual, even a parent, to threaten a child. For example, a few parents have been heard to say, "You be good or I'll have the nurse give you a shot." It is appropriate to interrupt this parent.

Conveying Respect

It is easy for adults to impose their own wishes on a child. Respecting a child's right to feel and to express feelings appropriately is important. Providing truthful answers is a hallmark of respect. When interacting with the older child, using the concept of mutuality will promote respect and should foster more positive and lasting health care outcomes. Confidentiality needs to be maintained unless the nurse judges that revealing information is necessary to prevent harm to the child or adolescent. In such cases, the child needs to be advised of the disclosure.

Providing Anticipatory Guidance to the Child

The nursing profession advocates education for children, as do pediatricians. The American Academy of Pediatrics has published suggestions for giving caretakers health promotion information at appropriate ages. There is an increased focus on the role a child can assume in being responsible for his or her own health care. It is never too early to begin. For example, written handouts for incorporating violence prevention can be incorporated into well-child visits. A shift in placing responsibility for good health practices onto the individual is in line with recommendations in *Healthy People 2020*. In fact, one of the stated objectives is to increase the proportion of time that the health care worker provides needed information.

FORMING HEALTH CARE PARTNERSHIPS WITH PARENTS

Having an ill child is stressful for parents. Evidence shows that loss of the ability to act as the child's parent, to alleviate their child's pain, and to offer comfort is more stressful than factors connected with the illness, including coping with uncertainty over the outcome. Studies point to a lack of needed information and support from professionals as being a top stressor. It is essential that we work in partnership with families, especially if we assess risk factors that endanger the child. Most parents want to participate

BOX 18.4   Representative Nursing Problem: Dealing With a Frightened Parent

During report, the night nurse relates an incident that occurred between Mrs. Smith, the mother of an 8-year-old admitted for possible acute lymphocytic leukemia and the night supervisor. Mrs. Smith told the supervisor that her son was receiving poor care from the nurses and that they frequently ignored her and refused to answer her questions. While you are making rounds after the report, Mrs. Smith corners you outside her son's room and begins to tell you about all the things that went wrong during the night. She goes on to say, "If you people think I'm going to stand around and allow my son to be treated this way, you are sadly mistaken."

Problem

Frustration and anger caused by feelings of being without power to effect son's hospitalization and possible leukemic condition.

Nursing Goals

Increase the mother's sense of control and problem-solving capabilities; help the mother to develop adaptive coping behaviors.

Method of Assistance

Guiding; supporting; providing developmental environment

Interventions

1. Actively listen to concerns with as much objectivity as possible; maintain eye contact, use minimal verbal activity, allow opportunities for expression of concerns and fears.
2. Use reflective questioning to determine levels of understanding and the extent of information obtained from health team members.
3. Listen for repetitive words or phrases that may serve to identify problem areas or provide insight into fears and concerns.
4. Reassure parents, when appropriate, that their child's hospitalization is indeed frightening and it is all right to be scared; remember to demonstrate interest, and use listening responses (e.g., "It must be hard not knowing the results of all these tests.") to create an atmosphere of concern.
5. Avoid communication blocks, such as giving false reassurance, dictating what to do, or ignoring concerns; such behavior effectively cuts off therapeutic communication.
6. Keep parents continually informed regarding their child's progress.
7. Involve family in care; do not overwhelm them or make them feel they must give care; watch for cues about readiness "to do more."
8. Acknowledge the effect this illness may have on the family; involve the health team in identifying ways to reduce fears and provide for continuity in the type of information presented to family members.
9. Assign a primary nurse to give care and act as a resource. Identify support systems in the community that might provide help and support.

From M. Michaels, University of Maryland School of Nursing, Baltimore.

in their child's care during acute hospitalizations but need information, advice, and clarification as to their role (i.e., what is okay to do). They need to feel valued but not pressured into doing tasks they are uncomfortable with or do not want to do. Parents often have questions about discussing their child's illness or disability with others. Telling siblings and friends the truth is important. For one thing, it provides a role model for the siblings to follow in answering the curious questions of their friends. More frustrating to nurses are parents who are critical of the nurse's interventions, displacing the anger they feel about their own powerlessness onto the nurse (Box 18.4). The nurse may be tempted to become defensive or sarcastic or simply to dismiss the comments of the parent as irrational. However, a more helpful response would be to place oneself in the parents' shoes and to consider the possible issues. Asking the parents what information they have or might need, simply listening in a nondefensive way, and allowing the parents to vent some of their frustrations may help to get at underlying feelings. Use of listening strategies is helpful. Sometimes a listening response that acknowledges the legitimacy of the parent's feeling is helpful: "I'm sorry that you feel so bad," or "It must be difficult for you to see your child in such pain." These simple comments acknowledge the very real anguish parents experience in health care situations having few palatable options. If possible, parental venting of feeling should occur in a private setting out of hearing range from the child. It is very upsetting to children to experience splitting in the parent-nurse relationship. Guidelines for communicating with parents are presented in Box 18.5.

Communicating With Parents of Special Health Care Needs Children

Many children have a chronic health condition requiring additional services. Caring for these children requires

BOX 18.5   Guidelines for Communicating With Parents

- Present complex information in informational chunks.
- Repeat information and allow plenty of time for questions.
- Keep parents continually informed of progress and changes in condition.
- Involve parents in determining goals; anticipate possible reactions and difficulties.
- Discuss problems with parents directly and honestly.
- Explore all alternative options with parents.
- Share knowledge of community supports; help parents to role-play responses to others.
- Acknowledge the impact of the illness on finances; on emotions; and especially on the family, including siblings.
- Use other staff for support in personally coping with the emotional drain created by working with very ill children and their parents.

parental time and alters family communication patterns. Studies show these families have less time for communication. Nurses need to provide care and information about the child's condition and time for discussions about balancing family needs with care for this child and suggest strategies for moving the child toward future independence. Refer parents to community resources. We need to recognize that as the child reaches developmental milestones, this can be a time of increased family stress, requiring additional support from us.

Community

Partnering with the family can be the best method you have to address the complex health care needs of children. Parents are the central figures in care planning, especially for chronically ill children. We need to help provide information about which community agencies, networks, and professionals will be mobilized to provide care to their child. For example, school nurses often act as case managers by communicating about the child's needs among parent, care providers, teachers, and other resource personnel. By law in the United States, children with special needs in the educational system are required to have an Individualized Education Program. A part of this may be the health plan for children who need medical intervention or treatment during school.

Anticipatory guidance in the community. Because the parents usually assume responsibility for the child's care after they leave the hospital, it is essential to encourage active involvement from the very beginning of treatment. Parents may also need facts about normal development and milestones to expect, as well as information about prevention of illness.

Community Support Groups

Community groups have organized to assist families. Often, information about the groups' meeting times can be obtained from health care providers, from the national or local organization, or the internet. For parents who cannot travel to meetings, internet support groups are available.

Nurse as Advocate for Children in the Community

Because children cannot communicate their needs to policy makers, we need to broaden our advocacy to fight for better child health at local and national levels. Children's access to health care is affected by their neighborhood, the level of their parent's education, their insurance status, and problems with referrals. Poverty is associated with poorer child health status, lack of a regular care provider, lack of dental care, and a myriad of other health problems. Part of our advocacy role is to become actively involved in improving access to care and to focus public attention on pediatric health problems. For example, *Healthy People 2020* has designated obesity and physical activity as priorities for action, stating that only 1 in 10 American youth meet national guidelines for exercise (1 hour per day). Child obesity is causing a huge increase in related health problems such as diabetes. Related nursing advocacy interventions include organizing campaigns to eliminate sale of junk food in schools, reinstituting recess and physical education opportunities, and joining community activist groups advocating restructuring of community neighborhoods to allow for increased exercise with sidewalks to school and safe bike paths.

SUMMARY

Communicating with ill children requires modification of standard communication skills to suit the children's developmental stage. Children's ability to understand and communicate with you is largely influenced by their cognitive understanding, vocabulary level, and their limited life experiences. We need to develop an understanding of feelings and thought processes from the child's perspective, and our adaptation of communication should reflect these understandings. Various strategies for communicating with children of different ages are suggested. Parents of ill children are under considerable stress. We need to form a trusting relationship and offer open, full communication. A marvelous characteristic of children is how well they respond to caregivers who make an effort to understand their needs and take the time to relate to them.

ETHICAL DILEMMA: What Would You Do?
You are caring for Mika Soon, a 15-year-old adolescent. She has confided to you that she is being treated for chlamydia. Her mother approaches you privately and demands to know if Mika has told you if she is sexually active with her boyfriend. Because Mika is a minor and Mrs. Soon is paying for this clinic visit, are you obligated to tell her the truth?

REVIEW QUESTIONS

1. Using the case in the ethical dilemma, describe any interventions you would use with this single mother.

2. Evaluate your pain assessment: how does it differ for an infant and a 5-year-old. Use text to support your answer.

REFERENCES

Bleser, W. K., Young, S. I., & Miranda, P. Y. (2017). Disparities in patient-family-centered care during US children's health care encounters: A closer examination. *Academic Pediatrics, 17*(1), 17–26.

Brown, A. B., & Elder, J. H. (2015). Communication in autism spectrum disorder: A guide for pediatric nurses. *Pediatrics Nurse, 40*(5), 219–225.

Erikson, E. H. (1963). *Childhood and society.* New York: Norton.

Jones, L., Taylor, T., Watson, B., & Dordic, T. (2015). Negotiating care in the special care nursery: Parents & nurses perceptions of nurse-parent communication. *Journal of Pediatric Nursing, 30*, e71–e80.

Kodjebacheva, G. D., Sabot, T., & Xiong, J. (2016). Interventions to improve child-parent-medical provider communication: A systematic review. *Social Science and Medicine, 166*, 120–127.

LaFond, C. M., Vincent, C., Oosterhouse, K., & Wilkie, D. J. (2016). Nurses beliefs regarding pain in critically ill children: a mixed-methods study. *Journal of Pediatric Nursing, 31*(6), 691–700.

Limke, C. M., Peabody, M., & Kullgren, K. (2015). Integration of mobile health applications into pain intervention on an inpatient psychology Consultation Liaison service. *Pediatric Pain Letter, 17*(2), 21–26.

Mullen, J. E., Reynolds, M. R., & Larson, J. S. (2015). Caring for pediatric patients' families at the child's end of life. *Critical Care Nursing, 35*(6), 46–55.

Piaget, J. (1972). *The child's conception of the world.* Savage, MD: Littlefield: Adams.

O'Toole, S., Lambert, V., Gallagler, P., Shahwan, A., & Austin, J. K. (2016). Talking about epilepsy: Challenges parents face when communicating with their children about epilepsy and epilepsy-related issues. *Epilepsy and Behavior, 57*, 9–15.

Quality and safety education for nurse (QSEN). www.qsen.org/competencies. Accessed 10.3.18.

Sparapani, V., Jacob, E., & Nascimento, L. C. (2015). What is it like to be a child with Type 1 diabetes mellitus? *Pediatric Nursing, 41*(1), 17–22.

Sposito, A. M., Silva-Rodrigues, F. M., Sparapani, V., Pfeifer, L. I., de Lima, R. A., & Nascimento, L. C. (2015). Coping strategies used by hospitalized children with cancer undergoing chemotherapy. *Journal of Nursing Scholarship, 47*(2), 143–151.

Twycross, A. (2015). Pediatric nurses' post-op pain management in hospital settings. *International Journal of Nursing Studies, 52*, 836–863.

US Department of Health and Human Services (DHHS). (2011). *Health Resources and Services Administration (HRSA).* www.HRSA.gov.

US Department of Health and Human Services (DHHS). In: Healthy People 2020. Adolescent Health. http://healthypeople.gov/2020/topicsobjectives2020/overview.aspx?topicid=2.

US Department of Health and Human Services (DHHS). (n.d.). Health Resources and Services Administration (HRSA). Maternal and Child Health Bureau. www.HRSA.gov.

World Health Organization (WHO). (n.d.). www.who.int/mediacentre/factsheets/fs150/en/. Accessed 07.01.17.

Young, V. B. (2017). Effective management of pain and anxiety for the pediatric patient in the emergency department. *Critical Care Nursing Clinics of North America, 29*, 205–216.

19

Communicating With Older Adults

Elizabeth C. Arnold

OBJECTIVES

At the end of the chapter, the reader will be able to:

1. Discuss concepts of normal aging.
2. Identify theoretical frameworks used in communicating with older patients and families.
3. Describe patient-centered assessment strategies for older adults.
4. Discuss supportive self-management care strategies with older adults.
5. Describe patient-centered care and communication strategies with cognitively impaired adults.

INTRODUCTION

Older adults are the fastest growing segment of the US population. They represent 14.5% of the population, compared with 4.1% in 1900 (Administration on Aging, 2015). Once fatal diseases have been replaced with chronic diseases as the major cause of disability and death; as people live longer and healthier lives (Institute of Medicine [IOM], 2007). These disorders require coordinated, long term care and attention.

This chapter addresses features of the aging process, identifies selected theory frameworks, and discusses how nurses can effectively communicate with older adults to promote their health and well-being. The chapter concludes with discussion of dementia and related communication strategies nurses can use with cognitively impaired patients.

BASIC CONCEPTS

Aging and Age-Related Changes

Aging represents a universal life process of "advancing through the life cycle, beginning at birth, and ending at death" (Pankow & Solotoroff, 2007, p. 19). Age 65 is commonly identified as the beginning of late adulthood (Narang, Kordia, Meena, & Meena, 2013). In part because people are living longer, the term "older adult" is broken down into three age cohorts: young old (65–74 years), old-old (75–84 years), and oldest-old (85 years and older)

(Moody & Sasser, 2017). Of those older than 65 years, 85% will have at least one chronic disease and 50% will have more than one chronic condition. Chronological age is only one measurement of old age. Old age is recognized as a significant social and psychological dimension of our lives. (Moody & Sasser, 2017, p. 3)

Aging is accompanied by changes in appearance and energy levels, diminishing organ functioning, a weaker immune system, sensory losses, and decreased functional capacity related to mobility. As people age, they experience diminished physiological reserve, which affects physical strength, stamina, and flexibility, to varying degrees. It often takes them more time to recuperate from an injury or illness, as their immune system may not respond as well. Ultimately, the effects of impaired mobility and functional decline may impact a person's ability to independently negotiate their physical environment. Preventing and reducing the major functional losses associated with aging is an essential wellness goal for older patients (Gray-Micelli, 2017).

How the aging process influences one's life reflects each person's genetic makeup, personality, motivation, life experiences, level of support, environmental and cultural factors, and engagement with health promotion activities. Limitations are to some extent preventable or reversible through careful self-management health strategies. Developing the resilience to prevent and/or to effectively self-manage chronic conditions is key to leading a meaningful life as an older adult (Ebrahimi, Wilhelmson, Moore, & Jakobsson, 2013).

Psychologically, changes in role responsibilities, and even the meaning of life, can force a reevaluation of how older adults choose to spend their time. As people age, role responsibilities and expectations change; some are desired and embraced. Becoming a grandparent can be an ongoing experience of joy and satisfaction. There is more free time to renew and enjoy friendships, to travel, and to do meaningful volunteer work contributing to the lives of others. Other age-related changes are not chosen. Limitations in mobility and function, loss of social supports through death or retirement, and significant changes in income can be stressful.

Case Example

Before he retired, Pat H. was a highly paid lawyer, well respected, and very busy. Now retired, he volunteers at his area public library to help young people learn English. He does this twice a week and derives a great deal of pleasure from his new work. Pat is making a difference in the lives of his "students." In the process, his own life has become enriched.

Successful Aging

Cotter and Gonzalez (2009) describe "*successful aging* as the ability to adapt flexibly to age-related changes without relinquishing the central components of self-definition" (p. 335). This definition invites older adults to take charge of their participation in a personally relevant aging process. Empowering older adults to restructure everyday life routines to accommodate and minimize deficits contributes to living a purposeful life, with optimal functioning. Helping older adults to enhance security in the home environment and encouraging regular social contacts and connectivity with others are essential supportive interventions for the older adult. Staying as active as possible, and as engaged in life with supportive relationships, is key to thriving as an older adult. Simulation Exercise 19.1, "What Will It Be Like to Be Old?" provides you with an opportunity to explore your personal ideas about aging and what this time of life might mean for you.

Fundamental aspects of successful active aging include the *autonomy* to make decisions. Also important is the capability to cope with daily life in line with personal preference and the capacity to *live independently* in the community, with little or no assistance from others (Constanca, Ribeiro, & Teixeira, 2012).

Staying actively engaged with chosen life activities and having regular social interactions with others are important dimensions of successful aging (Ebrahimi et al., 2013). Within the community, more nurses play a critical role in helping patients embrace new roles that allow them to make these types of creative life choices (Fig. 19.1).

SIMULATION EXERCISE 19.1   What Will It Be Like to Be Old?

Purpose:
To stimulate personal awareness and feelings about the aging process.

Procedure:
Think about and write down the answers to the following questions about your own aging process:
* What do you think will be important to you when you are 65 years of age?
* Prepare a list of the traits, qualities, and attributes you hope you will have when you are this age.
* What do you think will be different for you in terms of physical, emotional, spiritual, and social perceptions and activities?
* How would you like people to treat you when you are an older adult?

Discussion:
In groups of three to four students, share your thoughts. Have one person act as a scribe and write down common themes. Students should ask questions about anything they do not understand.
* In what ways did doing this exercise give you some insight into what the issues of aging might be for your age group?
* In what ways might the issues be different for people in your age group and for people currently classified as older adults?
* How could you use this exercise to better understand the needs of older adults in the hospital, long-term setting, or home?

Aging and Health

Chronic diseases have largely replaced acute infectious conditions as the major source of health care burden (Avolio et al., 2013).

Older adults are the largest users of health services (National Council on Aging, 2014). Age-related chronic diseases, such as cancer, macular degeneration, glaucoma, cognitive disorders, cardiac and circulatory problems, diabetes, stroke, and degenerative bone loss, occur with greater frequency as people live longer. Five functional syndromes associated with aging include falls, urinary incontinence, pressure ulcers, functional decline, and delirium. These are classified as "geriatric syndromes" in the literature (Brown-O'Hara, 2013; Gray-Miceli, 2017).

Barriers to Treatment

Initially described by Dr. Robert Butler in 1969, ageism is still an issue in health care. *Ageism* is described as discrimination against older adults. Older adults can experience discrimination in accessing health care, level of screening, and choice of treatment options. Health care providers are less likely to use extensive diagnostic testing or aggressive treatment with older adults for reasons of age rather than health or function. Kagan (2012) writes, "Discrimination on the basis of chronological age is perhaps the most pervasive unacknowledged prejudice in our society" (p. 60).

Other barriers that older adults face include navigating the complexity of an unfamiliar, multifaceted medical system composed of many interacting parts, and working with the current limitations or gaps in services for chronic health care conditions. This obstacle is particularly challenging for dementia patients and their families (Murray & Boyd, 2009).

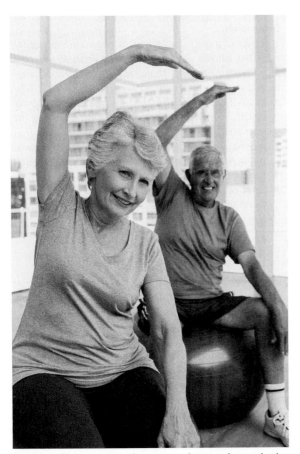

Fig. 19.1 Older adults who engage in exercise and other health promotion activities are better able to offset the ills of old age.

The decreasing number of physicians and other health care providers accepting Medicare patients is another factor. On a positive note, Medicare recently introduced initial preventative physical exams (IPPEs) and subsequent annual wellness visits (AWVs). These services, plus annual screening mammograms and pelvic exams, are exempt from deductibles and copays, which makes them available as disease prevention supports for older adults (Resnick, 2013).

Nurses are in a position to work with patients on strategies to prevent falls, which is a major cause of death and disability in the elderly. Having knowledge of community resources as a basis to recommend community-based strengthening programs such as Tai Chi, bone builders, and other exercise and general fitness classes for older adults is also helpful.

Health Assessment for Older Adults

The elderly represent a more health conscious and better-informed age group than even a decade ago. Many are living into their 90s because of advances in medicine, health screening, technology, and healthy behaviors. They eat better, exercise more, actively engage with life, and take personal responsibility for their health and well-being. Annual wellness exams, which are not subject to Medicare deductibles, and other changes brought about by the Patient Protection and Affordable Care Act have dramatically shifted the focus of the health care system from a disease focus to a wellness paradigm. This new emphasis requires older adults to assume greater responsibility for health promotion and disease prevention activities, and to better manage their health and well-being. In this

---

SIMULATION EXERCISE 19.2   Quality Health Care for Baby Boomers

Purpose:
To provide an understanding of changes needed to provide quality health care for baby boomers.

Procedure:
Break class into groups of four to six students. Allow yourself to go beyond the facts and think about your personal response.
Answer the following questions:
- How do you think the influx of baby boomers will affect health care?
- What types of challenges do you see the health care system facing with the anticipated dramatic increase in numbers of older adults?
- What are your ideas as a health professional to resolve the health care issues of the future related to care of older adults?

new health care design, self-management health strategies assume a primary emphasis. Nurses need to be prepared to perform nursing functions in both acute and community-based health care settings (Simulation Exercise 19.2).

PSYCHOLOGICAL MODELS THEORETICAL FRAMEWORKS

Erikson's Ego Development Model

Erikson's model addresses stage development in later adulthood. With older adults, ego integrity becomes the dominant ego strength. **Ego integrity** describes acceptance of "one's one and only life cycle as something that had to be and that by necessity permitted of no substitutions" (Erikson, 1980, p. 104). Ego integrity develops through self-reflection and dialogue with others about the meaning of one's life. Nurses

can help frame the older adult's illness story with recognition of social supports and patterns of psychosocial responses in ways that help them reflect on the personal meaning of life. Nursing strategies encouraging life review and reminiscence groups facilitate the process. **Ego despair** describes the failure of a person to accept one's life as appropriate and meaningful. Left unresolved, despair leads to feelings of emotional desolation and bitterness.

Wisdom is the virtue associated with this stage of ego development. It is a form of "knowing" about the meaning and conduct of life, and being willing to share one's wisdom with others. Le (2008) discusses two forms of wisdom: practical wisdom and transcendent wisdom. *Practical wisdom* emphasizes good judgment and the capacity to resolve complex human problems in the real world. *Transcendent wisdom* focuses on existential concerns and self-knowledge, which allows a person to transcend subjectivity, bias, and self-centeredness in relation to an issue. Wisdom allows older adults to share their understanding of life with those who will follow. Simulation Exercise 19.3, "The Wisdom of Aging," explores the relationship of life experiences to the development of wisdom.

Theoretical Understandings of the Older Adult

An older adult's quality of life correlates with his/her functional capacity and capacity to meet personal dependency needs (Miller, 2011). A functional consequences framework helps nurses assess patients across a continuum of functioning, from high functioning to frail older adults. This framework emphasizes interventions, which emphasize functional self-management. Activities considered essential to self-regulating functional capacity include self-care, mobility, interaction and relationships with others, cognitive reasoning ability, and engagement with life tasks.

Hierarchy of Needs Theory

Maslow's (1954) hierarchy of needs helps nurses prioritize nursing actions, beginning with basic survival needs. Physiological integrity, followed by safety and security, emerge as the most basic critical issues for older patients. They need to be addressed first. For example, Touhy and Jett (2015) note that an agitated patient with dementia looking for a toilet and not being able to find it will not respond to a nurse's comfort or redirection strategies until the toileting need is met. Love and belonging needs in older adults are challenged by increased losses associated with death of important people. Esteem needs, especially those associated with meaningful purpose, and independence remain important issues in later life. Abraham Maslow believed that self-actualization occurs more often in middle-aged and older adults (Moody & Sasser, 2017).

SIMULATION EXERCISE 19.3 The Wisdom of Aging

Purpose:
To promote an understanding of the sources of wisdom in the older adult.

Procedure:
- Interview an older adult (65 years or older) who, in your opinion, has had a fulfilling life. Ask the person to describe his or her most satisfying life events, and what he or she did to accomplish them. Ask the person to identify his or her most meaningful life experience or accomplishment. Immediately after the interview, write down your impressions, with direct quotes if possible to support your impressions.
- Reflect on the person's comments and your ideas of what strengths this person had that allowed him or her to achieve a sense of well-being, and to value his or her accomplishments.

Discussion:
- Were you surprised at any older adults' responses to the question about most satisfying experiences? Most meaningful experiences?
- On a blackboard or flip chart, identify the accomplishments that people have identified. Classify them as work-related or people-related.
- What common themes emerged in the overall class responses that speak to the strengths in the life experience of older adults?
- How can you apply what you learned from doing this exercise in your future nursing practice?

DEVELOPING AN EVIDENCE-BASED PRACTICE

Objectives:
The purpose of this study was to explore and access definitions of person-centered care (PCC) for older adults and to identify the important elements of PCC.

Methods:
Close to 3000 articles were examined, yielding 132 nonduplicative sources. Fifteen descriptors of PCC in older adults and 17 central principles were identified.

Results:
The most prominent domains of PCC were identified as holistic care, patient respect and value, choices respect for patient dignity, self-determination, and purposeful living.

Application to Your Clinical Practice:
This sweeping systematic study review of patient-centered care can inform your care of older adults in clinical settings. Findings from this study guided the development of a separate American Geriatrics Society expert panel statement used to develop a standardized definition and categorizing PCC elements for older adults with chronic conditions or functional impairment.

From Kogan, A., Wilber, K., & Mosqueda, L. (2016). Person-centered care for older adults with chronic conditions and functional impairment: A systematic literature review. *Journal of American Geriatric Society, 64*(1), e1–e7.

BOX 19.1 *Healthy People 2020*
Objectives Related to Care of Older Adults

1. Increase the proportion of older adults who use the Welcome to Medicare Benefit.
2. Increase the proportion of older adults who are up to date on a core set of clinical preventive services.
3. Increase the proportion of older adults with one or more chronic health conditions who report confidence in managing their conditions.
4. Reduce the proportion of older adults who have moderate to severe functional limitations.
5. Increase the proportion of older adults with reduced physical or cognitive function who engage in light, moderate, or vigorous leisure-time physical activities.

US Department of Health and Human Services. (2010). *Healthy People 2020.* Available online at: http://www.Healthypeople2020. Accessed July 19, 2013.

BOX 19.2 **Communication Guidelines for Assessment Interviews**

1. Establish rapport.
2. Use open-ended questions first, followed by focused questions.
3. Ask one question at a time.
4. Elicit patient perspectives first.
5. Elicit family perspectives, if indicated.
6. Invite ideas and feelings about diagnosis and treatment.
7. Acknowledge feelings and emotions.
8. Communicate a willingness to help.
9. Provide information in small segments.
10. Summarize the problem or condition discussed in the interview.
11. Validate with the patient and/or family for accuracy.
12. Provide contact information for further questions or concerns.

APPLICATIONS

Selected objectives from *Healthy People 2020* specifically address the health and well-being of older adults as identified in Box 19.1.

These guidelines emphasize a renewed focus on health promotion, disease prevention, and efficacy with self-management of chronic disorders. Self-management is fundamental to the chronic care model (CCM). The concept refers to decisions and behaviors that the person undertakes to independently manage his or her chronic condition on a day-to-day basis. Successful self-management of chronic disorders requires active partnership by the patient and family in collaboration with health care professionals to achieve desired outcomes (Lorig & Fries, 2006).

Guidelines for communication in assessment interviews are found in Box 19.2.

New situations can cause transitory confusion for older adults. Heightened anxiety can be true for any patient, but it is even more so for the elderly with multiple comorbidities.

Older adults are aware of stereotypes associated with aging and may be reluctant to expose themselves as inadequate in a new situation. So they wait and see how their comments will be received. Older adults may stumble over questions when unusually stressed because of anxiety or needing more processing time. Should this occur, the presence of family members can be helpful in giving the health care team a verbal picture of the patient's pre-illness state and normalizing care situations for the patient (Happ, 2010).

Older adults tend to be more responsive when time is taken to establish a supportive environment before conducting a formal assessment. Sensitive issues such as loneliness, abuse and neglect, caregiver burden, fears about death or frailty, memory loss, incontinence, alcohol abuse, and sexual dysfunction will only be discussed within a trustworthy relationship (Adelman, Greene, & Ory, 2000). Continuity of care with one primary caregiver, when possible, helps foster the development of a comfortable nurse-patient relationship.

Providing structure for history taking facilitates communication. You should begin by explaining what information is needed and why it is important.

Nurses need to get to know the patient as a person rather than categorically as an "older adult." Moody and Sasser (2017) maintains that old age "is shaped by a life time of experience" (p. 2).

Box 19.2 provides guidelines for communication strategies related to patient centered assessment interviews.

Assessment of older patients begins with their story of what brought them to the hospital or health care center. It is important to understand each patient within the context of his or her biographical narrative (Cenci, 2016). Letting a patient share a health history in his or her words with few interruptions provides information you might otherwise not get.

Asking patients to share something about themselves and their life history helps establish rapport and increases the patient's comfort level. Listen for the facts, but also pay attention to what the patient identifies as his or her most important concern(s). Look for value-laden psychosocial issues associated with the patient's need for medical consultation (e.g., independence, fears about the future, role changes, sensory and cognitive losses, loneliness, and vulnerability) and patient preferences. These issues can color the older adult's perception of overall health and well-being.

A person-centered approach to high quality health care for older adults is one, which supports a person's dignity and independence (AGS Expert Panel, 2016) (Fig. 19.2). Look for patient strengths and affirm them. Help patients identify their sources of social support, assess their personal and financial resources, and describe their coping strategies. Help family caregivers of patients find community support. Simulation Exercise 19.4, "The Story of Aging," provides a glimpse into the personal life stories of older adults.

Accommodating for Sensory Loss

Sensory changes occur with normal aging. Both hearing and vision changes can have a direct and significant impact on communication. Compensatory enhancements are essential to ensuring patient safety and staying connected with others (Bonder & Dal Bello-Haas, 2018). Because vision and hearing decline are accepted as normal facts of aging, their significance is not always addressed as vigorously as it should be. Sensory impairment can cause major confusion about the meaning of important health messages (Anderson, 2005).

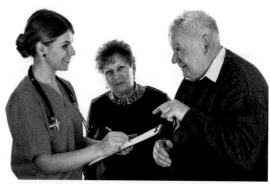

Fig. 19.2 Cognitively intact older adults are an important source of information about their health issues. (Copyright © Ocskaymark/iStock/Thinkstock.)

SIMULATION EXERCISE 19.4 The Story of Aging

Purpose:
To promote an understanding of older adults.

Procedure:
1. Interview an older adult in your family (minimum age, 65 years). If there are no older adults in your family, interview a family friend whose lifestyle is similar to your family's.
2. Ask this person to describe what growing up was like, what is different today from the way it was when he or she was your age, what are the important values held, and if there have been any changes in them over the years. Ask this person what advice he or she would give you about how to achieve satisfaction in life. If this person could change one thing about our society today, what would it be?

Discussion:
1. Were you surprised at any of the answers older adults gave you?
2. What are some common themes you and your classmates found that related to values and the type of advice older adults gave each of you?
3. What implications do the findings from this exercise have for your future nursing practice?

Hearing Loss

According to the National Institute on Deafness and Other Communication Disorders (NIDCD, 2013), one in three people older than 60 years of age, and half of those older than 85 years of age, will experience hearing loss. Hearing loss associated with normal aging begins after age 50 years, due to loss of hair cells (which are not replaced) in the inner ear. This change leads initially to a loss in the ability to hear high-frequency sounds (e.g., *f, s, th, sh, ch*), with later losses related to frequency vowel sounds (Gallo, 2000).

There is perhaps nothing more socially isolating than not being able to hear, and respond in social situations. Older adults with hearing loss have special difficulty in distinguishing sounds from background noises, understanding people talking with accents, and following fast-paced speech. Hearing problems diminish an older person's ability to interact with others, attend concerts and other social functions, and understand medical directions.

Communication difficulties related to hearing are frustrating for both speaker and listener. Difficulties can occur because of environmental factors such as background noise, half hearing or misinterpreting conversations, or incorrectly manipulating an ear piece (Pryce & Gooberman, 2012). This does not have to happen. There are hearing aid programs for people with limited income that can help with financial costs. The Department of Rehabilitation Services and nonprofit hearing aid programs have hearing aids available for free or at a discount (see http://savvysenior.org).

Adaptive communication strategies for hearing loss.
- Proactive strategies can minimize hearing loss in conversation. By positioning yourself at the same level as the patient, the patient is more likely to hear what you are saying. Speak slowly and distinctly. Annunciate your words. Repeat what you said if the patient looks confused or gives an unusual response. Remember that communication is a two-way street and that the most important element is mutual understanding of the conversation.
  Other strategies include the following:
- Address the patient by name before beginning to speak to focus attention.
- Maintain eye contact with the patient.
- If the patient has a "better" ear, sit or stand on the side with the more functional ear.
- If your voice is high-pitched, lower it.
- Make sure the patient can see your facial expression and/or read your lips to enhance comprehension. Keep the patient's view of your mouth unobstructed.
- Help patients adjust hearing aids; some may not be able to insert aids correctly to amplify hearing. Make sure hearing aids are turned on. If difficulties persist, check the batteries. Patients with hearing aids should always have extra batteries readily accessible.
- Keep background noise to a minimum (e.g., radio or television, competing conversations, high-activity locations, children running around, and sudden noises).

- Sometimes you can tell from a vague facial expression or inappropriate response that your message was misheard. Check in with the patient frequently. Solicit feedback to monitor how much and what the person has heard.

Age-Related Vision Loss

Vision normally declines as a person ages (Whiteside, Wallhagen, & Pettengill, 2006). Colors become dimmer and images less clear. Brighter lighting and larger print can help. More serious age-related vision problems such as cataracts, glaucoma, and age-related macular degeneration can cause blindness in the elderly, if left untreated. Loss of visual acuity is gradual, but progressive, associated with age-related changes in the support structures of the eye and the visual pathway (Mauk, 2010).

Guidelines for effective communication in assessment interviews are found in Box 19.2.

Poor vision has implications for effective communication, safety, and functional ability. Older adults with progressive vision loss may miss seeing you shaking your head or nodding, as these are subtle movements. They also may not see slight changes in emotional facial expressions, which can change the meaning of the communication.

Impaired vision can affect a person's ability to perform everyday activities (e.g., dressing, preparing meals, taking medication, driving, handling the checkbook, and seeing phone numbers). Poor vision disturbs functional ability to engage in hobbies or leisure activities requiring vision (e.g., reading, doing handwork, driving, or watching television).

Reduced visual acuity, loss of contrast sensitivity, and loss of depth perception create major safety issues related to falls. Lord (2006) notes that vision plays a significant role in postural stability because it provides the nervous system with information regarding the individual's position and movement in relation to the environment. Mobility slows as a person ages, and this combined with decreased vision can lead to increased risk for falling. Any patient with "balance" issues should avoid ice and uneven terrain.

Adaptive communication strategies for vision loss. Common adaptive devices that older adults use are prescription glasses and handheld magnifiers. Nurses can support the independence of the visually impaired patient with the following strategies:
- If eyeglasses are worn, make sure they are clean and in place. (Glasses can be cleaned with a soft cloth and water.)
- Check that the older adult's glasses prescription gets updated as vision decreases. Regularly scheduled eye exams are vital.
- "Mature" eyes undergo age-related structural changes that affect vision.
- Assist the older adult on steps (particularly descent), on curbs, and on uneven terrain.

- Eliminate all throw rugs.
- Caution patients about slippery or wet floors.
- Verbally note changes in the physical environment that could cause mobility problems *before* patients meet them.
- Face the patient directly when speaking. They may see your form even when features are indistinct.
- Verbally explain all written information, allowing time for the patient to ask questions.
- Provide bright lighting with no glare.
- When using written materials, consider font and letter size (14 point) for readability. Use upper and lowercase letters rather than all capitals. Use solid paper, with sharp contrasting writing, and a lot of white space.
- Encourage older adults to use audio books or electronic readers that can enlarge print.

Older adults may require more time to complete verbal tasks or to process unfamiliar information. It also is not uncommon for older adults to have trouble with digital communication if they have not been exposed to technology.

Older adults are more cautious. They may hesitate, become flustered, or may not be able to respond as well if they are under time pressure to perform. Otherwise, there should be no significant difference in the cognitive functioning of an older adult.

Assessing for Cognitive Changes

According to a worldwide study, "dementia is the greatest cause of years lost due to disability in developed countries and the second greatest worldwide" (UNFPA UNPF 2012, p. 62.). Approximately 6% to 8% of the population older than 65 years and more than 30% of those who reach the age of 85 years will experience profound progressive cognitive changes associated with dementia (Yuhas et al., 2006). Dementia is characterized by working memory loss, particularly for recent events, significant personality changes, and a progressive deterioration in intellectual functioning.

Appraisal of serious cognitive changes is a critical assessment with older adults, because it has such a significant effect on a person's ability to perform activities of daily living (ADLs) (Moody & Sasser, 2017). Performing a mental status assessment early in the interview helps with an accurate diagnosis. The Mini-Mental State Examination (Folstein, Folstein, & McHugh, 1975) measures several dimensions of cognition (e.g., orientation, memory, abstraction, and language). An abnormal score (<26) suggests dementia and the need for further evaluation of cognition. Guides for mental status testing are presented in Box 19.3.

Guidelines for conducting mental status assessments are found in Box 19.4.

BOX 19.3 Guide for Mental Status Assessment of Older Adults

- Select a standardized test such as the Mini-Mental State Examination.
- Administer the test in a quiet, nondistracting environment at a time when the patient is not anxious, agitated, or tired.
- Make sure the patient has eyeglasses and/or hearing aids, if needed, before testing.
- Ask easier questions first and provide frequent reassurance that the patient is doing well with the testing.
- Determine the patient's level of formal education. If the patient never learned to spell, it will be impossible to spell "world" backward. Saying the days of the week backward is a good alternative.
- Document your findings clearly in the patient's record, including the patient's response to the testing process, so that future comparisons can be made.

BOX 19.4 Working with Older Adult Groups

1. Affirm the dignity, intelligence, and pride of elderly group members.
2. Ask group members to introduce themselves and ask how they would like to be called.
3. Make use of humor, but never at the expense of an individual group member.
4. Keep the communication simple, but at an adult level.
5. Ask relevant questions at important points in a patient's story.
6. Call attention to the range of life experiences and personal strengths when they occur.
7. Allow group members to voice their complaints, even when nothing can be done about them, and then refocus on the group task.
8. Avoid probing for the release of strong emotions that neither you nor they can handle effectively in the group sessions.
9. Thank each person for contributing to the group and summarize the group activity for that session.

Adapted from Corey, M., & Corey, G. (2013). *Groups for the elderly* (9th ed.). Belmont, CA: Thompson/Brooks Cole.

COMMON ASSESSMENT ISSUES WITH OLDER ADULTS

Assessment of Functional Status

The ability to perform ADLs and Instrumental Activities of Daily Livings (IADLs) is an essential competency for older adults, especially for those who live alone.

Functional status refers to a broad range of purposeful abilities related to physical health maintenance, role performance, cognitive or intellectual abilities, social activities, and level of emotional functioning. Impaired functional status is a determinant of an older adult's ability to live independently.

Functional status rather than chronological age should be a stronger indicator of disability-related needs in older adults, as functional impairment is not associated solely with age. A chronically ill 50-year-old with no support system may have more disabling symptoms of aging than a healthy, active 75-year-old with a strong social support system in place (Burke & Laramie, 2004).

Evaluation of functional abilities helps determine the type and level of care an older adult requires. Essential ADLs refer to six areas of essential function: toileting, feeding, dressing, grooming, bathing, and ambulation (Miller, 2011).

Pain in Older Adults

Pain is a common concern of older adults, related to an increased number of chronic and acute medical conditions (Horgas, 2017). Moderate, episodic pain associated with chronic disorders of aging occurs more frequently than not and needs to be addressed.

Persistent pain is reported in more than 50% of the elderly (Herr, 2013). Pain limits an older adult's functional ability and compromises well-being. Although pain is a component of many chronic conditions associated with aging, it should not be considered a normal consequence of aging. Pain in the older adult is often underreported because people equate pain with being a natural part of the aging process (Cavalieri, 2005). Once identified, reducing pain to improve function should be a treatment goal (Herr, 2010). There is no more reason for an older adult patient to suffer with chronic pain than there is for younger patients.

Rowan and Faul (2007) label prescription drug abuse as one of the fastest growing public health problems among older adults in the United States. The elderly are frequently prescribed opiods to control chronic pain, and benzodiazapines for anxiety, and insomnia. Neither proscriber or patient considers this a potential addictive risk. Chronic coexisting disorders such as depression or dementia can also limit an older adult's ability to report and correctly interpret underlying causes of pain. Agitated cognitively impaired patients are often given benzodiazipines to calm their acute anxiety. For example, undiagnosed depression may present as neck or shoulder pain, severe enough to interfere with sleep or activity. Liberal dispensing of analgesics to older adults for pain relief without full assessment of the nature of the pain can lead to undesired outcomes. But an alternate system where patients can report when their pain interferes with daily functioning, identifying pain levels on a linear scale, can be more of a challenge for the elderly (Gloth, 2010).

A comprehensive pain assessment for older adults should ask the patient to:

- Specify the quality and nature of the pain. For example, is the pain constant, or is it associated with movement or position? Is it aching, burning, pressure, acute, or stabbing? (Some older adults will use the word *discomfort* instead of *pain*.)
- Identify when the pain occurs and under what circumstances.
- Identify specific pain patterns and/or changes in pain intensity.
- Describe how the pain affects the patient's physical, psychological, and social functioning.
- Define the area of the body where the pain occurs, whether it is deep or superficial, localized, or radiating (Feldt, 2008).
- Note possible contributing factors such as changes in the patient's caregiver, family, or social situation such as death or absence of an important support person.

Assessment of pain in cognitively impaired patients and in those who cannot communicate verbally is more difficult. It tends to be expressed in behavior instead of words. Behavioral observation of symptoms suggestive of pain include grimacing, tightened muscles, groaning, crying, agitation, lethargy, and an unwillingness to move. Older adults who are socially isolated or depressed can experience greater pain than those who remain connected with a social support system.

Ask about recent losses and changes. Loss is a reoccurring issue for older adults. Many will suffer losses of people, activities, and functions of importance to them during this life stage. Unlike symptoms of depression in younger people, somatization with vague physical complaints is often a presenting sign of depression (Arnold, 2005). Older adults, particularly white males, are at higher risk for suicide. Comments reflecting hopelessness such as "life doesn't hold much for me" or "sometimes I just wish God would take me" should never be taken lightly.

EMPOWERING OLDER ADULTS: COMMUNICATION STRATEGIES

Promotion of patient social connectedness are important dimensions of improved health-related quality of life (HRQoL). Whereas older adults can experience negative situational stressors, they also possess a lifetime of strengths.

General nursing care for cognitively intact older adult patients in community centers around discussion of supports related to self-management of chronic illness and promoting healthy lifestyles. Sometimes it is simply a lack of information that prevents older adults from pursuing possible options. Patients may not be aware of elder care services: transportation, meals on wheels, church-sponsored friendly visitors, and other aging in place initiatives. Others know of elder support services, but do not know how to access the available resources in their community. With encouragement, older adults may engage in an exercise program, attend senior center activities, or explore a Tai Chi program combining exercise and meditation. Programs such as bone builders and fall prevention classes often are free for elders in the community.

Studies indicate that many older adults experience higher psychosocial well-being compared with their younger counterparts (Windsor & Anstey, 2008). This sounds counterintuitive, but older adults are more likely to seek and enjoy emotionally meaningful activities in the present moment.

They are less competitive and less concerned with high achievement. Older adults appreciate short, frequent conversations. Like everyone else, the need to be acknowledged is paramount to older adults' sense of self-esteem.

The *level* of social support people use depends on personal preference, individual, financial, and social resources, plus what older adults have at their disposal and are willing and able to use. Asking questions such as "Can you tell me who visits you?," "Whom have you visited in the last couple of weeks?," or "If you needed immediate help, whom would you call?" are useful ways to introduce the importance of social support as a part of self-management strategies.

Heliker (2009) describes story sharing strategy as "a reciprocal give-and-take process of respectful telling and listening that focuses on what matters to the individual and minimizes the power of one over another" (p. 44). Stories become a shared experience, reminding patients of a valued social identity that goes beyond descriptions of their health. Each time older adults tell their story, they remember how they saw themselves as valued, productive members of society. Sharing the story with their nurse tells them they still are valuable. They know someone cares to listen. Nurses can teach and model this communication strategy for use by nursing assistants in long-term settings.

The conversational world for older adults may narrow for many reasons: mobility, social isolation, cognitive decline, death of friends, distance, or transportation. Current events to draw from as a means of starting a conversation are not as available, so even cognitively intact older adults repeat stories. In addition, family members need empathetic updates and tailored information about their family member that enables realistic decision-making with, and for the patient throughout the care experience (Van Vliet, Lindenberger, & Van Weert, 2015).

Each conversation becomes an opportunity to gain insight into the person, such as what the person values, what aspirations and dreams were fulfilled or unfulfilled, what contributions are valued, and what goals are yet to be attained. Focusing on what a person considers important enhances well-being among older adults, particularly the homebound.

Life Review and Reminiscence

Life review is a useful intervention with older adult patients. It can occur as an individual sharing. Gentle prompts and relevant questions for clarification are usually sufficient to keep the conversation going. Sharing recollections from youth or early adulthood days with a compassionate listener helps older adults review their life and/or re-establish its meaning. Sometimes telling the story provides useful reasons for older adults to resolve long-standing conflicts with important people in their lives (Bohlmeijer, Kramer, Smit, Onrust, & van Marwijk, 2009).

Reminiscence

Reminiscence is an empowerment strategy that reminds older adults of personal strengths and meaningful goals already achieved. Asking simple concrete questions about the older adult's life, where the person grew up, and what was most important to him or her is a prompt you can use to initiate conversation, or when communication stalls. Notice if the patient's face seems more animated at any point in the conversation. If so, then comment on it, with simple acknowledgment (for example, "It seems like this was a time that was important to you") and ask for more details.

A specialized group for older adults in long-term settings is the reminiscence group. Minardi and Hayes (2003) differentiate between life review, which explores life events in depth, and reminiscence groups. **Reminiscence groups** focus on sharing important life experiences as simple stories. They follow a structured format, with broad category themes decided on beforehand. Examples include special times in childhood or adolescence, child-rearing or work experience, and handling of a crisis. The leader guides the group in telling their stories, asking questions, and points out common themes to stimulate further reflections. In the process of remembering critical incidents, patients can reconnect with forgotten moments that held meaning for them, thus giving them a sense of continuity with their current circumstances (Jonsdottir, Jonsdottir, Steingrimsdottir, & Tryggvadottir, 2001). Guidelines for group work with older adults are presented in Box 19.4.

Encouraging Social and Spiritual Supports

Staying engaged with life and stimulating the mind is essential to the health and well-being of older adults (Reichstadt, Sengupta, Depp, Palinkas, & Jeste, 2010). Older adults have the same need for meaningful activity and personal relationships as younger adults (Potempa, Butterworth, & Flaherty-Robb Gaynor, 2010). Age-related changes in eyesight, hearing, and mobility make it more difficult to easily socialize with others. Because older adults can lose self-confidence and begin to disengage socially, they may need encouragement to make the additional effort needed to retain social connections. The amount of socialization depends to some extent on inclination and personality factors, but social isolation compromises the health and well-being of older adults (Strine, Chapman, Balluz, & Mokdad, 2008). In many cases, providing social support needs to be proactive due to mobility issues.

For people who have lost their "personal" support system for age-related reasons, a connection with a personal God or church community can become an important source of social and spiritual support. Bishop (2008) notes, "Social and spiritual ties share an interdependent link to positive psychological well-being in late adulthood" (p. 2).

Existential awareness of a shortened life span promotes thinking about death and the meaning of life. Spiritual interventions relevant to the care of older adults include instilling hope, prayer, use of spiritual hymns or readings, and talking about the patient's spiritual concerns. Helping patients cope with unfinished business is an important nursing intervention (Delgado, 2007). In the following case example, note the interaction between social and spiritual connections.

Case Example

Lois visits a patient with dementia weekly. The woman is mostly mute with little natural speech. One day Lois read her the 23rd Psalm. The woman spontaneously repeated the psalm from a different version, smiling broadly when finished. She could not respond in the present, but she could in the past about something familiar to her.

Supporting Independence

Independence is something most people take for granted as a younger adult; it becomes a significant issue for older adults and their caregivers. Corey and Corey (2006) note, "As we age, we have to adjust to an increasingly external locus of control when confronted with losses over which we have little control" (p. 403).

Nurses need to be sensitive to the often-unexpressed fears of older adults around surrendering their independence. For example, an older adult awaiting discharge from the hospital told his nurse that he had a bedside commode and no stairs in his home. When the nurse visited the home, there was no commode, and the patient's home had a significant number of stairs. The patient told her that he was afraid his nurse would insist he move to a nursing home if he revealed his real circumstances to her. This is not an uncommon fear of the elderly. "How could you respond if you were working with this patient?" Formal support services in the community, meals on wheels, home health aides, medical alerts, and informal family supports can be critical factors in enabling frail older adults to remain independent. Nurses can help older identify and access these supports.

Safety Supports

There often is a delicate balance between the older adult's perceived and actual need for safety in health care. Restrictions and supports needed for safety can and should be negotiated, not simply imposed. The personhood of the patient should always trump patienthood (Chochinov, 2013).

Interventions to promote quality of life while protecting safety and independence include the following:

- Respecting choices in food selection.
- Providing chair risers, walkers, and canes as needed.
- Safety modifications in the home (e.g., handrails on stairs, bathtub/shower grip bars, scatter rug removal, night lights). Increased frailty may make independent showering a safer option than a bath.
- Including older patients in decision making about health care and giving them the information they need to make responsible choices.
- Installing home security, health alarm monitors, giving trusted neighbors or relatives keys and emergency phone numbers.
- Providing information about low-cost Tai Chi, and other low impact exercise programs in the community. Inform patients about fall prevention programs for patients with balance.

Medication Supports

Medications in general have a stronger effect on the metabolism of older adults and take longer to eliminate from the body. Poly-pharmacy is a fact of life for many older adults related to multiple chronic conditions. Older adults are at risk for medication side effects and drug interactions because of the variety of meds they take and age-related changes in metabolism (Kim, Kocilja, & Nielsen, 2018). Successful self-management requires consistent coordinated and active participation of the patient, family, and other health professionals to achieve positive health outcomes.

Unmonitored poly-pharmacy is a major contributor to falls and hip fractures, and medication mismanagement is often a formal reason for hospital or nursing home admissions. Nurses perform important coordinating functions with helping older adults self-manage their medications and treatments. With limited knowledge of a patient's full profile, including over-the-counter medications, dangerous interactions can occur. Important questions you can ask include:

- What do you take each medication for?
- How and when do you take it?
- What kind of problems are you having? (Gould & Mitty, 2010, p. 294).

Encourage older adults and their family members to keep a written list of all medications, including over-the-counter and natural remedies, to be shared with each provider. Do not think of herbal supplements only as add-ons; they too can spike interactions if not understood. Ownby (2006) recommends using an open-ended question, such as "Tell me how you take your medications," rather than asking, "Are you taking your medication as prescribed?" (p. 33). Box 19.5 covers key areas for medication assessment.

Ask about medications, including over-the-counter and herbal or natural medications. You should ask the essential safety questions during initial assessment and during each medical contact or health-related home visit. Reasons for poor self-management of medications include complexity of taking multiple medications, difficulty removing safety tops, using incorrect techniques, improper medication storage, level of health literacy, cost of medications factors, and poor eyesight. Using a teach-back strategy to assess this information is helpful. Visually checking medications with the patient and talking about how the medication is working with the patient and/or primary caretaker is essential in home care.

Health teaching helps patients establish and maintain appropriate self-management of medications. Simplifying the medication regimen and regular checking of expiration dates enhance medication management and lessen the possibility of adverse reactions. The adage "start low, and go slow" (Miller, 2011), plus regular communication with prescribers, is essential. Careful instruction as to the purpose, dosage, anticipated outcomes, and side effects can increase medication compliance. Establish a system with the patient or family for medication administration, for example, prefilled

---

BOX 19.5   Teaching Medication Self-Management

Areas of Assessment

- List of current and previously taken medications, herbal and over-the-counter medications
- Medications taken episodically for insomnia, pain, intestinal upsets, colds, and coughs
- Allergies (include exact symptoms)
- Determine if the patient knows what each medication is for, storage, what to do for missed doses, drug interactions, side effects.
- Ability to read medication labels or printed instructions
- Motor difficulties with appropriate medication administration
- Expiration dates, brown bag syndrome (having older adult bring all medications in a brown bag for clinic visit observation)
- Determination of family responsibility, and availability if medication administration support is needed

---

medication dispensers or a medication calendar. Use a teach-back strategy to ensure that instructions are understood and the patient or family feels comfortable with their knowledge and capacity to implement administration.

Elder Abuse

Box 19.6 identifies fundamental rights of older adult. Elder abuse represents a major threat to the safety and well-being of older adults; this term refers to the mistreatment of vulnerable older adults, usually at the hands of caregivers, including professional personnel.

The most common form of elder abuse is neglect. Active neglect is deliberate. Passive neglect occurs when patients, most notably those with dementia, lack properly supervised care or essential supports related to implementing instrumental or basic ADL.

Elder abuse is a difficult problem to identify and treat. Many older adults are dependent on their caregivers. For those with diminished mental capacity, a patient may not even understand what is happening, let alone take constructive actions to stop the abuse or to use any community services available to them (Nerenberg, 2008). Pride, embarrassment, and a desire to protect family members prevent vulnerable older adults from wanting to prosecute a family member for abuse or neglect. If the nurse identifies abuse or neglect, it must be reported to appropriate social and legal protective services.

BOX 19.6   Fundamental Older Adult Rights

Older adults need to be able to:

- Live in safe and appropriate living environments.
- Establish and maintain meaningful relationships and social networks.
- Have equal access to health care, legal, and social services consistent with their needs.
- Have the right to make decisions about their care and quality of life.
- Have their rights, autonomy, and assets protected.
- Have appropriate information to make reasoned decisions.
- Have their personal, cultural, and spiritual values, beliefs, and preferences respected.
- Participate in all aspects of their care plan, including care decisions, to the fullest extent possible.
- Expect confidentiality of all communication and clinical records related to their care.
- Be involved in advocacy and the formulation of policies that directly impact their health and well-being.

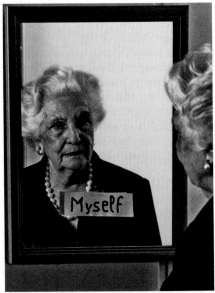

Fig. 19.3 One of the most disabling chronic conditions experienced by older adults is Alzheimer's disease. (Copyright © Syldavia/iStock/Thinkstock.)

Advocacy Support

Fundamental rights of older adults in health care settings are identified in Box 19.5. Nurses have an important role in explaining treatment to patients and families, helping them frame questions for physicians and hospitalists, and arranging for continuity of care with community agencies (see also Chapter 24). Role modeling is an indirect form of advocacy, which nurses provide in institutional settings. Treating older patients with respect, not becoming impatient with primitive behaviors, and providing excellent care is noted by family and nonprofessionals. Holding nursing assistants accountable for maintaining quality care is a nursing responsibility.

HEALTH PROMOTION FOR OLDER ADULTS

Health-damaging behaviors such as poor nutrition, inactivity, alcohol, and tobacco abuse contribute heavily to the onset of disability in the elderly. The Centers for Disease Control and Prevention (CDC) recommends an integrated health promotion approach to address common risk factors and comorbidities in older adults (, Moore, Harris, & Anderson, 2005). Older adults benefit from health promotion activities tailored to their stage of life. It is never too late to practice good nutrition; engage in healthful exercise such as strength training, walking, and yoga; connect with social relationships on a regular basis; and improve safety factors. Most urban communities have groups specifically for older adults (Fig. 19.3).

BOX 19.7   Areas of Relevant Health Promotion Activities

- Health protection: public health approaches promoting flu vaccines
- Health prevention: environmental or home assessments to prevent falls
- Health education: information about healthy eating and exercise
- Health preservation: promoting optimal levels of functioning by increasing the control older adults have over their lives and health

Adapted from Bernard, M. (2000). *Promoting health in old age.* Buckingham, England: Open University Press; Sanders, K. (2006). Developing practice for healthy aging. *Nursing Older People, 18*(3), 18–21.

At the same time, healthy older adults have special needs. Health requirements change as a person ages; their nutrition, exercise, sleep, and other health needs are different. Health promotion strategies need to be modified to meet the unique requirements of aging adults (Nakasato & Carnes, 2006). Box 19.7 identifies areas of relevant health promotion activities for older adults.

Nurses can engage older adults in health promotion activities by appealing to their interests, and by incorporating cultural values in the presentation. Examples of relevant activities can include:

- Preparing examples of healthy ethnic food (e.g., "soul cooking the healthy way")
- Assigning blocks of time for preventive screening, specifically for older adults
- Combining multiple prevention services into one clinical visit
- Providing free flu and pneumonia immunizations at convenient times in traditional and nontraditional settings (Lang et al. 2005; Penprase, 2006).

Health Teaching

Moody and Sasser (2017) notes that health teaching for the elderly is critical if they are to master the tasks of old age and maintain their health. Healthy older adult learning

---

SIMULATION EXERCISE 19.5 Health Promotion Teaching for Older Adults

Purpose:
To provide a health teaching segment for an older adult.

Procedure:
1. Develop a step-by-step mini teaching plan related to fall prevention for a cognitively intact older adult.
   a. Consider what person-centered information you will need from the patient to effectively provide tailored content.
   b. Identify specific content you will need to include in your presentation.
   c. Describe teaching strategies you will use.
   d. What accommodations will you need to make?
   e. How will you evaluate the patient's understanding of the material?
2. Implement the teaching plan.
3. Share your experience with other students in small groups of three to six students.

Discussion:
1. Were there any similarities/differences in themes, or patient responses to the teaching session?
2. Were you surprised at anything you found in preparing for the teaching session versus what occurred during the session?
3. If you had to provide patient education on another topic relevant to the older adult, what would you do differently, if anything?
4. What did you learn from doing this exercise that you could use in future practice with older adults?

---

capabilities remain intact for needing more time to think about how they want to handle a situation. The sensitive nurse observes the patient before implementing teaching for the purpose of matching teaching strategies to the individual learning needs of each patient. Four aspects of successful aging, fall prevention, adequate nutrition, socialization, and medication management, lend themselves to health teaching formats.

Simulation Exercise 19.5 provides an opportunity to think about health teaching for older adults.

Assuming that cognitively intact older adults lack the capacity to understand instructions is a common error. Health care providers often direct instruction to the older adult patient's younger companion, even when the patient has no cognitive impairment. This action invalidates the patient and diminishes self-worth. Mauk (2006) identifies simple modifications to reduce age-related barriers to learning when teaching older adults. Suggestions include:

- Explain why the information is important to the patient.
- Use familiar words and examples in providing information.
- Draw on the patient's experiences and interests when creating an action plan.
- Make teaching sessions short enough to avoid tiring the patient and frequent enough for continuous learning support.
- Speak slowly, naturally, and clearly.

COMMUNICATING WITH COGNITIVELY IMPAIRED OLDER ADULTS

Mild cognitive impairment (MCI) and dementia are neurological disorders characterized by a progressive decline in intellectual and behavioral functioning. When a person suffers with dementia, many people tend to focus on the cognitive and behavioral deficits and overlook the psychosocial, emotional, and spiritual personality components that make up the whole person (MacKinlay, 2012).

Symptoms of cognitive impairment and communication difficulties in older adults can appear similar to those in patients suffering from depression, delirium, and dementia, so accurate diagnosis is important. Communicating with a patient suffering from dementia requires a different set of strategies than those for the patient with depression. Table 19.1 identifies important differences between the three disorders in older adults. Secondary clinical depression and/or delirium can be superimposed on dementia, making a difficult situation even more challenging. Simulation Exercise 19.6 provides an opportunity to distinguish between dementia, delirium, and depression, using a case study.

TABLE 19.1   Sorting Out the Three D's: Delirium, Dementia, Depression

Disorder	Delirium	Dementia	Depression
Onset	Acute, over hours, days	Insidious, over months, years	Relatively rapid, over weeks to months
Acuity	Acute symptoms, medical emergency	Chronic symptoms, progresses slowly	Episodic symptoms, coincides with losses
Course	Short term; resolves with identification of cause, treatment	Gradual, progressive deterioration, memory loss	Self-limiting; recurrent symptoms; resolves with treatment
Duration	Lasts hours to weeks, resolves with treatment	Progressive and irreversible, ends in death	At least 2 weeks, may last months to years, responds to treatment
Alertness or consciousness	Fluctuates, intervals of lucidity and confusion, worse at night	Clear, stable during day, sundown syndrome	Clear, thinking may appear slowed; decreased alertness because of lack of motivation
Attention	Trouble focusing, short attention span, fluctuates	Usually unaffected	Minimal deficit, difficulty concentrating
Orientation	Disoriented to time and place, but not to person	Impaired as disease progresses; inability to recognize familiar people or objects, including self	Selective disorientation
Memory	Recent and immediate impaired	Impaired memory for immediate/recent events; unconcerned about memory deficits	Selective impairment, concerned about memory deficits
Thinking	Incoherent, global disorganization	Impoverished, inability to learn, trouble word finding	Intact, negative themes
Perception	Gross distortions; illusions, visual, tactile hallucinations	Prone to hallucinations as disease progresses	Intact, but colored by negative themes
Speech	Incoherent, disorganized, loud, belligerent	Impoverished, tangential, repetitive, superficial, confabulations	Quiet, decreased, can be irritable, language skills intact
Sleep/wake cycle	Disturbed; changes hourly	Disturbed; day/night reversal	Disturbed; early morning wakening, hypersomnia during day
Contributing factors	Underlying medical cause; toxicity, fever, tumor, infection, drugs	Degenerative disorder associated with age, cardiovascular deficits, substance dependence	Significant or cumulative loss; drug toxicity, diabetes, myocardial infarction

Adapted from Arnold, E. (2005). Sorting out the three D's: Delirium, depression, dementia. *Holist Nursing Practice, 19*(3), 99–104.

Supporting Adaptation to Daily Life

Box 19.8 outlines early cognitive changes seen with dementia. Memory loss is a consistent finding. Structure and consistency in the environment are important themes to consider. In the early stages, nurses can help patients develop reminder strategies such as making notes to themselves and using colored labels, alarms, or calendars. Focusing on what the patient can do, rather than on deficits; taps into the functions still available to the patient and decreases feelings of hopelessness (Cotter, 2009).

Apraxia, defined as the loss of the ability to take purposeful action even when the muscles, senses, and vocabulary seem intact, is a common feature of dementia. The person appears to register on a command but acts in ways that suggest he or she has little understanding of what transpired verbally. In the following case example, the caregiver observes the patient's difficulty. Notice how her response supports his ability to function.

SIMULATION EXERCISE 19.6   Distinguishing Between Dementia, Delirium, and Depression in the Older Adult

Developed by AM Spellbring, PhD, RN, FAAN, February 9, 2010.

Purpose:
To differentiate between the 3 D's.

Mrs. S. is a recently widowed 78-year-old woman living alone in a senior apartment complex in a suburban community. Her son and his wife live nearby and visit weekly. Over the last month, the family has noticed that Mrs. S. "has not been herself." Once a meticulous dresser, she shows no current interest in dressing and grooming. She has had difficulty keeping doctor appointments and getting medications refilled. When approached by the family regarding her change in behavior, Mrs. S. says that she "doesn't know—if I could just get a good night's sleep, I would feel better."

Discussion:
1. What distinguishing alterations in cognition does Mrs. S. exhibit to suggest a depression or a dementia?
2. What additional questions would you like to ask to support your observations?
3. What screening tools are appropriate?
4. What approaches would you suggest for communicating with Mrs. S.?
5. Identify ways to improve Mrs. S.'s ability to function safely and independently.
6. What sources of support can you identify to help Mrs. S. and her family cope?

BOX 19.8   Signs of Early Cognitive Changes With Dementia

- Difficulty remembering appointments
- Difficulty recalling the names of friends, neighbors, and family members
- Using the wrong word when talking
- Jumbling words: mixing up or missing letters in words when talking
- Not following the conversation of friends or coworkers
- Not understanding an explanation or story
- Difficulty recalling whether a task was just completed the day or week before
- Difficulty keeping up with all the steps to a task
- Difficulty planning and doing an activity such as a board meeting or family reunion
- New difficulty filling out complicated forms such as income tax forms
- Different behavior: restless, quick to get angry, constant hunger (especially for sweets), quiet or withdrawn, and so forth
- Buying items and forgetting there is plenty at home
- Struggling with work or home tasks that used to be routine and easy
- Loss of interest in meeting with friends or doing activities

Case Example

The care staff member noticed I.A.'s restlessness as he struggled to figure out which shoes to put on. I.A. began looking around with darting eyes, quickly shifting his gaze from here to there. The care staff member said, "I am sorry. I have put two pairs of shoes here and it is confusing. Please put these on." I.A. looked relieved, put on the shoes, and moved to a table where the care staff member placed a box that had many small articles brought from I.A.'s company. The care staff member said, "Would you help us, president?" I.A. smiled and said, "Okay...I can see you need help here," as he began to organize the articles into piles. He did not wander on that day (Ito, Takahashi, & Liehr, 2007, p. 14).

Supporting Communication

Difficulty with purposeful communication is a hallmark of dementia. The patient's loss is a gradual process initially, so many patients can maintain superficial conversation, with empathetic support. Miller (2008) notes that dementia affects basic receptive (decoding and understanding) and expressive (conveying information) forms of communication. These deficits influence the person's capacity to think abstractly and solve problems. Although patients may speak in fragments, they are still capable of interacting with prompts, and especially when given your full attention.

Difficulty with word retrieval can reflect short-term memory impairment. Patients may stop midsentence and look confused. They may ask for help with a word, or continue with phrases that have little to do with the intended conversation (Mace & Rabins, 2017).

Providing *verbal cues* helps older adults with short-term memory impairment. Nurses can support patients by suggesting a missing word or providing a simple meaning. Check with the patient that your interpretation is accurate.

Sometimes you can grasp what the word might be from its context.

Case Example

In a conversation with her nurse, Carol Buret could not could not retrieve the word "Halloween." Instead she said, "When people dress in costumes." The nurse said, "You mean like Halloween?" The patient said yes, and the conversation continued.

You also can ask the patient to point to an object or describe something similar if you do not understand what the patient is referencing (Miller, 2008).

Short-term memory allows people to follow a conversation when the topic changes. Cognitively impaired patients lack short-term memory, so topic transitions can be difficult (McCarthy, 2011). Restate ideas using simple words and sequence and validate the meaning of a patient's response. Using words directly applicable to daily routines, such as "before lunch," can anchor the patient's recognition of time frames better than saying a specific time such as 11:00 a.m.

Use plain language and simple questions that can be answered with a yes or no for patients. Be aware that the patient is acutely aware of your body language and may consider it as a measure of your acceptance. Your goal is to try and make each conversation a "person-centered" verbal connection. Box 19.9 summarizes communication guidelines for communicating with cognitively impaired patients.

Cognitively impaired patients often have trouble following instructions consisting of multiple steps. Breaking instructions into single steps helps these patients master tasks that otherwise are beyond their comprehension. Keep the conversation simple and focused only on one step at a time.

Case Example

A young woman in a dementia support group for family members spoke of a meaningful experience with her grandmother. As she went to make a tuna fish sandwich for her grandmother, she decided to involve her in the process. She gave her grandmother step-by-step verbal instructions (e.g., "Get the tuna fish out of the cabinet," "Get the knife from the drawer"), all of which her grandmother was able to do with structured guidance. As the granddaughter was spreading the mayonnaise, her grandmother said, "Now don't forget the onions." It was a priceless moment of connection for the granddaughter.

Do not explain why or what will happen if the directions are not followed. Scolding usually worsens confusion. Unlike children who can learn from a mistake, the

---

BOX 19.9 Communication Do's and Don'ts With Dementia Patients

Communication Do's

- Simplify environmental stimuli before beginning to converse.
- Look directly at the patient when talking.
- Ask the patient what he or she would like to be called.
- Try to identify the emotions behind the patient's words or behavior.
- Identify and minimize anything in the environment that creates anxiety for the patient.
- Watch your body language; convey interest and acceptance.
- Repeat simple messages slowly, calmly, and patiently.
- Give clear, simple directions one at a time in a step-by-step manner.
- Direct conversation toward concrete, familiar objects.
- Communicate with touch, smiles, calmness, and gentle redirection.
- Structure the environment and routines, to allow freedom within limits.
- Use soft music or hymns when the patient seems agitated.

Communication Don'ts

- Don't argue or reason with the patient; instead, use distraction.
- Avoid confrontation.
- Don't use slang, jargon, or abstract terms.
- If attention lapses, don't persist. Let the patient rest a few minutes before trying to regain his or her attention.
- Don't focus on difficult behavior; look for the underlying anxiety and redirect.
- Avoid hand restraints if at all possible.
- Avoid small objects that could be a choking hazard.

---

patient with dementia cannot. If the patient does not do a task or follow directions incorrectly, keep the words simple. Proactively state a next step in pleasant calm tones, for example, "Let's see if we can..." (followed by a one-step directive).

Patients with dementia often retain many of their social skills, even when their cognitive memory significantly declines, especially in the early stages (Mace & Rabins, 2017). Asking mild to early moderate cognitively impaired older adults about their past life experiences is a way to connect verbally with those who might have difficulty telling you what they had for breakfast 2 hours ago. Remote memory (recall of past events) is retained longer than memory for recent events. For the patient, the experience of connecting with another person is more important than having an in-depth conversation. Giving a compliment helps. Family members can be encouraged to reminisce with dementia patients. Even if the patient cannot respond verbally, sometimes behaviors will show through facial expression or garbled words an appreciation for the connection. Sometimes this occurs when least expected.

Case Example

Mary was visiting her sister with dementia. She had traveled from Ohio to Maryland to visit her. Her sister was unresponsive to her, and Mary was upset that she did not seem to realize that she was her sister. A few days after Mary returned home, her sister told the nurse, "You know, my sister Mary was here last week." Things register with dementia patients that are not always visible. This is important information to share with family members.

Touch

Touch is something patients with dementia can no longer ask for, create for themselves, or tell another of its meaning. Older adults generally experience gentle touch "not only physically as sensation, but also affectively as emotion and behavior" (Kim & Buschmann, 2004, p. 35). Touch is a form of communication that immediately acknowledges a dementia patient's stress, calms an agitated patient, and provides a sense of security, particularly if accompanied by a smile, or a compliment, and a gentle approach. As dementia progresses, informal and professional caregivers can use gentle touch to gain a patient's attention, to guide a person toward an activity, or simply as an expression of caring.

In general, patients with dementia appreciate the use of touch. But to some, it can be frightening, particularly if you move in too fast. Before using touch, make sure that the patient is open to it. You can usually tell when a patient thinks you are entering his or her personal space by looking at the patient's body language and facial expression. Touch, used in direct care such as putting lotion on dry skin, giving back rubs, and warming cold hands or feet, can be meaningful to the patient. When a person is no longer able to recognize familiar caregivers by name, nurturing touch provides a touchstone with the physical reality of someone who cares about the patient.

Reality Orientation Groups

Patients experiencing memory loss may forget exactly where they are, what time it is, who they are with, and in the later stages, even who they are, particularly if they are in a new setting. Using simple prompts in conversation can decrease anxiety and promote interpersonal comfort. Helping patients focus on their immediate personal environment and providing visual prompts (clocks, calendars, name ID on room doors, and photos) connect the patient with a personal environment. Calling the patient by name, putting the names of caregivers on white boards, and repeating information about time or place also strengthens recognition.

Reality orientation groups are used with older adults experiencing moderate cognitive impairment. These groups keep people in touch with time, place, and person. The group leader introduces the topic for the day and then goes around the group for patient responses. Topics can include landmarks in the dining room; routes to the dining room or bathroom; the date, time, and weather; what people would like to wear; and so on. Reality orientation groups may be conducted daily or weekly with three to four patients (Minardi & Hayes, 2003).

Validation Therapy

Validation describes a therapeutic communication process used in later stages of dementia. Developed by Naomi Feil, validation recognizes that a patient is responding to a different reality related to time, place, or person (Minardi & Hayes, 2003). Rather than confronting dementia patients with "facts"—that people they knew or places they have lived are no longer available to them—focus on the personal meaning events and people hold for the patient. For example, you might say, "Tell me about Chris," or "What was it like living on M street?"

Attending to the Special Needs of Dementia Patients

Catastrophic Reactions

Older adults with memory loss lack the cognitive ability to develop alternatives. They may emotionally overreact to situations, and can have what look like temper tantrums in response to real or perceived frustration. These behavioral outbursts are called **catastrophic reactions**. Usually there is something in the immediate environment that precipitates the reaction. Fatigue, multiple demands, overstimulation, misinterpretations, or an inability to meet expectations are often contributing factors (Mace & Rabins, 2017). Keep in mind that the emotion may be appropriate, even if the way it is expressed is not. Warning signs of an impending catastrophic reaction include agitation or restlessness, body stiffening, verbal or nonverbal refusals, and general uncooperativeness. Instead of focusing on the behavior, try to identify and eliminate the cause(s) (Hilgers, 2003).

You can use distraction to move the patient away from the offending stimuli in the environment: for example, with a simple statement, "I really need your help over here, or use postponement"; or, for example, say, "We will do that later; right now, it's time to go out on the porch," while gently leading the person away. Direct confrontation and an appeal for more civilized behavior usually serve to escalate, rather than diminish, the episode. Your tone of voice in supplying the distraction is important. A calm, kind tone gets the best results.

Sundowning

Sundowning is a term used to describe agitated behavioral symptoms, usually occurring later in the day with dementia patients. Common behaviors include fretfulness, anxiety, and demanding behaviors. Days and nights are reversed. This behavior can be very difficult for family members because their sleep is disturbed. Keeping the patient active during the day helps. Small doses of medication are used to alleviate symptoms. Caution is needed to avoid oversedating the patient and preventing medication buildup, which can occur because medications are metabolized more slowly in the elderly.

Legal Issues

Patients with early dementia can still make simple decisions, if they are supported and are patiently respected.

Decisional capacity refers to the capability of a person to:

- Understand and process information about diagnosis, prognosis, and treatment options.
- Weigh the benefits, burdens, and risks of the proposed options.
- Apply a set of personal values to the analysis.
- Arrive at a decision that is consistent over time.
- Communicate the decision (Farber Post & Boltz, 2016, p. 44).

If a patient is unable to make a cogent decision about type of application of personal health care, he or she can designate a health power of attorney to make realistic health decisions, including do not resuscitate decisions.

Mental competence represents a medico-legal determination, related to injury, disease, or intellectual disability of a person's ability to manage his or her personal legal affairs. By contrast with decisional capacity, **mental incompetence** occurs when a person lacks the capacity to negotiate legal

tasks such as making a will, entering into a contract, or making certain legal decisions.

The time to execute legal documents to patient rights is **before** patients become unable to cognitively assign decision-making authority to someone they trust. Patients in the early stages of dementia usually have sufficient mental competence to participate in legal decisions regarding their health care and finances. The criterion is that the patient has to understand what he or she is signing. Mand be in agreement with the course of action as it is presented in the document. Later, as the patient loses significant cognitive capacity, this same patient may be unable to lawfully execute legal documents.

Consultation with a lawyer regarding wills, durable and health power of attorney, and living wills should be accomplished while the patient is still legally competent. Once cognitive capacity is lost, a court procedure is necessary to establish a conservatorship or guardianship. This action is costly and emotionally painful for most families because it requires legally certifying the person as incompetent (Arnold, 2005).

Advocating for the Patient With Dementia: Advance directives and a durable power of attorney for health care (proxy) provide direction for the patient's health care wishes. For financial and property manners, the patient needs a durable power of attorney, a living trust, and/or a will. Power of attorney documents are subject to state laws and are only in effect when people are unable to manage their own affairs. Under federal guidelines, state laws determine qualifications for Medicaid and property distribution if a person dies with no will or trust. Medicaid qualifications may be important for families needing long-term care for a family member.

Nurses should refer patient family members to local Alzheimer disease and related dementia support groups. These support groups provide a place to talk about the challenges of caring for their family members. The *36-Hour Day* (Mace & Rabins, 2017), developed from the insights of family members coping with dementia in a loved one, is a classic understandable resource for family members.

CARING FOR PATIENTS WITH ADVANCED DEMENTIA

Dementia is a progressive disease; patients gradually lose control over body functions and the capacity to handle even simple tasks. Meaningful verbal communication terminates. Attempts to communicate through behavior are primitive and not easily understood.

Is the self still there? The answer is yes, but as the dementia progresses, patients have increasingly limited ways to connect with their environment and people in a meaningful way (Fig. 19.3). Touch, smiling, gentle kind approaches are meaningful. Just think what that would be like if you could no longer communicate with your words. Family members often speak of two deaths they experience with a dementia-afflicted family member—"the death of self and the actual death" (Nolan, personal communication, 2002).

Rabins et al. (2016) identifies care of the dementia patient as consisting of four pillars;
1. Treating the disease
2. Treating the symptoms
3. Supporting the patient
4. Supporting the caregiver (p. 100).

Since dementia attacks short-term memory first, talking or asking questions about past memories may stimulate conversations that otherwise would not be available to the dementia patient in the early to middle stages.

Treatment goals for patients with advanced dementia should emphasize dignity, quality of life, and supportive comfort strategies (Rabins, Lyketsos, & Steele, 2016). Table 19.2 identifies common neuropsychiatric symptoms associated with advanced dementia, with suggested behavioral communication interventions.

TABLE 19.2 Symptoms of Dementia With Suggested Behavioral Communication Interventions

Dementia Symptom Pattern	Suggested Intervention
Agitation	• Identify and remove cause • Assess for physical problems • Reduce stimuli, suggest a walk • Use simple repetitive activities: folding towels, rolling socks • Use soothing music, Bible verses • Look for patterns that trigger agitation
Aggression: grabbing, hitting	• Recognize that the patient is frightened • Decrease stimuli, move patient to a quiet place • Do not take the patient's behavior personally • Respect and enlarge the patient's personal space • Identify and minimize cause • Make eye contact; speak in a calm voice • Acknowledge frustration; do not reprimand • Check medications
Withdrawal: decreased socialization, apathy, social isolation	• Use simple activities • Find simple socialization opportunities and support patient involvement
Refusal or resistance to suggestions	• Drop the topic or activity and reintroduce it later
Disturbed motor activity: wandering, pacing, raiding waste cans, shadowing caregiver	• Keep the environment safe • Remove trash • Use medical alert bracelets • Label drawers, room (photos help) • Use locks on doors at home
Sleep disturbances: day/night sleep reversal, calling out/moaning in sleep	• Keep active during the day • Toilet patient as needed during night without conversation • Control wandering at night; lead back to bed; avoid use of restraints
Hallucinations, delusions, illusions	• Respond to the emotion, not content • Reduce stimuli • Use good nonglare lighting • Use distraction (e.g., walk, simple activity) • Use touch, reassurance, postponement

Continued

TABLE 19.2   Symptoms of Dementia With Suggested Behavioral Communication Interventions—cont'd

Dementia Symptom Pattern	Suggested Intervention
Disinhibition: inappropriate speech, touching, improper body exposure, entering other people's space	1. Do not reprimand 2. Respond to the emotion 3. Redirect patient to other activities
Incontinence: urine, feces, eliminating in wrong places	1. Check for bladder infection, fecal impaction 2. Note elimination pattern; establish corresponding toileting timetable 3. Schedule toileting at frequent intervals 4. Toilet before bedtime 5. Take patient to bathroom, verbally cue 6. Use washable clothing, Velcro closings
Swallowing difficulty: choking, stuffing mouth, not swallowing	1. Cut food into small pieces, offer small quantities of liquid at one time 2. Check medications for size, modify as needed 3. Sit with patient while eating 4. Verbally cue to chew and swallow
Agnosia: difficulty recognizing faces, including one's own	1. Remove or cover mirrors if patient is frightened by self-image 2. Verbally identify familiar people and their relationship to the patient

SUMMARY

Statistics reveal that older adults constitute the fastest growing population group in the United States. Aging is a universal life process with distinctive features. Typically there is a progressive decline in sensory and motor functions with appropriate supports; older adults can expect to live longer and enjoy a better quality of life than in previous generations.

Erikson's theory of psychosocial development identifies ego integrity versus despair as the central maturational crisis of old age. People who believe that their lives have purpose and meaning, and that they have few or no regrets about a well-lived life, demonstrate the ego strength of integrity. Supportive communication and empowerment strategies assist patients in maximizing their health and well-being.

This chapter presents current understandings about the course of dementia and discusses related communication strategies with patients and families. Differential assessment of depression, delirium, and dementia is important, as symptoms can appear similar. Communication strategies with patients with dementia emphasize verbal supports. Helping patients tell their story, promoting patient autonomy, using a proactive approach in conversations, acting as a patient advocate, and treating older adults with dignity are proposed. Health promotion activities that take into account the unique needs and cultural values of older adults are more likely to be successful. As a primary provider in long-term care and in the community, the nurse is in a unique role to support and meet the communication needs of older adult patients.

ETHICAL DILEMMA: What Would You Do?

Mrs. Allan is an accomplished 82-year-old woman, living alone. She treasures her independence. While she realizes she is more frail, she does not want to leave her home or lose her independence. Her daughter is worried about her and wants her to move to assisted living. During your initial assessment for a recent fall, Mrs. Allan confides that while she does have "some" memory lapses, she can't bear the idea of what assisted living will mean for her independence and quality of life. She asks you to keep her confidence. You can understand Mrs. Allan's concerns but you also know that keeping silent may not be in her best interest. How could you balance the ethical concept of beneficence with your patient's concerns? What would you do?

DISCUSSION QUESTIONS

- What are some examples of ageism affecting older adults?
- How is ageism perpetuated?

- From an advocacy perspective, how could you as a nurse help create a more positive image of older adults?

REFERENCES

Adelman, M., Greene, M., & Ory, M. (2000). Communication between older patients and their physicians. *Clinics Geriatric Medicine, 16*(1), 1–24.

American Geriatrics Society Expert Panel on Person Centered Care. (2016). Person-centered care: A definition and essential elements. *Journal of the American Geriatrics Society, 64*(1), 15–18.

Anderson, D. (2005). Preventing delirium in older people. *British Medical Bulletin, 73–74*, 25–34.

Arnold, E. (2005). Sorting out the 3 D's: Delirium, dementia, depression: Learn how to sift through overlapping signs and symptoms so you can help improve an older patient's quality of life. *Holistic Nursing Practice, 19*(3), 99–104.

Avolio, M., Montagnoli, S., Marino, D., Basso, D., Furia, G., Ricciardi, W., et al. (2013). Factors influencing quality of life for disabled and nondisabled elderly population: The results of a multiple correspondence analysis. *Current Gerontology and Geriatrics Research, 258*–274.

Bishop, A. (2008). Stress and Depression among older residents in religious monasteries: Do friends and God matter? *International Journal of Aging & Human Development, 67*(1), 1–23.

Bohlmeijer, E., Kramer, J., Smit, F., Onrust, S., & van Marwijk, H. (2009). The effects of integrative reminiscence on depressive symptomatology and mastery of older adults. *Community Mental Health Journal, 45*, 476–484.

Bonder, B. R., & Dal Bello-Haas, V. (2018). *Functional performance in older adults* (4th ed.). Philadelphia: FA Davis.

Brown-O'Hara, T. (2013). Geriatric syndromes and their implications for nursing. *Nursing, 43*(1), 1–3.

Burke, M., & Laramie, J. (2004). *Primary care of the older adult: A multidisciplinary approach* (2nd ed.). St. Louis: Mosby.

Buron, B. (2008). Levels of personhood: A model for dementia care. *Geriatric Nursing, 29*(5), 324–332.

Cavalieri, T. (2005). Management of pain in older adults. *The Journal of the American Osteopathic Association, 105*(3), 12S–17S.

Cenci, C. (2016). Narrative medicine and the personalization of treatment for elderly patients. *European Journal of Internal Medicine, 32*, 22–25.

Chochinov, H. M. (2013). Dignity in care: Time to take action. *Journal of Pain and Symptom Management, 46*, 756–759.

Constanca, P., Ribeiro, O., & Teixeira, L. (2012). Active ageing: An empirical approach to the WHO model. *Current Gerontology and Geriatrics Research, 382*–972. https://doi.org/10.1155/2012/382972.

Corey, M., & Corey, G. (2006). M. Corey & G. Corey. (Eds.). *Groups for the elderly. Groups: Process and practice* (7th ed.). Belmont, CA: Thompson Brooks/Cole.

Cotter, V. (2009). Hope in early-stage dementia: A concept analysis. *Holistic Nursing Practice, 23*(5), 297–301.

Cotter, V., & Gonzalez, E. (2009). Self-concept in older adults: An integrative review of empirical literature. *Holistic Nursing Practice, 23*(6), 335–348.

Delgado, C. (2007). Meeting patients' spiritual needs. *Nursing Clinical North America, 42*(2), 279–293.

Ebrahimi, Z., Wilhelmson, K., Moore, C., & Jakobsson, A. (2013). Health despite frailty: Exploring influences on frail older adults experiences of health. *Geriatrics Nursing, 34*, 289–294.

Ellison, D. (2015). Communication skills. *Nursing Clinical North America, 50*, 45–57.

Erikson, E. (1980). *Identity and the life cycle.* New York: Norton.

Feldt, K. (2008). Pain assessment in older adults. In M. M. Jansen (Ed.), *Managing pain in older adults* (pp. 35–54). New York: Springer.

Farber-Post, L., & Boltz, M. (2016). Health care decision making. Chapter 4. In M. Boltz, E. Capezuti, T. Fulmer, & D. Zwicker (Eds.), *Evidence based geriatric nursing protocols for best practice* (5th ed.). (pp. 43–49).

Folstein, M., Folstein, S., & McHugh, P. R. (1975). Mini-mental state: A practical method for grading cognition state of patients for the clinician. *Journal of Psychiatric Research, 12*, 189–198.

Gallo, J. (2000). *Handbook of geriatric assessment* (3rd ed.). Gaithersburg, MD: Aspen.

Gentleman, B. (2014). Focused assessment in the older adult. *Critical Care Nursing Clinics, 26*, 15–20.

Gloth, F. (2010). *Handbook of pain relief in older adults* (2nd ed.). Totowa, NJ: Humana Press.

Gould, E., & Mitty, E. (2010). Medication adherence is a partnership, medication compliance is not. *Geriatric Nursing, 31*, 290–298.

Gray-Miceli, D. (2017). Impaired mobility and functional decline in older adults. Evidence to facilitate a practice change. *Nursing Clinical North America, 52*, 469–487.

Happ, M. B. (2010). Individualized care for frail older adults: Challenges for health care reform in acute and critical care. *Gerontological Nursing, 31*(1), 63–65.

Healthy People. (2016). *2020: Older adults.* Retrieved from: http//www.healthpeople.gov/2020/topics-objectives/topic/older adults.

Heliker, D. (2009). Enhancing relationships in long-term care: Through story sharing. *Journal of Gerontological Nursing, 35*(6), 43–49.

Herr, K. (2010). Pain in the older adult: An imperative across all health care settings. *Pain Management Nursing, 11*(Suppl. 2), S1–S10.

Herr, K. (2013). *Retooling pain assessment for older adults. Presentation at the american pain society, 32nd Annual Scientific Meeting.* New Orleans: LA.

Hilgers, J. (2003). Comforting a confused patient. *Nursing, 33*(1), 48–50.

Horgas, A. (2017). Pain assessment in older adults. *Nursing Clinical North America, 52*(3), 375–378.

Institute of Medicine (IOM). (2008). *Retooling for an aging America: Building the health care workforce.* Washington, DC: National Academies Press.

Ito, M., Takahashi, R., & Liehr, P. (2007). Heeding the behavioral message of elders with dementia in day care. *Holist Nursing Practice, 21*(1), 12–18.

Jonsdottir, H., Jonsdottir, G., Steingrimsdottir, E., & Tryggvadottir, B. (2001). Group reminiscence among people with end-stage chronic lung diseases. *Journal of Advanced Nursing, 35*(1), 79–87.

Kagan, S. (2012). Gotcha! Don't let ageism sneak into your practice. *Geriatric Nursing, 33*(1), 60–62.

Katz, S., & Calasanti, T. (2015). Successful aging: Critical perspectives on successful aging: Does it "appeal more than it illuminates"? *The Gerontology, 56*(1), 26–33.

Kelly, K., Reinhard, S. C., & Brooks-Danso, A. (2008). Professional partners supporting family caregivers. *The American Journal of Nursing, 108*(9), 6–12.

Kim, E., & Buschmann, M. (2004). Touch—stress model and Alzheimer's disease. *Journal of Gerontological Nursing, 30*(12), 33–39.

Kim, L., Koncilja, K., & Nielsen, C. (2018). Medication management in older adults. *Cleveland Clinic Journal of Medicine, 85*(2), 129–135.

Lang, J., Moore, M., Harris, A., & Anderson, L. (2005). Healthy aging: Priorities and programs of the Centers for Disease Control and Prevention. *Generations, 29*(2), 24–29.

Le, T. (2008). Cultural values, life experiences, and wisdom. *International Journal of Aging and Human Development, 66*(4), 259–281.

Lord, S. (2006). Visual risk factors for falls in older people. *Age Ageing, 35*(Suppl. 2), ii42–ii45.

Lorig, K., & Fries, J. F. (2006). A tested self-management program for coping with arthritis and fibromyalgia. *The arthritis help book* (6th ed.). DeCapo Press.

Mace, N., & Rabins, P. (2017). *The 36-hour day: A family guide to caring for people with Alzheimer's disease, other dementias, and memory loss* (6th ed.). Baltimore, MD: Johns Hopkins University.

Machiels, M., Metzelthin, S., Hamers, P., & Zwakhalen, S. (2017). Interventions to improve communication between people with dementia and nursing staff during daily nursing care: A systematic review. *International Journal of Nursing Studies, 66*, 37–46.

MacKinlay, E. (2012). Resistance, resilience, and change: The person and dementia. *Journal of Religion, Spirituality & Aging, 24*, 80–92.

Maslow, A. (1954). *Motivation and personality.* Harper & Row: New York.

Maslow, A. (1975). *Motivation and personality.* New York: Harper & Row.

Mauk, K. L. (2006). Healthier aging: Reaching and teaching older adults. *Holist Nursing Practice, 20*(3), 158.

Mauk, K. L. (2010). *Gerontological nursing: Competencies for care.* Boston: Jones & Bartlett.

McCarthy, B. (2011). *Hearing the person with dementia: Person centered approaches.* Philadelphia, PA: Jessica Kingsley.

Miller, C. (2008). Communication difficulties in hospitalized older adults with dementia. *American Journal of Nursing, 108*(3), 58–66.

Miller, C. (2019). *Nursing for wellness in older adults.* Philadelphia, PA: Wolters Kluwer.

Minardi, H., & Hayes, N. (2003). Nursing older adults with mental health problems: Therapeutic interventions—part 2. *Nursing of Older People, 15*(7), 20–24.

Moody, H., & Sasser, J. (2017). *Aging: Concepts and controversies* (9th ed.). Thousand Oaks, CA: Pine Forge Press.

Murray, L. M., & Boyd, S. (2009). Protecting personhood and achieving quality of life for older adults with dementia in the U.S. health care system. *Journal of Aging Health, 21*, 350–373.

Nakasato, Y., & Carnes, B. (2006). Health promotion in older adults: Promoting successful aging in primary care settings. *Geriatrics, 61*(4), 27–31.

Narang, D., Kordia, K., Meena, J., & Meena, K. (2013). Interpersonal relationships of elderly within the family. *International Journal of Social Sciences & Interdisciplinary Research, 2*(3), 132–138.

National Council on Aging. (2014). Healthy aging facts. Available at: http//www.NCOA.org/.

National Institute on Deafness and Other Communication Disorders (NIDCD). (2013). Hearing loss and older adults. Available at: www.nidcd.nih.gov/health/hearing/older.asp. Accessed August 23, 2014.

Nerenberg, L. (2008). *Elder abuse prevention: Emerging trends and promising strategies.* New York: Springer.

Ownby, R. (2006). Medication adherence and cognition: Medical, personal and economic factors influence level of adherence in older adults. *Geriatrics, 61*(2), 30–35.

Pankow, L. J., & Solotoroff, J. M. (2007). Biological aspects and theories of aging. In J. A. Blackburn, & C. N. Dulmus (Eds.), *Handbook of gerontology: Evidence-based practice approaches to theory, practice, and policy* (pp. 19–57). Hoboken, NJ: John Wiley & Sons.

Penprase, B. (2006). Developing comprehensive health care for an underserved population. *Geriatrics Nursing, 27*(1), 45–50.

Potempa, K., Butterworth, S., & Flaherty-Robb Gaynor, W. (2010). The healthy ageing model: Health behaviors for older adults. *Collegian, 04*(008), 51–55.

Pryce, H., & Gooberman, R. (2012). There's a heal of a noise: Living with a hearing loss in residential care. *Age Ageing, 41*, 40–46.

Rabins, P., Lyketsos, C., & Steele, C. (2016). *Practical dementia care* (3rd ed.). New York: Oxford University Press.

Reichstadt, M., Sengupta, G., Depp, C., Palinkas, L., & Jeste, D. (2010). Older adults' perspectives on successful aging. Qualitative interviews. *American Journal of Geriatric Psychiatry, 18*(7), 567–575.

Rowan, N., & Faul, A. A. (2007). Substance abuse. In J. Blackburn, & C. Dulmus (Eds.), *Handbook of gerontology: Evidence-based approaches to theory, practice, and policy* (pp. 309–332). Hoboken, NJ: Wiley.

Resnick, B. (2013). New and exciting opportunities to promote health among older adults. *Geriatric Nursing, 34*, 9–11.

Scholder, J., Kagan, S., & Schumann, M. J. (2004). Nursing competence in aging overview. *The Nursing Clinics of North America, 39*, 429–442.

Strine, T., Chapman, D. D. P., Balluz, L., & Mokdad, A. H. (2008). Health-related quality of life and health behaviors by social and emotional support: Their relevance to psychiatry and medicine. *Social Psychiatry and Psychiatric Epidemiology, 43*, 151–159.

Touhy, T., & Jett, K. (2015). *Ebersole and Hess' Toward healthy aging: Human needs and nursing response* (9th ed.). St. Louis, MO: Elsevier.

UNFPA, U. N. P. F. (2012). *Ageing in the 21st Century: A Celebration and a Challenge*. Available at: http://www.unfpa.org/publications/ageing-twenty-first-century.

US Department of Health and Human Services (DHHS). (2010). *Healthy People 2020*. Available at: http//www.Healthypeople2020. Accessed July 19, 2013.

Van Vliet, E., Lindenberger, E., & Van Weert, J. (2015). Communication with older, seriously ill patients. *Clinical Geriatric Medicine, 31*, 219–230.

Whiteside, M., Wallhagen, M., & Pettengill, E. (2006). Sensory impairment in older adults: Part 2: vision loss. *American Journal of Nursing, 106*(11), 52–61.

Windsor, T., & Anstey, K. (2008). Volunteering and psychological well-being among young-old adults: How much is too much. *Gerontologist, 48*(1), 59–70.

Yuhas, N., McGowan, B., Fontaine, T., Czech, J., & Gambrell-Jones. (2006). Psychosocial interventions for disruptive symptoms of dementia. *Journal of Psychosocial Nursing, 44*(11), 34–42.

20

Communicating With Patients in Crisis

Pamela E. Marcus

INTRODUCTION

The purpose of this chapter is to describe communication strategies nurses can use with patients and families experiencing a crisis situation. The chapter describes the nature of crisis and identifies its theoretical foundations. The application section provides practical guidelines nurses can use with patients in crisis and during mental health emergencies and disaster management.

BASIC CONCEPTS

Definitions

Crisis

Flannery and Everly (2000) state, "A *crisis* occurs when a stressful life event overwhelms an individual's ability to cope effectively in the face of a perceived challenge or threat" (p. 119). People in a crisis state experience an actual or perceived overwhelming threat to self-concept, an insurmountable obstacle or a loss that conventional coping measures cannot handle. Unabated, the resulting tension continues to increase, creating major personality disorganization and a crisis state.

The word *crisis* comes from the Greek root word *krinen*, meaning "to decide, and in Latin, crisis means the turning point of a disease" Vroomen, Bosmans, van Hout,

and de Rooij (2013, p. 10). Personal responses to crisis can be adaptive or maladaptive. Nurses can help patients with restorative coping strategies to lessen the damaging impact of crisis. Successfully working through a crisis has the potential to strengthen people's coping responses and encourage a sense of self-efficacy. Maladaptive responses can result in the development of acute or chronic psychiatric symptoms.

Crisis State. Everly (2000) defines a **crisis state** as an acute but *normal* human response to severely abnormal circumstances. A crisis state is *not* a mental illness, although individuals with mental illness can experience a crisis state associated with their disorder. Crisis is a complex concept, which can defy easy cause/effect explanations (James, 2008). Because a crisis state represents a personal response, two people experiencing the same crisis event will respond differently to it. Understanding the patient's personal response to a crisis rather than an objective crisis stressor is critical to successful crisis intervention.

A crisis state creates a temporary disconnect from attachment to others, loss of meaning, and disruption of previous mastery skills (Flannery & Everly, 2000). Individuals feel vulnerable. Crisis intervention strategies are designed to help support people experiencing crisis achieve psychological homeostasis. A favorable outcome depends on the person's combined interpretation of the crisis, perception of coping ability, resources, and level of social support (Loughran, 2011).

Types of Crisis
Developmental Crisis

A crisis is classified as developmental or situational. Erikson's (1982) stage model of psychosocial development forms the basis for exploring the nature of developmental crisis. Developmental crisis can occur as individuals negotiate developmental age-related milestones in their lives, for example becoming a parent or retiring from long-term employment. Normative psychosocial crises are used as benchmarks for assessing signs and symptoms of developmental crisis. When a situational crisis is superimposed on a normative developmental crisis, the crisis experience can be more intense. For example, a woman losing a spouse at the same time she is going through menopause can experience a more intense impact.

Situational Crisis

A situational crisis refers to an unusually stressful life event, which exceeds a person's resources and coping skills. Examples include unexpected illness or injury, rape, a car accident, the loss of a home or spouse, or being laid off from a job. When the crisis impacts a large number of people simultaneously, for example, a disaster, it is referred to as an *adventitious crisis* (Michalopoulos & Michalopoulos, 2009). A situational crisis is *not* defined by the life event itself, but by the individual's personal response to it (Hoff, 2009). How successfully a person responds to a crisis can depend on the following:

- previous experience with crises, coping, and problem solving;
- perception of the crisis event;
- level of help or obstruction from significant others;
- developmental level and ego maturity; and
- concurrent stressors.

Loughran (2011) emphasizes determining how the individual involved in the incident identifies the crisis. It may be that the patient does not recognize this event as a crisis, whereas others may perceive the same occurrence as having crisis proportions. To provide individual care, it is important to determine the type of crisis and how the individual is experiencing the events as being a crisis.

Behavioral Emergencies

James and Gilliland (2013) state that a *behavioral emergency* occurs "when a crisis escalates to the point that the situation requires immediate intervention to avoid injury or death" (p. 8). Examples include any type of violent interpersonal behavior, psychotic crisis, suicide, or homicide. A behavioral emergency describes any type of thinking or behavior that places an individual in an immediate potentially injurious or lethal situation. A behavioral emergency is always an emotionally charged, unpredictable situation (Kleespies, 2009). In addition to assessing patient risk characteristics, it is important to evaluate the environmental features and other factors that can either increase or decrease suicidal risk, When this patient is discharged from the hospital, the family and patient should be provided suicide prevention information, for example crisis hotline (Joint Commission, 2017a, 2017b).

Crisis Intervention

Crisis intervention represents a systematic application of theory-based problem-solving strategies designed to help individuals and families resolve a crisis situation quickly and successfully. The desired clinical outcome is a return to an individual's pre-crisis functional level (Roberts & Yeager, 2009). Crisis intervention strategies should be adapted to fit each patient's preferences, beliefs, values, and individual circumstances. As a nurse, you cannot always change the nature of a crisis situation, but you can help defuse a patient's emotional reaction to it with compassionate professional support and guidance.

Crisis intervention is a *time-limited* treatment. Four to six weeks is considered the standard time frame for crisis resolution. Interventions should be present-focused and action-oriented. The emphasis is on *immediate problem solving* and *strengthening the personal resources* of patients and their families. Full recovery can take a much longer period of time, particularly from a disaster crisis (Callahan, 1998). Nurses function as advocates, resources, partners, and guides in helping patients resolve crisis situations, usually as part of a larger crisis intervention team.

THEORETICAL FRAMEWORKS

Lindemann (1944) and Caplan (1964) developed the most widely used models of crisis and crisis intervention. Lindemann's (1944) study of bereavement provides a frame of reference for understanding the stages involved in resolving emotional crisis and bereavement. His findings suggest, "roper psychiatric management of grief reactions may prevent prolonged and serious alterations in the patient's social adjustment, as well as potential medical disease" (p. 147).

Caplan broadened Lindemann's model to include developmental crisis and personal crisis (Roberts, 2005). Although the focus of crisis intervention is on secondary prevention because the crisis state is already in motion, Caplan's model of preventive psychiatry starts in the community. He introduced practical crisis intervention strategies, for example, crisis telephone lines, training for community workers, and early response strategies. He viewed nurses as key service providers in crisis intervention.

Caplan discusses a crisis response pattern. He identifies a person's initial response to a crisis state as *shock,* with varied emotions, ranging from anger, laughing, hysterics, crying, and acute anxiety to social withdrawal. An extended period of adjustment follows the state of shock with a period of *recoil,* which can last from 2 to 3 weeks. Behavior appears normal to outsiders, but patients describe nightmares, phobic reactions, and flashbacks of the crisis event.

Restoration or reconstruction describes the final phase of crisis intervention. This phase involves developing a plan and taking constructive actions to resolve the crisis situation. If successfully negotiated, the person returns to a pre-crisis functional level, which is the desired clinical outcome. Maladaptive coping strategies, such as drug or alcohol use, violence, or avoidance, prevents restoration and places the patient at risk for further problems. Exercise 20.1 is designed to help you to understand the nature of crisis.

Nursing Model

The nursing model developed by Aguilera (1998) approaches crisis intervention from a balancing perspective between a crisis situation and a patient's capacity to resolve it. The model proposes that a crisis state develops because of a distorted perception of a situation or because the patient lacks the resources to cope successfully with it. Balancing factors include a realistic perception of the event, the patient's internal resources (beliefs or attitudes), and the patient's external (environmental) supports. These factors can minimize or reduce the impact of the stressor, leading to resolution of the crisis.

Absence of adequate situational support, lack of coping skills, and a distorted perception of the crisis event can result in a crisis state, leaving individuals and families feeling overwhelmed and unable to cope. Interventions are designed to increase the balancing factors needed to restore a patient to pre-crisis functioning. Exercise 20.1 provides insight into the nature of crisis.

DEVELOPING AN EVIDENCE-BASED PRACTICE

Purpose
The Joint Commission has identified that death by suicide is the second most common sentinel event that is reported in an inpatient hospital setting (The Joint Commission, 2016). Several factors have been identified as causes for the problem.

Method
Neville and Roan (2013) conducted an extensive review of literature on this topic while formulating their research. It was determined that nurses had negative attitudes toward patients who had attempted suicide while hospitalized in a medical surgical setting. Their research study was aimed at determining common nurse's attitudes toward suicidal patients and comparing this to demographic information. The Joint Commission established that accurately assessing an individual for risk of suicide is determined by the nurse's attitude toward the patient.

Findings
This study was done as a descriptive replication study of a convenience sample of 45 nurses. Demographic information was gathered about each nurse: gender, hospital unit, age, nursing degree and educational level, years of experience, race, certification in discipline, and religion.

Each participant filled out a research tool, the Attitudes Towards Attempted Suicide Questionnaire (ATAS-Q) (Ouzouni & Nakakis, 2009). This tool has been shown to be highly reliable and valid. In this sample, the nurses were well educated, and 21 of these nurses were certified in their discipline. There was a statistically significant inverse relationship between positive feelings toward the patient and religion. The participants of this study who identified as Protestants were most positive toward their patients who were at risk for suicide. The highest mean score were the nurses who identified as Jewish and Orthodox Christian. These last two groups had a small sample size, and therefore more research needs to be done to determine if this will occur in another nurse samples. Nurses who were younger (aged 20 to 45) were more positive towards their patients who were suicidal than the older nurses (aged 46 to 65+). Nurses who had a higher education level were more positive than those nurses with an associate or BSN degree.

Application to Your Clinical Practice
Nurses need more education on assessment and intervention for the patient who is suicidal. During this education, it would be helpful for the nurse to evaluate and explore how their attitudes may influence assessment and identification of the risk for suicide. Discussing how to assess the individual and what steps to take when the patient endorses feeling at risk for suicide will assist the nurse in evaluating their practice and help them improve on their skills.

From Neville, K., & Roan, N. M. Suicide in hospitalized medical-surgical patients: Exploring nurses' attitudes. *Journal of Psychosocial Nursing & Mental Health Services, 2013, 51*(1), 35–43. https://doi.org.ezproxy.pgcc.edu/10.3928/02793695-20121204-01

EXERCISE 20.1   Understanding the Nature of Crisis

Purpose

To help students understand crisis in preparation for assessing and planning communication strategies in crisis situations in professional patient care situations.

Procedure

1. Describe a crisis you experienced in your life. There are no right or wrong definitions of a crisis, and it does not matter whether the crisis would be considered a crisis in someone else's life.
2. Identify how the crisis changed your roles, routines, relationships, and assumptions about yourself.
3. Apply a crisis model to the situation you are describing.
4. Identify the strategies you used to cope with the crisis.
5. Describe the ways in which your personal crisis strengthened or weakened your self-concept and increased your options and your understanding of life.

Discussion

1. What did you learn from doing this exercise that you can use in your clinical practice?

BOX 20.1   Field Expedient Tool to Assess Dangerousness to Self or Others

- **D**epression/suicidal
- **A**nger/agitation, aggressive
- **N**oncompliance with requests/taking medication
- **G**eneral appearance/inappropriate dress/poor hygiene
- **E**vidence of self-inflicted injury
- **R**esponding/reacting to delusions or hallucinations
- **O**wns/displays weapon(s)
- **U**norganized thoughts/appearance/behavior
- **S**peech pattern/substance/rate (too fast, too slow, jumps all over)
- **P**aranoid
- **E**rratic or fearful behavior
- **R**ecent loss of job/loved one/home
- **S**ubstance abuse
- **O**rientation to date/time/location/situation/insight into illness
- **N**umber and type of previous contacts with police, mental health, or crisis workers

From Officer Scott A Davis, Crisis Intervention Tea (CIT) Coordinator: *Field expedient tool to assess dangerousness to self or others,* Rockville, MD, February 2010a, Montgomery County Police Department.

APPLICATIONS

The goal of crisis intervention is to return the patient to his or her previous level of functioning. This goal is evidenced by:

- stabilization of distress symptoms,
- reduction of distress symptoms,
- restoration of functional capabilities to pre-crisis levels, and
- referrals for follow-up support care, if indicated (Everly, 2000, pp. 1–2).

STRUCTURING CRISIS INTERVENTION STRATEGIES

Roberts (2005) provides a seven-stage sequential blueprint for clinical intervention, which can be used to structure the crisis intervention process in nurse-patient relationships. This model is compatible with the nursing process sequence of assessment, planning, implementation, and evaluation.

Step 1 (Assessment): Assessing Lethality and Mental Status

Initially, assessment should focus on determining the severity of a patient's current danger potential—both to

self and to others. Box 20.1 presents a field expedient tool for initial assessment of a potential behavioral emergency. Crisis intervention teams (CIT) developed and use this tool to assess potential dangerous patient behaviors. CIT is collaboration between law enforcement officers and mental health providers that assist individuals in the community who are exhibiting a mental health crisis (Browning, Van Hasselt, Tucker, & Vecchi, 2011; Davis, 2014a, 2014b).

Psychotic individuals, and those under the influence of drugs, who are severely agitated or temporarily out of control for medical reasons, require immediate triage to stabilize their physical and mental conditions. Crisis states complicated by delirium or nonlethal self-harm necessitate high-priority medical attention before addressing crisis intervention issues. With the downturn in the economy and an increase in community anxiety, more patients are presenting in the community as mental health emergencies.

Step 2: Establishing Rapport and Engaging the Patient

Once the initial triage assessment of a patient in crisis is completed, the nurse performs a more comprehensive crisis appraisal. This assessment should be specific to the patient's current state and circumstances. Patients in crisis look to health professionals to structure interactions. Introduce yourself briefly, and quickly orient the patient to the purpose of the crisis questions and how the information will be used. Health Insurance Portability and Accountability Act (HIPAA) of 1996 regulations require confidentiality. If patients expect family members to give or receive information to health providers when the patient is not present, the patient needs to sign a consent form.

Patients experiencing a crisis state require a compassionate, flexible, but clearly directive calm approach from nurses. Place the patient in a quiet, lighted room with no shadows, away from the mainstream of activity. Avoid the use of touch, as the patient may be supersensitive to any form of unexpected response from a health professional. If there is a need to restrain a patient temporarily, explain what is happening simply and directly. Use fewer rather than more words to explain. Utilize a clear, concrete communication style, with an emphasis on attending to the patient's needs.

Only a minimum number of people should be involved with the patient, until the patient is emotionally stabilized. If the patient is unable to cooperate, for safety reasons, more than one professional may be needed to stabilize the situation. Depending on the nature of the crisis and the patient's personal responses, a trusted family member may be included.

Speak calmly and use short, clear, direct phrases and questions. James and Gilliland (2013) advocate the use of closed-ended questions in the *early* stages of crisis intervention related to safety issues, requesting specific information and eliciting a patient commitment to immediate action needed to stabilize the crisis situation.

Careful, accurate listening skills are essential. It is important to discover the patient's perception of the crisis—how it developed, how it impacts the patient's life, etc. One way to ask assessment questions can be as follows: "Is this the first time you have experienced a crisis like this? Have you had other crises? What were they like? How did you understand what was happening to you? How did you problem-solve these crises?

Questions to assess the patient's perception of his or her emotional coping strength are important. James (2008) suggests asking question such as, "How were you feeling about this before the crisis got so bad?" "Where do you see yourself headed with this problem?" (p. 51).

Use reflective listening responses to identify feelings (e.g., "It sounds as if you are feeling very sad [angry, lonely] right now."). You can help patients focus on relevant points by repeating a phrase, asking for validation or clarification to focus the discussion. Family and significant others can provide essential data related to the patient's current crisis state (e.g., documenting changes in behavior, ingestion of drugs, or medical history) if the patient is unable to do so.

Exercise 20.2 offers an opportunity to understand reflection as a listening response in crisis situations.

EXERCISE 20.2   Using Reflective Responses in a Crisis Situation

Purpose
To provide students with a means of appreciating the multipurpose uses of reflection as a listening response in crisis situations.

Procedure
Have one student role-play a patient in an emergency department situation involving a common crisis situation (e.g., fire, heart attack, auto accident). After this person talks about the crisis situation for 3 to 4 minutes, have each student write down a reflective listening response that they would use with the patient in crisis. Have each student read their reflective response to the class. (This can also be done in small groups of students if the class is large.)

Discussion
1. Were you surprised at the variety of reflective themes found in the students' responses?
2. In what ways could differences in the wording or emphasis of a reflective response influence the flow of information?
3. In what ways do reflective responses validate the patient's experience?
4. How could you use what you learned from doing this exercise in your clinical practice?

Step 3 (Assessment): Identifying Major Problems

Keep the focus on the here and now. Questions should be short and relevant to the crisis.

Request more specific details (e.g., ask who was involved, what happened, and when it happened) if this information is needed.

Ask about the feelings associated with the immediate crisis.

Responses to patients should be brief, empathetic, and clearly related to the patient's story.

Note changes in expression, body posture, and vocal inflections as patients tell their story and at what points they occur. Be alert for any escalation of agitation or verbal outbursts. If the patient shows signs of agitation, ask what would be helpful right now? Ask the patient if he or she needs a brief break from talking about the crisis? What thoughts may help the patient feel better; such as thinking about a favorite prayer, song, or story? The break may assist the person to gather their emotional resources to further cope with the crisis.

Identify central emotional themes in the patient's story (e.g., powerlessness, shame, stigma, hopelessness) to provide a focus for intervention.

- Proceed slowly with a calm tone and direct communication.
- Affirm patient efforts and offer encouragement.
- Summarize content often and ask for validation so that you and your patient are on the same page, with a comprehensive understanding of major issues.
- Periodically ask the patient to summarize thoughts.
- Check for personal reservations about part or the entire care plan.

Identifying Feelings

Patients can have difficulty putting crisis emotions into words because of high anxiety. Nurses can help patients clarify important feelings with observations about patient responses (e.g., "I wonder if because you think your son is using drugs [precipitating event], you feel helpless and confused [patient emotional response] and don't know what to do next [patient behavioral reaction].")."Does that capture what is going on with you?" Checking in with a patient helps to ensure that your interpretations represent the patient's truth.

Patients in crisis tend to develop tunnel vision (Dass-Brailsford, 2010). Often, they feel there is no solution. Losing sight of personal assets and potential reserves, which could be used to defuse the crisis, some patients are frightened by the intensity of their emotional reactions. Patients appreciate hearing that most people experience powerful and conflicting feelings in crisis situations. The message you want to get across is "you are not alone, and together we can come up with a plan to deal with this difficult situation." Global reassurance is not helpful, but specific supportive comments that recognize patient efforts can help patients to de-escalate a crisis event to workable proportions.

Affirming Personal Strengths

When combined with social supports and community resources, professional compassionate witnessing of the situation and calling attention to personal strengths can significantly enhance coping skills. For example, financial resources and knowledge about accessing health care services are critical assets people lose sight of in crisis situations. Reinforce personal strengths as you observe them or as the patient identifies them. Exercise 20.3 provides an opportunity to experience the value of personal support systems in crisis situations.

Providing Explicit Information

Being truthful about what is known and unknown and updating information as you learn about it helps build

---

EXERCISE 20.3 Personal Support Systems

Purpose

To help students appreciate the breadth and importance of personal support systems in stressful situations.

Procedure

All of us have support systems we can use in times of stress (e.g., church, friends, family, coworkers, clubs, recreational groups).

1. Identify a support person or system you could or do use in a time of crisis.
2. Reflect on why you would choose this person or support system.
3. What does this personal support system or person do for you (e.g., listen without judgment; provide honest, objective feedback; challenge you to think; broaden your perspective; give unconditional support; share your perceptions)? List all relevant reasons.
4. What factors go into choosing your personal support system (e.g., availability, expertise, perception of support)? Which is the most important factor?

Discussion

1. What types of support systems were most commonly used by class or group members?
2. What were the most common reasons for selecting a support person or system?
3. After doing this exercise, what strategies would you advise for enlarging a personal support system?
4. What applications do you see in this exercise for your nursing practice?

---

trust with patients in crisis. Even with unknowns, people cope better when uncertainty is briefly acknowledged, rather than not mentioned. Explain what is going to happen, step by step. Letting patients know as much as possible about progress, treatment, and the consequences of choosing different alternatives allows patients to make informed decisions and reduces the heightened anxiety associated with a crisis situation.

Step 4 (Planning): Exploring Alternative Options and Partial Solutions

Step 4 strategies focus on broadening the patient perspective by looking at partial solutions. Breaking tasks down into small, achievable parts empowers patients. Proposed strategies should accommodate both the immediate problems and patient resources.

It is important to encourage the patient to make autonomous choices, rather than giving advice. You can assist patients in discussing the consequences, costs, and benefits of choosing one action versus another (e.g., "What would happen if you choose this course of action as compared with...?" or "What is the worst that could happen if you decided to...?"). Making choices helps patients reestablish control. Even a small decision encourages patients to become invested in the solution-finding process and hopeful about finding a resolution to a crisis situation.

Involving Immediate Support Systems and Community Resources

Accessing immediate social supports and available community resources provides a buffer and can act as a source of information and a sounding board for individuals in a crisis state. Support networks provide practical advice and a sense of security. They are a source of encouragement that can reaffirm a patient's worth and help defuse anxiety associated with the uncertainty of a crisis situation. In addition to inquiring about the number and variety of people in the patient's support network, find out, "who does the patient and/or family trust" and "who would the patient be most comfortable telling about their situation." It is helpful to learn when the patient and/or family last had contact with the identified person. In crisis situations, many patients and families temporarily withdraw from natural support systems and may need encouragement to reconnect.

Step 5 (Planning): Develop A Realistic Action Plan

Crisis intervention *"is action-oriented and situation focused"* (Dass-Brailsford, 2010, p. 56). Formulating a realistic action plan starts with prioritizing identified problems and related essential action steps. An effective crisis plan should have a practical, here-and-now, therapeutic, short-term focus and should reflect the patient's choices about best options (Loughran, 2011, p. 89). Stabilization of the patient through guidance, careful listening, and developing small viable plans helps to defuse the sense of helplessness in a crisis situation.

Focus on the Present

Help your patients to think in terms of short-term intervals and immediate next steps (e.g., "What can you do with the rest of today just to get through it better?"). Examples include getting more information, gathering essential data, taking a walk, calling a family member, and/or taking time for self. When people begin to take even the smallest step, they gain a sense of control, and this stimulates hope for future mastery of the crisis situation. Thinking about crisis resolution as a whole is counterproductive.

Incorporate Previously Successful Coping Strategies

Looking at past coping strategies can sometimes reveal skills that could be used in resolving the current crisis situation. Ask, "What do you usually do when you have a problem?" or "To whom do you turn when you are in trouble?" Explore the nature of tension-reducing strategies that the patient has used in the past (e.g., aerobics, Bible study, calling a friend, participating in a hobby). If the patient seems immobilized and unable to give an answer about usual coping strategies, you can offer prompts, such as, "Some people talk to their friends, pray, go to church..." Usually, with verbal encouragement, patients begin to identify successful coping mechanisms, which can be built on, for use in resolving the current crisis.

Step 6 (Implementation): Developing an Action Plan

Developing Reasonable Goals

Crisis offers patients an opportunity to discover and develop new self-awareness about things that are important to them. Developing realistic goals is a critical component of crisis intervention. This process includes becoming aware of choices, letting go of ideas that are toxic or self-defeating, and making the best choice among the viable options. Goal-directed activities should reflect the patient's strengths, values, capabilities, beliefs, and preferences. Tangible, achievable goals give patients and families hope that they can get to a different place with resolving their crisis. Goals with meaning to the patient are more likely to be accomplished.

Designing Achievable Tasks

Help patients choose tasks that are within their capabilities, circumstances, and energy level. Achievable tasks can be as simple as getting more information or making time for self. You can suggest, "What do you think needs to happen first?" or "Let's look at what you might be able to do quickly." Engaging patients in simple problem solving reduces crisis-related feelings of helplessness and hopelessness. Problem-solving tasks that strengthen the patient's realistic perception of the crisis event, incorporate a patient's beliefs and values, and integrate social and environmental supports offer the best chance for success. Loughran (2011) suggests that helping patients tap into and use their personal resources to achieve goals facilitates crisis resolution and provides individuals with tools for further personal development.

Providing Structure and Encouragement

Patients need structure and encouragement as they perform the tasks that will move them forward. Setting time limits and monitoring task achievement is important. Resolving a crisis state is not a straightforward movement. There will be setbacks. Patients need ongoing affirmation of their efforts. Supportive reinforcement includes validation of the struggles that patients are coping with, anticipatory guidance regarding what to expect, and discussion of ambivalent feelings, uncertainty, and fears surrounding the process. Comparing progressive functioning with baseline admission presentations helps nurses and their patients mutually evaluate progress, foresee areas of necessary focus, and monitor progress toward treatment goals.

Providing Support for Families

Crisis intervention strategies should include support for family members. A crisis affects family dynamics, such that each family member is coping with some sort of emotional fallout brought about by the patient's crisis. Additionally, there may be issues requiring family response to an unstable home environment created by the patient's absence or an inability to function in their previous roles. There may be legal or safety issues that family members also have to address.

Individual family members experience a crisis in diverse ways, so different levels of information and support will be required. Bluhm (1987) suggests picturing the family as "a group of people standing together, with arms interlocked. What happens if one family member becomes seriously ill and can no longer stand? The other family members will attempt to carry their loved one, each person shifting his weight to accommodate the additional burden" (p. 44). Giving families an opportunity to talk about the meaning of the crisis for each family member and offering practical guidance about resources they can use to support the patient and take care of themselves are important strategies nurses can use with families. Communication strategies the nurse can use to help families in crisis are presented in Box 20.2.

Step 7 (Evaluation): Developing A Termination and Follow-Up Protocol

Patients should receive verbal instructions, with *written* discharge or follow-up directives and phone numbers to call for added help or clarification. Although acute symptoms subside with standard crisis intervention strategies, many patients will need follow-up for residual clinical issues.

Mobilize community resources to provide essential supports. Some patients are reluctant to use social services, medications, or mental health services, even in the short term, because of the stigma they feel about their use (Coleman, Stevelink, Hatch, Denny, & Greenberg, 2017). Others are cautious about the need for follow up. Nurses can help patients and families sort out their concerns, assess their practicality, and develop viable contacts. If indicated, nurses can facilitate the referral process by sharing information with community agencies and by giving patients enough information to follow through on getting additional assistance. Having written referral information available regarding eligibility requirements, location, cost, and accessibility can make a difference in patient interest and adherence. Exercise 20.4 provides an opportunity to practice crisis intervention skills.

MENTAL HEALTH EMERGENCIES

Mental health emergencies present significant challenges for nurses. Whether encountered in the community or with patients admitted to an emergency department, these patients often present as a danger to themselves or others. They present with chaotic distress behaviors, which are not under the patient's control. The fact that they are not easily controllable makes them particularly distressing for.

In addition to mental health emergencies, nurses should be aware of the presentation of co-occurring disorders. A person with a co-occurring disorder presents with both a mental illness and a substance use disorder (SUD). Often these patients will stop taking their prescribed psychotropic medications and instead self-medicate with other, non-prescribed medications (sometimes from other family members or friends) or illicit drugs or alcohol. Patients may feel that their psychiatric symptoms have subsided or even gone away for a while when they self-medicate. The problems arise with the propensity of overdose and the possibility of going into drug-induced delirium (also known in the law enforcement field as "excited delirium") or other somatic (cardiac problems) or drug-induced effects (difficulty driving, impulsive behavior, etc.). Nurses should be aware that these patients may present at the emergency department sometimes seeking legitimate care for their symptoms or may present to obtain medications (narcotics, benzodiazepines) that they are either out of, or abuse regularly, which, in turn, can counter or repress their psychiatric symptoms (Davis, 2014b; Vierheller & Denton, 2014).

Mental health emergencies require an *immediate* coordinated response designed to alleviate the potential for harm and restore basic stability. Examples of a mental health emergency include suicidal, homicidal, or threatening behavior, self-injury, severe drug or alcohol impairment, and highly erratic or unusual behavior associated with serious mental disorders. Unpredictability, acute emotions, and acting-out behaviors increase the intensity of mental health emergencies. Myer and Conte (2006) describe a triage assessment system (TAS) for mental health

BOX 20.2   Suggested Nursing Interventions for Initial Family Responses to Crisis

Anxiety, Shock, Fear

- Give information that is brief, concise, explicit, and concrete.
- Repeat information and frequently reinforce; encourage families to record important facts in writing.
- Determine comprehension by asking family to repeat back to you what information they have been given.
- Provide for and encourage or allow expression of feelings, even if they are extreme.
- Maintain a constant, nonanxious presence in the face of a highly anxious family.
- Inform family as to the potential range of behaviors and feelings that are within the "norm" for crisis.
- Maximize control within hospital environment, as possible.

Denial

- Identify what purpose denial is serving for family (e.g., Is it buying them "psychological time" for future coping and mobilization of resources?).
- Evaluate appropriateness of use of denial in terms of time; denial becomes inappropriate when it inhibits the family from taking necessary actions or when it is impinging on the course of treatment.
- Do not actively support denial, but do not dash hopes for the future (You might say, "It must be very difficult for you to believe your son is nonresponsive and in a trauma unit.").
- If denial is prolonged and dysfunctional, more direct and specific factual representation may be essential.

Anger, Hostility, Distrust

- Allow for venting of angry feelings, clarifying what thoughts, fears, and beliefs are behind the anger; let the family know it is okay to be angry.
- Do not personalize family's expressions of these strong emotions.
- Institute family control within the hospital environment when possible (e.g., arrange for set times and set person to give them information in reference to the patient and answer their questions).
- Remain available to families during their venting of these emotions.
- Ask families how they can take the energy in their anger and put it to positive use for themselves, for the patient, and for the situation.

Remorse and Guilt

- Do not try to rationalize away guilt for families.
- Listen and support their expression of feeling and verbalizations (e.g., "I can understand how or why you might feel that way; however...").
- Follow the "howevers" with careful, reality-oriented statements or questions (e.g., "None of us can truly control another's behavior"; "Kids make their own choices despite what parents think and want"; "How successful were you when you tried to control _____'s behavior with that before?"; "So many things happen for which there are no absolute answers").

Grief and Depression

- Acknowledge the family's grief and depression.
- Encourage them to be precise about what it is they are grieving and depressed about; give grief and depression a context.
- Allow the family appropriate time for grief.
- Recognize that this is an essential step for future adaptation; do not try to rush the grief process.
- Remain sensitive to your own unfinished business, and hence comfort or discomfort with family's grieving and depression.

Hope

- Clarify with families their hopes, individually and with one another.
- Clarify with families their worst fears in reference to the situation. Are the hopes/fears congruent? Realistic? Unrealistic?
- Support realistic hope.
- Offer gentle factual information to reframe unrealistic hope (e.g., "With the information you have or the observations you have made, do you think that is still possible?").
- Assist families in reframing unrealistic hope in some other fashion (e.g., "What do you think others will have learned from _____ if he doesn't make it?" "How do you think _____ would like for you to remember him/her?").

Adapted from Kleeman K. (1989) Families in crisis due to multiple trauma. *Critical Care Nursing Clinics of North America, 1*(1), 25.

EXERCISE 20.4 Interacting in Crisis Situations

Purpose

To give students experience in using the three-stage model of crisis intervention.

Procedure

1. Break the class up into groups of three. One student should take the role of the patient and one the role of the nurse; the third functions as the observer.
2. Using one of the following role-plays or one from your current clinical setting, engage the patient, and use the crisis intervention strategies presented in this chapter to frame your interventions.
3. The observer should provide feedback.

(This exercise can also be handled as discussion points rather than a role-play with small-group or class feedback as to how students would have handled the situations.)

Role-Play

Julie is a 23-year-old graduate student who has been dating Dan for the past 3 years. They plan to marry within the next 6 months. Last summer she had a brief affair with another graduate student while Dan was away but never told him. She is seeing you in the clinic having just found out that she has herpes from that encounter.

Sally is a 59-year-old postmenopausal woman who has been admitted for diagnostic testing and possible surgery. She has just found out that her tests reveal a malignancy in her colon with possible metastasis to her liver. You are the nurse responsible for her care.

Bill's mother was admitted last night to the intensive care unit (ICU) with sepsis. She is on life support and intravenous antibiotics. Bill had a close relationship with his mother earlier in his life, but he has not seen her in the past year. You are the nurse for the shift but do not yet know her well.

Discussion

1. What would you want to do differently as a result of this exercise when communicating with the patient in crisis?
2. What was the effect of using the three-stage model of crisis intervention as a way of organizing your approach to the crisis situation?

BOX 20.3 De-escalation Tips for Mental Health Emergencies

- Use a nonthreatening stance—open, but not vulnerable. Have them "take a seat."
- Eye contact—not constant, brief to show concern.
- Commands—brief, slow, with simple vocabulary, only as loud as needed, repeat as needed.
- Movement—not sudden, announce actions when possible, keep hands where they can be seen.
- Attitude—calm, interested, firm, patient, reassuring, respectful, truthful.
- Acknowledge legitimacy of feelings, delusions, hallucinations as being real to the patient "I understand you are seeing or feeling this, but I am not."
- Remove distractions, upsetting influences.
- Keep the patient talking/focused on the here and now.
- Ignore rather than argue with provocative statements.
- Allow verbal venting within reason.
- Be sensitive to personal space/comfort zone.
- Remove patient to a quiet space; remove others from immediate area (avoid the "group spectators").
- Give some choices or options, if possible.
- Set limits if necessary.
- Limit interaction to just one professional and let that person do the talking.
- Avoid rushing—slow things down.
- Give yourself an out; do not put the patient between yourself and the door.

Adapted from Davis, S. A. (2010b). *Crisis Intervention Team (CIT) Coordinator: De-escalation tips.* Rockville, MD: Montgomery County Police Department.

patient anger, fear, or sadness. Box 20.3 provides de-escalation tips for use with patients presenting in the community with mental health emergencies.

Model respect while communicating with mentally ill patients experiencing acute anxiety to avoid retraumatizing individuals already experiencing a chaotic, distressed state. Mentally ill patients respond best to respectful, calmly presented suggestions rather than commands.

It is helpful to provide additional personal space for individuals who have experienced a crisis and who have a mental illness. Keep communication calm, short, compassionate, and well defined. Do not indicate that you feel threatened or argue the logic of a situation. Avoid intimidating the patient, but set reasonable limits. Proceed slowly with purpose. Avoid sudden movements. Whenever possible, offer simple choices with structured coaching. Psychiatric emergency patients usually require medication for stabilization of symptoms and close supervision.

crises that can help nurses understand a patient's responses across three domains: affective, behavioral, and cognitive. The research on this tool is very positive. All three response domains are interrelated, but Meyer suggests that clinicians first focus on the patient's affective reaction, for example,

Types of Mental Health Emergencies

Violence

Violence is a mental health emergency, which creates a critical challenge to the safety, well-being, and health of the patients and others in their environment. Nurses should always assume an organic component (drugs, alcohol, psychosis, or delirium) underlying the aggression in patients presenting with disorganized impulsive or violent behaviors, until proven otherwise (Penterman & Nijman, 2011).

Patient body language offers clues to escalating anxiety, particularly agitation, threatening gestures, or darting eye movements. Table 20.1 presents indicators of increasing tension as precursors to violence. A history of violence, childhood abuse, substance abuse, neurodevelopmental disorders, problems with impulse control, and psychosis, particularly when accompanied by command hallucinations, are common contributing factors.

Treatment of violent patients consists of immediately providing a safe, nonstimulating environment for the patient. Often patients reduce the possibility of aggression if taken to an area with less sensory input. The patient should be checked thoroughly for potential weapons and physically disarmed, if necessary. Short-term medication usually is indicated to help defuse potentially harmful behaviors. The nurse should briefly identify why the medication is being given, and the patient should be carefully monitored for physical and behavioral responses.

Sexual Assault

Sexual assault and rape are serious forms of interpersonal victimization, which violate the core of self, in ways that are probably only second to murder. The patient's subjective stress is intense and long lasting. In the immediate aftermath of a sexual assault, everything should be done to help the patient feel safe and supported. The patient should be taken to a private room and should not be left alone. Evidence, if it is to be collected, requires that the patient not shower or douche prior to being examined. Larger emergency departments have a Sexual Assault Nurse Examiner (SANE) program, staffed by a specially trained nurse who provides first-response medical care and crisis intervention (James & Gilliland, 2013).

Adapting psychological first aid (PFA) to rape and sexual assault victims is a helpful comprehensive action-oriented intervention (Eifling & Moy, 2015; Forbes et al., 2011). PFA consists of eight core actions:
1. Contact and engagement
2. Safety and comfort
3. Stabilization
4. Information gathering
5. Practical assistance
6. Connection with social supports
7. Information on coping support
8. Linkage with collaborative services

TABLE 20.1	**Behavioral Indicators of Potential Violence**
Behavioral Categories	**Potential Indicators**
Mental status	Confused
	Paranoid ideation
	Disorganized
	Organic impairment
	Poor impulse control
Motor behavior	Agitated, pacing
	Exaggerated gestures
	Rapid breathing
Body language	Eyes darting
	Prolonged (staring) eye contact or lack of eye contact
	Spitting
	Pale, or red (flushed) face
	Menacing posture, throwing things
Speech patterns	Rapid, pressured
	Incoherent, mumbling, repeatedly making the same statements
	Menacing tones, raised voice, use of profanity
	Verbal threats
Affect	Belligerent
	Labile
	Angry

Data adapted from Keely, B. (2002). Recognition and prevention of hospital violence. *Dimensions of Critical Care Nursing, 21*(6), 236–241. Luck, L., Jackson, D., & Usher, K. (2007). Behavioral indicators of potential violence in the ED, and components of observable behavior indicative of patient violence in emergency departments. *Journal of Advanced Nursing, 59*(1), 11–19. In this study, five observable behaviors (staring, volume and tone of voice, heightened anxiety, mumbling, and pacing alerted nurses to potential for violence in the ED (Luck, Jackson, & Usher, 2007).

In a sexual assault situation, there should be no blame or conjecture about the victim's role in the attack. Sexual assault is always an act of violence and control. It is not a voluntary sexual act, even if the perpetrator and victim are known to each other. Follow-up referral to a mental health professional can help the patient cope with stress symptoms, shame, and the intrusive thoughts that frequently develop in the days and weeks following the assault.

Psychosis

An acute psychotic break represents a serious mental health behavioral emergency. Psychotic and delirious patients have disorganized thinking, reduced insight, and limited personal judgment. Patients experiencing "command" hallucinations, defined as *hallucinations* that direct the person to carry out an act, are at a higher risk for suicide and aggression. Medication is almost always indicated to manage acute psychotic symptoms, and one-to-one supervision is required (Randall et al., 2017). Allow the patient sufficient space to feel safe, and never try to subdue a patient by yourself. Remain calm and positive. Use less, rather than more words. An open expression, eye contact, a calm voice, and simple concrete words invite trust. Do not use touch, as it can be misinterpreted.

Suicide

Suicide is the 10th leading cause of death in the United States, and for every person who commits suicide, there are 25 other non-fatal suicide attempts (American Association of Suicidology [AAS], 2017). Suicide is defined as any self-injurious behavior that results in the death of an individual. This is classified as a behavioral emergency. The World Health Organization (WHO) describes suicide as a public health priority (WHO, 2016). The Joint Commission (2017b) identifies suicide as a "*sentinel event*" and calls for appropriate screening in behavioral care units, medical surgical units, and the emergency department to avert a death. People turn to suicide as an option in times of acute distress, when under the influence of drugs or when they believe there are no other alternatives. Impulsivity and hopelessness often go together with suicidal behaviors. Behavioral indicators of escalating suicidal ideation include a noteworthy change in behavior, often characterized by a burst of energy. Examples of changes in behavior of an individual who died by suicide include:

- A father gave away all of his deceased wife's jewelry 2 weeks before his death.
- An 18-year-old young man went door to door in his neighborhood apologizing for his "past" erratic behavior 3 days before he shot himself.
- A chronically mentally ill outpatient shared personal information and talked extensively in group therapy for the first time the week before he jumped off a bridge.

Impact of Suicide on Others

An individual who dies by suicide creates long-lasting effects for families, friends, coworkers, and the larger community. Individuals who are suicidal are often hesitant to talk about their feelings, due to stigma and hopelessness. They can be quite isolative and/or hard to engage in meaningful relationships. It is hard for family members or friends to know how to respond. People who talk about harming themselves are not necessarily at less risk, but there is more opportunity to prevent suicide. Every suicidal statement, however indirect, should be taken seriously. Even with patients who indicate that they are "just kidding," the fact that they have verbalized the threat places them at greater risk.

Passive suicidal wishes and actions, such as not taking medications, not practicing safe sex, drinking too much, driving too fast, and not caring if you are in an accident, warrant exploration. Pay attention to statements such as "I don't think I can go on without...," "I sometimes wish I could just disappear," or "People would be better off without me," as they are examples of suicidal ideation. Such statements require further clarification (e.g., "You say you can't go on without... Can you tell me more about what you mean?"). *Nurses should ask directly:*

"Do you have any thoughts of hurting yourself?" (include frequency and intensity of thoughts). Do you have a plan? Individuals with a detailed plan and the means to carry it out are at greatest risk for suicide. If the patient answers yes, you should **assess the lethality of the plan and inquire about the method and the patient's knowledge and skills about its use , along with the accessibility of the means to facilitate the suicide attempt** (Roberts, Monferrari, & Yeager, 2008).

You should also ask the following questions if you have any concerns about suicidal intent:

- Have you ever rehearsed the plan for suicide? What was that like? How did you interrupt the rehearsal?
- What do you hope to accomplish with the suicide attempt? (look for *hopelessness,* including severity and duration)
- Have you thought about when you might do this? (immediate vs. chronic thinking)
- Have you ever attempted suicide in the past? What happened? What type of care did you receive? How was it helpful?
- Has anyone in your family ever attempted or died by suicide?
- Who are you able to turn to when you are in trouble? (social support)
- What thoughts or activities help you to interrupt thoughts of suicide? (Jacobs, Brewer, & Klien-Benheun, 1999; Shea, 2009a, 2009b)

Risk Factors

Patients with mental illnesses, particularly depression, bipolar disorder, schizophrenia with command hallucinations, panic disorder, and comorbidity with substance abuse are more at risk for suicide. Although psychiatric diagnosis is a risk factor for suicide, many patients who have died by suicide have no previous psychiatric history and no evidence of prior suicide attempts (Rittenmeyer, 2012). WHO (2017) identified individuals who are unable to deal with life stresses, experience a break up of a relationship, or experience chronic pain and/or illness as having a possibility of an impulsive suicide attempt. Individuals who are isolated, experienced conflict, disaster, violence, abuse or loss are also at risk (WHO, 2017).

Suicide rates are greater for individuals aged 45 to 54 than among any other age group as reported in the USA Suicide: 2015 Official Final Data by Centers for Disease Control and Prevention (CDC, 2016). Caucasian men have the highest suicide rate followed by Caucasian women; African American women have the lowest rate of suicide (CDC, 2016).

In the USA, official data gathered by the CDC (2016) reported that there are 3.3 male deaths to each women who died by suicide. Women attempt three times to every one of the reported non-fatal attempts by men. Other high-risk factors include:

- Previous attempts or family history of suicide
- Family history of child abuse
- History of alcohol and substance abuse
- Major physical illness
- Social isolation, lack of social support
- Recent major loss
- History of trauma
- A sense of hopelessness
- Local epidemics of suicide
- Easy access to lethal means
- Not obtaining help due to stigma (CDC, 2016)
- Within the first few weeks of discharge from a psychiatric hospital
- Within 72 hours of discharge from a hospital, including the Emergency Department (ED) (The Joint Commission, 2016)

Stabilization of symptoms and patient safety are the most immediate concerns with patients experiencing a suicidal crisis. Possible weapons (e.g., mirrors, belts, knitting needles, scissors, razors, medications, clothes hangers) should be removed.

Explain in a calm, compassionate manner the reason why the items should not be in the patient's possession and where they will be kept. Patients need to be assured that the items will be returned when the danger of self-harm is resolved. Connectedness with others is considered a key protective factor in suicide prevention (Rodgers, 2017).

In the general hospital, death by suicide occurs more frequently than one would suppose. Patients experiencing intense pain, a terminal prognosis, substance abuse, or a recent bereavement are at higher risk. Patients have greater access to potentially lethal means to commit suicide, and health personnel do not immediately think of suicide in medical health situations. The Joint Commission has determined that 1089 deaths from suicide occurred between the years 2010 to 2014 within 72 hours of discharge from

a hospital setting, including the emergency department. This has been attributed to the health care staff not completing a comprehensive assessment for suicide (The Joint Commission, 2016). Documentation of a suicidal risk assessment, interventions, and patient responses are essential. Included in the documentation should be quotes made by the patient, details of observed behavior, a review of identified risk factors, and patient responses to initial crisis intervention strategies. The names and times of anyone you notified and contacts with family should be documented. Protective measures, such as individuals who the patient can call in a time of crisis, ways the patient can reduce their desire to die, and available telephone numbers for help, are important to assess and document. The Joint Commission requires that any death that is not consistent with a patient's disease process, or any permanent loss of function occurring as a consequence of an attempted suicide in a hospital, be reported as a sentinel event (The Joint Commission, 2017a).

Most psychiatric inpatient settings and emergency departments have written suicide precaution protocols that must be followed with patients presenting with suicidal ideation. Patients exhibiting high-risk behaviors require constant one-to-one staff observation; a potentially suicidal patient should never be left alone. Monitoring of suicidal patients ranges from constant 1:1 observation, to 15- or 30-minute observational checks. Less restrictive checks can include supervised bathroom visits, unit restriction or restriction to public areas, and supervised sharps (Jacobs, 2007). The frequency and type of observation is dependent on the suicidal assessment of the patient.

Consistent with a high risk for suicidal behavior is a sense of hopelessness, lack of meaningful connection with others, and the feeling of being a burden to others (AAS, 2017; CDC, 2017a). Acceptance of the patient is a critical element of rapport. Nurses need to explore their own feelings about suicide behaviors as the basis for understanding the patient in danger of self-injury.

Suicidal ideation waxes and wanes, so careful observation is critical even after the acute crisis has subsided.

The American Nurses Credentialing Center Competencies

In 2015, the American Psychiatric Nurses Association wrote the Psychiatric-Mental Health Nurse Essential Competencies for Assessment and Management of Individuals at Risk for Suicide. This document is a guide for practice based on extensive literature review and peer review. The nine essential competencies are:

- The psychiatric nurse understands the phenomenon of suicide.
- The psychiatric nurse manages personal reactions, attitudes, and beliefs.

- The psychiatric nurse develops and maintains a collaborative, therapeutic relationship with the patient.
- The psychiatric nurse collects accurate assessment information and communicates the risk to the treatment team and appropriate persons (i.e., nursing supervisor, on duty MD., etc.).
- The psychiatric nurse formulates a risk assessment.
- The psychiatric nurse develops an ongoing nursing plan of care based on continuous assessment.
- The psychiatric nurse performs an ongoing assessment of the environment in determining the level of safety and modifies the environment accordingly.
- The psychiatric nurse understands legal and ethical issues related to suicide.
- The psychiatric nurse accurately and thoroughly documents suicide risk (APNA, 2015).

Assessments should be repeated whenever changes in behavior are noted and again before discharge. The patient and nurse should develop a safety planning intervention (Stanley & Brown, 2012). This document is not a contract for safety, but rather, a collaborative plan that empowers the patient to determine ways to reduce the drive to die by suicide. The safety planning intervention helps the patient to identify the following:

- warning signs of suicide;
- internal coping strategies: the patient identifies what he/she can do to interrupt thoughts about suicide;
- people or social settings that can assist the patient to distract from the drive to commit suicide;
- people in the patient's life that can be called to assist the patient to maintain safety;
- professionals or agencies that the patient can call during a crisis; including 1-800-273-TALK (8255) #1 for veterans; and
- making the environment safe by removing all available means to commit suicide.

The nurse and the patient should discuss these items together. Following that each discussion, the patient should write down the relevant safety plan information that was discussed so the patient can refer to this safety plan at a later date. The safety planning intervention should begin after the patient has had an assessment for suicidal intent, and it should be revisited by the nurse after each assessment.

Crisis Intervention Teams

In the community, police with special training are important first responders in behavioral health emergencies (Miller, 2010). Community-based CIT offers a successful model of collaborative interventions between specially trained law enforcement officers and mental health care providers designed to treat rather than incarcerate mentally ill patients with comorbid behavioral emergency

(Davis, 2014a, 2014b) symptoms (Watson & Fulambarker, 2012). Emergency nurses are important stakeholders and collaborators with CIT-trained law enforcement officers (Ellis, 2011; Ralph, 2010). Officer Davis (2014a, 2014b), CIT coordinator with the Montgomery County Police Department, shares a field expedient tool, using the acronym "DANGEROUS PERSON" (see Box 20.1), to assess dangerousness to self or others in patients presenting as a mental health emergency.

Patients experiencing mental health emergencies may perceive necessary medical procedures as being intrusive and threatening. It is important to adhere to a nursing principle that before starting any procedure, you should tell the patient exactly what you are going to do and why the procedure is necessary, with a request to cooperate. If the patient refuses, do not insist, but explain the reason for doing the procedure in a calm, quiet voice. If you can help patients regain a sense of control, they are more likely to cooperate with you. Your movements should be calm, firm, and respectful.

DISASTER MANAGEMENT

Disaster and Mass Trauma Situations

A **disaster** is defined as "a calamitous event of slow or rapid onset that results in large-scale physical destruction of property, social infrastructure, and human life" (Deeny & McFetridge, 2005, p. 432). Recent years have borne witness to more natural disasters, terrorism, and war than the world has seen in many decades. Major hurricanes in Texas, Puerto Rico, and Florida all within the same year, fires in California, terrorist attacks spontaneously occurring in many areas of the world, and the threat of nuclear war from adversarial nations have heightened attention and tension. Terrorist attacks have stimulated a fresh awareness of the need for community and national planned responses to disaster events. These events can happen anywhere and at any time to innocent masses of people. Webb (2004) identifies the components of mass trauma events in Table 20.2.

Planning for Disaster Management

In the United States, the Federal Emergency Management Agency (FEMA) is responsible for setting forth recommendations related to creating an effective disaster plan. FEMA recommendations provide guidelines for the creation of local disaster planning teams (FEMA, 2017). Community-based governments and businesses, first responders, hospitals, and health providers are expected to be actively involved in community disaster planning. Around the globe, tsunamis in Indonesia, earthquakes occurring in rapid succession in China, Iceland, and South America, the threat of nations developing nuclear weapons, pandemic flu, and

TABLE 20.2　Assessing Elements of Mass Trauma Events

Element	Example
Single vs. recurring traumatic event	Type I (acute) trauma
	Type II (chronic or ongoing) trauma
Proximity to the traumatic event	Onsite
	On the periphery
	Through the media
Exposure to violence/injury/pain	Witnessed and/or experienced
Nature of losses/death/destruction	Personal, community, and/or symbolic loss
	Danger, loss, and/or responsibility traumas
	Loved one, missing or no physical evidence
	Death determined by retrieval of body or fragment
	Loss of status/employment/family income
	Loss of a predictable future
Attribution of causality	Random
	Act of God or deliberate
	Human-made

From Webb, N. (2004). The impact of traumatic stress and loss on children and families. In: Webb N (Ed.) *Mass trauma and violence: Helping families and children cope* (p. 6). New York: Guilford, reprinted with permission.

severe acute respiratory syndrome (SARS) remind us of the need for a global approach to emergency preparedness. The Sendai Framework was adapted by the United Nations (UN) to promote a prevention-based approach to international disasters. The emphasis in the Sendai Framework is on early warning when a disaster may take place; predicting the event and needs for prevention of causalities; recovery after the disaster; and rehabilitation once recovery of the disaster takes place. The Sendai Framework goals will be implemented and utilized between the years of 2015–2030 (Aitsi-Selmi & Murray, 2016).

Strategies for creating and sustaining community-wide emergency preparedness are published by The Joint Commission (2015). These plans include the following:

- exploring ethical considerations, including legal authority and environmental concerns;
- education and information sharing;
- provider and community engagement;
- development of clinical processes and operations, performance improvement;
- hospital care, outpatient care, Emergency Medical Sevices (EMS), public health, and public safety; and
- local, state, and federal government emergency-management standards (The Joint Commission, 2015).

Disaster planning can act as a deterrent to terrorist activity and as an immediate resource in a disaster situation. Disaster management requires providing immediate physical and emotional first aid. Instead of initially eliciting details of the experience, Everly and Flynn (2006) stress promotion of adaptive functioning and stabilization as a first response. They use the acronym BICEPS, which stands for brevity, immediacy, contact, expectancy, proximity, and simplicity to describe the type of PFA needed in mass disaster situations.

Critical Incident Debriefing

Disasters, deliberate violence, and terrorist attacks are random events producing permanent changes in people's lives and shaking their perception of being in charge of their lives. Critical incident stress management (CISM) is used to help people who have witnessed or experienced a crisis event externalize and process its meaning. Guided sharing of the crisis experience by those most impacted by it can be healing. CISM may be done on an individual basis, if indicated by the incident. The debriefing allows the people involved in a traumatic situation to achieve a sense of psychological closure. The debriefing team also teaches participants about the nature of distress reactions and offers helpful hints to reduce their effects (Everly & Mitchell, 2017).

Critical Incident Stress Debriefing Process

A specially trained professional generally leads the debriefing. The leader introduces the purpose of the

CISM and assures the participants that everything said in the session will be kept confidential. People are asked to identify who they are and what happened from their perspective, including the role they played in the incident. After preliminary factual data are addressed, the next step is to explore feelings. The leader asks participants to recall the first thing they remember thinking or feeling about the incident. Participants are asked to discuss any stress symptoms they may have related to the incident. The final discussion focuses on the emotional reactions associated with the critical incident. This part of the session is followed by psychoeducational strategies to reduce stress. Any lingering questions are answered, and the leader summarizes the high points of the critical incident debriefing for the group (Everly & Mitchell, 2017).

Critical incident debriefings are used with families witnessing a tragedy involving a family member, for children and adolescents dealing with the death of a classmate, mass murders, robberies, or environmental disasters. A critical incident stress debriefing offers people an opportunity to externalize a traumatic experience through being able to vent feelings, discuss their role in the situation, develop a realistic sense of the big picture, and receive peer support in putting a crisis event in perspective (Everly & Mitchell, 2017).

Critical Incident Debriefing for Health Care Providers

Research indicates that health care providers who assist or witness critical incidents can be vulnerable to experience "secondary traumatization" similar to that experienced by direct survivors of the incident. Principles of critical incident debriefing can also be applied to strengthen the emotional coping skills of staff working in clinical settings on units with frequent or unexpected loss. Support for nurses, first responders, and emergency health care providers include the use of employee assistance programs (EAP). Some organizations have assistance at the national level, such as the National Fallen Firefighters Foundation (NFFF) Stress First Aid (Jones, 2017).

Community Response Patterns

The Joint Commission (2015) explicitly portrays disaster management and emergency preparedness as a community responsibility. When disaster strikes, the existence and function of the community are significantly impaired. Initially people are confused and stunned. Emotions vary as the extent of the impact is realized. The closer the person is to the crisis event, the more intense the impact. The immediate concern is protection of self and those closest to them. By preparing for a disaster, the community is more resilient and able to recover faster (Zukowski, 2014).

Disaster Management in Health Care Settings

All hospitals are required to form disaster committees composed of key departments within the hospital, including nursing. Nurses interested in emergency volunteer activities should become aware of credentialing requirements to ensure their participation as part of a national emergency volunteer system for health professionals. Hospital and community disaster planning must be coordinated so all phases of the disaster cycle are covered. Designated hospital personnel must receive training to carry out triage at the emergency department entrance. Protocols should contain the capability to relocate staff and patients to another facility if necessary, and a plan must be in place detailing mechanisms for equipment resupply. Policies regarding notification, maintenance of accurate records, and establishment of a facility control center are required (The Joint Commission, 2016).

Citizen Responders

Unsolicited responders play a large role in sudden onset, large-scale disasters. Emergency plans should anticipate the presence of unsolicited individuals who respond to the disaster, wishing to assist. As part of a comprehensive community disaster plan, an infrastructure for coordinating their efforts should be developed. Public education related to the citizen role in disaster management is essential.

Citizen Corps Programs, developed by FEMA, is a grassroots crisis intervention strategy that can provide community volunteers with a program to develop emergency preparedness and first-aid skills. The web site (www.ready.gov/citizen-corps) provides training and tool kits to help improve the on-site care of disaster victims. It also provides links to information for families interested in developing emergency-preparedness plans.

HELPING CHILDREN COPE WITH TRAUMA

Children do not have the same resources when coping with traumatic events as adults do. Preexisting exposure to traumatic events and lack of social support increases vulnerability. It is not unusual for children to demonstrate regressive behaviors as a reaction to crisis. While helping the child work through the emotional aspects of the trauma, utilize language appropriate to the child's level of development and cognitive ability. Assess how the child perceives the stressor, and determine the child's self-perception of how they are able to problem-solve (Pfefferbaum, Noffsinger, & Wind, 2012).

Children will look for cues from key adults in their lives and tend to mirror their adult caregivers, so it is essential to communicate calmly and with confidence. More than anything else, children need reassurance that they and the people who are important to them are safe. Encourage the family to maintain regular routines. Parents need to provide children with opportunities both to talk about the crisis and to ask questions. Repetitive questions are to be expected. This often reflect the child's need for reassurance. Offering factual information helps dispel misperceptions.

HELPING OLDER ADULTS COPE WITH TRAUMA

Reducing anxiety is especially important for the older adult disaster victim. Even the most capable older adult can appear confused and vulnerable in a disaster situation. Actions nurses can take include the following:

1. Initiate contact and take the older adult to as safe a place as possible.
2. Speak calmly and provide concrete information about what is happening and what you need the older adult to do in simple terms.
3. Assess for mobility, and provide assistance where needed.
4. Older adults may need warmer clothing because of compromised temperature regulation.

Functional limitations associated with compromised physical mobility, diminished sensory awareness, and pre-existing health conditions create special issues for older patients impacted by a disaster. Older adults have more injury and greater disaster-related deaths than adults in other age groups. Within the older population, special attention should focus on those who require medical or nursing care and those receiving services, care, or food from health, social, or volunteer agencies.

Disaster management for older adults needs to be pro-active (Johnson, Ling, & McBee, 2015). The following core actions can make a difference in helping older adults weather a disaster event successfully. Proactive planning includes working with patients:

- Identify a support network that can be used in an emergency situation. Facilitate connections with social support systems and community support structures. Have this information readily available for use in an emergency situation.
- Older adults with a disability should wear tags or a bracelet to identify their disability. Keeping extra eyeglasses and hearing aid batteries on hand and identifying any assistive devices is essential.
- Identify the closest special needs evacuation center.
- Develop a written list of all medications, with any special directions, for example, crushing pills, hours of administration, and dietary restrictions.
- Identify physicians and social support contacts, including someone apart from people in the local area who can be contacted.

Other actions, such as ensuring the safety, meeting mobility needs, and medication administration, need special attention during the course of actual disaster management.

SUMMARY

Crisis is defined as an unexpected, sudden turn of events or set of circumstances requiring an immediate human response. People experience a crisis as overwhelming, traumatic, and personally intrusive. It is an unexpected life event challenging a person's sense of self and his or her place in the world. The most common types of crisis are situational and developmental crises. Most health crises are situational. Crisis can be private, involving one person, or public, involving large numbers of people.

Theoretical frameworks guiding crisis intervention include Lindemann's (1944) model of grieving and Caplan's (1964) model, based on preventive psychiatry concepts. Aguilera's (1998) nursing model explores the role of balancing factors in defusing the impact of a crisis state. Erikson's (1982) model of psychosocial development provides a framework for exploring developmental crises.

Crisis intervention is a time-limited treatment, which focuses on the immediate crisis and its resolution. Roberts' (2005) seven-stage model, used to guide nursing interventions, consists of assessing lethality, establishing rapport, dealing with feelings, defining the problem, exploring alternative options, formulating a plan, and follow-up measures. The goal of crisis intervention is to return the patient to his or her pre-crisis level of functioning.

Mental health emergencies require immediate assessment interventions and close supervision. The most common types are violence, suicide, and a psychotic break. Guidelines for communication with patients experiencing mental health emergencies (e.g., violence and suicide) focus on safety and rapid stabilization of the patient's behavior. CITs represent a new model of collaboration between local law enforcement and mental health services designed to treat rather than punish individuals experiencing mental health emergencies in the community (Davis, 2014a; Watson & Fulambarker, 2012).

As the world becomes more dynamically unstable, nurses will need to understand the dimensions of disaster management and develop the skills to respond effectively in disaster situations. Disaster management is a special kind of crisis intervention applied to large groups of people. The Joint Commission (2015) requires hospitals to develop and exercise disaster-management plans at regular intervals. CISM is a crisis intervention strategy designed to help those closely involved with disasters process critical incidents in health care, thereby reducing the possibility of symptoms occurring.

ETHICAL DILEMMA: What Would You Do?

Sara Murdano is only 20 years old when she arrives at the mobile intensive care unit (MICU), but this is not her first hospital admission. She has been treated for depression previously. She states she is determined to kill herself be-

cause she has nothing to live for and that it is her right to do so because she is no longer a minor. As she describes her life to date, you cannot help but think that she really does not have a lot to live for. How would you respond to this patient from an ethical perspective?

DISCUSSION QUESTIONS

- What would you identify as the essential knowledge, skills, and attitudes required of a nurse confronted with a patient who is at high risk for a suicide attempt?
- What questions would you ask Sara to determine her level of risk and protective measures?

- How would you apply The Joint Commission safety standards in the emergency department?
- What would you document regarding Sara's assessment and interventions?

REFERENCES

Aguilera, D. (1998). *Crisis Intervention: Theory and Methodology* (7th ed.). St Louis: Mosby.

American Psychiatric Nurses Association (APNA). (2015). *Psychiatric-Mental Health Nurse Essential Competencies for Assessment and Management of Individual at Risk of Suicide.* Retrieved from: www.apna.org.

Aitsi-Selmi, A., & Murray, V. (2016). Protecting the health and well-being of populations from disasters: Health and health care in the sendai framework for disaster risk reduction 2015-2030. *Prehospital and Disaster Medicine, 31*(1), 74–78. https://doi.org/10.1017/S1049023X15005531.

American Association of Suicidology (AAS). (2017). *Suicide in the USA Based on 2015 Data.* http://www.suicidology.org.

Bluhm, J. (1987). Helping families in crisis hold on. *Nursing, 17*(10), 44–46.

Browning, S. L., Van Hasselt, V. B., Tucker, A. S., & Vecchi, G. M. (2011). Dealing with individuals who have mental illness: the crisis intervention team (CIT) in law enforcement. *British Journal of Forensic Practice, 13*(4), 235–243. https://doi.org.ez-proxy.pgcc.edu/10.1108/14636641111189990.

Callahan, J. (1998). Crisis theory and crisis intervention in emergencies. In P. M. Kleespies (Ed.), *Emergencies in mental health practice: Evaluation and management.* New York: Guilford Press.

Caplan, G. (1964). *Principles of Preventive Psychiatry.* New York: Basic Books.

Centers for Disease Control and Prevention (CDC). (2017a). National Violent Death Reporting System. *CDC MMWR Surveillance Summaries.* http://www.cdc.gov/ViolencePreven-tion/intimatepartnerviolence/consequences.html.

Centers for Disease Control and Prevention (CDC). (2017b). *Web-based injury statistics query and Reporting System (WISQARS).* http://www.cdc.gov/injury/wisquars/index.html.

Coleman, S. J., Stevelink, S. A. M., Hatch, S. L., Denny, J. A., & Greenberg, N. (2017). Stigma-related barriers and facilitators to help seeking for mental health issues in the armed forces: A

systematic review and thematic synthesis of qualitative literature. *Psychological Medicine, 47*(11), 1880–1892. https://doi.org.ezproxy.pgcc.edu/10.1017/S0033291717000356.

Dass-Brailsford, P. (2010). *Crisis and Disaster Counseling: Lessons Learned from Hurricane Katrina and Other Disasters.* Thousand Oaks, CA: Sage Publications.

Davis, S. (2014a). *CIT Teams: Unpublished Manuscript.*

Davis, S. (2014b). De-escalation tips in crisis situations. In *Montgomery county.* Rockville, MD: MD Police Department.

Deeny, P., & McFetridge, B. (2005). The impact of disaster on culture, self, and identity: Increased awareness by health care professionals is needed. *Nursing Clinics of North America, 40*(3), 431–444.

Eifling, K. M. D., & Moy, H. P. M. D. (2015). Evidence-based EMS: Psychological first aid. *EMS World, 44*(7), 32–34. https://ezproxy.pgcc.edu/login?url=https://search-proquest-com.ezproxy.pgcc.edu/docview/1708156049?accountid=13315.

Ellis, H. A. (2011). The crisis intervention team—A revolutionary tool for law enforcement: The psychiatric-mental health nursing perspective. *Journal of Psychosocial Nursing and Mental Health Services, 49*(11), 37–43. https://doi.org.ezproxy.pgcc.edu/10.3928/02793695-20111004-01.

Erikson, E. (1982). *The Life Cycle Completed.* New York: Norton.

Everly, G. (2000). Five principles of crisis intervention: Reducing the risk of premature crisis intervention. *International Journal of Emergency Mental Health, 2*(1), 1–4.

Everly, G., & Flynn, B. (2006). Principles and practical procedures for acute first aid training for personnel without mental health experience. *International Journal of Emergency Mental Health, 8*(2), 93–100.

Everly, G. S., & Mitchell, J. T. (2017). *Critical incident stress management (CISM): A practical review.*

Federal Emergency Management Agency (FEMA): 2017. https://www.fema.gov/recover-directorate/crisis-counseling-assistance-training programs. (Assessed 14.01.015).

Flannery, R., Jr., & Everly, G., Jr. (2000). Crisis intervention: A review. *International Journal of Emergency Mental Health, 2*(2), 119–125.

Forbes, D., Lewis, V., Varker, T., et al. (2011). Psychological first aid following trauma: Implementation and evaluation framework for high-risk organizations. *Psychiatry, 74*(3), 224–239. https://doi.org.ezproxy.pgcc.edu/101521psyc2011743224.

Hoff, L. (2009). People in crisis: cultural and diversity perspectives. In *Routledge* (6th ed.). New York: Taylor & Francis Group.

Jacobs, D. (2007). *Screening for Mental Health: a Resource Guide for Implementing the Joint Commission on Accreditation of Health Care Organizations (CAHO) 2007 Patient Safety Goals on Suicide.* Wellesley Hills: Screening for Mental Health Inc.

Jacobs, D., Brewer, M. I., Klien-Benheun, et al. (1999). Chapter 1: Suicide assessment: An overview and recommended protocol. In G. Douglas (Ed.), *The Harvard Medical School guide to suicide assessment and intervention* (pp. 3–39). San Francisco, CA: Josey-Bass Publishers.

James, R. (2008). *Crisis Intervention Strategies* (8th ed.). Belmont CA: Thompson Brooks/Cole.

James, R., & Gilliland, B. (2013). *Crisis Intervention Strategies* (7th ed.). Belmont CA: Thomson Brooks/Cole.

Johnson, H. L., Ling, C. G., & McBee, E. C. (2015). Multidisciplinary care for the elderly in disasters: An integrative review. *Prehospital and Disaster Medicine, 30*(1), 72–79. https://doi.org.ezproxy.pgcc.edu/10.1017/S1049023X14001241.

Jones, S. (2017). Describing the mental health profile of first responders: A systematic review. *Journal of the American Psychiatric Nurses Association, 23*(3), 200–214.

The Joint Commission. (2015a). Emergency management: Getting started with crisis standards of care. Part 1. *Environ care news, 18*(11). http://www.jointcommission.org.

The Joint Commission. (2015b). Emergency management: Getting started with crisis standards of care. Part 2. *Environ Care News, 18*(12). http://www.jointcommission.org.

The Joint Commission. (2016). Sentinel event alert: Detecting and treating suicidal ideation in all settings. *Issue, 56.* http://www.jointcommission.org.

The Joint Commission: National patient safety goals effective January 2017a behavioral health care accreditation program, *Goal 15 NPSG 15.01.01.* http://www.jointcommission.org.

The Joint Commission: *Sentinel events: comprehensive accreditation manual for behavioral health care (CAMBHC)* E-dition, July 1, 2017b. http://www.jointcommission.org.

Keely, B. (2002). Recognition and prevention of hospital violence. *Dimensions of Critical Care Nursing, 21*(6), 236–241.

Kleeman, K. (1989). Families in crisis due to multiple trauma. *Critical Care Nursing Clinics of North America, 25*(1).

Kleespies, P. M. (2009). *An Evidence Based Resource for Evaluating and Managing Risk of Suicide, Violence, and Victimization.* Washington DC: American Psychological Association.

Lindemann, E. (1944). Symptomatology and management of acute grief. *American Journal of Psychiatry, 101*, 141–148.

Loughran, H. (2011). *Understanding Crisis Therapies: An Integrative Approach to Crisis Intervention and Post Traumatic Stress.* London: Jessica Kingsley Publishers.

Luck, L., Jackson, D., & Usher, K. (2007). STAMP: Components of observable behaviour that indicate potential for patient violence in emergency departments. *Journal of Advanced Nursing, 59*(1), 11–19.

Michalopoulos, H., & Michalopoulos, A. (2009). Crisis counseling: be prepared to intervene. *Nursing, 39*(9), 47–50.

Miller, L. (2010). On-scene crisis intervention: Psychological guidelines and communication strategies for first responders. *International Journal of Emergency Mental Health, 12*(1), 11–19.

Myer, R., & Conte, C. (2006). Assessment for crisis intervention. *Journal of Clinical Psychology, 62*(8), 959–970.

Neville, K., & Roan, N. (2013). Suicide in hospitalized medical-surgical patients: Exploring nurses' attitudes. *Journal of Psychosocial Nursing and Mental Health Services, 51*(1), 35–43. https://doi.org.ezproxy.pgcc.edu/10.3928/02793695-20121204-01.

Ouzouni, C., & Nakakis, K. (2009). Attitudes towards attempted suicide: The development of a measurement tool. *Health Science Journal, 3*, 222–231.

Penterman, B., & Nijman, H. (2011). Assessing aggression risks in patients of the ambulatory mental health crisis team. *Community Mental Health Journal, 47*(4), 463–471. https://doi.org.ezproxy.pgcc.edu/10.1007/s10597-010-9348-7.

Pfefferbaum, B., Noffsinger, M. A., & Wind, L. H. (2012). Issues in the assessment of children's coping in the context of mass trauma. *Prehospital and Disaster Medicine, 27*(3), 272–279. https://doi.org/10.1017/S1049023X12000702.

Ralph, M. (2010). The impact of crisis intervention team programs: Fostering collaborative relationships. *Journal of Emergency Nursing, 36*(1), 60–62.

Randall, J., Chateau, D., Bolton, J. M., Smith, M., Katz, L., Burland, E., et al. (2017). Increasing medication adherence and income assistance access for first-episode psychosis patients. *PLoS One, 12*(6), e0179089. https://doi.org.ezproxy.pgcc.edu/10.1371/journal.pone.0179089.

Rittenmeyer, L. (2012). Assessment of risk for in-hospital suicide and aggression in high dependency care environments. *Critical Care Nursing Clinics of North America, 24*, 41–51.

Roberts, A. (2005). *Crisis Intervention Handbook: Assessment, Treatment and Research.* New York: Oxford University Press.

Roberts, A., & Yeager, K. (2009). *Pocket Guide to Crisis Intervention.* New York: Oxford University Press.

Roberts, A., Monferrari, I., & Yeager, K. (2008). Avoiding malpractice lawsuits by following risk assessment and suicide prevention guidelines. *Brief Treatment and Crisis Intervention, 8*, 5–14.

Rodgers P, Suicide Prevention Resource Center: *Understanding risk and protective factors for suicide: A primer for preventing suicide.* Retrieved from: www.sprc.org/library_resources/items/understanding-risk-and-protective-factors-suicide-primer-preventing-suicide (Accessed 23.08.17).

Shea, S. D. (2009a). Suicide Assessment Part 1: Uncovering suicidal intent a sophisticated art. *Psychiatric Times* (26), 1–6.

Shea, S. D. (2009b). Suicide Assessment Part 2: Uncovering suicidal intent using the Chronological Assessment of Suicide Events (CASE Approach). *Psychiatric Times* (26), 1–26.

Stanley B, Brown GK: Safety planning intervention: A brief intervention to mitigate suicide risk. *Cognitive and Behavioral*

Practice 19(2012): 256–264. http://www.suicidesafety-plan.com; www.sciencedirect.com. (Accessed 30.07.17).

Vierheller, C. C., & Denton, M. (2014). When mental health and medicine collide: Maintaining safety in the emergency department. *Journal of Nursing Education and Practice*, 4(2), 49–55. https://dx.xoi.org/10.5430/jnep.v4n2p49.

Vroomen, J. M., Bosmans, J. E., van Hout, H. P., & de Rooij, S. E. (2013). Reviewing the definition of crisis in dementia care. *BMC Geriatrics*, 13(10). https://doi.org/10.1186/1471-2318-13-10.

Watson, A., & Fulambarker, A. (2012). The crisis intervention team model of police response to mental health crises: A primer for mental health practitioners. *Best Practice Mental Health*, 8(2), 71–77.

Webb, N. B. (Ed.). (2004). *Mass trauma and violence: helping families and children cope.* New York: Guilford Press.

World Health Organization (WHO) (2016): Preventing suicide: *A community engagement toolkit. Pilot version 1.0.* License: CC BY-NC-SA 3.0 IGO, http://www.who.int/mediacentre/fact-sheets/fs398/en/ (Accessed March 2017).

Zukowski, R. S. (2014). The impact of adaptive capacity on disaster response and recovery: Evidence supporting core community capabilities. *Prehosp Dis Med*, 29(4), 380–387. https://doi.org/10.1017/S1049023X14000624.

SUGGESTED READING

Davis, S. (2015). Field expedient tool to assess dangerousness in self and others. In *Montgomery county*. Rockville, MD: MD Police Department.

21

Communication Approaches in Palliative Care

Elizabeth C. Arnold

OBJECTIVES

At the end of the chapter, the reader will be able to:

1. Discuss the concept of loss.
2. Identify theory-based concepts of grief and grieving.
3. Describe the nurse's role in palliative care.
4. Discuss key issues and approaches in end-of-life (EOL) care.
5. Identify cultural and spiritual needs in EOL care.
6. Describe supportive strategies for children.
7. Discuss strategies to help patients achieve a good death.
8. Identify stress issues for nurses in EOL care.

INTRODUCTION

- Structure and process of care
- Physical aspects of care
- Psychological and psychiatric aspects of care
- Social aspects of care
- Spiritual, religious, and existential aspects of care
- Cultural aspects of care

The purpose of this chapter is to introduce palliative care approaches that nurses can use to effectively communicate with patients (and families) in the last stage of life. The chapter identifies selected theoretical frameworks related to loss, stages of dying, and the process of grief and grieving. The application section highlights communication and care issues nurses face in providing patient/family palliative care. Helping clinicians recognize and cope with the high stress of providing quality EOL care is also addressed.

BASIC CONCEPTS

Loss, Grief, and Bereavement

Corless (2001) defines **loss** as "a generic term that signifies absence of an object, position, ability or attribute" (p. 352). Important losses occur as part of everyone's personal experience. Anything or anyone in whom we invest time, energy, or a part of ourselves creates a sense of loss when it is no longer available to us. When people *suffer the loss of* someone or something important to them, there is a loss of their sense of "wholeness," and a break in the person's expected life story (Attig, 2004). The passage of time never fully erases this sense of loss.

The feelings associated with each loss differ only in the intensity with which one experiences them. Mark Twain noted: "Nothing that grieves us can be called little; by the eternal laws of proportion a child's loss of a doll and a king's loss of a crown are events of the same size" (Mark, 2002). Only the person experiencing the loss can appreciate the unique void and strength of feelings that each loss entails. Some losses are gradual; others occur concurrently, or sequentially.

One loss can precipitate other losses. For example, a patient with Alzheimer disease doesn't simply lose memory. Accompanying cognitive deficits are accumulating losses of role, communication, independence, and gradual loss of identity. Simulation Exercise 21.1 is designed to help you understand the dimensions of personal loss.

Multiple Losses

Acknowledging differences between single and multiple loss helps patients put the enormity of multiple losses into perspective (Mercer & Evans, 2006). Older adults typically experience the deaths of friends and family members with greater frequency. Others lose multiple friends to AIDS, military action, and natural or man-made disasters. A car accident can wipe out an entire family or group of friends.

Multiple losses intensify the grief experience and it usually requires more time to resolve grief feelings. From a communication perspective, helping patients to focus on one relationship at a time instead of trying to address the losses together works best. Otherwise, bereavement can be overwhelming. Patience with oneself is critical to successfully working through difficult emotions associated with multiple losses. Bereavement takes time, and one should not rush the process.

DEATH: THE FINAL LOSS

Death represents a tangible loss in that the *physical* presence of the lost person can never be replaced. More than a biological event, death has spiritual, social, and cultural features that help people make sense of its meaning.

Regardless of primary medical diagnosis, patients experience many different emotions, ranging from anger or sadness to a sense of peace about a life well lived with few regrets as they approach death.

For some people, a significant family member is snatched away in an instant. For others, there are precious time-limited opportunities to say good-bye, and to find a sense of closure. Being able to actively participate in helping a loved one achieve the peace of having a good death is comforting. Sharing in an end-of-life (EOL) process with a loved one is meaningful, especially if family members receive support with the process. The memory of this time together is critically important to those left behind.

Death is a normal part of the life order for everyone. It is not a failure. No one can tell you how it will be for you based on his or her experience. Pashby (2015), an expert hospice nurse, states that most patients identify fear of pain, losing control, and dying alone as their principal fears. Nurses are an important resource in providing practical support and offering meaningful presence to patients and families coping with life-limiting illnesses.

THEORETICAL FRAMEWORKS

Elisabeth Kübler-Ross's (1969) five-stage model provides an evidence-based framework for the study of death and dying (Keegan & Drick, 2011). Not every person experiences each stage. Some people remain in the denial stage until the very end of their illness. Their right to do so should be respected.

Denial

Kübler-Ross (1969) characterizes the denial stage as the "No, not me" stage. Nurses should be sensitive to the patient's need for denial.

Anger

Anger is characterized as the "Why me?" stage. This stage can produce feelings about the unfairness of life or anger with God. Feelings often get projected on those closest to the patient. Family members need support to recognize that the anger is not a personal attack (although sometimes it feels that way to the family member).

Bargaining

Kübler-Ross refers to the bargaining stage as the "Yes, me, but … I need just a little more time." Bargaining is not a futile exercise. Sometimes the extra energy a person gets by focusing on living long enough to attend a graduation, a birth, or a wedding is meaningful to all involved in making it happen. By supporting hope and avoiding challenges to the patient's reality, the nurse facilitates the process of living while dying.

Depression

The "Yes, me" stage of dying is expressed through depressive feelings and mood swings. You can help family members understand that this is a "normal" response to anticipating loss. Review of significant life events and relationships helps patients consider unfinished business that could be reworked. Serving as an empathetic listening witness to the pain that patients and families experience in this stage helps them work through this stage.

Acceptance

The acceptance stage is characterized by an acknowledgment of an inevitable end to physical life. There is a gradual detachment from the world; the patient experiences being almost "void of feeling" (Kübler-Ross, 1969, p. 124). Ideally, patients experience a personal sense of peace and letting go. To outsiders, the patient is straddling between two world realities: the organic and the existential.

Grief

Eric Lindemann (1994 [1944]) pioneered the concept of grief work based on interviews with bereaved persons suffering a sudden tragic loss. He described patterns of grief and identified physical and emotional changes associated with significant loss. Lindemann observed that grief can occur immediately after a loss, or it can be delayed. He summarized three components of support: (a) open, empathetic communication; (b) honesty; and (c) tolerance of emotional expression as being important in grieving. When the symptoms of grief are exaggerated over a period of time, or absent, it is considered pathological or complicated grief. People experiencing complicated grief may require psychological treatment to resolve their grief and move into life again.

Engel's Contributions

George Engel's (1964) concepts build on Lindemann's work. He described three sequential phases of grief work: (a) shock and disbelief, (b) developing awareness, and (c) restitution.

In the shock and disbelief phase, a newly bereaved person may feel alienated or detached from normal—"literally numb with shock; no tears, no feelings, just absolute numbness" (Lendrum & Syme, 1992, pp. 24–25). Seeing or hearing the lost person or sensing his or her presence is a temporary altered sensory experience related to the loss, which should not be confused with psychotic hallucinations.

The developing awareness phase occurs slowly as the void created by the loss fully enters consciousness. Patients experience a loss of energy, not the kind that requires sleep, but rather recognizing that one lacks the functional energy to engage fully in normal everyday responsibilities.

The restitution phase is characterized by adaptation to a new life without the deceased. There is a resurgence of hope and a renewed energy to fashion a new life. With successful grieving, the loss is not forgotten, but the pain diminishes, and is replaced with memories that enrich and give energy to life.

Case Example

"Throughout the year following my mother's death, I was aware of a persistent feeling of heaviness— not physical heaviness, but emotional and spiritual. It was as if a dark cloud hung over my heart and soul. I tired easily, with little energy to do anything but the most essential activities, and even those frequently received perfunctory attention. My usual pattern of 'sleeping like a log' was disrupted, and in its place, I experienced uneasy rest that left me feeling as if I had never closed my eyes" (Anonymous).

Listening, identifying feelings, and having an empathetic willingness to repeatedly hear the patient's story without needing to give advice or interpretation offer presence without demands.

Contemporary models

Florczak (2008) states, "The newer worldview considers loss to be a unique, intersubjective process in which the individual maintains connections with the absent and the meaning of the experience continually changes" (p. 8). Contemporary authors Neimeyer (2001) and Attig (2001) emphasize meaning construction as a central issue in grief work. The past is not forgotten. Instead, there is a continuous spiritual connection with the deceased, which illuminates different features of self, and possibilities for fuller engagement with life. Features of past experiences with the loved one are transformed and rewoven into the fabric of a person's life in a new form. The concept of a palliative approach to care represents an "integrative model, which can guide the care of persons at any stage of chronic illness, dispelling the myth that palliative care is only for EOL.

GRIEF AND GRIEVING

The concept of **grief** describes a holistic, adaptive process that a person goes through following a significant loss. Grief is an adaptive process, which is different for each person (Jeffreys, 2011). There is an ebb and flow to the intense feelings that a death or significant loss stimulates in those who remain. Awareness of the loss creates recurring, wave-like feelings of memories and sadness. People describe it as "feeling unexpectedly punched in the gut." Intense feelings are particularly inclined to surface when the griever is alone, for example, while driving. Certain situations, holidays, and anniversaries, particularly during the first few years, make feelings of grief more poignant.

Case Example

"I would think I was doing okay, that I had a handle on my grief. Then without warning, a scent, a scene on television, an innocuous conversation would flip a switch in my mind, and I would be flooded with memories of my mother. My eyes would fill up with tears as my fragile composure dissolved. My grief lay right under the surface of my awareness and ambushed me at times and in places not of my choosing" (Anonymous).

Over time, grief feelings usually diminish in intensity, but there is no magic time frame. Grief over the loss of a child can be particularly pervasive, sometimes lasting a lifetime. Variables affecting the intensity and timeframe for the grieving process following a death include:

- "Cultural beliefs and rituals
- Nature of relationship with the deceased
- Previous losses
- Spiritual and religious background
- Support system available" (Keegan & Drick, 2011, p. 113).

As people work through their grief, they are more open to the spiritual continuance of a relationship with the deceased, occurring as cherished memories or supportive remembrances of "what the deceased person might say or do in the situation." These shared moments provide an affirming spiritual union with the deceased, and a personal knowing of self in relationship. They offer a unique legacy, which will continue to influence the behaviors of future generations.

John Thomas (2011) describes his sense of successfully making the journey through grief with a stronger sense of self. He states, "I want to be known as one who

- Is identified with life and love rather than loss and grief.
- Walks with the stride of renewal rather than the shuffle of grief.
- Still embraces life knowing that the pain of loss is intense.

- Has one foot planted firmly in this life and is developing an equally firm footing in the spiritual realm.
- Is confident about the future without needing a tangible GPS.
- Can be alone without being lonely.
- Faced grief head-on, and reached a deeper core of self, faith, and spirituality.
- Has much to give in many arenas living a life that honors my past, and shares the blessings derived from it …" (Thomas, 2011, pp. 202–203).

PATTERNS OF GRIEVING

Acute Grief

Acute grief occurs as "somatic distress that occurs in waves with feelings of tightness in the throat, shortness of breath, an empty feeling in the abdomen, a sense of heaviness and lack of muscular power, and intense mental pain" (Lindemann, 1994, p. 155). Acute grief is intense, and the emotional pain can be beyond imagination. It lasts a short time, and gradually subsides, as the bereaved person begins to re-engage in meaningful activities (Zisook et al., 2010).

Suicide survivors are at a disadvantage, made worse by their reluctance to discuss death details because of shame or perceived stigma. Survivors usually need more support; often they get less because people are uncomfortable about suicide or do not know how to talk about it with those most intimately involved (Harvard Women's Health Watch, 2009). Suicide survivor support groups can offer the specialized help that many survivors need after a suicide (Feigelman & Feigelman, 2008).

Anticipatory Grief

Anticipatory grief is an emotional response that occurs before the actual death around a family member with a degenerative or terminal disorder. A person thinking about his or her own death also can experience anticipatory grief. Grief symptoms are similar to those experienced after death but are often accompanied by colored by ambivalent feelings.

Case Example

Marge's husband, Albert, was diagnosed with Alzheimer disease 5 years ago. Albert is in a nursing home, unable to care for himself. Marge grieves the impending loss of Albert as her mate. At the same time, she would like a life of her own. Her "other feelings" of wishing it could all be over cause her to feel guilty. Simulation Exercise 21.2 helps you explore grief from a personal perspective.

SIMULATION EXERCISE 21.2   A Personal Grief Inventory

Purpose:
To provide a close examination of one's history with grief.

Procedure:
Complete each sentence and reflect on your answers:
The first significant experience with grief that I can remember in my life was _____.
The circumstances were _____.
My age was _____.
The feelings I had at the time were_____.
The thing I remember most about that experience was _____.
I coped with the loss by _____.
The primary sources of support during this period were _____.
What helped most was _____.
The most difficult death for me to face would be _____.

Adapted from Carson, V. B., & Arnold, E. N. (1996). *Mental health nursing: The nurse-patient journey* (p. 666). Philadelphia: WB Saunders.

Chronic Sorrow

Chronic sorrow is defined as "a normal grief response associated with an ongoing living loss that is permanent, progressive, recurring, and cyclic in nature" (Gordon, 2009, p. 115). Many parents of children with a physical, developmental, emotional, or chronic disorder experience chronic sorrow. Families need nurses to affirm their coping efforts and acknowledge the legitimacy of their sadness. Providing timely support for families when there is an exacerbation of symptoms can make the situation more manageable.

Complicated Grieving

Complicated grieving represents an intense expression of grief, which is significantly longer in duration and emotionally incapacitating. A history of depression, substance abuse, death of a parent or sibling during childhood, prolonged conflict or dependence on the deceased person, or a succession of deaths within a short period predispose a person to complicated grief. Statements such as "I never recovered from my son's death" or "I feel like my life ended when my husband died" can alert the nurse to potential complicated grief.

Complicated grief can also present as an absence of grief in situations where it would be expected, for example, a marine who displays no emotion over the deaths of war comrades. When deaths and important losses are not mourned, the feelings do not just disappear; they reappear in unexpected ways sometimes years later. Simulation Exercise 21.3 provides a personal opportunity to reflect on the relevance of memories in significant relationships.

DEVELOPING AN EVIDENCE-BASED PRACTICE This qualitative descriptive study was designed to explore family perceptions of nursing strategies, which are helpful to them when a family at high risk for dying is in the ICU. A purposive sample of family members with a family member at high risk for dying were asked to identify specific strategies nurses used to support their decision making.

Results: Study narratives identified four nursing approaches as being helpful: Demonstrating concern, demonstrating professionalism, providing factual information, and supporting their decision-making. These strategies helped them to have more confidence in their decision-making skills, and to better prepare for and accept the impending death of their relative.

Implications for Clinical Practice: Knowledge of therapeutic approaches important to family members and most likely to improve their ability to make decisions and their well-being in EOL care lays a foundation for choosing therapeutic interventions.

From Adams, J., Anderson, R., Docherty, S., Tulsky, J., Steinhauser, K., & Bailey, D. (2014). Nursing strategies to support family members of ICU patients at high risk of dying. *Heart Lung, 43*(5), 406–415.

APPLICATIONS

Palliative Care: Nursing Care at the End of Life
Structure and Process of Palliative Care

Palliative care is patient-centered care, with an emphasis on care of patients with diagnosed, progressive, life-limiting health conditions (Sawatzky, 2016). Palliative care emphasizes supports rather than curative actions, with comfort measures increasing and curative activities diminishing as the patient prepares for the EOL. Treatment goals progress from disease control to maintaining a good quality of life, comfort, and pain and other symptom control. Care directives may have to be revisited, especially if there is a change in prognosis and the potential for quality of life diminishes significantly (Guido, 2010).

Palliative care is unique in that it considers care for the patient *and* the family as a single integrated care unit.

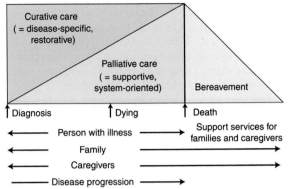

Fig. 21.1 Model of Curative and Palliative Care for Progressive Illness.

From World Health Organization. (2008). *WHO Definition of Palliative Care.* Retrieved from http://www.who.int/cancer/palliative/definition/en/. Accessed February 28, 2009.

> **BOX 21.1   Dimensions of Palliative Care**
>
> - Provides relief from pain and other distressing symptoms
> - Affirms life and regards dying as a normal process
> - Intends neither to hasten nor postpone death
> - Integrates the psychological and spiritual aspects of patient care
> - Offers a support system to help patients live as actively as possible until death
> - Offers a support system to help the family cope during the patient's illness and in their own bereavement
> - Uses a team approach to address the needs of patients and their families, including bereavement counseling if indicated
> - Will enhance quality of life, and may also positively influence the course of illness
> - Is applicable early in the course of illness, in conjunction with other therapies that are intended to prolong life such as chemotherapy or radiation therapy, and includes those investigations needed to better understand and manage distressing clinical complications

As a patient's life-limiting condition progresses, palliative care supports "living while dying" as comfortably as is possible as displayed in Fig. 21.1. Symptom management for the patient and practical support for the family as they negotiate the last stage of life becomes the priority. Unlike hospice, patients admitted to palliative care services can still receive active treatment for their disease process to control symptoms and improve quality of life (McIlfatrick, 2007). Primary dimensions of palliative care identified by the World Health Organization (WHO) are presented in Box 21.1.

The overarching goal of palliative care is to help patients improve function and quality of life, regardless of stage of disease or the presence of other treatments, and to prevent or relieve suffering (Kogan, Cheng, Rao, DeMocker, & Nelson, 2017). Palliative care strategies are designed to help critically ill patients and their families understand the dying process as a part of life, and to maximize a patient's quality-of-life options in the time left to them.

The basic axiom for palliative care is to follow what patients want for themselves (Silveira & Schneider, 2004). After a patient's death, palliative care offers bereavement support for family members.

Nursing Initiatives: End-of-Life Care

Nurses have been at the forefront of developing guidelines for quality EOL care for many years, beginning with the original work of Dame Cicely Saunders, Florence Wald, and others. In 2006, the National Consensus Project for Palliative Care was established to develop standards and guidelines for quality palliative care.

Nationally recognized nursing experts, funded by the American Association of Colleges of Nursing (AACN) and the City of Hope, developed the End-of-Life Nursing Education Consortium (ELNEC), a national education initiative to improve EOL care in the United States. To date, over 17,500 nurses and other health professionals have received training through these national courses (AACN, 2014). Specific EOL training allows nurses to teach others and to enter into the lives of many more people facing EOL as skilled, compassionate professionals with specialized care tools (Malloy, Paice, Virani, Ferrell, & Bednash, 2008).

Palliative Care Team Approaches

Palliative care is a team effort, designed to "assess and manage patients' and families' care needs across physical, psychological, social, spiritual, and information domains" Bruera and Yennarajalingam (2012, p. 268). An *interdisciplinary palliative care team* usually consists of nurses, physicians, social workers, and clergy specially trained in palliative care. Patients are enrolled in palliative care, which operates as a 24-hour resource, providing comprehensive, holistic services to patients and families in hospitals, people's homes, nursing homes, and community settings. The therapeutic focus in palliative care is on patient comfort, pain control, management of physical symptoms, and easing the psychosocial and spiritual distress experienced by families and patients as they come to terms with coping with a life-limiting illness. In addition to practical, spiritual, and supportive care for patients and families, team members provide education and consultation about EOL care for hospital staff. Palliative comfort care can be used concurrently with disease-modifying treatment. The level of comfort care increases according to patient need (Savory & Marco, 2009).

Nurses play a pivotal role as professional coordinators, direct providers of care, and advocates for patient autonomy, dignity, and control in EOL care. They are in a key position to help the family maintain its integrity, to support their efforts in managing the process of living while dying, and in preparing families for the death of their loved one. The palliative care model is displayed in Fig. 21.1.

Pain assessment. Pain is a complex phenomenon with sensory, emotional, cognitive, and behavioral dimensions (Wilkie & Ezenwa, 2012). Pain is a subjective experience, assessed verbally with the patient and/or observed in patient behavior (see Fig. 21.2). This tool can be used with children, aged 3 and older, for pain assessment only. Nurses perform screenings for pain, focused on:

- Onset and duration of pain
- Location of the pain
- Character of the pain (sharp, dull, burning, persistent, changes with movement, direct or referred pain)
- Intensity—using a 0 to 10 numerical rating scale, with 0 being no pain and 10 being unbearable pain (use the Wong–Baker FACES Pain Rating Scale for children and people with limited health literacy)
- History of substance dependence (needed to determine potential crossover tolerance)
- Aggravating factors such as difficulty breathing or turning
- Relief factors such as distraction with visitors, food or fluids, reassurance

Small children usually cannot meaningfully measure their pain level. Instead, look for behavioral indicators of pain in children such as abrupt changes in activity, crying, inability to be consoled, listlessness or unwillingness to move, rubbing a body part, wincing, or facial grimacing (Atkinson, Chesters, & Heinz, 2009). The same is true for patients with cognitive slippage related to delirium, dementia, or changes in consciousness. Behavior changes, particularly when associated with agitation, can indicate pain in cognitively impaired patients. Observation of behavioral distress indicators is particularly important with older adults.

Estimates of older adults having significant pain range from upwards of 40%. Some are able to evaluate their pain, using the suggestions above, but those with even mild cognitive changes may not be able to do so accurately when stressed.

Chronic pain related to cancer, diabetic neuropathy, osteoporosis, or arthritis may not readily respond to pain medication. Guido (2010) maintains that pain in older patients can be undertreated because it is assumed that they cannot tolerate strong pain medications, or that their pain is due to chronic, persistent conditions which will not be as responsive. Misperceptions about addiction and medication strength can result in inadequate pain management for children and mentally ill patients.

Patients needing palliative care often experience moderate to severe levels of pain. Having appropriate pain control for moderate-to-severe pain usually requires the use of opioids. Misperceptions about pain-relieving opioids are a major, unnecessary barrier to adequate pain control. According to Pashby (Pashby, N., (Expert Hospice Nurse), personal communication, Odenton, MD, March 2014) nurses need to educate patients and families about pain control, including the differences between pain associated with disease progression and adverse effects related to opioids. For example, some patients do not want to take opioids for fear of "feeling loopy" or not being able to think clearly.

A second barrier is fear of addiction (Clary & Lawson, 2009). All patients, including addicts, are entitled to appropriate and adequate pain management of severe pain. People do not become addicted from taking legally prescribed opioid medications for pain associated with terminal illness. There is a fundamental difference between taking essential medication for pain control on a prescribed scheduled basis, and addictive use. Addicted patients

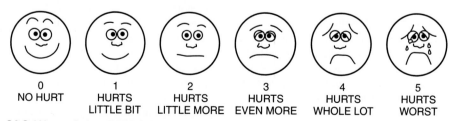

Fig. 21.2 Wong–Baker FACES Pain Rating Scale. (From Used with permission, Wong-Baker Foundation (2016). www.WongBakerFaces.org. Originally published in *Whaley & Wong's Nursing Care of Infants and Children.* Copyright, Elsevier.)

may require larger doses of pain medication because of cross-tolerance. Other barriers include a belief that suffering should be tolerated (stoicism) or is an unavoidable part of the dying process. Limited capacity to accurately describe pain intensity, or seeing pain as a weakness, also represent obstacles.

Families sometimes attribute signs and symptoms of approaching death—such as increased lethargy, confusion, and declining appetite—to side effects of opioids. This is not usually true. With or without pain medication, actively dying patients become less responsive as death approaches. Although patients may experience drowsiness with initial dosing, this side effect quickly disappears. Once patients and families understand the mechanisms and goals of pain control and are assured that the patient will not die or become addicted from appropriate pain control, most will support its use in palliative care. Patients approaching death can experience "breakthrough" pain, which occurs episodically as severe pain spikes. When breakthrough pain occurs, rescue medications, which are faster acting, can be used. Touch and light massage are helpful adjuncts for pain relief. *The bottom line is that no patient should suffer from preventable pain.*

KEY ISSUES AND APPROACHES IN END-OF-LIFE CARE

Self-Awareness

Self-awareness is a critical foundation for effective palliative nursing practice. Nurses must be aware of their personal feelings about death and previous EOL experiences, including attitudes, expectations, and feelings about death and the process of dying. Nurses are not immune to fears of being alone at time of death, or of feeling stress when helping patients cope with unrelenting pain. You may find it difficult to maintain a balance between your own sensitivity to a patient's death and providing the empathy and support needed by patients and families. Self-awareness about death and dying issues is critical in palliative care.

As the body begins to shut down in preparation for imminent death, the gold standard for EOL care is to restrict nutritional support (Kim & Seo, 2016). However, a teaspoon of ice chips and mouth care can be a comfort measure. Patient preferences often change over time. Care directives often must be revisited, especially if there is a change in prognosis and the potential for quality of life diminishes significantly (Guido, 2010).

Supporting End-of-Life Decision Making

Thelan (2005) defines **EOL decision making** as "the process that health care providers, patients, and patients'

families go through when considering what treatments will or will not be used to treat a life-threatening illness" (p. 29). Patients and families face difficult, irreversible decisions in the last phase of life. Preference decisions related to discontinuation of fluids, antibiotics, blood transfusions, and ventilator support require a clear understanding of a complex care situation. These are emotional issues with adaptive components for families. Much more than simple clinical explanation is needed (Adams, Bailey, Anderson, & Galanos, 2013). Families need support in meeting the adaptive challenges EOL decisions present, which cannot be resolved with technical intervention or clear-cut solutions. Box 21.2 presents principles guiding decisions about EOL care.

EOL decisions should be transparent, meaning that all parties involved in the decision should fully understand the implications of their decision. For example, to make an informed decision about use of life supports for terminal patients, patients and families need to know whether further treatments will enhance or diminish quality of life, their potential impact on life expectancy, and whether the treatment is known to be effective or is an investigative treatment.

BOX 21.2 Principles Guiding End-of-Life Care Decision Making

- Discussions of medical futility with patients and family will be more effective if they include concrete information about treatment, its likelihood of success, and the implications of the intervention and nonintervention decisions.
- Effective decision making at the end of life can be improved with the use of advance directives and surrogate decision makers.
- Ethnic and cultural traditions and practices influence the use of advance directives and health care decision-making surrogates.
- Taking the time to explore the patient's perceptions about quality of life at the end of life is a core component of clinical assessment and is essential to ensuring optimal outcomes.
- The cost of failing to offer patients and families a full range of end-of-life care options, services, and settings is incalculable in terms of quality of life and utilization of appropriate health care resources at the end of life.

Modified from Bookbinder, M., Rutledge, D. N., Donaldson, N. E., Bennett, C., & Brown, D. S. (2001). End-of-life care series: Part I: principles. *Online Journal of Clinical Innovations, 4*(4), 1–30, with permission. © 2001, Cinahl Information Systems.

Family members need to understand the potential implications of choosing one option over another. Making unrealistic hypothetical choices without carefully considering the longer-term potential impact on quality of life and financial considerations helps no one. For example, keeping a patient in a permanent unconscious condition alive on a ventilator can be harmful to the patient—and family. This and other futile "curative" treatments can cause needless pain and physical symptoms. Additionally, they can create noteworthy quality-of-life issues, health cost issues, and unnecessary anxiety for patients and families.

Ethical and Legal Issues

Families and patients must consider a number of legal issues as patients approach the EOL. Below is information about the legal protections patients need related to finances and choices about medical care.

Advance Directives

In 1990, the *Patient Self-Determination Act* was passed into law. This law requires that adult patients be given information about advance directives. Advance directives are written instructions detailing a "process by which patient, together with their families and health care practitioners, consider their values and goals and articulate preferences for future care" (Tulsky, 2005, p. 360).

Advance directives specify a person's right to participate in and direct personal health care decisions, including do not resuscitate (DNR) directives. This information should be documented and made available for review by caregivers directly involved in the patient's care. An advance directive is not permanently binding; if the patient chooses to later revoke the document, the patient can do so. Timing is important. Advance directives completed too far in advance or too close to death may not truly reflect patient goals or preferences (Billings & Bernacki, 2014).

The nurse's role is to provide the patient with full information about risks and benefits of prolonging life and to serve as patient advocate in support of the person's right to make decisions about treatment and care (American Nurses Association [ANA], 1991; Erlen, 2005). When patients are decisionally competent, they should be key decision makers. If a patient is not competent, or is unable to articulate his/her wishes, a responsible family member or significant person can be designated to legally assume the responsibility of surrogate spokesperson. Here, the conversation can start with asking the family "what would this patient prefer under the circumstances if the patient was able to speak for himself?" (Adams et al., 2013).

Family Conferences

Getting everyone's input is important as a source of information, explanation, and support for the patient. Formal family meetings held with the palliative care team provide an essential opportunity for providing the same information to all involved family members at the same time, thereby ensuring full disclosure with opportunities to ask questions.

Much more than simple clinical explanation is needed. Families need supportive information about meeting the adaptive challenges that EOL decisions present as they usually present with limited palatable options (Adams et al., 2013). If an essential family member cannot be physically present, having that person available by phone may be the next best option. What is helpful in many situations is to have one family person identified as the point of contact for follow-up issues.

Durable Power of Attorney for Health Care

Competent adults can choose to appoint a surrogate decision maker (durable power of attorney for health care) in the event that they cannot make important health decisions on their own behalf. This designation includes the surrogate's authority to accept or refuse treatment on the patient's behalf.

Some patients have neither power of attorney for health nor advance directives. Box 21.3 provides guidelines for talking with families about care options at EOL when an advance directive or durable power of attorney is not in effect.

Pain Assessment and Management

Pain assessment and management control is an essential component of quality palliative care. The American Pain Society (APS), Joint Commission, and Veterans Administration identify pain as the fifth vital sign to be assessed with standard vital signs (temperature, pulse, respiration, and blood pressure). Standards for pain management established by the Joint Commission (2010) require that every inpatient be routinely assessed for pain, with documentation of appropriate monitoring and pain management.

Communication in End-of-Life Care

Curtis (2004) suggests that communication skill is equal to or supersedes clinical skill in EOL care. Everyone experiences a death differently; it is the uniqueness of each person's experience that the nurse attempts to tap into and facilitate discussion of through conversation (Mok & Chiu, 2004). Conversations with patients and families provide nurses with insights about personal values and preferences regarding EOL care and provide a forum to

BOX 21.3 Talking With Families About Care Options

If neither durable power of attorney nor written directive is in effect, nurses can facilitate the process by helping to:

- Determine who should be approached to make the decisions about care options.
- Determine whether any key members are absent. (Try to keep those who know the patient best in the center of decision making.)
- Find a quiet place to meet where each family member can be seated comfortably.
- Sit down and establish rapport with each person present. Ask about the relationship each person has with the patient and how each person feels about the patient's current condition.
- Try to achieve a consensus about the patient's clinical situation, especially prognosis.
- Provide a professional observation about the patient's status and expected quality of life—survival vs. quality of life. Ask what each person thinks the patient would want.
- Should the family choose comfort measures only, assure the family of the attention to patient comfort and dignity that will occur.
- Seek verbal confirmation of understanding and agreement.
- Attention to the family's emotional responses is appropriate and appreciated.

Adapted from Lang, F., & Quill, T. (2004). Making decisions with families at the end of life. *American Family Physician, 70*(4), 720.

answer difficult questions in a supportive environment. There is some evidence that if clinicians discuss patient preferences, and if they are documented, they are more likely to be fulfilled (Cox, Moghaddam, Almack, Pollock, & Seymour, 2011).

The quality of the relationship between nurse, patient, and family members is a key factor contributing to creating an environment to support a good death (Mok & Chiu, 2004). EOL interactions help people find meaning, achieve emotional closure, and provide the best means for helping patients and families make complex life decisions. Understanding patient and family *perceptions* of their EOL experience is essential to developing a patient centered approach to palliative care interventions.

Schim and Raspa (2007) believe that the process of dying is a narrative: "Life-altering happenings are expressed

through stories" (p. 202). Personal reflections are critical sources of assessment data. Once rapport is established, Pashby (2015) suggests nurses can ask patients how they learned of their diagnosis. She notes that a terminal diagnosis is usually a "Technicolor Moment" that the person remembers vividly and appreciates talking about. Other questions such as "What has changed for you since the diagnosis?" or "What is it like for you now?" provide additional data. Giving voice to the experience helps patients to consider its personal meaning and provides the nurse with a more complete picture of each person's distinctive concerns and goals.

Most patients know intuitively when their time is getting shorter, but the exact time frame may not be apparent until very close to death. It is not unusual for a patient to ask in the course of conversation, "Am I going to die?" or "How much longer do you think I have?" Before answering, find out more about the origin of the question. A useful listening response is, "What is your sense of it?" Box 21.4 provides guidelines for communicating with palliative care patients.

Morgan (2001) identifies a protective coping and adjustment response that nurses can use with palliative care patients. This is a two part intervention, which involves nursing conversations that 1. protect, maintain and support individual patient integrity, and 2. Explore the patient's preferences and values in end of life care.

Communicating With Families

Family members have different levels of readiness to engage in discussions about the dying process. It is "normal" for an impending death to have a different impact on each family member, because each has had a unique relationship with the dying person. Conversations with families need not be long in duration, but regularity is important.

Common concerns include discontinuing life support; conflicts among family members about care; tensions between the patient, family, and/or physician and family about treatment; where death should occur (home, hospital, hospice); and if/when hospice should be engaged. The clear goal of palliative care is to improve the quality of life of patients through the management of their symptoms, whether medical, emotional, spiritual, or psychosocial" (Fox, 2014, p. 40).

Creating Family Memories

Patients and families need to talk about things other than the disease process and treatments. Nurses can help make this happen. There are spiritual stories, cultural stories, funny stories, developmental stories, narratives of advocacy, and family stories. Each reinforces the

SIMULATION EXERCISE 21.3 Reflections on Memory Making in Significant Relationships

Purpose:

To provide students with an opportunity to see the value of memory making as a strategy for facilitating the grieving process.

Procedure:

1. Write a letter to someone who has died or is no longer in your life. Before writing the letter, reflect on the meaning this person had for you and the person you have become.
2. In the letter, tell the person what they meant to you and why it is that you miss them.
3. Tell the person what you remember most about your relationship.
4. Tell the person anything you wished you had said but didn't when the person was in your life.

   With a partner, each student should share his or her story without interruption. When the student finishes his or her story, the listener can ask questions for further understanding.

Discussion:

1. What was it like to write a letter to someone who had meaning in your life and is no longer available to you?
2. Were there any common themes?
3. In what ways was each story unique?
4. How could you use this exercise in your care of patients who are grieving?

BOX 21.4 Guidelines for Communicating With Patients

- Avoid automatic responses and trite reassurances.
- Each death is a unique, deeply personal experience for the patient and should be treated as such.
- Avoid destroying hope. Reframe hope to what can happen in the here and now.
- Let the patient lead the discussion about the future. Be comfortable with focusing on the here and now. (This discussion is not a one-time event; openings for discussion should be encouraged as the patient's condition worsens.)
- Relate on a human level. Show humor as well as sorrow.
- Use your mind, eyes, and ears to hear what is said, as well as what is not said.
- Respect the individual's pattern of communication and ways of dealing with stress. Support the patient's desire for control of his or her life to whatever extent is possible.
- Maintain a sense of calm. Use eye contact, touch, and comfort measures to communicate.
- Do not force the patient to talk. Respect the patient's need for privacy, be sensitive to the patient's readiness to talk, and let him or her know that you will be available to listen.
- Humility and honesty are essential. Be willing to admit when you do not know the answer.
- Be willing to allow the patient to see some of your fears and vulnerabilities. It is much easier to open up to someone who is "human and vulnerable" than to someone who appears to have all the answers.

bonds and affirms the depth of meaning a family holds with a dying person. The moments of laughter, foibles, and shared experiences are connections that need to be remembered.

Case Example

Evelyn was an 83-year-old woman diagnosed with terminal lung cancer. During a guided imagery exercise, the nurse asked her to recall a time when she felt relaxed and happy. Evelyn described in vivid detail being with her family at a picnic near a lake many years ago. When her family came to visit that night, Evelyn related the story again, and the entire family talked about their parts in the remembered event. It was one of their last conversations, one that reinforced family bonds in the initial telling and later as her family remembered Evelyn after her death. Later, her daughter made a special point of letting the nurse know how important sharing this story was to the patient and family.

Providing Information

Nurses are key informants about patient status and changes in the patient's condition. There are fundamental differences in the level of information an individual or family will desire. The response of the patient should determine the content and pace of sharing information. Talking with families about care details and potential outcomes should happen often, but even more frequently when the patient's health status begins to decline or show a change.

Ideally, one nurse serves as the primary contact for the patient and family and acts as a liaison between providers and patients. This nurse keeps other health team members informed of new issues and shares their input into planning and evaluation of care with the family. Using precise language, giving full and truthful information about the patient's condition, and admitting to uncertainty, when it exists, are important dimensions of EOL information giving.

Family Conferences

Family conferences are effective tools to alleviate family anxiety about the dying process, reduce unnecessary conflict between family members, and assist family members with important decision-making processes. Gavrin (2007) notes, "the analog of informed consent is informed refusal" (p. S86). This concept becomes important to patients and families as a component of decision making related to withdrawing or withholding life support in EOL care. Although a physician commonly leads the discussion, nurses often present data and answer questions. Data sharing should be compassionate, accurate, and presented in language understandable to the family (Ambuel & Weissman, 2005).

Contradictory recommendations and incomplete information add to a family's confusion and cause unnecessary distress (Wright et al., 2009). A coordinated approach prevents fragmentary and inconsistent care.

Curtis (2004) recommends that there be a higher ratio of family member-to-health care provider speaking time, with follow-up communication. Helping patients and families understand the importance of advance directives and DNR orders can prevent later conflicts when tensions arise near the time of death (Boyle, Miller, & Forbes-Thompson, 2005). Nurses are invaluable resources in clarifying meanings with patients or individual family members after the conference.

ADDRESSING CULTURAL AND SPIRITUAL NEEDS

Incorporating Cultural Differences

Different cultures have distinctive communication and care standards for patients with life-threatening conditions (Searight & Gafford, 2005). Box 21.5 presents cross-cultural variations found in palliative and EOL care.

Cultural distinctions focus on (a) type of care that provides comfort to the dying person; (b) understanding of the causes of illness and death; (c) appropriate care of the body and burial rites; and (d) expression of grief responses (Doolen & York, 2007; LaVera et al., 2002).

Asking patients/families directly about their cultural values and issues as a starting point helps ensure cultural safety for patients and families. Chovan, Cluxton, and Rancour (2015) note, "The transition from life to death is as sacred as the transition experienced at birth" (p. 49). The dying process, grief, and death itself herald a spiritual crisis—a crisis of faith, hope, and meaning for many people.

BOX 21.5   Cross-Cultural Variations in End-of-Life Care

- Emphasis on autonomy vs. collectivism
- Attitudes toward advance directives
- Decision making about life support, code status guidelines
- Preference for direct vs. indirect disclosure of information
- Individual vs. family-based decision making about treatment
- Disclosure of life-threatening diagnoses
- Provider's choice of words in verbal exchanges
- Reliance on physician as the ultimate authority
- Specific rituals or practices performed at time of death
- Role of religion and spirituality in coping and afterlife
- Views about suffering

Adapted from Searight, H., & Gafford, J. (2005). Cultural diversity at the end of life: Issues and guidelines for family physicians. *American Family Physician, 71*(3), 515–522.

Spiritual pain occurs when a person's sense of purpose is challenged or one's existence is threatened (Millspaugh, 2005). For many cultures, spirituality is significantly embedded in a person's culture, and many cultures have special rituals at EOL. A simple question such as "Can you tell me about how your family/culture/spiritual beliefs views serious illness or treatment?" provides a framework for discussion. When cultural differences are considered, it is important to avoid stereotyping, as each person's interpretation of their culture is unique. Once cultural needs are identified, every effort should be taken to honor their meaning to patients and families by incorporating them in care (see Chapter 7).

Attending to Spiritual Needs

Spirituality becomes a priority for many people at EOL (Williams, 2006). It is not unusual for patients who have previously declined spiritual interventions to desire them as they move into the final phase of life. Spiritual beliefs and religious rituals provide a tangible vehicle for individuals and families to express and experience meaning and purpose. Religious practices and rituals relevant to EOL can be important to patients even if the person no longer formally practices the religion. Facilitating these practices touches the patient's inner core and helps the person move toward a peaceful death (Bryson, 2004).

Most people welcome an inquiry about their spiritual well-being (Morrison & Meier, 2004). To elicit more information about its nature, an appropriate question is: "Is there anything I should know about your spiritual or religious views?" The answer can tell you what is important related to their current circumstances. Steinhauser et al. (2006) suggest using the probe "Are you at peace?" as a useful way to initiate a conversation about spiritual concerns without being intrusive. Nurses can ask the patient and/or family if they would like a visit from an appropriate clergy or hospital chaplain.

Not all people attach their concept of spirituality to a particular belief system. Instead, they define their spirituality from an existential perspective. Attig (2001) describes this sense of spirituality as follows:

> That within us that reaches beyond present circumstances, soars in extraordinary experiences, strives for excellence and a better life, struggles to overcome adversity, and searches for meaning and transcendent understanding. (p. 37)

When individuals frame their spirituality from an existential perspective, it is appropriate to explore spirituality sources in terms of meaningful relationships. Asking a question such as "Can you tell me about the relationship you had with someone whom you loved who has died?" helps start the conversation. A follow-up question relates to how the patient feels about the person now. The value of this intervention is that it emphasizes that the person's life held meaning for this other person. This line of questioning indirectly tells the person that they too will be remembered after death (Pashby, 2015).

People benefit from telling stories about how they view their life, and to validate its meaning. A life review helps people consider the deeper values and purpose of their lives, the experience of joy and sorrow. As one person stated, "I lived my life as best I could. I have no regrets." A follow-up listening response to help the person put into words what he or she reflect on the meaning of a life well lived might be: "Tell me more about this."

Clary and Lawson (2009) suggest that the EOL offers a final opportunity for people to experience spiritual growth. The most important intervention nurses can provide is to actively and respectfully listen to each patient's search for clarity about their spirituality with compassion and a desire to understand. Helping patients think through spiritual preferences and assisting them in identifying resources that can give them strength, courage, purpose, and encouragement to cope with their situation is highly valued. Providing explicit attention to inclusion of appropriate spiritual advisors, prayer, and scripture reading can be helpful to faith-based patients and families coping with a terminal condition.

Spiritual issues that (Baird, 2010) trouble patients relate to forgiveness, unresolved guilt issues, expressions of love, saying good-bye to important people, and existential questions about the meaning of life, the hereafter, and concern for their family. Nurses need to take an honest look at their own spirituality. Self-awareness allows nurses to enter their patient's spiritual world from an authentic position, without imposing personal values and beliefs.

PALLIATIVE CARE FOR CHILDREN

It is not the natural order of things for a child to die. People are supposed to live into adulthood. When a child is diagnosed with a life-limiting condition, the effect on parents is devastating; it influences role functioning, friendships, and treatment of siblings (Hinds, Schum, Baker, & Wolfe, 2005). Children are such an integral part of their parents' identity that issues of parental protectiveness, guilt, responsible caregiving, balancing family demands, and helplessness parents feel should be part of the discussion. In addition to providing appropriate symptom management medications to make the child more comfortable, the following interventions are supportive to children with a life-limiting illness.

1. Encourage visits from family and friends.
2. Involve and inform the child of everything that is going on, with developmentally appropriate language and content.
3. Encourage the family to keep the child's life as normal as possible.
4. Suggest ways to enhance family functioning with attention paid to making special time for siblings and involving them in care discussions.
5. Arrange respite for parents and encourage special parent times.
6. Encourage families to maintain or adapt cultural, family, and religious traditions.
7. Encourage families to seek emotional support: support groups, extended family, friends (Field & Behrman, 2002).

Parents are a major anchoring force for children. They need to be recognized as the expert and a primary advocate for their child. Here are some ways that nurses can help. Take the time to explore with the parents how they conceptualize quality of life for their child, and what is important for the nurse to know about the child's preferences. Nurses can identify situations in which there is a mismatch between a child's condition and a parent's understanding of that condition (Field

& Behrman, 2002). This is important information that needs to be shared with the palliative care team. By observing the child you can begin to note preferences. Children also value being asked about likes and dislikes. There should be no surprises. You need to talk with the child and the parents about each procedure in language they can understand. Giving a child a sense that you and the parents are on the same page provides security and comfort. Critical to parent satisfaction is the knowledge that everything possible was done for their child; that they received accurate, timely information and support; and that preventable suffering was not permitted.

Grief Issues

Children grieve within the context of the family, but they do not grieve in the same ways. Nurses can help parents talk with their children about the impending death of a significant person in their lives. Encourage parents to explain what is happening in a concrete, direct way using clear, concrete language suitable to the child's developmental level. Questions should be answered directly and honestly at the child's developmental level of comprehension, free of medical jargon. This type of discussion should *not* be a one-time event, and parents may need to be proactive in initiating the conversation.

Sometimes a family will want to exclude young children from contact with or knowledge about a person who is likely to die soon. Sometimes it is a judgment call as to whether visitation is a good idea. Drawing a picture or sending a note card is another way for a child to connect with a critically ill relative if visitation is not an option. With preparation, adolescents can benefit from being allowed to visit with terminal patients.

Case Example
Brendan and his grandfather had a close relationship. Earlier in life, they would stroke each other's thumbs as part of a "special handshake." Now, at 15, his grandfather was close to death and unresponsive. As Brendan sat next to him, stroking his thumb in the remembered way, he felt sure that his grandfather had squeezed his hand more than once. It was a weak squeeze, but it was a meaningful connection for Brendan.

Death of a significant person is difficult for children because they have neither the cognitive development nor the life experiences to fully process its meaning. A child younger than 5 years has no clear concept of what death means.

Until children reach the formal operations stage of cognitive development, they can have fantasies about the circumstances surrounding the death and their part in it.

How a Child Grieves

Children do not express their grief in the same way adults do. Unpredictable acting-out behaviors, withdrawal, anger, fear, and crying are common responses. One minute the child may be playing, the next he is angry or withdrawn. Preschoolers may repeatedly ask when someone close to them will be coming home even if parents tell them that person has died. Developmentally, they do not understand the permanence of death. Elementary school children accept the permanence of death but view it in a concrete manner.

Case Example
A short time after 5-year-old Aidan's grandfather died, he asked his grandmother where his grandfather had gone. She told him that grandpa died and was in heaven, to which Aidan said, "Oh no, grandma, he's in that brown box in the ground."

The National Cancer Institutes of Health (2010) identifies common concerns children may have about the death of someone important to them:
1. Did I cause the death to happen?
2. Is it going to happen to me?
3. Who is going to take care of me?

Parents can *create* opportunities for children to ask these questions. Asking the child about potential concerns can elicit a conversation that will not happen otherwise.

Maintaining daily routines in the child's life after the death of a parent or primary caregiver is critical. Children need to know that they are safe and will be taken care of by the remaining adults in their life. If changes are needed, children should have the opportunity to discuss the reasons for them and time to absorb this information if at all possible.

Adolescents are particularly vulnerable to unresolved grief. They are often expected to act grown up and model the grieving process for younger siblings. It is unfair to have this expectation. Adults expect adolescents to grieve a death more as an adult than as a child, but they lack the life experience to do so.

Sometimes adolescents will not openly ask questions because they do not want to interfere with parental grief. They may not know how to frame important questions, or they are not sure of the reaction. Any or all of these feelings are normal. Nurses can help parents to gently and proactively offer lead-ins to relevant concerns. Even if the child cannot respond at the moment, having an adult reach out can be very meaningful to a child or adolescent.

At the other extreme, the remaining parent may be unable to fully connect with a child's grief because their own grief is overwhelming. Expectations that an adolescent will step up to the plate and perform household or childcare are common. Without a place to talk about their feelings, an adolescent may bury feelings that are necessary to process for healing. Adolescents need physical contact, reassurance, and many relevant discussions about the person who has died. If parents are unable to provide the level of communication an adolescent needs, nurses can help them with appropriate referrals.

ACHIEVING QUALITY CARE AT END-OF-LIFE

Death is a deeply personal experience. The Institute of Medicine (2014) defines a **good death** as "one that is free from unavoidable distress and suffering for patients, families, and caregivers; in general accord with patients' and families' wishes; and reasonably consistent with clinical, cultural, and ethical standards" (p. 82). Pain and symptom relief, transparent decision making, preparation for death, affirmation of the whole person, and the sense of contributing to others are identified in other research (Steinhauser et al., 2000). In the example below, a nurse helps a terminally ill patient achieve a sense of spiritual completion.

Case Example

George was in the last stages of his end-of-life journey. He had repeatedly refused to have spiritual visits and had no desire for the sacrament of the living (a religious rite in the Catholic church). His nurse said the priest was on the floor at the hospital and asked him if he would like to receive communion. He answered, "Yes, but nothing else." The priest gave him communion, after which the patient asked him to hear his confession and requested the last rites. This would not have happened without the collaborative efforts of this nurse's advocacy. After the priest left, George told his nurse, "You always seem to know what to do, and when to do it; thank you."

Simulation Exercise 21.4 provides you with the opportunity to personally think about what constitutes a good death.

SIMULATION EXERCISE 21.4   What Makes for a Good Death?

Purpose:
To help students focus on defining the characteristics of a good death.

Procedure:
1. In pairs or small groups, think about, write down, and then share briefly examples of a "good" and a "not-so-good" death that you have witnessed in your personal life or clinical setting.
2. What were the elements that you thought contributed to its being a "good" or "not-so-good" death?

Discussion:
Were there any common themes found in the stories as to what constitutes a "good" death? How could you use the findings of this exercise in helping patients achieve a "good" death?

What to Expect: Anticipatory Guidance

Dying is a normal life process and most family members feel privileged to be present. But, as death approaches, communication becomes more challenging. Anticipatory guidance and nursing presence become important interventions. Family members look to the nurse for information about the dying process, and for emotional support (Wittenberg-Lyles, Goldsmith, Ferrell, & Ragan, 2013). Unsupported, the process of watching someone die can be a frightening experience for the family.

Family members appreciate anticipatory guidance about what is happening and what to expect, with concrete suggestions about ways to connect with their loved one. With some patients, the dying process is swift. With others, there is gradual downward spiral. Common symptoms include long periods of sleeping or coma, decreased urinary output (dark urine), changes in vital signs, disorientation, restlessness and agitation, dyspnea (breathlessness), cheyne stokes breathing, picking at bed clothes, plus skin temperature, and color changes. All of these changes are normal findings as a person prepares to leave this world. Dying patients experience profound weakness such that they cannot independently complete even basic hygiene.

You can help family members understand that as death approaches, there are significant changes in the patient's capacity to connect with others or to participate in conversation. Physically touching the patient can be comforting as can holding the person's hand.

Most patients will stop eating as death approaches (Reid, McKenna, Fitsimons, & McCance, 2009). This is a natural

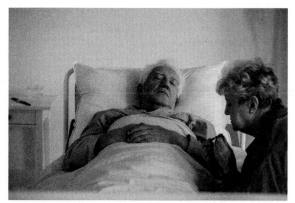

Fig. 21.3 Nurses can facilitate meaningful family "presence" at life's ending, even when verbal communication is limited. (Copyright © KatarzynaBialasiewicz/iStock/Thinkstock.)

part of the body's effort to shut down; it is important to not force food. Giving very small amounts of ice chips or using glycerin mouth swabs can keep the patient comfortable. The extremities may become colder to touch and appear mottled. This also is normal. Oxygen can help with breathing and usually is available even in home settings if the patient has hospice care. Patient comfort should be the number one consideration. The American Cancer Society web site provides an excellent description of typical changes in the patient when death is near and offers a clear outline of what caregivers can do to provide comfort to the patient.

A nurse's calming *presence* is perhaps the most important form of communication and emotional support for dying patients *and* families (Fig. 21.3). Most patients cannot carry on an in-depth conversation as death approaches. Flexibility in allowing family and/or significant others open access to the patient can reduce family anxiety and can be comforting for all concerned. At the same time, as patients approach death it becomes an effort for the patient to respond to family and friends. Telling the family that it is their presence that matters and to use gentle touch or simple words without expecting much verbal communication in return is a helpful intervention, Box 21.6 identifies family communication needs when death is imminent.

Case Example

"I remember standing next to my mom's bed. We had gone to her room to pay our last respects. A young nurse stood near to me and reached out gently and touched my shoulder. Softly she said, 'I'll just stay here with you in case you need something.' When I looked at her I saw eyes brimming with tears and a profound sadness on her face. Her presence meant so much; I was grateful for her open expression of sorrow. It confirmed the pain we were all experiencing" (Anonymous).

BOX 21.6 Imminent Death: Family Communication Needs

- Honest and complete answers to questions; repetition and further explanation if needed
- Updates about the patient's condition and changes as they occur
- Clear, understandable explanations delivered with empathy and respect
- Frequent opportunities to express concerns and feelings in a supportive, unhurried environment
- Information about what to expect—physical, emotional, spiritual—as death approaches
- Discussion of whom to call, legal issues, memorial or funeral planning
- Conversation about cultural and/or religious rituals at time of and after death
- Appreciation of the conflicts that families experience when the illness dictates that few options exist; for example, a frequent dilemma at end of life is whether life support measures are extending life or prolonging the dying phase
- Short private times to be present and/or minister to the patient
- Permission to leave the dying patient for short periods with the knowledge that the nurse will contact the family member if there is a change in status

Family members often find it difficult to leave a dying patient, even when it would be in their best interest to take a short respite. Assuring family members that the nurse will check on the patient frequently and will call the family immediately if change occurs gives families permission to take a brief respite from the patient's bedside.

Caring for the Patient After Death

Respect for the dignity of the patient continues after death. If the family is present at time of death, allowing uninterrupted private time with the patient before initiating postmortem care is important. If the family is not present, all excess equipment and trash should be removed from the room. You can offer presence and emotional support as you escort the family into the room. Some families will want privacy; others will appreciate having the presence of the nurse or chaplain. Family preference should be honored.

The tone of the room and the positioning of the patient should "give a sense of peace for the family" (Marthaler, 2005, p. 217). Provide soft lighting, chairs for the family, and tissues. The patient's head should be elevated at a 30-degree angle, in a natural position. Hair should be combed, exposed body parts cleaned, and dentures replaced if possible. It is important for the nurse to allow the family as much time as they need with the patient. The nurse can obtain signatures to release the patient to the funeral home *after* the family has spent some time with the patient.

STRESS ISSUES FOR NURSES IN PALLIATIVE CARE SETTINGS

Nurses become invested in the care and comfort of patients and families facing immediate death; it is an emotional time for everyone involved. **Disenfranchised grieving** is a term applied to the grief nurses can experience after the death of a significant patient (Brosche, 2007). Unlike their patients, who live through one loss at a time, nurses can experience several losses a week while caring for terminally ill patients and their families (Brunelli, 2005).

Nurses can experience **compassion fatigue**, a syndrome associated with serious spiritual, physical, and emotional depletion related to caring for patients that can affect the nurse's ability to care for other patients (Worley, 2005). Unrelieved compassion fatigue can result in burnout and a nurse's decision to leave nursing.

Case Example

Barbara was a new graduate, selected as a nursing intern on a research oncology unit, providing care for seriously ill pediatric oncology patients. She had a de-

gree in another field and an excellent job, but always wanted to pursue nursing. Her original preceptor left the hospital and was replaced by an efficient nurse without much empathy. The stress of weekly deaths, severe symptomatology, and lack of empathetic support led Barbara to leave nursing entirely after less than a year. She returned to her former position.

Developing Self Compassion

All nurses, but particularly those working on high intensity units, need to actively pursue ways to experience self-compassion. Self-compassion encourages nurses to balance care for others with care for self. Reflecting on the meaning of connections with dying patients and becoming aware not only of your personal strengths but also your limitations are essential forms of the self-awareness needed for self-compassion. Regular self-reflection allows you to know yourself and gives you more options in relating to patients, families, and other members of the health care team (Wittenberg-Lyles et al., 2013). Support groups for nurses in which they can successfully address and resolve the secondary stress of continuously caring for terminally ill patients and some of the ethical issues involved with that care are helpful to nurses. See also the strategies presented in Chapter 16 related to burnout prevention.

SUMMARY

This chapter describes the stages of death and dying, and theory frameworks of Eric Lindeman and George Engel for understanding grief and grieving. Palliative care is discussed as a philosophy of care and an emerging discipline focused on making EOL care a quality life experience. A good death is defined as a peaceful death experienced with dignity and respect; one that wholly honors the patient's values and wishes at the EOL. Nurses can offer compassionate communication, presence, and anticipatory guidance to ease the grief of loss.

Nursing strategies are designed to help patients cope with the secondary psychological and spiritual aspects of having a terminal illness such that they achieve the best quality of life in the time left to them. Talking with patients

about advance directives is a professional responsibility of the nurse, and it reduces unnecessary conflict among family members at this critical time in a person's life. Talking with children about terminal illness or death of a relative or in coping with a terminal diagnosis themselves should take into consideration the child's developmental level. Questions should be answered honestly and empathetically.

As death approaches, nurses can help families understand the physiological changes signaling the body's natural shutdown of systems. Providing support for clinicians is considered a quality indicator in EOL care. When not addressed, the disenfranchised grief that nurses experience with providing EOL care to multiple patients can lead to compassion fatigue, burnout, and moral distress.

ETHICAL DILEMMA: What Would You Do?

Francis Dillon has been on a ventilator for the past 3 weeks. He is not decisionally competent, and he is not able to communicate. Although he has virtually no chance of recovery, his family refuses to take him off the ventilator because "there is always the chance that he might wake up." What do you see as the ethical issues, and how would you, as the nurse, address this problem?

REVIEW QUESTIONS

1. What is meant by the statement, "There is potential for healing and meaning even in the face of impending death"?
2. Describe your most challenging EOL experience. How did you cope with it?
3. What does the concept "quality of life" mean in EOL care?
4. How do you care for yourself when working with seriously ill patients and what would you recommend to avoid burnout?

REFERENCES

Adams, J., Bailey, D., Anderson, R., & Galanos, A. (2013). Adaptive leadership: A novel approach for family decision making. *Journal of Palliative Medicine, 16*(3), 326–329.

Ambuel, B., & Weissman, D. E. (2005). Moderating an end-of-life family conference. In *Fast Facts and Concepts* (2nd ed.). Retrieved from: http://www.eperc.mcw.edu/EPERC/Fast-FactsIndex/ff_016.htm.

American Academy of Hospice and Palliative Medicine: www.aahpm.org.

American Association of Colleges of Nursing (AACN). (2014). *End-of-Life Nursing Education Consortium (ELNEC) fact sheet.* Washington, DC: Author. Retrieved from: http://www.aacn.nche.edu/ELNEC/about.htm.

American Nurses Association (ANA). (1991). *ANA position statements: Nursing and the patient self-determination acts.* ANA Nursing World. Retrieved from: www.nursingworld.org/readroom/position/ethics/etsdet.html.

Atkinson, P., Chesters, A., & Heinz, P. (2009). Pain management and sedation for children in the emergency department. *British Medical Journal, 339*, b4234.

Attig, T. (2001). Relearning the world: Making and finding meanings. In R. Neimeyer (Ed.), *Meaning reconstruction and the experience of loss* (pp. 33–53). Washington, DC: American Psychological Association.

Attig, T. (2004). Meanings of death seen through the lens of grieving. *Death Studies, 28*, 341–360.

Baird, P. (2010). Spiritual care interventions. In B. R. Ferrell, & N. Coyle (Eds.), *Oxford textbook of palliative nursing* (3rd ed.) (pp. 663–671). New York: Oxford University Press.

Barclay, L., & Lie, D. (2007). New guidelines issued for family support in patient-centered ICU. *Critical Care Medicine, 37*, 605–622.

Billings, J. A., & Bernacki, R. (2014). Strategic targeting of advance care planning interventions: The goldilocks phenomenon. *JAMA Internal Medicine, 174*(4), 620–624.

Boyle, D., Miller, P., & Forbes-Thompson, S. (2005). Communication and end-of-life care in the intensive care unit. *Critical Care Nursing Quarterly, 28*(4), 302–316.

Brosche, T. (2007). A grief team within a healthcare system. *Dimensions of Critical Care Nursing, 26*(1), 21–28.

Bruera, E., & Yennurajalingam, S. (2012). Palliative care in advanced cancer patients: How and when? *The Oncologist, 17*, 267–273.

Brunelli, T. (2005). A concept analysis: The grieving process for nurses. *Nursing Forum, 40*(4), 123–128.

Bryson, K. A. (2004). Spirituality, meaning, and transcendence. *Palliative & Supportive Care, 2*(3), 321–328.

Chovan, J., Cluxton, D., & Rancour, P. (2015). Principles of patient and family assessment. In B. Ferrell, & N. Coyle (Eds.), *Textbook of palliative nursing* (4th ed.). New York: Oxford University Press.

Clary, P., & Lawson, P. (2009). Pharmacologic pearls for end of life care. *American Family Physician, 79*(12), 1059–1065.

Corless, I. (2001). Bereavement. In B. Ferrell, & N. Coyle (Eds.), *Textbook of palliative nursing* (pp. 352–362). New York: Oxford University Press.

Cox, K., Moghaddam, N., Almack, K., Pollock, K., & Seymour, J. (2011). Is it recorded in the notes? Documentation of end-of-life care and preferred place to die discussions in the final weeks of life. *BMC Palliative Care, 10*(18), 1–9.

Crawley, L., Marshall, P., Lo, B., Koenig, B., & End-of-Life Care Consensus Panel. (2002). Strategies for culturally effective end of life care. *Annals of Internal Medicine, 136*(9), 673–677.

Curtis, J. R. (2004). Communicating about end-of-life care with patients and families in the intensive care unit. *Critical Care Clinics, 20*, 363–380.

Doolen, J., & York, N. (2007). Cultural differences with end of life care in the critical care unit. *Dimensions of Critical Care Nursing, 26*(5), 194–198.

Engel, G. (1964). Grief and grieving. *American Journal of Nursing, 64*(7), 93–96.

Erlen, J. (2005). When patients and families disagree. *Orthopaedic Nursing, 24*(4), 279–282.

Feigelman, B., & Feigelman, W. (2008). Surviving after suicide loss: The healing potential of suicide survivor support groups. *Illness, Crisis and Loss, 16*(4), 285–304.

Field, M., & Behrman, R. (2002). *When children die: Improving palliative and end of life care for children and their families.* Washington, DC: The National Academies Press.

Florczak, K. (2008). The persistent yet everchanging nature of grieving a loss. *Nursing Science Quarterly, 21*(1), 7–11.

Fox, M. (2014). Improving communication with patients and families in the intensive care unit: Palliative care strategies for the intensive care unit nurse. *Journal of Hospice & Palliative Nursing, 16*(2), 93–98.

Gavrin, J. (2007). Ethical considerations at the end of life in the intensive care unit. *Critical Care Medicine, 35*(2), S85–S94.

Gordon, J. (2009). An evidence-based approach for supporting parents experiencing chronic sorrow. *Pediatric Nursing, 35*(20), 115–119.

Guido, G. (2010). *Nursing care at the end of life.* Upper Saddle River, NJ: Pearson.

Harvard Women's Health Watch. (2009). *Left behind after suicide.* Retrieved from: www.health.harvard.edu.

Hinds, P., Schum, L., Baker, J., & Wolfe, J. (2005). Key factors affecting dying children and their families. *Journal of Palliative Medicine, 8*(Suppl. 1), S70–S78.

Institute of Medicine. (2014). *Dying in America: Improving quality and honoring individual preferences near the end of life.* Washington, DC: National Academy Press.

Jeffreys, J. (2011). *Helping grieving people—When tears are not enough: A handbook for care providers* (2nd ed.). New York: Brunner-Routledge.

Joint Commission. (2010). *The approaches to pain management: An essential guide for clinical leaders* (2nd ed.). Oakbrook Terrace, IL: Joint Commission Resources.

Keegan, L., & Drick, C. (2011). *End of life: Nursing solutions for death with dignity.* New York: Springer.

Kim, S., & Seo, M. (2016). Description of good patient care at end of life. *Applied Nursing Research, 32,* 245–246.

Kogan, M., Cheng, S., Rao, S., DeMocker, S., & Nelson, M. (2017). Integrative medicine for geriatric and palliative care. *Medical Clinics of North America, 101,* 1005–1029.

Kübler-Ross, E. (1969). *On death and dying: What the dying have to teach doctors, nurses, clergy, and their own families.* New York: Scribner.

Lang, F., & Quill, T. (2004). Making decisions with families at the end of life. *American Family Physician, 70*(4), 719–723.

LaVera M, Marshall, P, Lo B, Koenig B. (2002). End of life care consensus panel. Strategies for culturally effective end of life care. *Annals of Internal Medicine, 36*(9), 673–679.

Lendrum, S., & Syme, G. (1992). *Gift of tears: A practice approach to loss and bereavement counseling.* London: Routledge.

Lindemann, E. (1994). Symptomatology and management of acute grief. *The American Journal of Psychiatry, 151*(Suppl. 6), 155–160 (Originally published in 1944.).

Malloy, P., Paice, J., Virani, R., Ferrell, B. R., & Bednash, G. P. (2008). End-of life-nursing education consortium: 5 years of educating graduate nursing faculty in excellent palliative care. *Journal of Professional Nursing, 24*(6), 352–357.

Mark, T. (2002). *Mark Twain quotations, newspaper collections, & related resources.* Retrieved from: www.twainquotes.com.

Marthaler, M. T. (2005). End of life care: Practical tips. *Dimensions of Critical Care Nursing, 24*(5), 215–218.

McIlfatrick, S. (2007). Assessing palliative care needs: Views of patients, informal careers and healthcare professionals. *Journal of Advanced Nursing, 57*(1), 77–86.

Mercer, D., & Evans, J. (2006). The impact of multiple losses on the grieving process: An exploratory study. *Journal of Loss and Trauma, 11,* 219–227.

Millspaugh, D. (2005). Assessment and response to spiritual pain: Part I. *Journal of Palliative Medicine, 8*(5), 919–923.

Mok, E., & Chiu, P. (2004). Nurse-patient relationships in palliative care. *Journal of Advanced Nursing, 48*(5), 475–483.

Morgan, A. (2001). A grounded theory of nurse-patient interactions in palliative care nursing. *Journal of Clinical Nursing, 10*(4), 583–584.

Morrison, S., & Meier, D. (2004). Palliative care. *The New England Journal of Medicine, 350,* 2582–2590.

National Cancer Institutes of Health. (2010). *Children and grief.* Retrieved from: http://www.cancer.gov/cancertopics/pdq/supportivecare/bereavement/Patient/page9.

Neimeyer, R. A. (Ed.). (2001). *Meaning reconstruction and the experience of loss.* Washington, DC: American Psychological Association.

Pashby, N. (2015). *Expert hospice nurse.* Bethesda, MD.

Reid, J., McKenna, H., Fitsimons, D., & McCance, T. (2009). Fighting over food: Patient and family understanding of cancer cachexia. *Oncology Nursing Forum, 36*(4), 439–445.

Rushton, C. H., Reder, E., Hall, B., Comello, K., Sellers, D. E., & Hutton, N. (2006). Interdisciplinary interventions to improve pediatric palliative care and reduce health care professional suffering. *Journal of Palliative Medicine, 9,* 922–933.

Savory, E., & Marco, C. (2009). End of life issues in the acute and critically ill patient. *Scandinavian Journal of Trauma, Resuscitation and Emergency Medicine, 17,* 21.

Sawatzky, R. (2016). Conceptual foundations of a palliative approach: a knowledge synthesis. *BMC Palliative Care, 15:* 5.

Schim, S., & Raspa, R. (2007). Cross disciplinary boundaries in end-of-life education. *Journal of Professional Nursing, 23*(4), 201–207.

Searight, H., & Gafford, J. (2005). Cultural diversity at the end of life: Issues and guidelines for family physicians. *American Family Physician, 71*(3), 515–522.

Silveira, M., & Schneider, C. (2004). Common sense and compassion: Planning for the end of life. *Clinics in Family Practice, 6*(2), 349–368.

Steinhauser, K. E., Clipp, E., McNeilly, M., Christakis, N. A., McIntyre, L. M., & Tulsky, J. A. (2000). In search of a good death: Observations of patients, families, and providers. *Annals of Internal Medicine, 132*(10), 825–832.

Steinhauser, K. E., Voils, C., Clipp, E., Bosworth, H. B., Christakis, N. A., & Tulsky, J. A. (2006). Are you at peace? One item to probe spiritual concerns at the end of life. *Archives of Internal Medicine, 166*(1), 101–105.

Thelan, M. (2005). End of life decision making in intensive care. *Critical Care Nurse, 25*(6), 28–37.

Thomas, J. (2011). *My saints alive: Reflections on a journey of love, loss and life.* Charlottesville, VA: CreateSpace Independent Publishing Platform.

Tulsky, J. (2005). Beyond advance directives: The importance of communication skills at the end of life. *JAMA, 293*(3), 359–365.

Wilkie, D., & Ezenwa, M. (2012). Pain and symptom management in palliative care and at end of life. *Nursing Outlook, 60*(6), 357–364.

Williams, A. L. (2006). Perspectives on spirituality at the end of life: A meta-summary. *Palliative & Supportive Care, 4,* 407–417.

Wittenberg-Lyles, E., Goldsmith, J., Ferrell, B., & Ragan, S. (2013). *Communication in palliative nursing.* New York: Oxford University Press.

Worley, C. A. (2005). The art of caring: Compassion fatigue (from the editor). *Dermatology Nursing, 17*(6), 416.

Wright, B., Aldridge, J., Wurr, K., Sloper, T., Tomlinson, H., & Miller, M. (2009). Clinical dilemmas in children with life-limiting illnesses: Decision making and the law. *Palliative Medicine, 23,* 238–247.

Zisook, S., Simon, N., Reynolds, C., Pies, R., Lebowitz, B., Young, I. T., et al. (2010). Bereavement, complicated grief and DSM. *The Journal of Clinical Psychiatry, 71*(8), 1097–1098.

SUGGESTED READING

Block, S. (2006). Psychological issues in end of life care. *Journal of Palliative Medicine, 9*(3), 751–772.

Brajtman, S. (2005). Helping the family through the experience of terminal restlessness. *Journal of Hospice & Palliative Nursing, 7,* 73–81.

Bruera, E., & Yennurajalingam, S. (2011). *Oxford American handbook of hospice and palliative medicine.* New York: Oxford University Press.

Bulow, H., Sprung, C., Reinhart, K., Prayag, S., Du, B., Armaganidis, A., et al. (2008). The world's major religions' points of view on end-of-life decisions in the intensive care unit. *Intensive Care Medicine, 34,* 423–430.

Dahlin, C. (2010). Communication in palliative care: An essential competency for nurses. In B. R. Ferrell, & N. Coyle (Eds.), *Oxford textbook of palliative nursing* (3rd ed.) (pp. 663–671). New York: Oxford University Press.

Davies, B., Contro, N., Larson, J., & Widger, K. (2010). Culturally sensitive information sharing in pediatric palliative care. *Pediatrics, 4,* e859–e865.

Hui, D., De La Cruz, M., Mori, M., Parsons, H. A., Kwon, J. H., Torres-Vigil, I., et al. (2013). Concepts and definitions for "supportive care", "palliative care" and "hospice care" in the published literature, dictionaries, and textbooks. *Supportive Care in Cancer, 21*(3), 659–685.

Jevon, P. (2010). *Caring of the dying and deceased patient: A practical guide for nurses.* Oxford UK: Wiley-Blackwell.

LaPorte Matzo, M., & Witt-Sherman, D. (Eds.). (2006). *Palliative care nursing: Quality care to the end of life* (2nd ed.) New York: Springer.

Loomis, B. (2009). End of life issues: Difficult decisions and dealing with grief. *Nursing Clinics of North America, 44,* 223–231.

Marr, L. (2009). Can compassion fatigue? *Journal of Palliative Medicine, 12*(8), 739–740.

Miller, J. (2001). *The art of being a healing presence.* Ft. Wayne, IN: Willowgreen Publishing.

Moules, N., Simonson, K., Fleizer, A., Prins, M., & Glasgow, B. (2007). The soul of sorrow work: Grief and therapeutic interventions with families. *Journal of Family Nursing, 13*(1), 117–141.

Mularski, R., Curtis, J., Billings, A., Burt, R., Byock, I., Fuhrman, C., et al. (2006). Proposed quality measures for palliative care in the critically ill: A consensus from the Robert Wood Johnson Foundation Critical Care Workgroup. *Critical Care Medicine, 34,* S404–S411.

National Cancer Institutes of Health. (2011). *Grief, bereavement, and coping with loss.* Bethesda, MD: Author. Retrieved from: http://cancer.gov/cancertopics/pdq/supportivecare/bereavement/HealthProfessional.

Neimeyer, R., Currier, J., Coleman, R., Tomer, A., & Samuel, E. (2011). Confronting suffering and death at the end of life: The impact of religiosity, psychosocial factors and life regret among hospice patients. *Death Studies, 35,* 777–800.

Noyes, J., Hastings, R., Lewis, M., Hain, R., Bennett, V., Hobson, L., et al. (2013). Planning ahead with children with life-limiting conditions and their families: Development, implementation and evaluation of "My Choices." *BMC Palliative Care, 12*(1), Article 5, 1–17.

Perrin, K., Sheehan, C., Potter, M., & Kazanowski, M. (2012). *Palliative care nursing: Caring for suffering patients.* Sudbury, MA: Jones and Bartlett Learning.

Puntillo, K., Nelson, J., Weissmann, D., & Curtis, R. (2013). Palliative care in the ICU: Relief of pain, dyspnea, and thirst—A report from the IPAAL—ICU Advisory board. *Intensive Care Medicine.*

Sherman, D. (2010). Culture and spirituality as domains of quality palliative care. In M. Matzo, & D. W. Sherman (Eds.), *Palliative care nursing: Quality care at the end of life* (pp. 3–38). New York: Springer.

Smith, R. (2000). A good death. *British Medical Journal, 320,* 129–130.

Thomas, J. (2010). *My saints alive: A journey of life, loss, and love.* Charlottesville, VA: Unpublished Manuscript.

Volker, D., & Limerick, M. (2007). What constitutes a dignified death? The voice of oncology advanced practice nurses. *Clinical Nurse Specialist, 21*(5), 241–247.

Walczak, A., Butow, P., Bu, S., & Clayton, J. (2016). A systematic review of evidence for end of life communication interventions: Who do they target, how are they structured and do they work? *Patient Education and Counseling, 99,* 3–16.

World Health Organization (WHO). (2016). *WHO definition of palliative care.* Geneva: WHO. Retrieved from: http://www.who.int/cancer/palliative/definition/en/.

ADDITIONAL WEB RESOURCES

Center to Advance Palliative Care: www.capc.org.
Canadian Virtual Hospice: www.virtualhospice.ca.
Children's Hospice Palliative Care Coalition: www.chpcc.org.
Hospice and Palliative Nurses Association: www.hpna.org.
National Hospice and Palliative Care Organization: www.nhpco.org.

22

Role Relationship Communication Within Nursing

Kathleen Underman Boggs

OBJECTIVES

At the end of the chapter, the reader will be able to:

1. Discuss professional role relationships among nurses in health care.
2. Distinguish among the professional nursing role opportunities.
3. Describe the components of professional role socialization in nursing.
4. Construct a model of safe, supportive work environments you would work in.
5. Discuss the advocacy role in nurse-patient relationships.
6. Apply evidence-based role research to clinical practice situations.

Chapter 22 presents an overview of role relationships within professional nursing and their implications for professional communication, education, and practice. Being clear about your professional role is essential for meaningful functional relationships with others. Empirical evidence shows effective communication among members of the team reduces the potential for error and the consequences of error, aiding us in providing safe care (Amodo, Baker, Emery, & Hines, 2017). Applications address the process of professional nursing socialization, role development, mentorship, and communication with supervisors, peers, and nursing assistant personnel. Leadership competencies are discussed. Chapter 23 will address communication in interdisciplinary teams.

BASIC CONCEPTS

Role

Role is a multidimensional psychosocial concept defined as a traditional pattern of behavior and self-expression, performed by or expected of an individual within a given society. People develop social, work, and professional roles throughout life. Some roles are conferred at birth (ascribed roles), and some are attained through circumstance during a lifetime (acquired roles). Personal ascribed role performance standards reflect social, cultural, gender, and family expectations.

Clinical practice blends your knowledge, skills, and attitudes with patient care. Professional and work relationships have distinctive expectations for your role participation as a member of the organization. These expectations influence communication content and style of presentation (MacArthur, Dailey, & Vilagran, 2016). Work relationships have tangible and intangible structural elements that define communication. For example, nurses will communicate differently with their peers, supervisor, those they supervise, and their patients. Institutional norms also have an effect on the enactment of professional roles and vary according to the work environment. The ability to accurately interpret and negotiate role relationships in a work setting helps nurses to communicate more effectively.

BOX 22.1   Flexner's Criteria

- Members share a common identity, values, attitudes, and behaviors.
- A distinctive specialized substantial body of knowledge exists.
- Education is extensive, with both theory and practice components.
- Unique service contributions are made to society.
- Acceptance of personal responsibility in discharging services to the public.
- Governance and autonomy over policies that govern activities of profession members.
- A code of ethics that members acknowledge and incorporate in their actions.

Professionalism and Work Environment

Criteria that are characteristic of a "2" were initially developed by Flexner more than a century ago (1915). Box 22.1 offers an adaptation of these criteria. A nurse's professional relationships and work environment play a big part in satisfaction. Job dissatisfaction contributes to high turnover rates at a time when there is a worldwide nursing shortage (World Health Organization [WHO], 2010). Even in developed countries, new graduates leave their jobs and even the profession in high numbers. Job attrition is cited as running between 15% and greater than 60% in various countries, as cited by numerous articles (Phillips, Esterma, & Kenny, 2015; Shatto, Meyer, & Delicath, 2016). Could creating a supportive work place with open communication and respect promote better retention?

Professionalism in Nursing

Professional nurses comprise the largest professional group of health care providers. They spend more sustained professional time with patients and families than any other hospital care professional. Nursing roles have steadily evolved to include current expectations for nurses to assume leadership roles, to provide primary care, and to act as first-line providers in implementing health care reform initiatives.

Professional Nursing Roles

Direct patient care nurses are expected to exhibit competent care skills and also show competency in their communication skills. Contemporary professional nursing roles reflect the increasing complexities of health care, globalization, changing patient demographic characteristics and diversity, and the exponential growth of health information technology.

The bedside nurses' role consists of delivery and organization of care for multiple patients. This role includes quality control issues, problem solving, patient education, and coordination of communication among the many health team members (McKenna, Brooks, & Vanderheide, 2017). There is a strengthened focus on health promotion/disease prevention, and self-management of chronic disorders also echoes new economic realities and provider availability. Fig. 22.1 identifies the core professional **role competencies** required of contemporary nurses, identified by the Institute of Medicine (IOM, 2003; 2011). To deliver high-quality, safe, patient-centered care, the focus is on collaboration (Farrell, Payne, & Heye, 2015), a hallmark of role competence. We need to know our own role so we can work together smoothly. Read the Saretha case for an example of patient-centered care.

Case Example: Saretha

As a community nurse you make a home visit to Ms. Saretha, who has diabetes and multiple health issues. She lives in a trailer park in a remote area with no transportation. Her primary physician reports she does not follow the American Diabetic Association diet he prescribed. You discover that her only source of food is a fast food place on a nearby highway. After initial lack of success trying to locate alternative food supplies, you decide to adapt to this patient's lifestyle resources and, using the fast food menu, help her to select healthier, low fat foods from what is available to her.

Courtesy Connie Bowler, DNP, RN, Lakeland Community College, 2017.

The scope of practice for professional nurses continues to expand to include reimbursable health screening and promotion, risk reduction, and disease prevention strategies. Nurses increasingly provide care as part of interdisciplinary health care teams in hospitals and the community. All nurses are expected to advocate for health care transformation and to take a leadership role in addressing environmental, social, and economic determinants of health. Nurses are assuming public advocacy roles to inform policy makers, educators, and other health care providers about health-related issues. Nurses also provide leadership and coordination in health care improvement through education and participation in research. Simulation Exercise 22.1 is designed to help you look at the different role responsibilities of practicing nurses.

Technology

Competency in use of technology is a QSEN goal. Technology permits swift transactions, universal access, and levels of portability unanticipated 20 years ago. Defining aspects of caring and patient communication are supported, not led, by technology. Nurses are more responsible than ever to devise communication strategies that preserve the caring aspects of nursing. Chapter 25 and 26 provide in-depth discussions of communication and technology use issues.

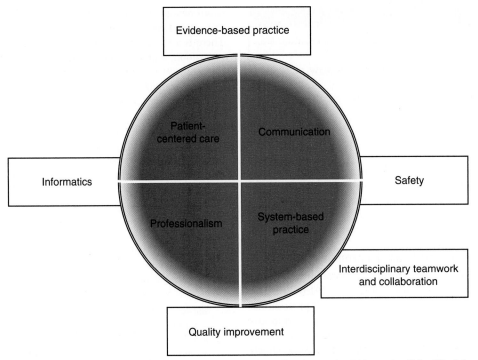

Fig. 22.1 Professional Nursing Role: Core Competencies for Health Professionals. (Modified from Institute of Medicine (IOM). (2003). *Health professions education: A bridge to quality* (pp. 45–46). Washington, DC: National Academies Press.)

Leadership

Hesburgh's (1971) description of leadership, and its relationship to caring, still holds true: The mystique of leadership, be it educational, political, religious, commercial or whatever, is next to impossible to describe, but wherever it exists, morale flourishes, people pull together toward common goals, spirits soar, order is maintained, not as an end in itself, but as a means to move forward together. Such leadership always has a moral as well as intellectual dimension; it requires courage as well as wisdom; it does not simply know, it cares (p. 764).

Role Clarity

Professional role clarity is an essential quality for working with health care teams. If nurses are not clear about their professional roles, it is difficult for them to communicate their value as health care providers to other professionals. Yet, a 2017 study found new graduates still lack knowledge about their role (McKenna, 2017). Role clarity about professional competencies is necessary to support patient safety initiatives that lead to improved client outcomes. Influencing change and making difficult decisions become easier when nurses have a clear vision of their professional role, because they are better able to stimulate confidence in others.

Competency

Competency is defined as "a set of capabilities, skills, aptitude, and experience" (Rick, 2014). In addition to development of technical nursing skills, technology, and communication skills, collaborative skills are needed to become a positive force in team-based health care.

New Differentiated Practice Roles

The IOM (2011) mandate to increase the number of professional nurses in advanced practice roles makes a strong statement in health care reform. An empowering aspect of the nurse role is the opportunity to evolve roles, change specialties of care, move into advanced roles, or take on new administrative roles. Nurses must put forth the value of nurses as skilled health care providers. Evolved scope of practice and professional standards serve as the foundation for practice accountability and decision authority in contemporary nursing practice.

Advanced Practice Nurses

An advanced practice nurse (APRN) is a licensed skilled practitioner holding a minimum of a master's degree in a clinical specialty, with the expert knowledge base, complex decision-making skills, and clinical competencies required

SIMULATION EXERCISE 22.1
Professional Nursing Roles

Procedure:

Ask a nurse whom you admire if you can have a 20-minute interview related to his or her role development as a registered nurse in clinical practice.

Ask the following questions:

1. What are the different responsibilities involved in his or her job?
2. What training and credentials are required for the nurse's position?
3. What is the type of patient population encountered?
4. What are the most difficult and rewarding aspects of the job?
5. Why did the nurse choose a particular area or role in nursing?
6. What opportunities does the nurse see for the future of nursing?
7. You are also encouraged to create your own explorative questions.

Discussion

1. Describe any surprises you had during the interview.
2. Compare similarities and differences in the results of your interview with your classmates.
3. Create a scenario implementing what you have learned in a future professional experience.

for expanded specialty practice. Box 22.1 identifies the four core categories of advanced practice nursing found in contemporary health care. Various countries have established many roles for Advanced Practice Nurses (APNs), including Nurse Practitioners, Clinical Nurse Specialists, Certified Nurse Midwives, Nurse Anesthetists, etc. Specialized training allows APRNs to diagnose and independently manage care, including prescriptive authority for some. In addition to clinical roles, APRNs function in research, educational, and administrative roles. A significant issue yet to be completely resolved is a lack of consistency that has lessened but still exists surrounding role responsibilities and scope of practice of APRNs.

The Clinical Nurse Leader

In response to the IOM (2001) report, the American Association of Colleges of Nursing (AACN) developed the clinical nurse leader (CNL) model as a Master's prepared generalist role to provide leadership at the bedside. The CNL's focus is on quality of care, bridging the gaps between members of the health team (AACN, 2003; Moore, Schmidt, & Howington, 2014). The CNL curriculum prepares students with a baccalaureate degree in another field

to become an advanced generalist nurse (Master's degree and eligibility for licensure as a registered nurse). Core competencies include clinical leadership skills, environmental management, and clinical outcome management (Bender, 2016). For CNLs to practice as an APRN in a specific *clinical specialty*, the CNL must complete further academic preparation.

The Doctor of Nursing Practice

In 2004 the AACN introduced the Doctor of Nursing Practice (DNP) as a *terminal practice* degree for professional nurses. The complexity of the nation's health care environment served as a major impetus for promoting transitions to practice doctorates, as did the need to position nursing professionally on a par with other major health professions, all of which offer practice-focused doctorates. The curriculum combines advanced nursing practice skill proficiency with a solid foundation in the clinical sciences, evidence-based practice methods, system leadership, information technology, health policy, and interdisciplinary collaboration (AACN, 2004).

The PhD-Prepared Nurse Researcher

Doctoral research degree programs in nursing have grown substantially in developed countries. These nurses are prepared to conduct original research, to be primary investigators seeking substantial grants, working not only in university settings but in many health care corporations.

Trends in education which develop communication skills

Experiential learning. Experiential learning is defined as active participation in learning scenarios, with self-reflection to analyze learning components. Contemporary health care education depends on experiential learning for developing both technical care skills and communication proficiency. Its competency-based goal is to provide students with the knowledge, skills, and attitudes needed to effectively collaborate and improve the quality of health care. Students use case study analyses, role play, exercise activities, computer simulations, standardized patient models, etc. The most vital part of the experiential learning process is the final activity of **reflection analysis** to recap what was learned and strategize about how to correct mistakes made.

Clinical Simulations

Problem-based learning scenarios provide innovative opportunities for students to analyze and find solutions in a safe, controlled environment. Clinical simulation is a preferred learning strategy because it allows interdisciplinary students to give close attention to all aspects of the clinical environment and to actively problem solve solutions from a collaborative team perspective. Students construct and develop "live" understanding of interdisciplinary health team functioning through shared reflection on their actions and interactions with each other in collectively meeting identified patient-centered goals.

Interdisciplinary Courses

Interdisciplinary education is defined as educational occasions when two or more professions learn from and about each other to improve collaboration and the quality of care. Introducing interdisciplinary coursework early in the curriculum helps students to understand nursing roles and communication across other professionals. It gives some insight into the "mind set" of other professionals and encourages a pattern of collaboration. Cultivating interdependence between health professionals required for quality care in an era of cost containment is noted as being critical to success in meeting national health goals (IOM, 2003). Students gain firsthand understanding of the professional values held by other disciplines. In clinical scenarios the decision-making process with team approaches is more complex than with single discipline methods, *acknowledging* and *respecting* the unique expected behaviors and skill sets of each health discipline fosters understanding. Frequent communication is essential to good results.

Examples of shared interdisciplinary electives include ethics, death and dying, culture, quality improvement (QI), genomics, emergency preparedness, gerontology, health policy, and legal issues. Clinical simulation courses open to students from multiple health disciplines provide unique opportunities for students in the health care professions to work together in the clinical management of complex disease health conditions.

Case Example

A multidisciplinary learning opportunity is being offered in collaboration with the University of Maryland and Montgomery County's Department of Health and Human Services involving nursing, pharmacy, and social work students. The students will be engaged in seeing patients and participating in collaborative discussions with faculty preceptorship related to their care at the Mercy Health Clinic. This outpatient clinic serves those without medical insurance and has a large culturally diverse clientele. The goals of the project are:

1. To expose students to interdisciplinary collaborative practice in a community setting with diverse client values and needs.
2. To enhance the quality of care for clients with complex medical, cross-cultural, and social issues through interdisciplinary collaboration

---

DEVELOPING AN EVIDENCE-BASED PRACTICE

The American Medical Association's seven communication techniques were applied to the role of Advanced Practice Nursing in rural clinics assessing dental health. Koo, Horowitz, Radice, Wang, and Kleinman (2016) used a Likert-scale instrument to survey 1410 Maryland APNs, reaping a 20% response rate.

Results: More than half of nurses reported using each of the seven communication techniques, and more than three-quarters of respondents believed these techniques to be effective in communicating with patients.

Communication Technique	Percent of Time Techniques Used by APN
Speaks slowly	80%
Uses simple words	95.5%
Limits teaching to 2 or 3 concepts	80%
Uses the "teach-back" method where patient repeats how they will do procedure, etc.	54%
Uses handouts of printed information	74%
Gives printed instructions	73.7%
Underlines key points on instruction sheet	56.7%

Application to Your Clinical Practice

Many of these communication techniques could be used in your patient teaching. In the teach-back method the nurse asks patients how they will follow the treatment instructions just taught. When they repeat back correctly, you have assessed their understanding of the material. If handing out written material and highlighting key points is an effective communication technique, why are we not doing so more often?

Koo, L. W., Horowitz, A. M., Radice, S. D., Wang, M. Q., Kleinman, D. V. (2016). Nurse practitioners' use of communication techniques: Results of the Maryland oral health literacy study. *PLoS ONE, 11*(1), e0146545.

APPLICATIONS

Professional Role Socialization

Professional role socialization is a complex, continuous, interactive educational process through which student nurses acquire the knowledge, skills, attitudes, norms, values, and behaviors associated with the nursing profession (de Swardt, van Rensburg, & Oosthuizen, 2017;

Strouse & Nickerson, 2016). Beginning nurses acquire their professional identity. Role identity is thought to mitigate the negative effects of stress, helping you avoid "burnout" (Sun, Gau, Yang, Zang, & Wang, 2016). Transmission of the cultural value system inherent in the nursing profession is seen as the key element in role socialization. For example, beginners learn that nurses value their patients and their autonomy (Thomas, Jenks, & Jack, 2015). Building on Lenninger's ideas (1991) about the culture of nursing, we identify the process of mastering the knowledge, skills, and attitudes on our role. Although we still need greater understanding of the transition process, we know role modeling by academics and especially by expert clinicians is vital (Baldwin, Mills, Birks, & Budden, 2014). Some say the clinical area is where we are really socialized (Thomas et al., 2015).

Acquiring the Profession's Culture

This involves internalizing the values, standards, and role behaviors associated with professional nursing. As students begin to try out new professional behaviors, they receive feedback and support for their efforts from clinical staff, faculty, and clients. Positive feedback empowers students by acknowledging their clinical judgments and encourages them to perform successfully.

Academic Role Models as Socializing Agents

Initially, nursing students are absorbed in learning basic knowledge and skills. They depend on textbooks, instructors, and simulation labs to help them. As students become comfortable with foundational nursing knowledge, they interact with clinical staff. With increased experience, students begin to trust their reasoning in making clinical judgments.

Clinical Nurses as Socializing Agents

Nursing faculty, clinical preceptors, and nursing mentors serve as important socializing agents, helping students learn the values, traditions, norms, and competencies of the nursing profession (Felstead & Springett, 2016).

Clinical Preceptors

In a formalized, goal-directed clinical orientation relationship, the clinical preceptor is an experienced nurse, chosen for clinical competence and charged with supporting, guiding, and participating in the evaluation of student or new graduate clinical competence on a one-to-one basis. Perhaps designated by employers or by virtue of being on a career ladder, clinical preceptors' model professional behaviors, give constructive feedback, and promote clinical thinking in the novice nurse or nursing student.

Mentors

Mentoring describes a commitment to help another nurse become the best professional they can be. Mentors are expert nurses who act as advisors for less experienced nurses, generally over a long time period. They can be a sounding board for career option discussions and for providing guidance in looking at the whole picture, while considering what will fit in with our personal responsibilities. *Every nurse should seek out a career mentor, someone whose experience can help to guide your career.*

Orientation

Accrediting agencies now recommend formal "residency" programs to orient and guide new graduate nurses, suggesting that to be effective, such programs need to be at least a year in length. Such programs combine some didactic instruction with clinical guidance by one or more preceptors. Expectations about profession communication skills and agency goals, rules and communication styles are imparted (MacArthur et al., 2016). The attitudes, actions, and directed support of the preceptor encourages students to adopt clinically appropriate professional behaviors. On the other hand, a clinical mentor who does not follow good communication strategies, such as the tools provided by the TeamSTEPPS program, can negate all that the mentored nurse has learned in the classroom (Amodo et al., 2017). In addition to clinical preceptors, other informal socializing agents include patients, families, and peers. They promote understanding of the professional nursing role from a consumer perspective.

Employment Transition

Employer socialization: professional skill acquisition and role development. Transitioning to a new role is always stressful, even for experienced nurses. Personality traits that include resilience and inquisitiveness aid this transition. The Bauer and Erdogan (2011) "socialization model" as well as organizational theories have been applied to understand what makes a nurse effectively transition from student to novice nurse to competent practitioner (Phillips et al., 2015).

Internationally, several authors developed models designed to describe the role transition process undergone by all new nurses during their first year of work (Benner, 2001; Duchscher, & Kramer, 2012; Schoessler & Waldo, 2006). In her classic work discussing the theory-practice gap and subsequent "reality shock," Benner describes five developmental stages of formative role development in professional nursing. Based on the *Dreyfus and Dreyfus model (1980)* of skill acquisition, each developmental stage demonstrates increasing proficiency in implementing the professional nursing role: novice, advanced beginner, competence, proficiency, and expert.

1. Novice. The first stage is referred to as the *novice stage.* Initially students have limited or no nursing experience to perform required nursing tasks. Novice

nurses need structure and exposure to the objective foundations upon which to base their nursing practice. They tend to compare clinical findings with the textbook picture because they lack the practice experience to do otherwise. Theoretical knowledge and confidence in the expertise of more practiced nurses and faculty serve as guides to practice. Schoessler and Waldo's model suggests that in the first 3 months of employment, the new graduate nurse struggles to develop organizational skills, master technical skills, and deal with coping with mistakes or the fear of making them.

2. Advanced *beginner*. In this stage, nurses understand the basic elements of practice and can organize and prioritize clinical tasks. Although clinical analysis of health care situations occurs at a higher level than strict association with the textbook picture, the advanced beginner is able to only partially grasp the unique complexity of each patient's situation. Preceptors can make a difference in helping new nurses cope with the uncertainty of new clinical situations and to hone their skills. They act as a "guide by the side" in helping new nurses gain nursing proficiency (Dracup & Bryan-Brown, 2004). The new nurse's patients are also an important resource. For example, patients can help us to develop a greater appreciation for the complexity of social, psychological, and physical aspects of chronic disease as a result of their interactions. By paying close attention to their patients, and what seems to work best, advanced beginner nurses learn the art of nursing. In the Schoessler and Waldo model, this time is referred to a "neutral zone," the phase in which communication with others, including physicians or patients, is still problematic, while feeling more comfortable with organization and knowledge. After the first year and before 18 months, the new nurse enters a "new beginning" phase of feeling comfortable with nursing activities.

3. *Competence*. This stage occurs 1 to 2 years into nursing practice. The competent nurse is able to easily manage the many contingencies of clinical nursing (Benner, 2001). Nurses begin to practice the "art" of nursing. They view the clinical picture from a broader perspective and are more confident about their roles in health care.

4. *Proficiency*. This stage occurs 3 to 5 years into practice. Nurses in this stage are self-confident about their clinical skills and perform them with competence, speed, and flexibility. The proficient nurse sees the clinical situation as a whole, has well-developed psychosocial skills, and knows from experience what needs to be modified in response to a given situation (Benner, 1984).

5. *Expert*. This last stage is marked with a high level of clinical skill and the capacity to respond authentically and creatively to patient needs and concerns. Expert nurses "have confidence in their own ability and rarely panic in the face of a breakdown" (Benner, 2001, p. 115). They can recognize the unexpected and work creatively with complex clinical situations. Expert nurses demonstrate mastery of technology, sensitivity in interpersonal relationships, and specialized nursing skills in all aspects of their care giving. Being an expert nurse is not an end point; nurses have the professional and ethical responsibility to continuously upgrade and refine their clinical skills through professional development and clinical skill training. Table 22.1 identifies behaviors associated with different levels of Benner's model.

Continuing Education

Professional development represents a lifelong commitment to excellence in nursing and requires regular upgrading of skills. As QSEN experts say "No patient wants a nurse who still practices only what she learned 10 years ago." Standard means of continued professional development include relevant continuing education presentations, staff development modules, conference attendance, academic education, specialized training, and research activities. Professional development also occurs through informal means such as consultation, professional reading, experiential learning, giving presentations, and self-directed learning activities such as internet-based modules. The Profession and Governmental Licensure Bureaus encourage and, in some areas, require nurses to annually complete a certain level of continuing education activities to maintain licensure or certification. These offer unique opportunities to access new information and to network, share expertise, and learn different perspectives from others in the field.

Strategic Career Planning

Serious career plans should reflect careful appraisal of values, skills, interests, and different career possibilities. Mentors can be helpful in this area.

Role Relationships within Nursing

It is inevitable that you will encounter some communication and collaboration problems with nurse colleagues. If managed appropriately, these difficulties can become opportunities for innovative solutions and improved relationships. A number of strategies discussed in Chapter 23 are useful in dealing with fellow nurses.

TABLE 22.1　Benner's Stages of Clinical Competence

Nurse Competency Level	Description of Behaviors
Advanced beginner	• Enters clinical situations with some apprehension • Sees task requirements as central to the clinical context, whereas other aspects of the situation are seen as background • Requires knowledge application to meet clinical realities • Perceives each clinical situation as a personal challenge • Are typically dependent on standards of care, unit procedures
Competent	• Focuses more on clinical issues in contrast to tasks • Can handle familiar situations • Expects certain clinical trajectories on the basis of the experience with particular patients • Searches for broader explanations of clinical situations • Has enhanced organizational ability, technical skills • Focuses on managing patients' conditions
Proficient	• Responds to particulars of clinical situations in a broader way • Requires an experiential base with past patient populations • Understands patient transitions over time • Learns to gauge involvement with patients and families to promote appropriate caring
Expert	• Has increased intuition regarding what are important clinical factors and how to respond to these • Engages in practical reasoning • Anticipates and prepares for situations while remaining open to changes • Performs care in a "fluid, almost seamless" manner • Bonds emotionally with patients and families depending on their needs • Sees the big picture, including the unexpected • Works both with and through others

From Norman, V. (2008). Uncovering and recognizing nurse caring from clinical narratives. *Holistic Nursing Practice, 22*(6), 324–335, by permission.

Peers

The nurse-patient relationship occurs within the larger context of your professional relationships with coworkers. Issues will arise. However, if we ignore relationship problems, others may unconsciously "act out" and undermine care. Historically, newly hired staff nurses encountered as much "hazing" as they received support. Bullying is discussed in Chapter 23. Occasionally you may have to work with a peer with whom you develop a "personality conflict." Stop and consider what led up to the current situation. In general, it is due to the accumulation of small annoyances that occur over time. The best method is to verbalize occurrences rather than ignoring them until they become a major problem. Avoid "the blame game," and discuss in a private, calm moment what you both can do to make things better. Modeling positive interactions may assist in resolution. Holding an "intervention" or "crucial conversation" discussion is

needed. Blair (2013) suggests using the mnemonic CRIB to guide the conversation:

C = Commit to seeking a mutual purpose (to move toward resolution of the conflict).

R = Recognize the purpose (can use a mentor to help)

I = Invent a mutual purpose (agree to a win-win purpose)

B = Brainstorm new strategies (agree to work together differently to move forward).

Whenever there is covert conflict among nurses, it is the patient who ultimately suffers the repercussions. The level of trust a patient has in the professional relationship is compromised until the staff conflict can be resolved. Getting accepted and building congenial working relationships take time and some energy.

Supervisors

Negotiating with persons in authority can be stressful, even threatening, because such people have control over your future as a staff nurse or student. Supervision implies shared responsibility in our overall goal of providing safe, high-quality care to patients. The wise supervisor is able to promote a nonthreatening environment in which all aspects of professionalism are allowed to emerge. In the supervisor-nurse relationship, conflict may arise when performance expectations are unclear or when the nurse is unable to perform at the desired level. Communication of expectations often occurs after the fact, within the context of employee performance evaluations. Effective management means these job expectations are known from the first day. Frequent feedback and performance reviews are used to let you know about areas needing improvement, as part of an ongoing, constructive relationship. When a supervisor gives constructive criticism, it should be in a caring, nonthreatening manner.

Supervision of Staff

Use of open communication techniques already discussed are effective in supervising others. If a problem occurs, use the same communication techniques described in Chapter 13: state your concern, state expectations, and mention outcomes that will occur if the problem behavior persists. There are two categories of personnel you as a staff nurse might be responsible for supervising: unlicensed and licensed personnel.

Unlicensed Assistive Personnel

Our nursing workload demands have given rise to employment of several types of unlicensed personnel, such as nursing assistants and orderlies. Although we are ultimately responsible for the quality and safety of care given under our supervision, we delegate less complex tasks to assistants. Delegation is defined as the transfer of responsibility for the performance of an activity from one individual to another while retaining accountability. Whether delegating to a peer or unlicensed assistive personnel (UAP), the nurse is only transferring a task, not responsibility for care (ANA, 1994). Delegation can free a nurse for attending to more complex care needs (ANA, 2005). In the current health care environment, some UAPs possess minimal knowledge or experience skills, whereas others have excellent abilities. Refer to your licensure organization for guidelines.

Licensed Nurses

There are several categories of nurses who, while licensed, have a more limited scope of practice and may require your supervision. In some countries, these nurses are known as licensed practical nurses (LPNs) or licensed vocational nurses (LVNs). Role overlap, lack of clear distinctions in roles, power factors, and pay inequality still lead some to struggle with maintaining collegial relationships (Limoges

& Jagos, 2015). Appropriate use of delegation can facilitate your ability to meet these challenges. More often than not, novice nurses are inadequately prepared for the demands of delegation. Reflect on Monica's case.

Case Example: Monica Lewis, RN

After receiving the report of her patient assignments, Ms. Lewis assigns a newly hired nursing assistant Sally (UAP) to provide routine care (morning bath, assistance with breakfast, vital signs, fingerstick for glucose level) to several patients, including Ms. Jones, who was admitted yesterday for exacerbation of her type 2 diabetes mellitus. While on rounds, Monica finds that Mrs. Jones is unresponsive, cold, and clammy, with a heart rate of 110 beats/min. Her record shows that the 8 a.m. fingerstick reading of a glucose level was 60 mg/dL, as performed by Sally. Thinking that Mrs. Jones is experiencing hypoglycemia, Monica requests Sally obtain another glucose reading. While preparing to administer glucose intravenously, Monica observes Sally make several errors obtaining an accurate blood glucose test. Sally admits she was never taught the procedure but says she thought reading the instructions was sufficient. Monica had wrongly assumed all UAPs underwent training on principles of obtaining accurate fingersticks

---

Inherent in effective delegation is an adequate understanding of the skills and knowledge of UAPs, as well as of legal parameters such as the Nurse Practice Act in the location in which you are nursing. Nurse Practice Acts clearly state what and what not can be delegated and to what type of personnel these actions can be delegated. The employing agency and the nurse need to reinforce the UAP's knowledge base, assess current level of abilities, oversee tasks, and evaluate outcomes. This is a costly process both in time and energy. Practice of Simulation Exercise 22.2 should help you to consider the principles of delegation.

Self-Awareness

Self-awareness is defined as the capacity to accurately recognize emotional reactions as they happen and to understand your responses to different people and situations. Self-awareness helps nurses to work from their strengths and cope more effectively to minimize personal weaknesses in interactions with others. Developing self-awareness allows nurses to make higher-quality decisions because decisions are more likely to be based on facts than personal feelings.

SIMULATION EXERCISE 22.2   Applying Principles of Delegation

Purpose:
To help students differentiate between delegating nursing tasks and evaluating outcomes.

Procedure:
Divide class into two groups. Reflect on the following case study of a typical day for the charge nurse in an extended-care facility. Group A is to describe the nursing tasks they would delegate to assistants and the instructions they would give. Group B is to describe the responsibilities of the professional nurse related to the delegated work.
   Reflective analysis and discussion: identify goals.

Case:
Anne Marie Roach, RN, is the day shift charge nurse at Shadyside extended care facility. Today the unit census is 24 and her staff includes four nursing assistants (NAs) and two Certified Medicine Aides (CMAs) who are allowed to administer oral medications. The NAs are qualified to give morning baths; assist with feeding; obtain and record vital signs, intake, and output; do fingersticks for blood glucose readings; and turn and reposition bed-bound patients and assist the others to ambulate. They also change decubitus dressings for the three needing this care. Of the residents, 12 are bed bound, requiring full baths and feeding assistance. The remaining 12 need some assistance with morning care and ambulation to the dining room. Nine residents need glucose levels; seven have weakness recovering from strokes. All residents are at risk for falls. Night shift reported all residents' conditions as stable. Time to make today's assignments.

Reflective Analysis
Discuss and evaluate groups responses.

It is not always easy to be completely honest about one's personal weaknesses, values, and beliefs. However, this level of self-awareness is a crucial component of effective professional leadership development. Self-awareness directly affects self-management and how we professionally respond to others. Professional self-awareness promotes recognition of the need for continuing education, the acceptance of accountability for one's own actions, the capacity to be assertive with professional colleagues, and the capability of serving as a patient advocate when the situation warrants it, even if it is uncomfortable to do so.

BOX 22.2   Key Messages of the Institute of Medicine Report

Future of Nursing: Leading Change, Advancing Health

- Nurses should practice to the full extent of their education and training.
- Nurses should achieve higher levels of education and training through an improved education that promotes seamless academic progression.
- Nurses should be full partners, with physicians and other health professionals, in redesigning health care in the United States.
- Effective workforce planning and policy making require better data collection and an improved information infrastructure.

Nurses have Rights

In addition to significant responsibilities, you as a nurse have rights in your professional relationships with colleagues and patients (see Box 22.2).

Think about your professional collegial relationships and your dual professional commitment to self and others. How can you balance your legitimate responsibilities to self and your responsibilities to patients and coworkers?

Transformational leadership. Leadership plays a pivotal role in setting expectations regarding scope of practice, collaboration, optimal interdisciplinary teamwork, and empowered knowledge partnerships in professional nursing practice. Transformational leadership requires engaging the hearts, as well as the minds, of those in the workforce. The transformational leader is self-actualized, stays focused on group processes, influences others in a warm, trusting climate, inspires trust, challenges the status quo, and empowers others. Simulation Exercise 22.3 provides an opportunity to examine nurse leadership behaviors.

Demonstration of transformational leadership is required for **magnet hospital** status designation (Schwartz, Spencer, & Wilson, 2011). Transformational leadership qualities include a clear vision and commitment to excellence, with a willingness to take reasonable risks, consult with others, and persistent dedication to task completion. They understand leadership as a communication process, not an event or position. Transformational leaders are energetic, positive thinkers, who act as visible role models in helping other nurses to develop leadership skills (Rolfe, 2011).

SIMULATION EXERCISE 22.3
Characteristics of Exemplary Nurse Leaders

Purpose:

To help students distinguish leadership characteristics in exemplary leaders and managers encountered in everyday nursing practice. Identifying leadership characteristics helps students become aware of professional behaviors associated with achieving the mission of professional nursing.

Procedure

This exercise is most effective when the reflections take place prior to class time and findings are discussed in small groups of four to six students.

1. Reflect on the professional characteristics and behaviors of a professional nurse you admire as a leader in your work or educational setting.
2. Write down what stood out for you about this person as a leader in your mind. What specific characteristics framed this person as a leader? How did this person relate to other health professionals including students?
3. Share and discuss your findings with your small group. Have one student act as a scribe. Identify commonalities and differences in student perceptions.
4. Share small group findings with your larger class group.

Discussion

1. Describe specific behaviors associated with effective leadership.
2. Distinguish ways nurses can demonstrate leadership in contemporary health care.
3. Evaluate ways nursing leadership is a dynamic, interactive process.
4. What are some of the ways nurses can demonstrate leadership in contemporary health care?

Structural empowerment. Structural empowerment is a concept that describes the organizational commitments and configurations that give informational and supportive power to health care workers to accomplish their work effectively in significant ways. Complex health care issues require different types and levels of expertise, working together to achieve an outcome greater than the sum of individual efforts. Communication among health professionals is open, and there is an appropriate mix of health care personnel to ensure quality care.

Communicating to Creating Safe, Supportive Work Environments

We are in a time of increasing nurse shortages but increasing acuity for hospitalized patients. Measures need to be implemented that attract nurses and improve clinical outcomes for patients. Improving work environments in health care shapes *both* nursing and patient outcomes (Bianco, Dudkiewicz, & Linette 2014). The literature suggests attention to:

Physical Space

Agency administrators have tried various strategies to promote healthy work environments which support easier communication among staff. Batch and Windsor's 2015 study found use of space integral to effective communication. For example, arranging in-patient beds and storing supplies in patient rooms to decrease the number of steps nurses walk. Communication devices such as smartphones or hands-free models such as VOCERA allow nurses to locate other personnel more easily. Computers or tablets at bedsides promote easier record keeping. Refer to Chapters 25 and 26.

Climate

Beyond the physical arrangements, the work environment is patient centered not person centered. There is a supportive atmosphere with a commitment to seek solutions, value nurses, and provide quality patient-centered care. Likewise, nurses who are good communicators, competent, dependable, adaptable, and responsible are key variables in creating a satisfying, quality work environment.

Open Communication

Collaborative relationships characterized by open communication are directly linked to optimal patient outcomes. Goals that focus on improvement rather than punitive measures are important to prevent future errors. Embracing use of technology also helps to reduce errors, such as bar coding for medicines or for lab specimens.

Team Collaboration

Components of collaboration include working with other nurses who are clinically competent, with a supportive manager, and with team members who respect each other's roles and respond to errors in a facilitative, nonpunitive manner.

Manageable Workload

Safe work environments include safe staffing levels, provisions for adequate off-unit breaks, ongoing education, nurse

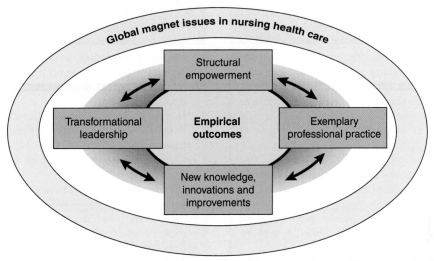

Fig. 22.2 **Magnet model components.** (Developed from Morgan, S. (2009). The magnet (TM) model as a framework for excellence. *Journal of Nursing Care Quality*, 24(2), 106.)

autonomy and accountability, and adherence to standards of care with evidence-based interventions (Amir, 2013).

Magnet Hospitals

In an effort to develop and support quality work environments favorable to nurses, the ANA through its credentialing center developed the Magnet Recognition Program in 1993, to recognize nursing role excellence. Characteristics of a magnet culture include:

- Active support of education
- Clinically competent nurses
- Positive interdisciplinary professional relationships
- Control over and autonomy in nursing practice
- Client-centered care for clients and families
- Adequate staffing and nurse-manager support (ANCC, 2014a, 2014b) Fig. 22.2.

Networking Roles

Networking is an essential component of professional role development and ultimately of advancing the status of professional nursing roles in health care delivery systems. Professional networking is defined as establishing and using contacts for information, support, and other assistance to achieve career goals (Puetz, 2007). Nurses can use networking when they are in the market for a new job, need a referral, want to receive or share information about an area of interest, or need assistance with making a career choice. Networking is a two-way interactive process. As a form of communication, networking offers valuable professional opportunities for developing new ideas and receiving feedback that might not otherwise be available. Have your business cards with you. Follow up

with contacts by sending a text, e-mail, etc. Participating in activities of nursing organizations or continuing education events provides fertile opportunities. Networking with health professionals from other disciplines is also important.

Patient Advocacy Roles

The goal of client advocacy support is to empower clients and to help them attain the services they need for self-management of health issues. Nurses are advocates for patients every time they protect, defend, and support a patient's rights and/or intervene on behalf of patients who cannot do so for themselves. The ANA (2015) affirms advocacy as an essential role in its Code of Ethics for Nurses. Patients who benefit from advocacy fall into two categories: those who need advocacy because of vulnerability caused by their illness and those who have trouble successfully navigating the health care system. Nursing patient advocacy includes facilitating access to essential health care services for patients and acting as a liaison between patients and the health care system to ensure quality care, improve health, and reduce health deviations. Skill sets associated with patient advocacy are identified in Box 22.3. For more information on nurse involvement in community-based advocacy, see Chapter 24.

Advocacy should support autonomy. Patients need to be in control of their own destiny, even when the decision reached is not what you as the nurse would recommend. Referrals to community resources should be chosen, based on compatibility with the patient's expressed need, financial resources, accessibility (time as well as place), and ease of access.

BOX 22.3 American Nurses Association's Bill of Rights for Registered Nurses

- Nurses have the right to practice in a manner that fulfills their obligations to society and to those who receive nursing care.
- Nurses have the right to practice in environments that allow them to act in accordance with professional standards and legally authorized scopes of practice.
- Nurses have the right to a work environment that supports and facilitates ethical practice, in accordance with the Code of Ethics for Nurses and its interpretive statements.
- Nurses have the right to freely and openly advocate for themselves and their patients, without fear of retribution.
- Nurses have the right to fair compensation for their work, consistent with their knowledge, experience, and professional responsibilities.
- Nurses have the right to a work environment that is safe for themselves and their patients.
- Nurses have the right to negotiate the conditions of their employment, either as individuals or collectively, in all practice settings.

Reprinted from American Nurses Association (2002). Know your rights: ANA's bill of rights arms nurses with critical information. *American Nurses, 34*(6), 16, with permission.

BOX 22.4 Knowledge Base Needed for Patient Advocacy

- Patient values, beliefs, and preferences
- Alignment with treatment goals
- Informed consent procedures, patient's third-party insurance
- Nurse's personal, professional, and cultural biases
- Print materials, and online resources relevant to patient needs
- Organizational system variables related to service delivery
- Current laws, service delivery policies, and regulations
- Community resources including referral processes, eligibility, and access requirements
- Effective communication strategies related to consultation and collaboration
- Understanding of required documentation, management, and interpretation of patient records

Reprinted from American Nurses Association (2002). Know your rights: ANA's bill of rights arms nurses with critical information. *American Nurses, 34*(6), 16, with permission.

Nurse-Patient Role Relationships

Nurse. Professional performance behaviors in the nurse-patient relationship include a sound knowledge base (Box 22.4), technical competency, and interpersonal competency, as well as caring. On a daily basis, nurses must collect and process multiple, often indistinct, pieces of behavioral data. They problem solve with patients and families to come up with workable, realistic solutions. Through words and behaviors in relationship with other health care providers and agencies, nurses provide quality care and act as advocates for patients and for the nursing profession.

Currently, nurses function in a high-tech, managed health care environment in which the human caring aspects of nursing are easier to overlook. Unique challenges to the nurse-patient relationship in clinical practice include shorter in-patient contacts, technology, and lower levels of trust in relation to these factors. The nurse-patient relationship will become increasingly important in helping patients feel cared for in a health care environment that sometimes neglects their psychosocial needs in favor of cost effectiveness.

Patient role. In the current health care environment, patients are expected to take an active role in self-management of their condition to whatever extent is possible. The relational expectation is for an equal partnership, having shared power and authority as joint decision makers in their health care. Is the patient-centered model of health care delivery actually true? Is every decision related to diagnosis and treatment based on combined input and joint responsibility for implementing the recommendations? Use of the patient's self-knowledge and inner resources allows nurses to more effectively respond to their needs.

SUMMARY

How nurses perceive their professional role and how they function as a nurse in that role has a sizable effect on the success of their interpersonal communication. The professional nursing role should be evidenced in every aspect of nursing care but nowhere more fully than in the nurse-patient relationship. A professional nurse's first role responsibility is to the patient. Because hospitals no longer are the primary settings for nursing practice, nurse practice roles take place in nontraditional and traditional community-based health care settings. Expanded nursing roles were described. Emphasis on

health team roles and communicating with interdisciplinary team members will be further described in Chapter 23.

Socialization theory was described to explain the transition to the professional role. Among other theorists, focus was given to Benner's five developmental stages of increasing proficiency to describe the nurse's progression from novice to expert. Professional development as a nurse is a lifelong commitment. Mentorship and continuing education assist nurses in maintaining their competency and professional role development.

ETHICAL DILEMMA: What Would You Do?

As a new nurse on the unit, you witness diminished patient care quality due to poor communication and lack of provider continuity. If you raise the issue in a staff meeting with your supervisor and coworkers, you fear your opinion will not be taken seriously because the others have been working together for a much longer time. What should you do?

DISCUSSION QUESTIONS

1. Identify the critical indicators of professionalism in nursing.
2. Classify the skills you consider the most important in developing a collaborative team approach to clinical care.
3. Evaluate the statement "Every nurse should be a leader," and explain how this idea might be realized in contemporary health care.

4. What do you conjecture as the distinct and collaborative contributions of different professional roles to patient care and health care delivery?

REFERENCES

American Association of Colleges of Nursing (AACN). (2003). Competencies and curricular expectations for clinical nurse leader education and practice. Retrieved from: www.aacnnursing.org/cnl. (Accessed 10/3/18).

American Association of Colleges of Nursing (AACN). (2004). AACN position statement on the practice doctorate in nursing. Washington, DC, American Association of Colleges of Nursing. Retrieved from: www.aacnnursing.org/DNP. (Accessed 10/3/18).

American Nurses Association (ANA). (2002). Know your rights: ANA's bill of rights arms nurses with critical information. *American Nurses Association*, 34(6), 16.

American Nurses Association (ANA). (2015). *Code of Ethics*. Retrieved from: www.nursingworld.org.

American Nurses Credentialing Center (ANCC). (2014a). Magnet application manual. Silver Spring, MD: Author.

American Nurses Credentialing Center (ANCC). (2014b). Magnet recognition program model. Retrieved from: www.truthaboutnursinf.org/faq/magnet.html. (Accessed 10/3/18).

Amir, K. (2013). *Quality and safety for transformational nursing: Core competencies.* Upper Saddle River, NJ: Pearson Education, Inc.

Amodo, A., Baker, D., Emery, D., & Hines, S. (2017). *TeamSTEPPS National Conference.* June 5, 2017.

Baldwin, A., Mills, J., Birks, M., & Budden, L. (2014). Role modeling in undergraduate nursing education: an integrative literature review. *Nurse Education Today, 34*(6), e18–e26.

Batch, M., & Windsor, C. (2015). Nursing casualization and communication: A critical ethnography. *Journal of Advanced Nursing, 71*(4), 870–880.

Bauer, T. N., & Erdogan, B. (2011). Organizational socialization: The effective on boarding of new employees. In S. Zedeck (Ed.), *APA handbook of industrial and organizational psychology* (Vol. 3) (pp. 51–64). Washington, DC: Author. https://doi.org/10.1037/12171-002.

Bender, M. (2016). Clinical nurse leader integration into practice: Developing theory to guide best practice. *Journal of Professional Nursing, 32*(1), 32–40.

Benner, P. (1984, 2001). *From novice to expert: Excellence and power in clinical nursing practice.* New York, NY: Prentice Hall.

Bianco, C., Dudkiewicz, P. B., & Linette, D. (2014). Building nurse leader relationships. *Nursing Management, 45*(5), 42–48.

deSwardt, H. C., van Rensburg, G. H., & Oosthuizen, M. J. (2017). Supporting students in professional socialization: Guidelines for professional nurses and educators. *International Journal of Africa Nursing Sciences, 6*, 1–7.

Dracup, K., & Bryan-Brown, C. W. (2004). From novice to expert to mentor: Shaping the future. *Americal Journal of Critical Care, 13*(6), 448–450.

Dreyfus, S. E., Dreyfus, H. L. (1980). *A five-stage model of the mental activities involved in directed skill acquisition.* Berkeley, CA: University of California at Berkeley.

Duchscher, J., & Kramer, M. (2012). *From surviving to thriving: Navigating the first year of professional nursing practice* (2nd ed.). Suskatoon, SK: Nursing The Future.

Farrell, K., Payne, C., & Heye, M. (2015). Integrating interprofessional collaboration skills into the advanced practice registered nurse socialization process. *Journal of Professional Nursing, 31*(1), 5–10.

Felstead, I. S., & Springett, K. (2016). An exploration of role model influence on adult nursing students' professional development: A phenomenological research study. *Nurse Education Today, 37*, 66–70.

Flexner, A. (1915). Is social work a profession? New York (paper presented at the National Conference on Charities and Correction, 1915). *Proceedings of the National Conference on Social Work, 581*, 584–588.

Hesburgh, T. (1971). Presidential leadership. *Journal of Higher Education, 42*(9), 763–765.

Institute of Medicine (IOM). (2001). *Crossing the quality chasm: a new health system for the 21st century.* Washington, D.C. National Academies Press.

Institute of Medicine (IOM). (2003). *Health professions education: A bridge to quality.* Washington, DC: National Academies Press.

Institute of Medicine (IOM). (2011). *The future of nursing: Leading change, advancing health.* Washington, DC: Author.

Limoges, J., & Jagos, K. (2015). The influences of nursing education on the socialization and professional working relationships of Canadian practical and degree nursing students: A critical analysis. *Nurse Education Today, 35*, 1023–1027.

MacArthur, B. L., Dailey, S. L., & Vilagran, M. M. (2016). Understanding healthcare providers' professional identification: The role of interprofessional communication in the vocational socialization of physicians. *Journal of Interprofessional Education and Practice, 5*, 11–17.

McKenna, L., Brooks, I., & Vanderheide, R. (2017). Graduate entry nurses' initial perspectives on nursing: Content analysis of open-ended survey questions. *Nurse Education Today, 49*, 22–26.

Moore, P., Schmidt, D., & Howington, L. (2014). Interdisciplinary preceptor teams to improve the clinical nurse leader student experience. *Journal of Professional Nursing, 30*(3), 190–195.

Phillips, C., Esterman, A., & Kenny, A. (2015). The theory of organizational socialization and its potential for improving transition experiences for new graduate nurses. *Nurse Education Today, 35*, 118–124.

Puetz, B. (2007). Networking. *Public Health Nurse, 24*(6), 577–579.

Quality and Safety Education for Nurses (QSEN). www.qsen.org/competencies/. (Accessed 10/3/18).

Rick, C. (2014). Competence in executive nursing leadership for the 21st century: The 5 eyes. *Nurse Leader, 12*(2), 64–66.

Rolfe, P. (2011). Transformational leadership theory: What every leader needs to know. *Nurse Leader, 9*(2), 54–57.

Schoessler, M., & Waldo, M. (2006). The first 18 months in practice: A developmental transition model for the newly graduated nurse. *Journal for Nurses in Staff Development, 22*(2), 47e–554e.

Schwartz, D., Spencer, T., Wilson, B., & Wood, K. (2011). Transformational leadership: Implications for nursing leaders in facilities seeking magnet status. *AORN Journal, 93*(6), 737–748.

Shatto, B., Meyer, G., & Delicath, T. A. (2016). The transition to practice of direct entry clinical nurse leader. *Nurse Education in Practice, 19*, 97e–103e.

Strouse, S. M., & Nickerson, C. J. (2016). Professional culture brokers: Nurse faculty perceptions of nursing culture and their role in student formation. *Nurse Education in Practice, 18*, 10–15.

Sun, L., Gau, Y., Yang, J., Zang, X., & Wang, Y. (2016). The impact of professional identity on role stress in nursing students: A cross-sectional study. *International Journal of Nursing Studies, 63*, 1–8.

Thomas, J., Jenks, A., & Jack, B. (2015). Finessing incivility: The professional socialization experiences of student nurses' first clinical placement, a grounded theory. *Nurse Education Today, 35*(12), e4–e9.

World Health Organization (WHO). (2010). *Framework for action on interprofessional education and collaborative practice.* Geneva, Switzerland: WHO. www.who.int/. (Accessed 10/3/18).

SUGGESTED READING

American Association of Colleges of Nursing (AACN). (2008). *The essentials of baccalaureate education for professional nursing practice.* Washington, DC: Author.

Benner, P. (2005). Using the Dreyfus model of skill acquisition to describe and interpret skill acquisition and clinical judgment in nursing practice and education. *Bulletin of Science, Technology & Society, 24*(3), 188–199.

Farag, A., & Tullai-McGuinness, S. (2017). Do leadership style, unit climate, and safety climate contribute to safe medication practices? *The Journal of Nursing Administration, 47*(1), 8–15.

Leininger, M. (1991). *Culture of care diversity and universality: A theory of nursing.* New York: National League for Nursing.

23

Interprofessional Communication

Kathleen Underman Boggs

OBJECTIVES

At the end of the chapter, the reader will be able to:

1. Discuss application of Quality and Safety Education for Nurses (QSEN) and Team Strategies and Tools to Enhance Performance and Patient Safety (TeamSTEPPS) concepts of team communication and effects on safe care.
2. Identify communication barriers in interprofessional relationships, including disruptive behaviors.
3. Describe methods for handling conflict through interpersonal negotiation.
4. Discuss methods for communicating effectively with others in organizational settings (QSEN competency).
5. Discuss application of research to evidence-based clinical communication, including TeamSTEPPS approach.

The World Health Organization (WHO) says that in order to promote safety, patients need to take ownership of their health care (2016). To be effective as a nursing professional, it is not enough to be deeply committed to patient-centered care; proficient communication skills are necessary to function as a member of an interprofessional team to effectively provide quality care safely. QSEN criteria for effective interprofessional functioning propose development of skills to foster open communication, demonstrate mutual respect, and share in decision making (Pre-licensure Competency, n.d., www.QSEN.org).

An essential communication skill is the ability to adapt your own communication style to meet the needs of team members, and to mindfully and continually scan changing situations. This chapter will focus on principles of communication with other professionals. Strategies will be suggested that you can use to function more effectively as an interprofessional team member and leader. Specific ways to communicate with other health care professionals are described to help you remove communication barriers. Collaboration in health care teams will again be discussed in Chapter 24.

BASIC CONCEPTS

Many experts cite **effective communication** as a bedrock principle of quality care. Effective communication is timely, accurate, complete, unambiguous, and understood by the recipient. Communication breakdowns can negatively affect patient care. For example, the literature shows that the greatest determinant of intensive care unit (ICU) death rates is how well nurses and physicians work together in planning and providing care. Effective communication prevents errors of all magnitudes. The Joint Commission (TJC) found that team communication breakdowns were the root cause of preventable sentinel events in 68% of cases (TJC, 2015). Communication challenges are substantial when many different providers are involved. Deliberate and mindful use of strategies to improve communication is part of a nurse's job (Perry, Christiansen, & Simmons, 2016).

STANDARDS FOR A HEALTHY WORK ENVIRONMENT

Shared mental model. Increasing complexity of care characterizes all health care workplaces, usually requiring interprofessional teamwork to provide comprehensive care. Every team member needs to "buy in" to the collaborative team concept. Team functioning, especially in increasingly complex health situations, requires effective teamwork to ensure patient safety (Mace-Vadjunec et al., 2015; Polis, Higgs, Manning, Netto, & Fernandez, 2017).

Open Communication. Open communication and trust are core elements for smooth and effective teamwork (Polis et al., 2017). For example, you trust team colleagues to communicate honest feedback about performance, such as occurs in the case example about F.R.O.G. (Friction Rubs Out Germs).

Case Example: Friction Rubs Out Germs Program

The Quality Analysis staff in a large hospital system instituted a Friction Rubs Out Germs **(F.R.O.G.)** hand hygiene in-service for all front line staff after attending the QSEN 2017 National Forum where Dr. Jane Barnsteiner quoted empirical findings indicating that staff nurses practice appropriate hand hygiene only 50% to 70% of the time. After attending, Liz observes Mr. Adam's nurse, Kay, forgetting to wash her hands before entering his room. She whispers the word "ribbit" into Kay's ear. Is this an effective but fun way to remind her about hand hygiene?

Collegiality. A culture of collegiality is essential for a work environment that is to provide high-quality patient care. The interprofessional team depends on an effective blending of the collective competencies of each provider to deliver quality health care. **Collaboration** begins with communicating an awareness of each other's roles, knowledge, and skills and continues with the development of shared values. If team members do not **trust** and **respect** each other and communicate in an open and respectful manner, they are more likely to make mistakes. Reflect on the following Surgical Unit case example.

Case Example: Conflict on a Surgical Unit

Two nursing teams work the day shift on a busy surgical unit. As nurse manager, Ms. Libby notices that both teams are arguing over computer use and have become unwilling to help cover the other team's patients. It now is taking longer to complete assigned work. To achieve a more harmonious work environment, she arranges a staff meeting to get the teams to communicate. Rather than just computer issues, multiple problems surface suggesting inadequate time management and work overload. Ms. Libby listens actively, responds with empathy, and provides positive regard and feedback for solutions proposed by the group. She asks the group to decide on two prioritized solutions. Recognizing that her staff feels unappreciated and knowing that compromise is a strategy that produces behavior change, she resolves to offer more frequent performance feedback,

such as weekly evaluations via email, and providing specific data on overtime. She herself assumes responsibility for requesting an immediate computer upgrade using the unit budget's emergency funding allocation. A team member who serves on the employee relations committee assumes responsibility for requesting that the human services department schedule an in-service training on time management and stress reduction within the next month. The group agrees to meet in 6 weeks to evaluate.

Collegiality is discussed in Chapters 13 and 22, as are aspects of healthy work environments.
- Nurses must be as efficient in communication skills as they are in clinical skills.
- Nurses must be relentless in pursuing and fostering true collaboration.
- Nurses must be valued and committed partners in making policy, directing and evaluating clinical care, and leading organizational operations.
- Staffing must ensure the effective match between patient needs and nurse competencies.
- Nurses must be recognized and must recognize others for the value each brings to the work of the organization.
- Nurse leaders must fully embrace the imperative of a healthy work environment, authentically live it, and engage others in its achievement.

Other professional nursing organizations have identified the following *elements* of a healthy workplace environment:
- Develop collaborative culture of trust
- Maintain respectful open communication and behavior
- Communication-rich culture that emphasizes trust and respect
- Clearly defined role expectations with accountability
- Adequate workforce
- Competent leadership
- Use shared decision making
- Participate in employee development
- Recognition of workers' contributions

Code of Behavior

The goal of collaboration is to communicate effectively with team members to provide safe, high-quality care. As part of creating a culture of teamwork where staff is valued, a standard across organizations should be zero tolerance for disruptive or bullying behaviors. To accomplish this, each organization needs one well-defined code of behavior applied consistently to all staff. TJC mandates

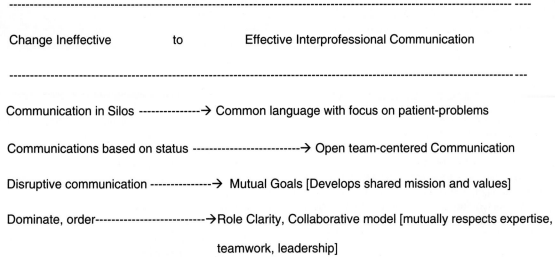

--- ----

Change Ineffective   to   Effective Interprofessional Communication

--- ---

Communication in Silos --------------→ Common language with focus on patient-problems

Communications based on status --------------------------→ Open team-centered Communication

Disruptive communication --------------→ Mutual Goals [Develops shared mission and values]

Dominate, order--------------------------→Role Clarity, Collaborative model [mutually respects expertise,

teamwork, leadership]

Fig. 23.1 Improve Interprofessional Communication.

that each health care organization has a code of conduct defining acceptable and unacceptable behaviors, as well as an agency process for reporting and handling disruptive behaviors, discrimination, or disrespectful treatment (TJC, 2008, 2010).

Collaboration. Collaboration definitions in the literature remain imprecise (Fewster-Thuente, 2015). Collaboration is a dynamic process in which work groups from different professional backgrounds cooperate and share expertise to deliver quality health care. This involves an integration of knowledge, skills, and attitudinal values. Complex health issues are best addressed by an interdisciplinary team approach (Farrell, Payne, & Heye, 2015). This coordinated form of care delivery was advocated by the Institute of Medicine (IOM) 2010 Report. Ideally, each team member understands the role of others and pools their own expertise with those of other team members.

An interprofessional expert panel has specified core competencies for interprofessional practice (Interprofessional Education Collaborative Expert Panel, 2011). These values include patient-centered, community-oriented, relationship-focused, process-oriented, and using common language, applicable across professions. The TeamSTEPPS program stresses the importance of developing a shared mental model (goal) for each patient's care.

Teamwork and Communication

Interprofessional team functioning is both a role-focused process and task-based skills focused process. Team members have unique personalities, egos, and skill sets, yet all must work together. Playing to each team member's strengths enhances the ability to deliver safe, quality care. Collaborating in joint decision making and care coordination requires knowing when to hold and when to let go of ideas and opinions.

According to the Agency for Healthcare Research and Quality (AHRQ), communication is central to team functioning (2017). This type of communication requires trust, mutual support, and thoughtful open communication. Information is shared for informed decision-making (Fig. 23.1). AHRQ (2017) refers to several models, but suggests a new "holacracy model" in which every team member's opinion is valued, generating an attitude of "no one wins unless everyone wins." This open communication is based on patient need and is undefined by status of team members. Overall treatment goals should be the guiding force in team conversation. To dramatize team function, try Simulation Exercise 23.1.

Barriers to Effective Team Communication

Barriers to effective team communication include not sharing information among team members; a hierarchical structure inhibiting some members from speaking up; variations in communication styles or vocabulary; complacency, defensiveness, and conflict (TeamSTEPPS, 2017). Note that studies show the vast majority of frontline staff report care not completed on the prior shift. Would open communication help resolve this?

SIMULATION EXERCISE 23.1   Zoom

Directions: Use one of the "Zoom" picture books (Banyai I. Zoom. NY: Viking: Penguin Books; available for purchase from Amazon).

Duplicate enough sets of photos for use by groups of 10. Place each photo into a manila folder. Mix up their order. Divide students into groups of 10 or so and give each group member a folder.

Activity Instructions: "Look at your photo but do not show it to anyone else. Verbally describe your photo. Group task or goal is to interpret." Allow 5–7 min.

Reflective Analysis: After activity completion, ask each group to apply team principles to describe their roles. Who was group leader?... Was there a clear goal?... Did each team member feel free to speak up?

BOX 23.1   Interpersonal Sources of Conflict in the Workplace: Barriers to Collaboration and Communication

1. Different expectations
   - Role ambiguity
   - Being asked to do something you know would be irresponsible or unsafe
   - Having your feelings or opinions ridiculed or discounted
   - Getting pressure to give more time or attention than you are able to give
   - Being asked to give more information than you feel comfortable sharing
   - Differences in language
2. Threats to self
   - Maintaining a sense of self in the face of hostility or sexual harassment
   - Being asked to do something concerning a patient that is in conflict with your personal or professional moral values
3. Differences in role hierarchy
   - Differences in education or experience
   - Differences in responsibility and rewards (payment)
   - Lack of support from leadership/administration
4. Clinical situation constraints
   - Emphasis on rapid decision making
   - Complexity of care interventions
   - Stressful workload

Conflict Antecedents

Ineffective communication often leads to disagreements, injured feelings, and unsafe care. Poor communication is one of several factors frequently cited in the literature as an underlying cause of conflict (Almost et al., 2016; Trepanier, Fernet, Austin, & Boudrias, 2016). Refer to Box 23.1 for others. Misfeldt, Suter, Oelke, Hepp, and Lait (2017) applied a sociological model to analyze the functioning of primary health care teams in Canada. Their model lists effective team characteristics as effective formal and informal communication; mutual respect; team leadership and vision; and role clarity and accountability. Problems in any of these areas can be reflected as disruptive behavior and can compromise patient safety.

Disruptive Behaviors

Conflict was defined in Chapter 13 as a hostile encounter. The nursing literature uses a variety of terms to refer to persistent uncivil behaviors in the workplace: bullying; verbal abuse; horizontal violence; lateral violence; "eating your young"; in-fighting; and mobbing, harassment, or scapegoating. The term we use in this book is disruptive behavior.

Definition. Disruptive behavior is defined as a lack of civility or lack of respect which occurs within professional relationships as frequently as weekly, and is repeated over time. Disruptive behaviors may include overt behaviors such as rudeness, verbal abuse, intimidation, put-downs; angry outbursts, yelling, blaming, or criticizing team members in front of others; sexual harassment; or even threatening physical confrontations. Other disruptive behaviors are more covert; these include passive-aggressive communication, withholding need-to-know information, withholding help, assigning excessively heavy workloads, refusing to perform assigned tasks, impatience or reluctance to answer questions, refusal to return telephone calls or pages, and speaking in a condescending tone. These behaviors threaten the well-being of nurses and the safety of patients (Castronovo, Pullizzi, & Evans, 2016; Koh, 2016).

Incidence. Disruptive behavior is fairly common in large organizations, especially hospitals. Ranging from half to three-quarters of all nurses report being subjected to disruptive behavior at some time, which they say compromised patient safety (Lyndon et al., 2015; Moore, Sublett, & Leahy, 2017). TJC cites ineffective communication between team members as contributing to 60% of errors (TJC, 2008). This also affects student nurses as seen in Tee's 2016 study in which half of student nurses reported experiencing bullying or harassment! Most studies have found that nurse-to-nurse disruptive behaviors occur more frequently than disruptive physician-nurse interactions and occur more often in high-stress areas such as surgical suites, psychiatric units, or emergency departments (Agency for Healthcare Research and Quality [AHRQ], n.d).

Patient Outcomes. Disruptive behavior is a barrier to effective health care (Kimes, Davis, Medlock, & Bishop, 2015). Subsequently, impaired communication compromises patient safety (AHRQ, n.d.) and decreases patient satisfaction (Mace-Vadjunec et al., 2015). For example, in Press and colleague's 2015 study, disruptive behavior was associated with increased levels of readmission to the hospital. Poor communication is associated with problems in patient safety. Good collaboration and communication have been shown to be associated with better patient outcomes, such as decreased infections, in a 2015 study by Boev and Xia.

Nurse Outcomes. As described earlier, failures in collaboration and communication among health team members are among the most common factors cited for nurse frustration, job stress, poor morale, job abandonment, lost productivity, loss of confidence, absenteeism, and task avoidance, and they adversely affect nurses' physical and mental health (Dzurec, Kennison, & Gillen, 2017; Eriksen, Hogh, & Hansen, 2016; Kimes et al., 2015).

Organization Outcomes. Costs to agency center on financial issues related to absenteeism, increased staff turnover, losses in productivity, as well as increases in care errors and even legal action. Other outcomes include decreases in care quality, increases in care errors, and adverse patient outcomes (Trepanier et al., 2016).

CREATING A COLLABORATIVE CULTURE OF REGARD TO ELIMINATE DISRUPTIVE BEHAVIOR

To deliver safe, high-quality health care, the corporate climate now emphasizes a **collaborative, patient-centered care model** in which the hierarchical power model is replaced by a model in which all team members are valued. Organizational support is essential for success. **Collaboration** is broadly defined as working with all members of the health care team to achieve maximum health outcomes for our mutual patient, and includes:

1. Common goal: Developing a **collaborative culture** in which all team members keep the delivery of safe, high-quality care foremost in mind requires that we trust and respect the decision making of all team members. Different professional groups were educated to hold differing beliefs and styles of communication. We need to develop an understanding of these various perspectives, not so we can change them, but so that we can utilize them.
2. Open, safe communication: Creating a communication-rich environment requires that all team members value open communication. We combine assertiveness (speaking up, giving and receiving feedback) with cooperation.
3. Mutual respect: Appreciation for each member's value. An important part of working together is developing mutual trust; you trust coworkers to "have your back."
4. Shared decision making: The IOM (2003) says nurses should be full partners with physicians and other health team members. Leadership is required to avoid duplication of tasks and to ensure that all tasks are completed.
5. Role clarity: Members of a team that have been working well together generally have developed complementary roles. We know our role and that of other team members and recognize when we need to call on their expertise.
6. Message clarity: Focusing on salient facts; avoiding inconsequential comments.

Collaboration is a dynamic process benefiting from ongoing practice and evaluation. In the past, some organizations tolerated disruptive workplace behaviors. Pressures on nurses exist to increase productivity and cost-effectiveness. Accrediting organizations encourage agencies to practice zero tolerance of these behaviors. Individually, we need to become aware of how to discourage disruptive behaviors as we work to develop a healthy, collaborative workplace atmosphere to ensure high-quality patient care (TJC, 2009). A hallmark of a professional is acceptance of accountability for one's own behavior. Preventing conflicts is accomplished by avoiding public criticism, cultivating a willingness to help attitude, and doing one's fair share.

Respect

Feeling respected or not is an integral part of how nurses rate the quality of their work environment. Three key factors to feeling respected are a positive climate of professional practice, a supportive manager, and positive relationships with other staff. Nurses say they feel respected and appreciated if their opinions are listened to attentively, and they receive feedback from authority figures as to the value of their work competence. When their opinions are discounted or ridiculed, they feel disrespected, angry, frustrated, and powerless. Such anger can be displaced toward others.

Factors that Affect Nurse Behavior toward Other Team Members

Team training has been instituted to educate all team members to work in a collaborative manner. But some factors may still negatively influence professional relationships.

Gender. Contemporary society is redefining traditional gender role behavior, negating some of the traditional gender stereotypical behaviors.

Hierarchy. Because health care authority traditionally was vested in a hierarchical structure, control rested with the physician. Changes in the physician-nurse communication process are occurring as nurses become more empowered, more assertive, and better educated. Most nurses still occasionally encounter problems in the physician-nurse relationship, however. Differences in power, perspective, education, status, and pay may be barriers to workgroup communication and care.

Communication Silos. Traditionally, each health care profession was educated separately, evolving their own unique vocabulary. If you encounter a conflict situation at work, reflect on whether the problem is due to differences in communication style.

Generational Diversity. As mentioned, members of older and younger generations differ in their preferred communication styles. It is suggested that nurses adapt their communication style based on communication method preferences of others.

Outcomes of Successful Team Training in Communication

Evidence from many studies on effects of team training shows improved efficiency and increased patient safety for the team approach to health care. Refer to the TeamSTEPPS web site for Team Strategies and Tools to Enhance Performance and Patient Safety (TeamSTEPPS) strategies. Each nurse team member needs to participate and be accountable for facilitating team communication.

APPLICATIONS

As nurses, we can help to establish and sustain a healthy workplace. This requires continuous assessment of our own and others' current communication practices and implementation of "best practices" to prevent and deal with conflict. Communication and conflict-resolution strategies can be learned but require continued reinforcement through ongoing communication training. Improving communication has been shown to improve patient safety. An essential component of communication in health care teams is leadership to set goals, provide feedback (care outcome data), and to facilitate conflict resolution.

CONFLICT RESOLUTION

As nurses we have the responsibility to work effectively with others to provide care. Yet, whenever people work together, conflicts inevitably arise. Many of the same resolution concepts described in Chapter 13 can be applied to conflicts occurring among staff. Refer to Table 8.6 in Chapter 8 to clarify the differences between groups and teams. System conflicts arising from agency or system policies also need attention.

TeamSTEPPS: Team Strategies and Tools to Enhance Performance and Patient Safety

When AHRQ adapted the Department of Defense team training program to use in health care settings, they gave it the TeamSTEPPS acronym. A main component of this free program is training to use a toolbox of communication strategies (AHRQ.gov). How many times do we say good communication is essential to effective team function? Effective communication skills convey accurate information and provide awareness of your role responsibilities. As a team member, you communicate to keep others informed as noted in Fig. 23.2.

Teamwork and collaboration are a major focus of both TeamSTEPPS and QSEN. Each team member shares a clear vision of expected outcomes for each patient. As described in Chapter 2, TeamSTEPPS creates a transformed health care model. Tools and strategies are provided which can be used to develop better system-wide communication knowledge, skills, and attitudes. Communication clarity is an important goal, as is the conciseness found on checklists. Chapter 2 described use of standardized communication tools such as SBAR (situation, background, assessment, recommendation), CUS assertive statements (see the CUS case study), the Two-Challenge Rule (stating your concern twice), check-backs (to verify that your communication message is understood accurately), briefs, debriefs, and huddles.

CUS Case Example

Mr. Michaels is scheduled for discharge today. During morning team rounds you notice redness at the intravenous (IV) site. Even though his temperature at 7 a.m. was recorded as 99.2°F, the resident wants to sign off on the discharge. You use the **CUS** assertive statements technique:

C = "I am concerned about possible sepsis."
U = "I am uncomfortable discharging him today."
S = "This is a safety issue."

When your CUS is ignored, you use the Two-Challenge Rule voicing your safety concern twice. The team leader acknowledges your concern, but if the discharge is still scheduled, you utilize your chain of command reporting this issue to your nurse supervisor.

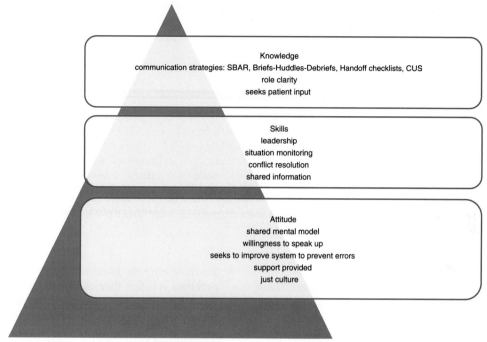

Fig. 23.2 Patient-Centered Care Team Collaboration.

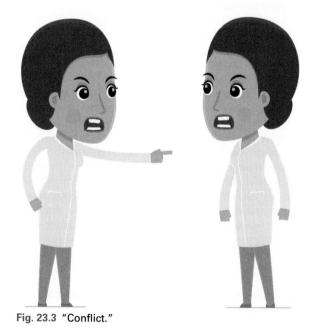

Fig. 23.3 "Conflict."

TeamSTEPPS teaches team members, including nurses, how to increase their competencies in leadership, situation monitoring, and use of mutual support strategies. Examples of leadership competency are clarifying team goals and roles. Competencies for situation monitoring include use of decision-making skills in emergent situations and providing corrective feedback. Mutual support skills include assisting others and using communication tools. Other team behaviors are discussed at the AHRQ web site. Table 23.1 lists their standards of effective communication for safer patient care outcomes.

CONFLICT RESOLUTION STEPS

Many of the same strategies for conflict resolution discussed for conflicts between patient and nurse can be applied to conflicts between the nurse and other health team members. Review the principles of conflict management in Fig. 13.1 in Chapter 13. As mentioned, conflict resolution can be a positive force for change. Instead of picturing a straight line of either you win or I win, envision the outcome of conflict resolution as a triangle with an outcome of mutual resolution as a peak, where you both have built something greater together (Fig. 23.3).

TABLE 23.1 TeamSTEPPS: Using a Team Training Program Improves Team Communication		
Essentials of Communication	**Sending Technique**	**Receiving Technique**
Clear	Common language/terminology used	Validate: use feedback or "talk back" to confirm understanding
Brief	Communicate only information essential for this situation	Clarify any nonverbal information
Timely	Verify message is received; respond quickly to requests for additional information; provide updates	Verify receipt of information
Complete	Give all relevant information; use standardized communication tools	Document: essential information validated, understood, and recorded

TeamSTEPPS, Team Strategies and Tools to Enhance Performance and Patient Safety. Adapted from Agency for Healthcare Research and Quality (AHRQ). *Curriculum/Instructors Guide*. http://www.ahrq.gov/professionals/education/curriculum-tools/teamstepps/instructor/fundamentals/module6/igltccommunication.pdf.

Step #1. Identify Sources of Conflict

Conflict often stems from miscommunication. Think through the possible causes of the conflict. Identify your own feelings about it and respond appropriately, even if the response is a deliberate choice not to respond verbally. Interpersonal conflicts that are not dealt with leave residual feelings that will reemerge in future interactions.

Step #2. Set Goals

Goals should be immediate, specific, and measurable.

Step #3. Implement Solutions

Your primary goal in dealing with workplace conflict is to find a high-quality, mutually acceptable solution: a win-win strategy. Remembering that we all share the ultimate goal of delivering high-quality patient-centered care may help us work together even if we personally do not like each other. In many instances, a better collaborative relationship can be developed through the use of the following conflict management communication techniques adapted from Johansen (2012):

- *Reframe* a clinical situation as a cooperative process in which the health goals and not the status of the providers becomes the focus.
- *Assume responsibility* for one's own behaviors and for maintaining a "blame-free" work environment.
- *Identify your goal.* A clear idea of the outcome you wish to achieve is a necessary first step in the process. Remember the issue is the conflict, not your coworker.
- *Obtain factual data.* It is important to do your homework by obtaining all relevant information about the specific issues involved—and about the individual's behavioral responses to a health care issue—before engaging in negotiation.

- *Intervene early.* Be assertive. The best time to resolve problems is before they escalate to a conflict. Create a forum for two-way communication, preferably meeting periodically. Structured formats have been developed for you to use in conflict resolution, especially in team meetings. Nielsen and Mann (2008) mention the format of *DESC* used by the TeamSTEPPS program:
- D = describe the specific behavior (the problem) using concrete data
- E = express your concerns, describing how this situation makes you feel
- S = specify a course of action, suggesting alternatives, and state consequences to patient goals
- C = obtain consensus
- *Avoid negative comments that can affect the self-esteem of the receiver.* Even when the critical statements are valid (e.g., "You do…" or "You make me feel…"), they should be replaced with "I" statements that define the sender's position. Otherwise, needless hostility is created and the meaning of the communication is lost.
- *Consider the other's viewpoint.* Having some idea of what issues might be relevant from the other person's perspective provides important information about the best interpersonal approach to use. In addition to dealing with your own feelings, you need an ability to deal with the feelings of the others. Be cooperative, acknowledging the team's interdependence and mutual goals.

Communicate to Promote Effective Collaboration: Avoid Barriers to Resolution

Refer to Box 23.2 for tips on how to turn conflict into collaboration.

Individual behaviors such as avoiding the use of negative or inflammatory, anger-provoking words, or avoiding

BOX 23.2 Strategies to Turn Conflict into Collaboration

1. Recognize and confront disruptive behaviors.
   * Use conflict-resolution strategies.
   * Take the initiative to discuss problems.
   * Use active listening skills (refrain from simultaneous activities that interrupt communication).
   * Present documented data relevant to the issue.
   * Propose resolutions.
   * Use a brief summary to provide feedback.
   * Record all decisions in writing.
2. Create a climate in which participants view negotiation as a collaborative effort.
   * Develop agency behavior policies with stated zero tolerance for disruptive or bullying behaviors.
   * Model communicating with staff in a respectful, courteous manner.
   * Participate in organizational interdisciplinary groups.
   * Solicit and give feedback on a regular, periodic basis.
   * Clarify role expectations.

phrases that imply coercion have been described. Examples include: "We must insist that…" or "You claim that…" Most individuals react to anger directed at them with a fight-or-flight response. Anyone can have a moment of rudeness, but monitor your own communications to avoid any pattern of abusive behaviors, including blaming or criticizing staff to others. When nurse supervisors become aware of how their behavior affects their nurses, they can increase the nurses' performance, increase their job involvement, and increase organizational identification. Participating in mentoring newly hired nurses, even helping sustain internship programs for novice nurses, may help to avert conflict (Weaver, 2013).

Physician-Nurse Conflict Resolution

Remarkable increases in safety in airline and space programs were achieved by creating a climate in which junior team members were free to question decisions of more senior, powerful team members. Health care is adopting a similar philosophy. The American Medical Association (American Medical Association [AMA], 2008) has specifically stated that codes of conduct define appropriate behavior as including a right to appropriately express a concern you have about patient care and safety. While this is being set forth as a medical code of conduct for physicians, should it also apply to nurses?

Nurses influence physician-patient communication. Nurses assess what physicians tell patients, encouraging

them to seek clarification, and support our patient's right to ask questions. This is an important aspect of our belief that the patient is a valued member of our health team. Do you think it is ever appropriate for a nurse to criticize a physician's actions to a patient? A common underlying factor in at least 25% of all malpractice suits is an inadvertent or deliberate critical comment by another health care professional concerning a colleague's actions.

Research has demonstrated that better collaboration and better communication are associated with safer care and better patient care outcomes, including reduced drug errors, reduced mortality, improved patient satisfaction, and somewhat with shorter hospital stays. There will be occasions when you have collaboration difficulties. Methods to improve safe communication are discussed in Chapter 2.

Make a Commitment to Open Dialogue. Listening should constitute at least half of a communication interaction. Foster a feeling of collegiality. Use strategies to defuse anger. During your negotiation, discussion should begin with a statement of either the commonalities of purpose or the points of agreement about the issue (e.g., "I thoroughly agree Mr. Smith will do much better at home. However, we need to contact social services and make a home care referral before we actually discharge him; otherwise, he will be right back in the hospital again."). Points of disagreement should always follow rather than precede points of agreement. Empathy and a genuine desire to understand the issues from the other's perspective enhance communications. Solutions that take into consideration the needs and human dignity of all parties are more likely to be considered as viable alternatives. Backing another health professional into a psychological corner by using intimidation, coercion, or blame is simply counterproductive. More often than not, solutions developed through such tactics never get implemented. The final solution derived through fair negotiation is often better than the one arrived at alone.

STRATEGIES TO REMOVE BARRIERS TO COMMUNICATION WITH OTHER PROFESSIONALS

Generally, conflict increases anxiety. When interaction with a certain peer or peer group stimulates anxious or angry feelings, the presence of conflict should be considered. Once it is determined that conflict is present, look for the basis of the conflict and label it as personal or professional. If it is personal in nature, it may not be appropriate to seek peer negotiation. It might be better to go back through the self-awareness exercises presented in previous chapters and locate the nature of the conflict through self-examination.

Sharing feelings about a conflict with others helps to reduce its intensity. It is confusing, for example, when nursing students first enter a nursing program or clinical rotation, but this confusion does not get discussed, and students commonly believe they should not feel confused or uncertain. As a nursing student, you face complex interpersonal situations. These situations may lead you to experience loneliness or self-doubt about your nursing skills compared with those of your peers. These feelings are universal at the beginning of any new experience. By sharing them with one or two peers, you usually find that others have had parallel experiences.

Individual Strategies to Deal With Workplace Conflicts

Consider using the behaviors listed in Table 23.2 when directly dealing with conflict in the workplace. Discussion of these behaviors may give you some ideas about how to implement them. Try Simulation Exercise 23.2.

TABLE 23.2	**Examples of Reframing Unclear Communication**	
Situation	**Cognitive Processes**	**Reframed to Improve Communication**
Low self-disclosure	No one knows my real thoughts, feelings, and needs. *Consequently:* I think no one cares about me or recognizes my needs. Others see me as self-sufficient and are unaware that I have a problem. *Consequently:* Others are unable to respond to my needs.	Attitude: • Respect • Value working with others • Willingness to collaborate Use skills: • Open communication—I verbalize aloud my needs clearly so others can have an opportunity to respond, to speak up. • Conflict-resolution strategies
Reluctance to delegate tasks	Other people think I do not believe that they can do the job as well as I can. *Consequently:* The others work at a minimum level. I do not expect or ask others to be involved. *Consequently:* Other people do not volunteer to help me. *Consequently:* I feel resentful, and others feel undervalued and dispensable.	Attitude: • Cooperate—I am part of a team. • Trust—I need to assign team members to do the tasks they can complete competently. Use skills: • Interdisciplinary communication
Making unnecessary demands	I expect more from others than they think is reasonable. *Consequently:* I feel the others are lazy and uncommitted and I must push harder. Others see me as manipulative and dehumanizing. *Consequently:* Others assume a low profile and do not contribute their ideas. *Consequently:* Work production is mediocre. Morale is low. Everyone, including me, feels disempowered.	Attitude: • Shared mental team model—accept team model and shared decision making • Willingness to listen • Acknowledge shared accountability—relinquish some autonomy Use skills: • Interdisciplinary communication strategies • Role clarity—I need to clearly define my expectations and capabilities; I need to set clear work goals and deadlines. • Develop situational awareness—crosscheck and offer assistance when needed. • Validation—I need to give feedback.

TABLE 23.2 **Examples of Reframing Unclear Communication—cont'd**		
Using communication styles unfamiliar to other disciplines	*Consequently:* Communication is unclear to others.	Attitude: • Willingness to reflect on personal communication style • Willingness to participate in conflict resolution Use skills: • Adapt own style to the needs of others on the health care team. • Use standardized communication tools, especially during emergent situations.

SIMULATION EXERCISE 23.2 Interprofessional Communication Case

Purpose:
To help students understand the basic concepts of patient advocacy, communication barriers, and peer negotiation in simulated nursing situations.

Procedure:
1. The following situation is an example of situations in which interprofessional communication barriers exist. Re-familiarize yourself with the concepts of professionalism, patient advocacy, communication barriers, and peer negotiation.
2. Formulate a response.
3. Compare your response with those of your classmates and discuss the implications of common and disparate answers. Sometimes dissimilar answers provide another important dimension of a problem situation.

Situation:
Dr. Tanlow interrupts Ms. Serf, RN, as she is preparing pain medication for 68-year-old Mrs. Gould. It is already 15 min late. Dr. Tanlow says he needs Ms. Serf immediately in Room 20C to assist with a drainage and dressing change. Knowing that Mrs. Gould, a diabetic, will respond to prolonged pain with vomiting, Ms. Serf replies that she will be available to help Dr. Tanlow in 10 min (during which time she will have administered Mrs. Gould's pain medication). Dr. Tanlow, already on his way to Room 20C, whirls around, stating loudly, "When I say I need assistance, I mean now. I am a busy man, in case you hadn't noticed."

If you were Ms. Serf, what would be an appropriate response?

Reflective analysis: This situation could be discussed in class, assigned as a paper, or used as an essay exam.
1. Construct the best possible response.
2. Justify your response using the concepts of professionalism, patient advocacy, communication barriers, and peer negotiation.

Model Behaviors That Convey Respect

Prevent conflict by behaving with respect. Just as you treat clients with respect, you have an ethical responsibility to treat coworkers with respect. In a survey by Costello, Clarke, Gravely, D'Agostino-Rose, and Puopolo (2011), 30% of surgical team respondents admitted to having treated coworkers with disrespect. Nurses need to be appreciated, recognized, and respected as professionals for the work they do. Unsupportive and uncivil coworkers and workplace conflicts negatively influence retention of nursing staff. Unprofessional communication can range from rudeness or gossip to overt hostile comments. Communication can become distorted rather than open when you are concerned about offending a more powerful individual. Strategies for dealing with disrespectful or disruptive behaviors include establishing common communication expectations and skills, teaching conflict resolution skills, and creating a culture of mutual respect within the health care system. Ideally, the system has ongoing education, leadership and team collaboration support, and policies to evaluate behavior violations.

Mentor New Nurses

Can it really be true that 50% of newly hired nurses leave within the first 3 years? A number of these transfer to other places, but many actually abandon the nursing profession entirely. Orientation of novice nurses is expensive for the institution. QSEN and IOM encourage agencies to establish internships or mentoring programs for the first 1 to 2 years of each novice nurse's employment.

Clarify Communications

Poor communication is repeatedly cited as an influential factor leading to conflict (Almost et al., 2016). You can use the tools and skills taught throughout this textbook to improve both the clarity of message content and the emotional tone of interactions. Communication problems lead to a large percentage of disruptive behaviors, especially telephone communication. If miscommunication occurs, seek clarity by owning your part in misunderstandings. Message clarity is enhanced when standardized formats such as SBAR, discussed in Chapter 2, are used: The nurse identifies self by name and position, the patient by name, diagnosis, the problem (include current problem, vital signs, new symptoms, etc.), and clearly states his or her request. In interprofessional communication, message clarity is crucial. Taking ownership of miscommunication allows recognition that no one is immune (Abourbih, Armstrong, Nixon, & Ackery, 2015).

Clarify Roles

Since role ambiguity is a factor frequently contributing to conflict (Almost et al., 2016), seek role clarity. Refer to Chapter 22 for an in-depth discussion of roles, so you can work toward role clarity.

Other Conflict-Resolution Strategies

Self-reflection. Self-awareness is beneficial in assessing the meaning of a professional conflict. The strategies for communicating with angry patients, as described in Chapter 13, can be applied when disrespect or anger is directed toward you from colleagues. First take a moment to reflect on your own behaviors. Have you inadvertently triggered inappropriate behavior in others? Take responsibility for how you communicate both verbally and nonverbally. Understand your own role. Do you value the role of other team members? Do you treat each of them in a courteous manner?

Take stress-reduction measures. Because we know that you are at higher risk for conflict if you are highly stressed, take whatever steps are needed to reduce personal stress.

Commit to a collaborative resolution process. Just as the agency should have a code of conduct defining respectful behavior, there should also be an established process for direct resolution of conflict issues, with support and even "coaches" who help staff resolve conflicts constructively (Box 23.3).

Process for responding to put-downs. In addition, you need to develop a strategy to respond to unwarranted put-downs and destructive criticisms. Generally, the person delivering them has but one intention—to decrease your

status and enhance the status of the person delivering the put-down. The put-down or criticism may be handed out because the speaker is feeling inadequate or threatened. Often it has little to do with the actual behavior of the nurse to whom it is delivered. Other times the criticism may be valid, but the time and place of delivery are grossly inappropriate (e.g., in the middle of the nurses' station or in the client's presence). In either case, the automatic response of many nurses is to become defensive, embarrassed, or angry.

Recognizing a put-down or unwarranted criticism is the first step toward dealing effectively with it. If a comment from a coworker or authority figure generates defensiveness

---

BOX 23.3 Steps to Promote Conflict Resolution Among Health Care Team Members

1. Set the stage for collaborative communication.
   - Self-reflection: Assume responsibility for own behavior.
   - Privacy: Meet in an appropriate venue, bringing together all involved groups.
   - Acknowledge the conflict problem using clear communication.
   - Allow sufficient time for discussion and resolution process.
2. Attitude: Maintain a respectful, nonpunitive atmosphere.
   - Solicit the perspective of each team member.
   - Define the problem issue and objectives clearly.
   - Stay focused while respecting the values and dignity of all parties.
   - Group members can be assertive but not manipulative.
   - Remember to criticize ideas, not people.
3. Be proactive: Initiate early discussion:
   - Use communication skills.
   - Identify the conflict's key points.
   - Have an objective or a goal clearly in mind.
   - Seek mutual solutions.
   - Have group members propose a solution: Identify the merits and drawbacks of each solution.
   - Be open to alternative solutions in which all parties can meet essential needs.
   - Depersonalize conflict situations.
4. Decide to implement the best solution.
   - Specify persons responsible for implementation (role clarity).
   - Establish timeline.
   - Decide on the evaluation method.
   - Emphasize common goal is a shared value of quality care.
   - Emphasize shared responsibility for team success.

or embarrassment, it is likely that the comment represents more than just factual information about performance. If the comment made by the speaker contains legitimate information to help improve one's skill and is delivered in a private and constructive manner, it represents a learning response and cannot be considered a put-down. Learning to differentiate between the two types of communication helps the nurse to "separate the wheat from the chaff." Reflect on the Student Nurse case.

Student Nurse Case

You examine a crying child's inner ears and note that the tympanic membranes (eardrums) are red. You report to your supervisor that the child may have an ear infection.

A. *Response:* When a child is crying, the drums often swell and redden. How about checking again when the child is calm? *(Learning response)*

Or

B. *Response:* Of course they are red when the child is crying. Didn't you learn that in nursing school? I haven't got time to answer such basic questions! *(Put-down response)*

Which response would you prefer to receive? Why? Whereas the first response allows the nurse to learn useful information to incorporate into practice, the second response serves to antagonize, and it is doubtful much learning takes place. What will happen is that the nurse will be more hesitant about approaching the supervisor again for clinical information. Again, it is the patient who ultimately suffers.

Once a put-down is recognized as such, you need to respond verbally in an assertive manner as soon as possible after the incident has taken place. Waiting an appreciable length of time is likely to cause resentment and loss of self-respect. It may be more difficult later for the other person to remember the details of the incident. At the same time, if your anger, not the problem behavior, is likely to dominate the response, it is better to wait a few minutes for the anger to cool a little and then to present the message in a reasoned manner. Preparing your response is a form of "cognitive rehearsal." You can respond to put-downs in the following way:

- *Address the objectionable or disrespectful behaviors first*. Briefly state the behavior and its impact on you. *Emphasize the specifics of the put-down behavior*. Once the put-down has been dealt with, you can discuss any criticism of your behavior on its own merits. Refer only to the behaviors identified.
- *Prepare a few standard responses*. Because put-downs often catch one by surprise, it is useful to have a standard set of opening replies ready. Exam-

ples might include the following:
- "I found your comments very disturbing and insulting."
- "I feel what you said as an attack. That wasn't called for by my actions."

Use Open Communication

Use standardized communication tools and standardized lists. These tools have been especially found effective during patient handovers. They are effective in improving interdisciplinary communication (Foronda, MacWilliams, & McArthur, 2016).

Criticize Constructively. Giving constructive criticism and receiving criticism is difficult for most people. Refer to Box 23.4. When a supervisor gives constructive criticism, some type of response from the person receiving it is indicated. Initially, it is crucial that the conflict problem be clearly defined and acknowledged. To help handle constructive criticism, nurses can do the following:

- Schedule a time when you are calm.
- Request that supervisory meetings be in a place that allows privacy.

BOX 23.4 Constructive Criticism Example

Steps in Giving:
1. Express sympathy. *Sample statement:* "I understand that things are difficult at home."
2. Describe the behavior. *Sample statement:* "But I see that you have been late coming to work 3 times during this pay period."
3. State expectations. *Sample statement:* "It is necessary for you to be here on time from now on."
4. List consequences. *Sample statement:* "If you get here on time, we'll all start off the shift better. If you are late again, I will have to report you to the personnel department."

Steps in Receiving:
1. Listen and paraphrase. If unclear, ask for specific examples. *Sample reply:* "You are saying being late is not acceptable."
2. Acknowledge you are taking suggestions seriously. *Sample comment:* "I hear what you are saying."
3. Give your side by stating supportive facts, without being defensive. *Sample comment:* "My car would not start."
4. Develop a plan for the future. *Sample plan:* "With this paycheck I will repair my car. Until then I'll ask Mary for a ride."

- Defuse personal anxiety.
- Listen carefully to the criticism and then paraphrase it.
- Acknowledge that you take suggestions for improvement seriously.
- Discuss the facts of the situation, but avoid becoming defensive.
- Develop a plan for dealing with similar situations; become proactive rather than reactive.
- Maintain open dialogue.

Document and Report Disruptive Behaviors

A crucial aspect of sustaining quality care is the ability to confront a team member whose behaviors violate accepted norms. Studies show that reporting a colleague to an authority figure without talking the objectionable behavior over with him or her is not effective in restoring harmony. Yet surveys show that the vast majority of physicians and nurses are reluctant to either confront or report. If your attempts to directly discuss behavior with the involved person fail to achieve behavior change, then you need to follow the agency's process and report the problem. In handling disruptive behavior occurrences, documentation is a key step. Hopefully the agency has a no-blame process, but remember that when pushed, many people will retaliate. Be aware!

Some agencies may hold "communication training sessions" after the offenses have been documented. Simulations such as Simulation Exercise 23.3 have you practice strategies to promote a healthy workplace.

SIMULATION EXERCISE 23.3
Communication to Promote a Healthy Work Environment

Suggestions include negotiating with nurse administrators to avoid being assigned to multiple shifts, or allowing small breaks every few hours to recharge; texting or posting affirmation (positive) messages for all the staff to read; saying or texting a message of "good job" or "thank you" to a team member; using humor; putting a smile on your face.

Purpose:
To brainstorm ideas about communicating with team members and administration to facilitate a healthier workplace.

Directions:
Gather in small groups to role play ways to communicate which might help promote a pleasant, healthy work environment.
Reflect, then compare ideas.

DEVELOP A SUPPORT SYSTEM

Collegial relationships are an important determinant of success for professionals. Since lack of support is associated with workplace conflicts (Almost et al., 2016), you need to make positive efforts to create a support system network. Don't just passively wait and hope it happens. Integrity, respect for others, dependability, a good sense of humor, and an openness to sharing with others are communication qualities people look for in developing a support system.

Positive Reinforcement

Everyone likes to be recognized for their efforts. Simple steps such as saying "thank you" or texting a "job well done" message to colleagues is appreciated. In organizations that have integrated team training and safety initiatives, participation in team activities is integrated into job evaluations. In some agencies, positive evaluations are tied to bonuses. Other organizations hold formal and informal affairs to recognize and celebrate efforts to improve communication and safety.

ORGANIZATIONAL STRATEGIES FOR CONFLICT PREVENTION AND RESOLUTION

Organizational climate. The American Nurses Association (ANA) Position Statement on "Incivility, Bullying, and Workplace Violence" (2015b) mandates that nurses and employers work to create a climate of respect using evidence-based strategies, including containing measures for accountability, negotiation, respect, and trust. Specific strategies mentioned by Dzurec et al. (2017), OSHA (2015), and many others include:

- Zero tolerance policy for disrespect (Organizations Code of Conduct)
- Continuing education programs to raise awareness and teach conflict intervention skills
- Accountability follow-up
- Creation of a corporate climate conveying respect for all workers.

Promote opportunities for interdisciplinary communication. Creating opportunities for interdisciplinary groups to get together is a highly effective strategy for enhancing collaboration and communication. Ideas for opportunities to get together include collaborative rounds, huddles, team briefings and debriefings, and committee meetings to discuss problems. Some studies associate daily team rounds and joint decision making with shorter hospital stays and lower hospital charges.

Promote understanding of the organizational system. Whenever you work in an organization, you automatically become a part of a system that has norms for acceptable behavior. Each organizational system defines its own chain of command and its rules about social processes in professional communication. Even though your idea may be excellent, failure to understand the chain of command, or an unwillingness to form the positive alliances needed to accomplish your objective, dilutes the impact.

Although sidestepping the identified chain of command and going to a higher or more tangential resource in the hierarchy may appear less threatening initially, the benefits of such action may not resolve the difficulty. Furthermore, the trust needed for serious discussion becomes limited. Some of the reasons for avoiding positive interactions stem from an internal circular process of faulty thinking. Because communication is viewed as part of a process, the sender and receiver act on the information received, which may or may not represent the reality of the situation.

Promote clear policies. As mentioned earlier, regulatory bodies are requiring that health care organizations have written codes of behavior and internal processes to handle disruptive behaviors.

Ongoing continuing education stressing awareness and safety training is advocated by OSHA (2015). Prevention strategies might include participation in assertiveness training, inservices, or participation in the TeamSTEPPS program. Educational interventions that increase staff awareness are extremely effective, as are simulations similar to the exercises in this book. It is not enough to offer an educational intervention once; team ongoing training is necessary. Literature recommends periodic reassessment of need, and offering reviews of communication skills and conflict management strategies.

SUMMARY

In this chapter the same principles of communication used with conflicts in the nurse-patient relationship are broadened to examine the nature of communication among health professionals on the health care team. Most nurses will experience conflicts with coworkers at some point during their careers. The same elements of thoughtful purpose, authenticity, empathy, active listening, and respect for the dignity of others that underscore successful nurse-patient relationships are needed in relations with other health professionals. Building effective communication with colleagues involves concepts of collaboration, coordination, and networking. Modification of barriers to professional communication includes negotiation and conflict resolution. Learning is a lifelong process, not only for nursing care skills but for communication skills. These will develop as you continue to gain experience working as part of an interdisciplinary health care team.

ETHICAL DILEMMA: What Would You Do?
You are working a 12-hr shift on a labor and delivery unit. Today, Mrs. Kalim is one of your assigned patients. She is fully dilated and effaced, but contractions are still 2 min apart after 10 hr of labor. Mrs. Kalim, her obstetrician, Dr. Mar and you have agreed on her plan to have a fully natural delivery without medication. However, her obstetrician's partner is handling day shift today. This new obstetrician orders you to administer several medications to Mrs. Kalim to strengthen contractions and speed up delivery because he has another patient across town to deliver. Your unit adheres to an empowering model of practice that believes in patient advocacy. How will you handle this potential physician conflict? Is this a true moral dilemma?

DISCUSSION QUESTIONS

1. Reflect on a time someone tried to intimidate or bully you. How did you feel? Assemble and support some productive strategies for responding in such situations.

2. Develop a list of strategies that seem to work best when communicating with team members from outside nursing to facilitate a collaborative environment.

DEVELOPING AN EVIDENCE-BASED PRACTICE: TEAM COMMUNICATION AND COLLABORATION The hospital's goal was to meet TJC requirements for using a standardized handoff process at change of shift, and to increase patient involvement in their care. The Agency determined that using bedside rounds for change of shift report would meet these requirements. After a prior implementation was unsuccessful, a new initiative involved quasi-experimental study was on two selected units. Based on Lewin's change theory, and with staff nurse input, the intervention team first identified nurse barriers. They then fostered nurse buy-in by educating staff

continued

regarding benefits, including Medicare financial incentives to the agency. The researchers addressed nurse-leader and staff nurse concerns including those about protecting patient privacy. They recommend related the use of the standardized shift report in SBAR format to increases in patient safety and satisfaction. The implementation team monitored compliance and a pre- and post-questionnaire measured patient satisfaction.

Results: Use of change of shift bedside rounds for report increased on both units as did patient satisfaction.

Application to Your Clinical Practice: It is well documented that collaborative strategies should include mutual goal setting, decision making and problem solving. Changing practice routines benefited from opening up communication between administrators and staff nurses, showing their concerns were understood or valued. Collaboration is a dynamic process. As the Misfeldt et al. (2017) report shows, on a team level, communication, relationships, and accountability are valued.

For fun, access some of the many videos on the Internet, such as www.bing.com/videos/browse (type in "communication of hospitals") and analyze communication processes. Google "Take the Bus" and reflect on what these cartoons can mean in relation to teamwork.

Example Research: Scheidenhelm, S., & Reitz, O. E. (2017). Hardwiring bedside shift report. *The Journal of Nursing Administration, 47*(3), 147–153.

REFERENCES

Abourbih, D., Armstrong, S., Nixon, K., & Ackery, A. D. (2015). Communication between nurses and physicians: Strategies to surviving in the emergency department trenches. *Emergency Medicine Australasia, 27*, 80–82.

Agency for Healthcare Research and Quality (AHRQ). (n.d.). *PSNet: Patient safety network. Patient safety primers: Disruptive and unprofessional behavior.* Retrieved from: http://psnet.ahrq.gov/primerHome.aspx. [click on disruptive behavior]. Accessed 10.05.18.

Agency for Healthcare Research and Quality (AHRQ). (2017). *TeamSTEPPS webinar Teams, TeamSTEPPS, and Team Structures: Models for Functional Collaboration.* Retrieved from: www.ahrq.gov/teamstepps/events/webinars/feb-2017.html. Accessed 26.09.18.

Almost, J., Wolff, A. C., Stewart-Pyne, A., McCormick, L. G., Strachan, D., & D'Souza, C. (2016). Managing and mitigating conflict in healthcare teams: An integrative review. *Journal of Advanced Nursing, 72*(7), 1490–1505.

American Medical Association (AMA). (2008). *Opinion 9.045 physicians with disruptive behavior.* Retrieved from: www.ama-assn.org/ama/pub/physician-resources/medical-ethics/code-medical-ethics/opinion9045.pageabout-ama/our-people or www.ama-assn.org/go/omss.

American Nurses Association (ANA). (2015b). *Position statements; incivility, bullying, and workplace violence.* Retrieved from: www.nursingworld.org/Bullying-Workplace-Violence. Accessed 10.05.18.

Boev, C., & Xia, Y. (2015). Nurse-physician collaboration and hospital acquired infections in critical care. *Critical Care Nurse, 35*(2), 66–72.

Castronovo, M. A., Pullizzi, A., & Evans, S. (2016). Nurse bullying: A review and a proposed solution. *Nursing Outlook, 64*(3), 208–214.

Costello, J., Clarke, C., Gravely, G., D'Agostino-Rose, D., & Puopolo, R. (2011). Working together to build a respectful workplace: Transforming OR culture. *AORN Journal, 93*(1), 115–126.

Dzurec, L. C., Kennison, M., & Gillen, P. (2017). The incongruity of workplace bullying victimization and inclusive excellence. *Nursing Outlook, 65*(5), 588–598. https://doi.org/10.1016/j.outlook.2017.01.012.

Eriksen, T. L., Hogh, A., & Hansen, A. M. (2016). Long-term consequences of workplace bullying on sickness absence. *Labour Economics, 43*, 129–150.

Farrell, K., Payne, C., & Heye, M. (2015). Integrating interprofessional collaboration skills into the advanced practice registered nurse socialization process. *Journal of Professional Nursing, 31*(1), 5–10.

Fewster-Thuente, L. (2015). Working together toward a common goal: A grounded theory of nurse-physician collaboration. *MedSurg Nursing, 24*(5), 356–362.

Foronda, C., MacWilliams, B., & McArthur, E. (2016). Interprofessional communication in healthcare: An integrative review. *Nurse Education in Practice, 19*, 36–40.

Institute of Medicine (IOM). (2003). *Health professions education: A bridge to quality.* Washington, DC: National Academies Press.

Interprofessional Education Collaborative Expert Panel. (2011). *Core competencies for interprofessional collaborative practice: Repost of an expert panel.* Washington, DC: Interprofessional Education Collaborative. Retrieved from: www.aacn.nche.edu/education-resources/ipecreport.pdf. Author.

Johansen, M. L. (2012). Keeping the peace: Conflict management strategies for nurse managers. *Nursing Management, 43*(2), 50–54.

Kimes, A., Davis, L., Medlock, A., & Bishop, M. (2015). 'I'm not calling him!': Disruptive physician behavior in the acute care setting. *MedSurg Nursing, 24*(4), 223–227.

Koh, W. M. S. (2016). Management of work place bullying in hospital: A review of the use of cognitive rehearsal as an alternative management strategy. *International Journal of Nursing Sciences, 3*(2), 213–222.

Lyndon, A., Johnson, M. C., Bingham, D., Napolitano, P. G., Joseph, G., Maxfield, D. G., et al. (2015). Transforming communication and safety culture in intrapartum care: A multi-organization blueprint. *JOGNN, 44*(3), 341–349.

Mace-Vadjunec, D., Hileman, B. M., Melnykovich, M. B., Hanes, M. C., Chance, E. A., & Emerick, E. S. (2015). The lack of common goals and communication within a Level I trauma system: Assessing the silo effect among trauma center employees. *Journal of Trauma Nursing, 22*(5), 274–281.

Misfeldt, R., Suter, E., Oelke, N., Hepp, S., & Lait, J. (2017). Creating high performing primary health care teams in Alberta, Canada: Mapping out the key issues using a socioecological model. *Journal of Interprofessional Education & Practice, 6*, 27–32.

Moore, L. W., Sublett, C., & Leahy, C. (2017). Nurse managers speak out about disruptive nurse-to-nurse relationships. *JONA, 47*(1), 24–29.

Nielsen, P., & Mann, S. (2008). Team function in obstetrics to reduce errors and improve outcomes. *Obstetrics and Gynecology Clinics of North America, 35*(1), 81–95.

OSHA. (2015). *Guidelines for preventing workplace violence for healthcare & social workers.* OSHA Publication No. 3148. Author.

Perry, V., Christiansen, M., & Simmons, A. (2016). A daily goals tool to facilitate indirect nurse-physician communication during morning rounds on a medical-surgical unit. *MedSurg Nursing, 25*(2), 83–87.

Polis, S., Higgs, M., Manning, V., Netto, G., & Fernandez, R. (2017). Factors contributing to nursing team work in an acute care tertiary hospital. *Collegian, 24*(1), 19–25.

Press, M. J., Gerber, L. M., Peng, T. R., Pesko, M. F., Feldman, P. H., Ouchida, K., et al. (2015). Post-discharge communication between home health nurses and physicians: Measurement, quality, and outcomes. *JAGS, 63*, 1299–1305.

Quality and Safety Education for Nurses QSEN Institute. (n.d.). *Pre-licensure KSAS.* Retrieved from: http://qsen.org/competencies/pre-licensure-ksas/. Accessed 22.09.18.

Quality and Safety Education for Nurses QSEN Institute. (n.d.). *Teamwork and collaboration QSEN learning module.* Retrieved from: www.qsen.org/ or www.aacn.nche.edu/qsen/workshop.details/new_orleans/EE-TWC.pdf. [click on Modules (learning module 10)]. Accessed 22.09.18.

Quality and Safety Education for Nurses/ (n.d.). Pre-licensure competency. www.QSEN.org.

TeamSTEPPS. (2017). *National TeamSTEPPS conference,* June 13, 2017. Cleveland, OH.

The Joint Commission (TJC). (2008). *Behaviors that undermine a culture of safety* (40). Sentinel Event Alert. Retrieved from: http://www.jointcommission.org/assets/1/18/SEA_40.pdf.

The Joint Commission (TJC). (2009). *Appendix A: Checklists to advance effective communication, cultural competence, and patient- and family-centered care for the lesbian, gay, bisexual, and transgender (LGBT) community.* A field guide, 35. Retrieved from: http://www.jointcommission.org/assets/1/18/LGBTFieldGuide.pdf. Accessed 10.05.18.

The Joint Commission (TJC). (2010). *Preventing violence in the health care setting* (45). Sentinel Event Alert. Retrieved from: http://www.jointcommission.org/assets/1/18/sea_45.pdf.

The Joint Commission (TJC). (2015). *Advancing effective communication, cultural competence, and patient- and family-centered care.* Retrieved from: http://www.jointcommission.org/Advancing_Effective_Communication/. Accessed 10.05.18 by clicking on the window].

Trepanier, S., Fernet, C., Austin, S., & Boudrias, V. (2016). Work environment antecedents of bullying: A review and integrative model applied to registered nurses. *International Journal of Nursing Studies, 55*, 85–97.

Weaver, K. B. (2013). The effects of horizontal violence and bullying on new nurse retention. *Journal for Nurses in Professional Development, 29*(3), 138–142.

World Health Organization (WHO). (2016). *Setting priorities for global patient safety.* Italy: Conference Florence. Retrieved from: www.who.int/patientsafety/. Accessed 10.05.18.

SUGGESTED READING

Agency for Healthcare Research and Quality (AHRQ). (2014). *TeamSTEPPS 2.0: Instructor manual: Table of contents.* Rockville, MD: Agency for Healthcare Research and Quality.

24

Communicating for Continuity of Care

Elizabeth C. Arnold

OBJECTIVES

At the end of the chapter, the reader will be able to:

1. Explain the concept of continuity of care (COC) in contemporary health care systems.
2. Describe current challenges in the health care system, related to COC.
3. Discuss applications of relational continuity in patient-centered care and interdisciplinary team collaboration.
4. Apply informational continuity concepts in transitional and discharge planning processes.
5. Discuss applications of management continuity related to case management, care coordination, and navigation of the health care system.

INTRODUCTION

The Cambridge dictionary defines a paradigm shift as "a time when the usual and accepted way of doing or thinking about something changes completely." Starting with the Institute of Medicine (IOM) report, Crossing the Quality Chasm in 2001, there has been the strong realization that health care systems organized around acute, episodic care no longer suffice as a primary service model. The complexity of contemporary health care requires a different care process to match new health realities (Mitchell et al., 2012). There are several reasons for the dramatic shift to community-based health models as a primary source of health care delivery. Examples include: longer life spans, demographics of the population with greater ethnic and racial diversity, skilled provider shortages, and cost.

Technology advances in diagnosis and treatment and discovery of novel medications and treatments have reduced the incidence of premature death from acute health conditions. Instead, chronic disorders account for people now self-managing previously untreatable cancers and other conditions as chronic health conditions with a good quality of life for longer periods of time as the rule rather than the exception. Thus attention has turned to chronic disease management, early detection, and interventions to enhance lifestyle health behaviors within a shared care process.

Patients are discharged earlier and sicker, often with complex medication and treatment regimens, which need to be followed in the community in primary care settings.

Chapter 24 explores the concept of continuity of care (COC) as the linchpin in collaborative health team functionality, central to its structure, and operations across contemporary health care systems. Three key features: relational, informational, and management continuity provide a conceptual framework the study and application of COC strategies (Haggerty et al., 2003). Addressing the role of communication in achieving the purposes of COC is essential to ensuring quality, safety, and patient satisfaction across contemporary health care systems.

BASIC CONCEPTS

Worldwide, chronic diseases account for up to 60% of deaths (Paquette-Warren et al., 2014). However, as people live longer, there is a higher incidence of chronic conditions requiring an array of supportive health care services. The focus on care provision has shifted from the hospital to the community and a public health focus using an integrated service framework (Cooke, Gemmill, & Grant, 2008; IOM, 2003). Providing a continuum of aggregated services offers the most comprehensive option for care of patients with chronic physical and mental conditions (Stans, Stevens, & Beurskens, 2013; Porter-O'Grady, 2014).

CONCEPTS

COC describes a multidimensional longitudinal process construct in health care, which emphasizes seamless provision and coordination of patient-centered quality care across clinical settings (Haggerty, Roberge, Freeman, & Beaulieu, 2013). COC operates across three dimensions: relational, informational, and management continuity. These dimensions are interdependent essential components of patient care (Schultz, 2009).

Haggerty et al. (2008) define **relational continuity** as "a therapeutic relationship with a practitioner that spans more than one episode of care and leads, in the practitioner, to a sense of clinical responsibility and an accumulated knowledge of the patient's personal and medical circumstances" (p. 118). Frequent team communication about all aspects of care helps to ensure relational continuity among treatment teams.

Informational continuity refers to the use of data to tailor current treatment and care to each patient's evidenced needs. The concept includes accurate record sharing and technology to allow real-time communication exchanges between providers and with patients in remote sites. It is a primary communication vehicle during care transitions and is used to help patients and families make quality patient care decisions.

Management continuity refers to a consistent, coherent patient-specific care management approach, which can be flexibly adjusted, as a patient's needs change. Care coordination and case management have emerged as significant methodologies associated with management continuity.

The COC process is concerned with the safety and quality of care. COC links acute care with primary care approaches for patients through coordinated, acute care, and community-based health services. The overarching goal of COC is to ensure reliable coordinated transition of patients from one health care setting to another, such that care in each setting continues to provide a secure trustworthy health safety net for individual patients and families that they can rely on for support and information.

Haggerty et al. (2003) suggest that COC contributes to the development of coordinated care through

- Increased accessibility to coordinated health care services with a smoother flow of care from one service area to another
- Personalization of care to meet a patient's changing needs across delivery systems
- Informational data sharing of various elements of personal and medical data electronically over time and place, which contribute to appropriate care delivery
- Health services provided in an organized, logical, and timely manner, using a shared management plan.

Sparbel and Anderson (2000) explain the COC construct as "a series of connected patient-care events both within a health care institution and among multiple settings" (p. 17).

COC decreases the potential for service duplication, conflicting assessments, and gaps in service. It reduces the use of preventable acute care services and lessens medication and treatment errors. Continuity provides timely follow-up and can ease transitions between care settings. For chronically ill and elderly patients, COC means that they are more likely to have health care providers familiar with their overall history, who can notice subtle changes in health status (Von Bultzingslowen, Eliasson, Sarvimaki, Mattsson, & Hjortdahl, 2006).

COC: Treatment Pathway of Choice for Chronic Conditions

COC is the treatment model of choice for chronic health conditions in primary care. The World Health Organization (WHO) (2002) defines *chronic health conditions* as "health problems that require ongoing management over a period of years or decades" (p. 11). Examples of chronic disorders include asthma, fibromyalgia, arthritis, osteoporosis, cancer, multiple sclerosis, diabetes, serious persistent mental disorders, chronic obstructive pulmonary disease (COPD), and congestive heart failure.

Chronic illness is a major cause of death and disability nationally and globally. The Agency for Healthcare Research and Quality (AHRQ, 2013) estimates that up to a third of all adults and 80% of older adults suffer from at least two comorbid chronic conditions. These conditions present symptoms that negatively impact health status, limit functional capacity or quality of life, and require health treatment. Chronic disorders typically have periods of exacerbations and remissions. They share a requirement for ongoing health support and self-care management (Wagner et al., 2001). Chronic disorders disrupt a person's personal life in multiple unexpected ways. Kleinman (1988) explains the impact in this way: "The undercurrent of chronic illness is like the volcano: it does not go away, it menaces. It erupts. It is out of control…confronting crises is only one part of the total picture. The rest is coming to grips with the mundaneness of worries…Chronic illness also means the loss of confidence in one's health and normal bodily processes" (pp. 44–45).

The COC construct is based on an expanded version of the Chronic Care Model, originally developed by Wagner and associates (2001). This model, as presented later, is designed to foster productive interactions between *informed patients and families* and prepared *proactive practice teams* to produce improved clinical outcomes. Application of the chronic care model within the primary health care system functions as a safety net and support by empowering individuals and families to assume primary responsibility for self-management of chronic illness in partnership with ongoing professional support from skilled providers across selected health care settings. This shared responsibility helps to bridge the gap between diminishing financial support for chronic care and its multifaceted care demands, which can last for years. Relevant primary care strategies focus on "patient-centered care, collaborative goal setting, problem solving, and coordinated follow-up" (Glasgow & Goldstein, 2008, p. 129).

Medical Home in Primary Care

Primary care, described as the hub of community-based care, provides a wide range of integrated health care services delivered in a single community-based setting. The *medical home* in primary care serve as the first point of entry for primary care patients. They offer diagnosis and treatment of common nonacute illnesses. Services also include health promotion education, preventive screenings, and health maintenance care. Community resource support, integrated decision backing, and information technology work together to strengthen patient-centered relationships and improve health outcomes (Coleman, Austin, Brach, & Wagner, 2009).

Key features of the medical home in primary care include

- *Person centeredness*, with sustained continuity of relationships between provider and patient
- Functions as a *first contact point* with easy access services for common health care problems
- *Comprehensive care*, which can meet many patient needs without referral
- A highly *personalized form of care* related to a stronger knowledge about individual health care needs and responses over time (IOM, 2012; Starfield & Horder, 2007).

DEVELOPING AN EVIDENCE-BASED PRACTICE

Purpose:
To identify measurable elements that recur over a variety of contexts and health conditions as the basis for developing a generic measure of management continuity.

Method:
This research examined 514 research studies from 1997 to 2007 related to continuity of care when patients see multiple clinicians; 33 studies were identified from the original scan, which matched study criteria of studies related to exploring patients' experiences of health care from various clinicians over time.

Findings:
Patients experienced continuity of care as security and confidence, rather than seamlessness, of care. Information about what to expect and having contingency plans provides security. Patients did not perceive the communication and coordination among clinicians as being direct dimensions of continuity with patients.

Implications for Clinical Practice:
Patients experience continuity through receiving information and having confidence and security in a relationship with a trusted clinician. The authors suggest that it is through gaps in COC services that patients become aware of the benefits of continuity.

From Haggerty, J., Roberge, D., Freeman, G., & Beaulieu, C. (2013). Experienced continuity of care when patients see multiple clinicians: A qualitative metasummary. *Annals of Family Medicine, 11*(3), 262–271.

APPLICATIONS

Coping with chronic conditions is embedded within the context of the larger life patterns and availability of health-related resources. "A common trap in primary care is to consider problems in isolation, failing to respect its multidimensional and longitudinal nature" (Ferrer & Gill, 2013, p. 301). COC recognizes the need to provide structured collaborative efforts in creating workable solutions for patients over time and space.

COC offers a care pathway to safeguard care stability and to provide a secure health safety net for individuals and families that they can rely on for support and information. Each dimension of COC—relational, informational, and management continuity—ideally works together to set directions and implement coordinated interventions throughout the health care system. Guilliford, Naithani, and Morgan (2006) advocate viewing COC from both patient and provider perspectives. This makes sense given the level of partnership needed to ensure continuity.

RELATIONAL CONTINUITY

Relational continuity refers to the interpersonal elements of the COC model across time and care settings. The term applies to nurse-patient and family relationships, team relationships, and relationships between health system providers, and community-based supports. The stronger the relationships, the greater are the potential for quality-coordinated care. Respect for patient and family values, beliefs, knowledge, cultural background, and preferences are fundamental aspects of patient-centered relational continuity. Trusting relationships with a primary provider or "medical home" health care team gives patients confidence that their care needs will be consistently met.

The goal of relational COC is to develop sustained patient-provider relationships in which informed, motivated patients interact with prepared, proactive professional health care teams to achieve identified health goals for chronic health conditions. Recent Joint Commission patient-centered communication standards include data on communication with physicians and nurses, responsiveness of staff, communication about medications, pain management, and discharge planning as measurable outcomes (The Joint Commission, 2013). Increasing the level of collaboration among health care professionals is identified as a primary strategy for improving the level of continuity needed for successful health care outcomes (San Martin-Rodriguez, D'Amour, & Leduc, 2008; Van Servellen, Fongwa, & Mockus D'Errico, 2006).

NEW ROLES IN CONTINUITY OF CARE

Continuity of care is described as "the connectedness between different stages in the health care system among the patient, health care professionals, and the organization" (Renholm, Suominen, Puukka, & Leino-Kilpi, 2016, p. 2). Health care reform has led to the development of new professional relational roles and service delivery approaches to better address the nation's health needs. Innovative roles include the hospitalist, the medical home, and collaborative interdisciplinary team-based care delivery. When thinking about COC, nurses and other health professionals should consider the health experience as a whole.

Hospitalist

A new professional role designed to improve COC in acute care settings is that of the "hospitalist" (Amin & Owen, 2006). The *hospitalist* may be a physician or nurse practitioner employed by the hospital to clinically manage a patient's medical care. The hospitalist specializes in medical care of hospitalized patients and assumes *full* responsibility for coordinating care, ordering, and integrating diagnostic test results, making decisions, presenting options to the patient and family, and communicating with other professionals who may be, or will become involved in the patient's care after discharge. The specific dimensions of the hospitalist role are determined by the care site rather than clinical specialty (Schneller & Epstein, 2006). Specialty physicians function as consultants.

Nurses play an important communication role with hospitalists. They function as key informants, skilled practitioners, patient advocates, and supporters of coordinated care in hospital settings. Patients do not have a prior relationship with the hospitalist prior to hospitalization and vice versa. As the patient's nurse, you are responsible for carrying out the hospitalist's orders. Nurses should be proactive by talking informally with hospitalists about their patients and presenting information formally in collaborative team meetings.

As a patient's condition changes, the hospitalist meets with the family to discuss changes, treatment options, and family concerns. Even in the best of circumstances, patient and family meetings with the hospitalist and/or health care team to discuss sensitive health issues such as discontinuing life support or transfer of patients can be intimidating. Nurses can help patients and families by continuing conversations after the hospitalist or health care team leaves, answering questions and providing support.

Medical Home

The *medical home* is considered a "concept" as well as a "place" in primary care. As a concept, it has particular relevance for increasing access to primary care in the public sector (Crabtree et al., 2010). A medical home accepts responsibility for providing regular, accessible, comprehensive primary care services for designated patients and families within a single familiar setting. It serves as a central first point of contact in primary care through which the majority of patient health needs are met (Grumbach & Bodenheimer, 2002; Keeling & Lewenson, 2013).

Patients depend on their medical home as a first-line treatment resource. Physicians, nurse practitioners, physician's assistants, nurses, social workers, dentists, and other health care providers can provide better-quality care because they have ongoing knowledge of the patient's medical and lifestyle issues. Subtle changes in the patient's situation or health status are recognized in subsequent care visits.

External coordination of health care services with specialists and community agencies expand the capabilities of the medical home. Because they are part of a larger health system in many cases, referrals are accomplished efficiently. Information passes swiftly and accurately between providers. There is less chance of duplicative or unnecessary medical appointments because care is coordinated through the patient's medical home. Of course, a critical element is that professional recipients of patient data have to carefully read the reports. Quality and safety are essential characteristics of primary care medical homes (see Chapter 2 for general principles associated with safety).

Relational Continuity on Collaborative Health Teams

Relational continuity on collaborative health teams describes an active, ongoing alliance between health care professionals from different disciplines who work together in complementary roles to provide integrated health care services. Each team

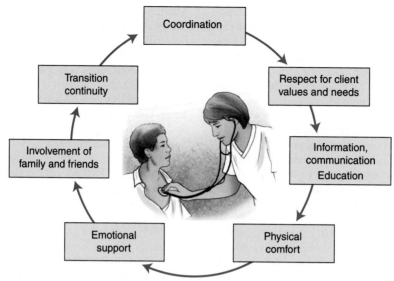

Fig. 24.1 Dimensions of patient-centered care in continuity of care (COC).

member brings skills to address different aspects of a patient's illness experience, but the team is expected to as a coordinated unit. Some functions overlap; others are complementary. All functions must be coordinated so that the team functions as an integrated unit. Team meetings allow skilled professionals to develop mutual understandings developed about common problems as a foundation for generating stronger innovative solutions. Professional health care team collaboration is an important contributor to total quality management and is identified as a nursing quality and safety in education and nursing competency (see Chapter 2).

SPECIAL FUNCTION TEAMS engage in coordinated activities to ensure that COC meets targeted patient-centered needs. Examples of special function teams include disaster response teams, acute care hospital teams, medical home–based and home care teams, mental health emergency teams, and palliative care teams (Mitchell et al., 2012). Collaborative health care teams are broadly classified as multidisciplinary, interdisciplinary, and transdisciplinary teams with the expectation that care will be provided through the combined collaborative efforts of two or more skilled clinical practitioners.

Interdisciplinary team relationships take into account the diverse standards and behaviors associated with each clinical discipline, while emphasizing a common mission of working together to resolve complex clinical problems (Clark, Cott, & Drinka, 2007; D'Amour & Oandasan, 2005). Team members are expected to value and respect diversity in the personal, cultural, and experiential backgrounds of each professional.

In formal meetings, relational continuity is encouraged by setting a direction, prioritizing agenda items and activities, and establishing realistic boundaries about care contributions. Members monitor potential relationship safety issues such as status differences and receptiveness to taking interpersonal risks, when others disagree. When interprofessional team members deal with relational group process issues successfully, members experience higher levels of learning and satisfaction with team care outcomes.

ESSENTIAL ELEMENTS OF RELATIONAL CONTINUITY

Development of therapeutic relationship with known providers offers a consistent fundamental communication channel patients can use to secure better health care services, which are tailored to their specific health needs. The interpersonal process relations required for relational COC involve the three C's: patient Centeredness, Collaboration, and Coordination in a shared enterprise of therapeutic care delivery across multiple systems (Stans et al., 2013).

Fig. 24.1 presents components of patient-centered care. Patients should be key informants, active negotiators, final decision makers, and engaged participants in evaluating treatment outcomes (Engebretson, Mahoney, & Carlson, 2008). They need to be actively involved in defining and updating realistic treatment goals. Patient centeredness is evidenced in a partnership characterized by mutual valuing and safeguarding of the legitimate interests of the provider and the patient in creating and managing health care decisions.

Shared decision making is a key element of relational continuity with patients and with the entire team. The decision-making process starts with providing each patient with sufficient information tailored to his or her unique circumstances to make an *informed* decision. The information must be in a format and language easily understandable to the patient. Information should be relevant to each patient's diagnosis, treatments, and treatment options. The first question you should consider is: What *essential* information does this patient need to have in order to make an informed decision? Some patients value knowing as much as possible; others want just the basic facts. Another may need to have essential information developed in steps and spread over several encounters. This accommodation allows for better processing and formulation of related questions. Cultural norms also can dictate levels of information and to whom the information should be given (see Chapter 7).

A second query is: What level of information does the patient *desire at this point in time?* For example, a patient with newly diagnosed terminal ovarian cancer focuses on a long trip she wants to take in the future. She suggests several times that she is going to make it and not die from her cancer. Empathetic acceptance of the patient as she is in processing a diagnosis is more helpful than presenting her with "facts" that she is not willing to accept in the current moment. Other professionals should be alerted to differences in patient informational needs and/or consulted so that all caregivers are on the same page.

To ensure that care decisions respect patient values, needs, and preferences, you need to observe and listen carefully to the patient description of his or her health experience. These data become the basis for providing patients and families with the tailored education and support they need to make reasoned health care decisions. Relevant information includes

- Detailed information on diagnosis
- Options for treatment and what to expect
- Risks and benefits of each treatment approach
- Anticipated clinical outcomes
- Treatment and care processes required to achieve desired clinical outcomes

Consistency of personnel over time allows patients and the professional team to share a stronger investment in achieving personalized quality health outcomes. Providers and patients learn to know, value, and respect each other. Box 24.1 identifies essential competencies for effective collaborative communication in team meetings.

COLLABORATION

The second C in relational continuity is collaboration. A goal of interprofessional relational collaboration is to

---

BOX 24.1 Essential Competencies for Effective Collaboration in Team Meetings

- Self-awareness of professional strengths and limitations, values, assumptions, biases, and expectations of self and others.
- Appreciate and accommodate for individual and professional diversity among team members, including gender-related communication style, different professional cultures, and differential professional perspectives.
- Develop professional tact and constructive conflict resolution skills to cope with contested professional barriers in delivery of collaborative care.
- Develop a synthesis of perspectives through negotiation, and work toward a creative integration of ideas acceptable to all interdisciplinary team members.
- Deliberately develop a sense of shared power to create win-win situations. Invite less verbal participants to express their opinion. Emphasize mutual exchange of ideas as the best way to develop shared power.
- Cultivate clinical competence, self-confidence, and assertiveness as professional attributes underlying your professional contributions. Seize all opportunities to present expertise as a way of building trust.
- Demonstrate knowledge of multiple interconnections associated with systems thinking and group dynamics. Develop the ability to view each clinical situation and collaborative processes within the larger organization and health care system.
- Be prepared and present (physically and mentally) throughout structured team meetings. Become aware of conflicting agendas and the diverse values of team members, so you can advocate effectively for patients.
- Become knowledgeable about timing and group development through group processes (see Chapter 7).
- Legitimize and incorporate opportunities for spontaneous collaborative conversations into more formal discussions.
- Respect the balance between autonomy and unity present in collaborative discussions.
- Remember that there is no "perfect" solution and that the patient is usually the final decision maker.
- Differentiate between problems requiring simple decisions and complex, challenging clinical situations requiring a collaborative, integrative solution. Collaboration is not required for all decisions.

Modified from Gardner, D. (2005). Ten lessons in collaboration. *Online Journal of Issues in Nursing, 10*(1), 2.

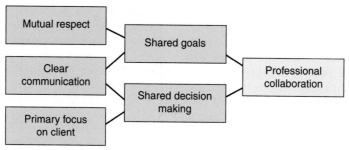

Fig. 24.2 Characteristics of Collaboration.

produce "a synthesis of the information such that the outcomes are more than additive" (Muir, 2008, p. 5). Patients need an integrated consistent flow of informed communication among providers and community agencies about their treatment and care.

Interdisciplinary collaboration enables practitioners to learn new skills and approaches and encourages synergistic creativity among professionals. As different disciplines work closely together, they build new understandings about each other's expertise and trust in each other to develop consensus about the best approaches to each patient's unique health care situation. Each discipline member is cognizant of unique and shared spheres of responsibility with team members from other disciplines. Structured team collaboration decreases fragmentation and duplication of effort and promotes safe quality care (see Chapter 2). Fig. 24.2 presents desired characteristics of relational interprofessional collaboration.

The level of collaborative team communication between patients and providers and between providers affects treatment outcomes and patient satisfaction. Receiving care within an ongoing therapeutic relationship with the same group of providers over time, with care that follows the patient across primary and secondary care setting enhances the patient's confidence. Mitchell et al. (2012) identify five principles of collaborative team effectiveness: "shared goals, clear roles, mutual trust, effective communication, and measurable processes and outcomes" (p. 6). Setting forth measurable process and outcome benchmarks from the outset of care planning helps all involved participants to keep an eye on the goal with formative evaluations along the way to correct for error.

COORDINATION

The third C of relational COC is coordination. Effective coordination depends on the development of dynamic relationships among involved professionals. Relationships are as important to success as content. Shared goals and basic knowledge regarding each provider's work such that each provider knows how that work fits together as a whole is key to understanding coordination and its role in facilitating positive clinical outcomes. Havens, Vasey, Gittell, and Lin (2010) suggest that relational understanding is particularly important as "participants from different disciplines often reside in different 'thought worlds' because of differences in training, socialization and expertise" (p. 928). The other knowledge requirement for active coordination relates to patient factors—preferences, financial resources, access to care, support systems, etc., because any of these can result in an unintended misalliance. Developing shared goals allows for effective coordination for treatment of chronic conditions.

Shared Goals

Shared goals are an essential product of effective patient-centered collaboration and coordination. The patient and family should be critical team members in determining, refining, and updating goals. Their inclusion as a collaborative team member allows for a more realistic assessment of a patient's needs, preferences, resources, and personal goals. They can provide important input into how things are going and can sensitize providers to realistic needs and priorities.

Patients and families are unique members of the care team. Usually they lack formal training in health care and may not always understand the medical language used in team meetings. Although the same team members interact with each other on a regular basis informally in the care of patients, this is not true of patient and/or members. Nurses are an essential resource in helping to orient and introduce nonprofessional team members to the roles and expectations of collaborative teamwork and to adapt medical language so that it easily understood (Mitchell et al., 2012).

Discussion at team meetings should focus on shared goals developed by the patient and professional team members. Carefully defining the patient's health problem and identifying possible contributing factors is an essential first step before moving on to brainstorming potential solutions. Unrelated data can compromise the concentration of the team on key patient/family needs and solutions.

Problem-solving communication should be respectful, accurate, timely, and frequent. Aim for developing share meanings rather than simple information exchanges. Mutual trust and respect for differences offer powerful reinforcement for open dialog. Once agreement is reached, the entire team, including the patient, needs to take full responsibility for implementing clearly described action plans.

Role Clarity

Role clarity is an essential prerequisite for relational continuity on interdisciplinary health care and community-based family care teams. Effective collaborative participation requires a clear understanding of one's own discipline's values and expected level of skill and scope of practice, *plus* a knowledge of and mutual respect for other team member discipline's roles, professional responsibilities, and expertise (Lidskog, Lofmark, & Ahlstrom, 2007).

Team members function both as an individual professional representing a distinct discipline *and* as a collaborative health care team member. Mosser and Begun (2014) note that "the roles, education and values of different health professions give each profession a distinctive character on teams" (p. 55). Each discipline has its own set of behavioral norms and professional ethics. Although they may be similar, they are neither identical in scope nor in implementation of care. Studies of provider perspectives on effective team functioning identify role understanding and interpersonal communication as being the most important variables affecting role functioning on interdisciplinary teams (Cramm & Nieboer, 2011).

Even when core personal and professional values, attitudes, and practices are not at odds with each other, professional training and interpretations of standards can shape how professional values are prioritized (D'Amour & Oandasan, 2005; Hall, 2005). Team role confusion, fueled by professional rivalries, territoriality, and lack of clarification about job responsibilities, is identified as a potential barrier to effective team communication (Sparbel & Anderson, 2000). Simulation Exercise 24.1, "Learning about Other Health Professions," offers an opportunity to understand roles of different health professions.

Mutual Trust

In time, health professionals from different disciplines learn to trust and rely on each other's competence and it becomes easier to support each other's efforts (Guilliford et al., 2006). This is unlikely to happen without regularly scheduled interdisciplinary team meetings. Unless there is a formal time and place for collaborative dialog, the necessary professional

---

SIMULATION EXERCISE 24.1 Learning About Other Health Professions

Purpose:
To familiarize students to differences and similarities in education and skill sets of key interdisciplinary health team members.

Procedure:
1. Break the class into teams of four to six students. Assign each student group a professional role to explore by describing the educational preparation and expected skill set of one of the following professional disciplines: physician, pharmacist, social worker, nurse practitioner.
2. (Initial research can be done as an out of class assignment.) Write a concise description about your assigned discipline, which can be easily explained to your team members.
3. Identify and agree upon 10 to 12 key descriptors related to your findings and the dominant features of the profession within your team group.
4. Each discipline team group should present its findings to the larger class group.

Discussion:
1. Compare and contrast similarities and differences in education and expected skill sets identified by each team.
2. In what ways might the skill sets of each discipline complement each other in patient-centered clinical care and decision making?
3. How could you use what you learned in this exercise to create better communication with other health care professionals?

---

connectivity for interdisciplinary collaboration will not take place in a meaningful way. Team meetings allow different disciplinary professionals to get to know each other. They also provide a forum for discussion of potential conflicts. Patients can sense when their care team is having conflicts. This tends to make the team's comments less credible, leading to potential confusion and adverse outcomes. Consistent consultations offer a scheduled opportunity to develop team-working processes, discuss potential conflicts, and reinforce commitment to delivering quality collaborative health care.

Effective Communication

Team communication skills are similar to those you would use in any professional health care situation. Added to these are specialized team communication skill sets, which include flexibility and openness, critical discernment skills, reading and writing proficiency, speaking, and nonverbal communication skills.

Interdisciplinary team meeting communication differs from other forms of work group communication, although similar group development processes occur (see Chapter 8). The focus of team group meetings is always on the immediate care issues of the patient. Each team member, including the patient, is personally accountable for sharing relevant patient information, listening to the comments of others, and actively participating in focused problem solving and decision discussions. In team group meetings, it is important to respect the diversity, professional values, and ideas of each team member even when you do not agree with them. It is important to respect and consider the input of other team members who may approach the same situation from a very different perspective.

Here are some simple tips you can use in team meetings to enhance communication in team and task groups:

- *Listen before you speak.* Attentive listening is one of the strongest collaborative communication skills. When you take a measured listening stance, you show respect for the speaker. As you hear the other person's words, visually attend to the attitudes and nonverbal behaviors of the speaker and other team members. These are important information-transmitting factors, which can influence understanding, so that you can respond appropriately.
- *Know what you are talking about.* When you share clinical observations and professional opinions in team meetings, be as informed, authentic, specific, and descriptive as possible. Honest feedback and genuine sharing builds trust and strengthens professional relationships, even when ideas are being challenged. Evidence-based data provide an underpinning for interdisciplinary discussions. Nurses can communicate a critical appraisal of a patient's presenting issues, health needs, preferences, values, and personal responses. This is your forte. Nurses spend the most time with patients and have the most "talking and observing" sustained contact with them.
- *Use your voice wisely.* Nurses' active participation in formal team meetings is essential. You do not have to comment on everything, but your input is unique and critical to the discussion. Information about the patient as a person and human responses to illness and treatment represents data nurses are best positioned to share.
- *Be open to different ideas.* A strong advantage of team communication is that it allows more than one viewpoint to bear on a health situation. Exploration of different ideas and perspectives enriches the problem-solving

approaches needed to develop a coordinated consistent and workable approach to difficult patient issues. Have knowledge of the differences in role responsibilities and common values of other disciplines so you can better frame messages and can understand their perspective. Recognize your limitations, as well as your strengths, and how you might be able to incorporate the expertise of other disciplines in total patient care.

- *Ask for feedback.* Encourage other team members with whom you interact to provide relevant feedback, for example, "I'd like to hear what you think about this." Analyze the information you receive, and ask relevant open-ended questions. Brainstorming and problem-solving processes are indispensable to developing the most workable solutions. Interdisciplinary team decisions should be negotiated, not dictated, with all members being mindful of working though their individual differences in a respectful manner. Consensus solutions work best and are more easily implemented.
- *Work within the system.* Although patients are the core focus of care, health care centers are part of much larger health care management systems, which influence team functions and outcomes (Ginter, Duncan, & Swayne, 2013). System factors beyond the control of the patient and the direct care team will influence what is and is not possible in a given health care situation. Valuable time is saved when team members are knowledgeable about the constraints and opportunities available within their delivery system.

CONTENT VERSUS COMMUNICATION PROCESSES IN TEAM MEETINGS

Content and process are interwoven in effective team meetings. Content should be focused, with each team member as fully prepared as possible. This means that you need to understand what you do know and what you do not know about the patient's situation. Scheduled team meetings should have clear agendas, with the time to be spent on each item identified. Structure keeps people on track. The agenda can be brief. Additional critical items can be added at the beginning of the meeting, if needed. Minutes taken at each meeting should highlight decisions made, identify action items to be completed, and specify individual team member responsibilities for tasks when indicated. Rotation of leadership and scribe roles help team members to share the workload and build a sense of collaborative team responsibility. Clarifying roles and expectations and identifying the scope of functional activities helps to direct attention to what is important and meaningful; it also helps to save time.

Sharing ideas with professional tact is an art. Skills can be learned. If someone makes a point that is particularly relevant, acknowledge its merit. If members have reservations about an idea, they should be encouraged to speak up. Presenting a concern or an alternative with a rationale is different from judging the rightness or wrongness of another team member's ideas, and it is easier to hear. Explain your rationale in neutral terms about the issue, not about the person. Learning to deal with conflict is as essential to team building as it is to individual professional collaborative conversations (see Chapter 23).

Smoothly run collaborative care meetings are those in which each team member understands and agrees to support the team mission of quality coordination of care. Time is a precious commodity for busy health care providers; team meetings should begin and end on time. An agenda keeps all team members focused on the business at hand. Simulation Exercise 24.2 provides an opportunity for students to understand collaboration skills in team decision making.

INFORMATIONAL CONTINUITY

Informational continuity refers to data exchanges among providers and provider systems and between providers and patients for the purpose of providing continuously coordinated quality care. Instant electronic transmission of data "links provider to provider, and health care event to health care event" (Pontin & Lewis, 2008, p. 1199). Ideally there is an uninterrupted flow of data and clinical impressions between health care providers and agencies, with patients and their families, over time and space. Specific information follows the patient from primary to secondary care settings, and vice versa. The same patient information is available to providers throughout the health care system (Agarwal & Crooks, 2008). Data about possible medication interactions, start and stop dates, and personal responses to specific medications are easily accessible.

Informational continuity is critical to providing safe, quality care. Gaps can occur as a result of misplaced clinical records, inadequate discharge planning or referral data, deficient or delayed authorization for treatment, and a lack of understanding by the patient about their illness, treatment, or self-management. Lack of information at time of transfer can result in treatment delays, which increases patient and family's anxiety unnecessarily.

Information continuity provides a safety net for patients who often become overwhelmed with the number of procedures, appointments, and providers involved with their care. The capacity to communicate directly with various providers and treatment centers—and feeling comfortable that everyone involved in their care has the same information—is one less thing patients and providers have to worry about.

SIMULATION EXERCISE 24.2
Collaborative Decision Making

Purpose:
To help students discover how they can work together to achieve consensus about an uncertain situation.

Procedure:
Break up the class into groups of three to four students. Identify one student for each group to act as scribe.
1. Each group member should present a real-time clinical scenario related to a patient with complex medical needs in one or two paragraphs.
2. Each student should present his or her scenario for group consideration. Other group members can ask questions.
3. The group should choose one of the scenarios and provide a rationale for its choice.

Discussion:
How did each group reach its decision?
What was it like to know you had to make a team decision about an issue for which there is no perfect answer?
What factors made collaborative discussion and decision making easier or harder?
What did you learn from doing this exercise about how people function as a team in making a difficult decision within a short time frame?

Immediate forms of informational continuity within hospital units include interdisciplinary team meetings, huddles, comfort rounds, and progress notes. Handovers, discharge plans, referral contacts, and patient summaries are used for patient transfers from one care setting to another.

In the community, informational continuity can empower patients through appointment reminders and call-back checks, careful instruction about diagnosis and care options, and accurate electronic health records (EHRs) shared with patients and providers. The goal for informational continuity is to help ensure that everyone involved in the care of a patient is on the same page. Sharing health and treatment information with patients and families should be consistent, complete, accurate, value neutral, and delivered in an easily understandable and supportive manner. Knowing what to expect, with contingency plans in place, increases patient security (Haggerty et al., 2013). Notifying the family of changes in the patient's condition or treatment recommendations is an essential part of ensuring informational continuity, particularly if the family is not in close contact with the patient. Informational COC facilitates effective and efficient transition of care from one clinical setting to another. Receiving consistent information from different providers bolsters patient confidence and is more likely to be believed.

Transition and Discharge Planning in Continuity of Care

Rhudy, Holland, and Bowles (2010) identify improving the quality of patient transitions across health care settings as a national priority. Patients with complex chronic conditions typically experience multiple care transitions in their health experience. Unfortunately, changeovers between care settings are associated with a larger number of "avoidable adverse events" and "near misses" (Mitchell et al., 2012). Accurate recording of information and sharing it between the giving and receiving institutions is part of information continuity, but there is a relational aspect too (Box 24.2).

In addition to time constraints imposed by insurance regulations, a transfer from one care setting to another often is precipitated by a change in health, functional status, or change in the complexity patient needs rather than

patient choice. Care transition, whether from the hospital to home or to a rehabilitation center, assisted living, or skilled care setting, or from a community setting to a hospital is an emotional as well as a physical event for patients and families. It is a vulnerable time. Patients and families caring for them are anxious because they do not know what to expect. Carr (2008) notes that "care transitions shouldn't be an abrupt end of care previously provided, but rather considered to be a coordinated changeover for the patient to a new team of involved caregivers" (p. 26).

NURSING ROLE IN TRANSITIONAL CARE

The Case Management Society of America (CMSA, 2008) makes a distinction between transitional care and care transitions. Transition of care refers to managing movement of patients between different levels of care and between health care locations or providers as patient care needs change. The American Geriatrics Society (2007) defines *transitional care* as "a set of actions designed to ensure the coordination and continuity of health care as patients transfer between

---

BOX 24.2   Core Functions for Transitional Sending and Receiving Teams

Both the **sending** and **receiving** care teams are expected to

- Shift their perspective from the concept of a patient discharge to that of a patient transfer with continuous management expectations.
- Begin planning for a transfer to the next care setting on or before a patient's admission.
- Elicit the preferences of patients and caregivers and incorporate these preferences into the care plan, where appropriate.
- Identify a patient's system of social support and baseline level of function (i.e., How will this patient care for himself or herself after discharge?).
- Communicate and collaborate with practitioners across settings to formulate and execute a common care plan.
- Use the preferred mode of communication (i.e., telephone, fax, e-mail) of collaborators in other settings.

The **sending** health care team is expected to ensure that

- The patient is stable enough to be transferred to the next care setting.
- The patient and caregiver understand the purpose of the transfer.
- The receiving institution is capable of and prepared to meet the patient's needs.
- All relevant sections of the transfer information form are complete.

- The care plan, orders, and a clinical summary precede the patient's arrival to the next care setting. The discharge summary should include the patient's baseline functional status (both physical and cognitive) and recommendations from other professionals involved with the patient's care, including social workers, occupational therapists, and physical therapists.
- The patient has a timely follow-up appointment with an appropriate health care professional.
- A member of the sending health care team is available to the patient, caregiver, and receiving health care team for 72 hours after the transfer to discuss any concerns regarding the care plan.
- The patient and family understand their health care insurance benefits and coverage as they pertain to the transfer.

The **receiving** health care team is expected to ensure that

- The transfer forms, clinical summary, discharge summary, and physician's orders are reviewed before or on the patient's arrival.
- The patient's goals and preferences are incorporated into the care plan.
- Discrepancies or confusion regarding the care plan, the patient's status, or the patient's medications are clarified with the sending health care team.

From HMO Work Group on Care Management. (2004). *One patient, many places: Managing health care transitions* (p. 7). Washington, DC: AAHP-HIAA Foundation.

different locations or different levels of care within the same location" (p. 30). Transitional care begins in the hospital and represents an expansion of the nurse's traditional role in hospital care. Successful transitions consider the combined needs of the patient and family, which are paired with the resources of an agency or health care provider to realistically identify and meet identified care needs. Table 24.1 identifies key elements in effective transitional care.

Acute care hospitals are intended for short-term stays. When patients require skilled medical and nursing care beyond a designated time period, they may be transferred to a long-term care or rehabilitation hospital. Patients and families need to know what parameters will be used for discharge as soon as this is known (The Joint Commission, 2013). Usually, the hospital has a care coordinator, but nurses are often involved in arranging for this person to see the patient and for working with follow-up concerns. All recommendations for transfer should be thoroughly discussed with the patient and family and included in the patient's treatment plan.

Nurses play a crucial role in planning transitions between care settings. Early planning for transition to a different care setting is essential. This planning time gives patients and significant caregivers a better chance to develop a realistic plan consistent with patient care needs, strengths, preferences, and financial mean—a plan that all those involved can feel is right and the best solution at the time. Follow-up plans are better negotiated if people have sufficient time to consider all aspects of potential choices, and to think them through carefully, before making significant decisions. Transition planning from a patient perspective also allows nurses to uncover hidden patient issues such as fear of being abandoned or of receiving substandard care in an unknown setting.

Nonroutine discharges in which the patient needs a postdischarge rehabilitative or subacute placement, additional health support services, and/or equipment at home require a more complex discharge planning process for optimum results. If the discharge is to home, involved family members should be part of the discussion and decision because they will be intimately involved in care provision.

A complex discharge planning process begins with a careful review of initial admission data and continues as a thread with each subsequent review. Starting early in the hospitalization allows time for both patients and families to become physically and emotionally prepared for transition and to have needed supports available post discharge.

Informal discussions can be introduced during routine care. Other times, patient education can be offered in a more concentrated way with teach-back and return demonstrations. Frequent check in with patients and families encourages them to ask questions and to express concerns in a supportive environment. Box 24.3 presents nursing actions associated with complex discharges.

Simulation Exercise 24.3 provides practice with discharge planning processes.

The goal of discharge planning is to provide patients and their families with the level and kind of information they need to secure their recovery and/or maintain health status during the immediate posthospital period. Research shows that having discharge plans tailored to individual patient needs seems to have an effect on reduced hospital stay and readmission rates and increases patient satisfaction (Shepperd et al., 2013).

If the patient is to be discharged to home, medication reconciliation, and teach-back strategies discussed in Chapter 15 should be part of the discharge planning. Specific instructions for postdischarge care and contact arrangements with external care providers should be shared with patients and families. Offering choices about

TABLE 24.1   Key Elements in Planning for Care Transitions

SUMMARY OF CARE ELEMENTS	
Activity	Components
Needs assessment	Medical and functional status, cognitive, emotional, and behavioral support needs, nature, and level of support system
Choose best next care setting	Nursing home Inpatient rehabilitation Assisted living Home, with home health care aide Home, with family or alone
Arrange services	Identify suitable agency(ies) and verify financial or insurance coverage
Clinical summary	Course (diagnosis and treatment) Key data (laboratory, radiographs, other) Care plan's main elements (how to care for the patient)
Medication reconciliation	Current medication list What was stopped and why What was started and why
Follow-up medical care	Appointments (names, times, dates, phone numbers)

Modified from Boling, P. (2009). Care transitions and home health care. *Clinics in Geriatric Medicine, 25,* 135–148.

BOX 24.3   Nursing Actions in Comprehensive Discharges

- Assess patients' understanding of the discharge plan by asking them to explain it in their own words.
- Advise patients and family of any tests completed at the hospital with pending results at time of discharge. Also notify appropriate clinicians of this contingency.
- Schedule follow-up appointments or tests after discharge, if needed. Provide relevant contact numbers.
- Provide information about home or health care services, if needed, or not initiated prior to discharge.
- Confirm the medication plan and ensuring that the patient and family understands any changes (e.g., medication in the hospital not available or accessible in the community).
- Review written summary care instructions with the patient and family and go over in detail what to do if a problem develops.
- Identify the responsible caregiver in the home and transportation arrangements.
- Expedite transmission of the discharge summary to health care providers and case managers accepting responsibility for the patient.

SIMULATION EXERCISE 24.3   Using a Discharge Planning Process

Purpose:
To provide an opportunity for students to develop an experiential understanding of a discharge planning process.

Procedure:
Using the guideline data, develop a simple discharge planning report for a newly admitted patient on your unit or use the following case study.

Jeff O'Connor is a 66-year-old man originally admitted to the emergency department with severe chest pain, shortness of breath, dizziness, and intermittent palpitations. He was diagnosed with a myocardial infarction and admitted to the coronary care unit. He was placed on oxygen and remained there for several days because his serum markers continued to rise. He received morphine for pain and sedatives to keep him comfortable. He is currently stabilized with digoxin, demonstrates a normal sinus rhythm, and is being transferred to the step-down unit this afternoon. His wife and daughter have visited him several times each day. His wife states she is exhausted but glad he is being transferred. Jeff has long-standing coronary artery disease and a family history of cardiac events. This is his first heart attack.

Discussion:
If this is the only information you have on Jeff, what other data might you need to develop a full transitional report using the SBAR (situation, background, assessment, recommendation) format described in Chapter 4?

Note: This exercise can be completed using a current patient transfer.

available and appropriate postacute providers represents a unique form of advocacy for patients and families (Birmingham, 2009).

Medication reconciliation is an important dimension of admission and discharge planning. The Joint Commission specifically identifies it as National Patient Safety Goal No. 8. Patients may come into a care setting on a wide variety of medications. Some medications may be changed or discontinued. Others may be added. When the patient is being discharged, a medication reconciliation, including the name of the medication, generic and prescribed name, dosage, frequency, and the time each medication was last taken should be entered into the EHR, with a computer-generated or written list given to the patient. Go over the list with the patient and designated caregiver, if applicable. Medication reconciliation also should be done periodically with the patient in primary care settings especially if the patient is seeing more than one provider.

Crucial questions are who in the patient's close support system is available to help the patient in the immediate postdischarge period and what arrangements are in place if additional care support is required. It is important to ask open-ended questions about the home environment and the support the patient is able to muster. This information needs to be precise. Just because a patient has family in the area does not mean that they would be available to the patient for direct support. You will need to identify the name of a primary support person and/or specific posthospital arrangements in the patient's EHR. Very important is asking patients about their concerns and expectations after discharge. Patients discharged to home and their caregivers need specific instruction to successfully self-manage recovery and chronic health problems at home, not just once, but several times. Written instructions should be verbally explained and given to each patient. Arrangements and/or referrals for essential support or training needs should be in place before discharge.

Discharge Summary

The Joint Commission (2013) mandates that discharge summaries be completed within 30 days of hospital discharge. A discharge summary should communicate diagnostic findings, hospital management, and plans for follow-up at the end of a patient's hospitalization (Kripalani et al., 2007). Content mandated for each patient's written discharge summary includes

- Reason for hospitalization
- Significant findings
- Procedures and treatment provided
- The patient's condition at discharge
- Patient and family instructions (as appropriate)
- Attending physician's signature

Nurses are accountable for verbally reviewing discharge summaries with the patient and/or caregiver, providing written instructions, and completing discharge documentation in the chart. Patients and/or their significant caregiver should be given a copy of the discharge summary and encouraged to keep it in a safe place. Patients should bring their discharge summary to initial follow-up appointments. Although the physician is responsible for initiating and signing discharge summaries and orders, nurses play a critical role in the discharge of patients.

Discharge instructions are not the same as discharge orders or discharge summaries. Specific *written* discharge instructions should include a basic follow-up plan identifying diet, activity level, weight monitoring, what to do if symptoms develop or worsen, and the contact numbers of relevant hospital and primary care providers. Written instructions should be simple and concrete—for example, "Call the doctor if you gain more than 2 pounds in 1 week." A written list of all medications prescribed at discharge, including prescription, over-the-counter medications, vitamins, and herbals, should be given to the patient and caregiver. Use teach-back methods (see Chapter 15) to ensure that your discharge home management instructions are understood. Relational continuity helps ensure that the coaching and health teaching, (presented in Chapter 15), gets shared across all involved agencies.

Subheadings help to organize and highlight pertinent information for follow-up care (Kripalani et al., 2007). Discharge documentation in the patient's chart should include the patient's condition or functional status at time of discharge, followed by a summarization of the treatment and nursing care provided and discharge instructions given to the patient/family and the patient's responses. Clearly identify the intermediate placement (nursing home, rehabilitation center) or home. You need to document that the patient and/or caregiver was physically given a copy of the discharge instructions.

MANAGEMENT CONTINUITY

The triple aim of transformational approaches required to overhaul the US health care system is designed to improve patient care experiences improving patient experiences of care (including quality and satisfaction), cultivate overall population health, and reduce the per capita cost of health care (Berwick, Nolan, & Whittington, 2008; Brandt, Luftiyya, King, & Chioresco, 2014).

Strong system-based management continuity facilitates self-care management. *Management continuity* is defined as a "consistent and coherent approach to the management of a health condition that is responsive to a patient's changing needs" (Al-Azri, 2008, p. 147). As a longitudinal approach to the clinical management of chronic disorders in the community, management continuity involves aligning patient needs with community supports through care coordination and case management. Care coordination is the term used to describe "management of interdependencies among tasks" (Yang & Meiners, 2014, p. 96).

CARE COORDINATION AND PATIENT SYSTEM NAVIGATION*

The basic goals of care coordination and patient system navigation are to proactively guide patients through the barriers in complex health systems, decrease fragmentation, coordinate services, and improve health outcomes. Care coordinators are responsible for ensuring that the plan of care developed by the provider is carried out in partnership with the patient. This process begins with developing a nonjudgmental collaborative relationship with a patient to identify health goals and any barriers that could impede success. Care coordinators are responsible for identifying an individual's health goals and coordinating services and providers to meet those goals. They must learn to be adept at navigating complex systems and communicating with patients, families, and professionals involved with the patient's care. Coordination activities include the following:

- Establishing relationships based on trust
- Communicating with patients, families, providers, and community resources that lead to shared expectations for communication and care
- Providing health education
- Assessing strengths, challenges, needs, and goals
- Implementing a proactive plan of care
- Monitoring progress and assisting with follow-up
- Supporting self-management goals
- Facilitating informed choice, consent, and decision making

---

* This section was developed by Mary Joseph, RN, 2014.

- Facilitating transitions in care
- Linking patients to community resources
- Aligning resources to meet the patient's needs
- Developing connectivity that provides pathways that encourage timely and effective information flow between all entities involved including the patient

Effectively establishing and maintaining professional boundaries are essential when working with patients and families to coordinate care. Boundaries provide the limits that enable care coordinators to maintain professionalism and to secure an environment where both patient and care coordinator are mutually respected. Listed next are some important tips on maintaining boundaries.

- Always work within the treatment recommendations of the patient's provider. The care coordinator should never give any recommendations contrary to the recommendations of the provider.
- The care coordinator is in a position of influence, and the patient is in a vulnerable position. Overinvolvement with a patient can be draining on the care coordinator and can interfere with the important tasks of the job.
- Assess your cultural ideas and prejudices. Know your community.

The success of care coordination depends to a large extent on the strength of the interpersonal relationships between individual clinicians and community support organization. Without familiarity and shared objectives, the administrative transfer of information will not occur or be sustained. Ongoing use of the broad stakeholder group (the medical neighborhood) and joint review of performance data at care coordination meetings can help to foster a community of continuous quality improvement among multiple providers. Routine performance measurement and reporting about the effectiveness and quality of care coordination are critical to understand if patients' needs are being met.

CASE MANAGEMENT

The CMSA (2009) defines **case management** as "a collaborative process of assessment, planning, facilitation and advocacy for options and services to meet an individual's health needs through communication and available resources to promote quality cost-effective outcomes." Case management has a strong record of success as a strategy to reduce fragmentation in health care delivery. It has been proven effective in reducing emergency department use and lower health costs (Woodward and Rice, 2015) Whether one works in the hospital or primary care setting, all nurses should have knowledge of how case management works and how it fits into COC.

Case management is a professional support intervention, which assists patients to self-manage their health (Nazareth et al., 2008; Saultz & Albedaiwi, 2004). AHRQ (2013)

advocates care coordination, team-based approaches, integration of behavioral and mental health with primary care, and stronger linkages with the community as the best means of improving the quality of health care delivery in the community. The goal of case management strategies is to help patients function at their highest possible level in the least restrictive environment. Case management strategies are designed with the following purposes:

- To enhance the patient's quality of life
- To decrease fragmentation and duplication of health delivery processes
- To contain unnecessary health care costs (Gallagher, Truglio-Londrigan, & Levin, 2009)

Case management allows patients with multiple or serious physical and mental chronic conditions to stay in their homes and function in the community (Ploeg, Hayward, Woodward, & Johnston, 2008). Patients need a case manager when they are unable to safely establish or maintain self-management of a chronic health condition in a consistent manner without external supports. Included in the population group served by case managers are frail elders, patients with mental illness or dementia, and patients with chronic mental illness or chronic physical disabilities affecting activities of daily living.

Carter (2009) notes, "Case management is a core component of what is needed to improve health care quality overall, while reducing costs" (p. 166). Knowledge of community resources to facilitate health care delivery in primary care settings allows case managers to consistently deliver the right care at the right time to the right patient and family. Standards of practice for case management related to quality of care, collaboration, and resource utilization are consistent with National Patient Safety goals developed by The Joint Commission (Amin & Owen, 2006).

Case Example

Ray Bolton is a 48-year-old man with severe chronic Crohn disease. He has a permanent ileostomy, is on multiple medications, and suffers from periodic exacerbations in his condition, resulting in hospitalization. Ray has Social Security Disability Insurance (SSDI) as his only source of income. He has neurological issues affecting his balance and gait and causing him significant pain. He cannot sleep and is socially isolated. He lives by himself with his cat. Apart from his 80-year-old mother who lives in another state, Ray has no support system except his physicians. He was referred for case management, following his latest hospitalization. Simulation Exercise 24.4 provides an opportunity to assess and plan for patient care using a case management approach.

CASE MANAGEMENT PRINCIPLES AND STRATEGIES

Case management strategies are designed to coordinate and manage patient care across a wide continuum of health care services and community supports. Case management models follow the nursing process as a structural framework. Strategies incorporate COC concepts related to communication, team building, and data sharing with all members of the multidisciplinary care team, including the patient and family caregivers.

Case finding is a proactive case management strategy to identify individuals at high risk for potential health problems (Thomas, 2009). The manner in which you approach the patient will determine the completeness of information you receive.

An intake assessment should include the names, addresses, and phone numbers of the patient's health care providers, social service representatives, school or work contacts, if applicable, and health insurance information. Availability of social supports and religious affiliations, previous hospitalizations, and history of treatment, current medications and allergies, advance directives and do not resuscitate (DNR) status, cognitive and mental status, mobility status, and functional assessment of activities of daily living are other pieces of case management assessment data. Identifying potential barriers to treatment adherence, including the impact that the patient's diagnosis has on family members and coworkers, is important. Case managers interact directly with all members of the collaborative health team, patients, and families on a regular basis. The case manager works with an assigned patient to identify the individual needs and health goals. Operationalizing patient self-management of chronic conditions requires special attention to empowering patients related to role and emotional self-management, as well as the patient's medical or behavioral management needs (McAllister, Dunn, Payne, Davies, & Todd, 2012). Case management treatment strategies are customized for each patient, based on personal needs, values, and preferences, using a rehabilitative strength-based focus. Because case management represents a longitudinal treatment management process, care plans will likely need adjustment from time to time to reflect changes in the patient's situation. Competent patients, capable of making valid judgments, should have final responsibility for decision making.

Case managers help patients to coordinate services and overcome barriers. They provide patients with the essential support to assume as much responsibility as possible in the self-management of their health issues. They meet with patients at scheduled intervals to monitor patient progress and provide suggestions, as needed. When single agency resources are insufficient to meet complex health needs, case managers help patients and families to identify and coordinate services with other agencies. Networking and communication with other health professionals involved with the patient help to prevent, or minimize, emergence of full-blown health problems. Strategies include guidance or referrals to social supports such as legal aid, social security benefits and disability, safe affordable housing, social services, and/or mental health and addiction services. To be effective, case managers need a strong understanding of community resources' strengths and weaknesses, including accessibility, availability, affordability, how systems work, and how patients and families can best make use of them.

Case managers have an advocacy role too. They educate community workers who work with disabled or chronically ill patients, about the social aspects of disability to facilitate understanding and acceptance of the patient's problems. Goodman (2014) suggests that the opportunities for

SIMULATION EXERCISE 24.5
Understanding the Role of a Family Caregiver

Purpose:
To help students understand the caregiver role from the perspective of family caregivers.

Procedure:
1. Interview the family caregiver of a patient with a long-standing chronic illness or mental disability, and write a summary of the caregiver's responses.
2. Use the following questions to obtain your data.
   a. Can you tell me why and how you assumed responsibility for caregiving?
   b. In what ways has your life changed since you became a caregiver for your parent, spouse, disabled child or adult, or mentally ill family member?
   c. What do you find most challenging about the caregiving role?
   d. What do you find rewarding about the caregiving role?
   e. How do you balance caring for your ill or disabled family member with caring for yourself?
   f. What advice would you give someone who is about to assume the caregiving role for a chronically ill or disabled family member?

Discussion:
- What was it like to get a picture of the caregiver role?
- Were you surprised by any of the caregiver's responses?
- What were the similarities and differences in caregiver responses?
- What are some of the reasons for any of the variants between student reports?
- How could you incorporate what you learned doing this exercise in your clinical practice?

nursing advocacy are boundless, depending on a nurse's personal interests and skills. For example, nurses often speak before legislative and other funding sources to advocate for essential services. Their testimony is believable because of their close relationship in caring for these vulnerable populations. Case managers sometimes negotiate on a patient's behalf with insurance companies and equipment suppliers, as a supportive adjunct when a patient is unable to do so.

Case managers evaluate outcomes in terms of patient satisfaction, clinical outcomes, and cost. Recommendations for treatment planning variations should correspond with observed changes in the patient's situation, health condition, or in health care resources. Documentation from external providers and agencies needs to be included in the patient's case management record, as do variances from the treatment plan, reasons for the variance, and plans for modification in care plans.

MANAGEMENT CONTINUITY RESOURCE FOR FAMILY CAREGIVERS

Case managers provide ongoing support and encouragement for family caregivers. Cott, Falter, Gignac, and Badley (2008) describe the medical home as "a unique clinical setting, different from acute care or institutional environments" (p. 19). Living with chronic illness increasingly is a home care responsibility, with family members as informal caregivers providing most of the care. Family caregiving is neither a career choice nor a role for which one can prepare. The caregiver has no "care map to lead the way," states Wright, Doherty, and Dumas (2009, p. 209). Simulation Exercise 24.5 offers insights into the role of family caregivers from the caregiver perspective.

Caring for patients with significant disability at home has positive and negative aspects. Being cared for at home offers stronger COC management because home is associated with personal identity, security, and relationships with people who genuinely care about the patient. Variation exists in a family member's capacity to be supportive, especially if the caregiver's health is not optimal, the care is labor intensive and time consuming, or the relationship with the patient is conflictual (Weinberg, Lusenhop, Gittell, & Kautz, 2007). Case managers can fill in essential information gaps for family caregivers through careful questioning, observation, validation about feelings and observations, and consultation about emerging health issues. Working with families should include providing educational information on medications, signs and symptoms of impending problems and potential adverse reactions and when to call a health care provider. Names, locations, and phone numbers of primary care and follow-up providers should be discussed and the information provided in written form to the caregiver.

CASE MANAGEMENT FOR CHRONICALLY MENTALLY ILL PATIENTS

COC is essential for effectively caring for chronically mentally ill patients in the community (Wierdsma, Mulder, de Vries, & Sytema, 2009). These patients find fulfilling even basic needs for shelter, food, clothing, and transportation to be quality-of-life issues. Chronically mentally ill and substance-dependent patients often function at a marginal level because of their symptoms. Many are homeless and in poor physical health. These patients often do not seek out help proactively. Yet, as A. C. Benson (n.d.) notes, "People seldom refuse help, if one offers it in the right way."

Case management for the chronically mentally ill is key to providing quality health care, particularly for youths and seniors in the public sector (Woodward J, Rice E, 2015). Case managers provide mentally ill individuals with mentoring, coaching, and referrals for job training services. They help patients to avert crisis relapses that precipitate rehospitalization. Case managers use recovery principles of care, such as linking patients with counseling and alternative treatment services, social services, and community networks.

COC for mentally ill and dually diagnosed patients includes formal wraparound support services for mentally ill children and families and case management for adults and children. Wraparound services use a strengths-based format, which involves the family, community, school, and service providers in the child's environment. Professionals work with the family and other social providers to promote adaptive functioning. Strengthening family ties to supportive people within the family's social environment is deliberately included in wraparound services to help strengthen social support (Walker & Schutte, 2004).

SUMMARY

COC is a dynamic, multidimensional concept, consisting of relational, informational, and management continuity and focused on assisting individuals and families with the resources they need to manage chronic illness within and across clinical settings. The goal of COC is to ensure a seamless continuum of quality care for patients, provided through coordinated, community-based health services. COC integrated delivery systems focus on what really matters to a patient and family and have the capacity to provide services to meet the patient's needs.

Relational continuity embraces collaborative relationships and shared decision making between health care providers and patients. Successful outcomes also depend on interdisciplinary collaboration and interprofessional team communication caring for the patient, who can be defined as an individual, a family, or a community in need of care.

Informational COC allows for an uninterrupted flow of data and clinical impressions between health care providers and agencies, with patients and their families, in a care experience that is connected and coherent over time. Informational COC is a critical component in effective transition and discharge planning.

Case management is a major vehicle in ensuring management continuity for individuals who otherwise might not be able to function independently in the community because of physical or mental disability. Care coordination and service navigation in public sector health care helps patients and families to get the support they need when multiple service providers are involved.

ETHICAL DILEMMA: What Would You Do?

Paul is ready to be discharged from the hospital, but it is clear that he can no longer live independently by himself. He has had several heart attacks in the past, with significant heart damage, and currently suffers from serious chronic obstructive pulmonary disease (COPD). His recent hospitalization was for uncontrolled diabetes. Paul has difficulty complying with diet restrictions and his need to take daily insulin. He is not an easy person to live with, but Paul is sure that his daughter will welcome him into her home because he is "family."

Although his daughter agrees to assume care for her father, she does so reluctantly. She has her own life and does not have a positive relationship with her father. She resents that he just assumes that she will take care of him. Without her support, Paul cannot live independently in the community. What would you do as the nurse in this situation to help them resolve this dilemma? What are the implications of this situation as an ethical dilemma?

DISCUSSION QUESTIONS

1. What do you see as facilitators and barriers for COC in your current care setting?
2. In what ways do different interdisciplinary roles influence and complement each other in complex clinical care situations?
3. In what ways does COC support the triple aim of effective health care? What do you understand better about COC as a result of reading this chapter?

REFERENCES

Agarwal, G., & Crooks, V. (2008). The nature of informational continuity in general practice. *British Journal of General Practice*, 58(556), e17–e24.

Agency for Healthcare Research and Quality (AHRQ). (2013). AHRQ updates on primary care research: Multiple chronic conditions research network. *Annals of Family Medicine*, 11(15), 485–486.

Al-Azri, M. (2008). Continuity of care and quality of care-inseparable twin. *Oman Medical Journal*, 23(3), 147–149.

American Geriatrics Society. (2007). *Improving the quality of transitional care for persons with complex care needs (American Geriatrics Society (AGS) position statement)*. Assisted Living Consult. March/April: 30–32, 2007.

Amin, A., & Owen, M. (2006). Productive interdisciplinary team relationships: The hospitalist and the case manager. *Lippincotts Case Management*, 11(3), 160–164.

Benson, A. C. (2013). *BrainyQuote.com, n.d.*, Retrieved October 27, 2013, from: BrainyQuote.com. http://www.brainyquote.com/quotes/quotes/a/acbenson101010.html.

Berwick, D. M., Nolan, T. W., & Whittington, J. (2008). The triple aim: Care, health, and cost. *Health Affairs*, 27, 759–769.

Birmingham, J. (2009). Patient choice in the discharge planning process. *Professional Case Management*, 14(6), 296–309; quiz 310–311.

Bodenheimer, T., Wagner, E., & Grumbach, K. (2002). Improving primary care for patients with chronic illness. *Journal of the American Medical Association*, 288(14), 1775–1779.

Boling, P. (2009). Care transitions and home health care. *Clinics in Geriatric Medicine*, 25, 135–148.

Bradway, C., Trotta, R., Bixby, M. B., McPartland, E., Wollman, M. C., Kapustka, H., et al. (2012). A qualitative analysis of an advanced practice nurse-directed transitional care model intervention. *Gerontologist*, 52(3), 394–407.

Brandt, B., Luftiyya, M., King, J., & Chioresco, C. (2014). A scoping review of interprofessional collaborative practice and education using the lens of the triple aim. *Journal of Interprofessional Care*, 28(5), 393–399.

Cambridge Dictionary. (2016). Retrieved from: http://dictionary.cambridge.org/ us/dictionary/english/ paradigm-shift%3E.

Carr, D. (2008). On the case: Effective care transitions. *Nursing Management*, 32(1), 25–31.

Carter, J. (2008). 2009 Finding our place at the discussion table: Case management and health care reform. *Professional Case Management*, 14(4), 165–166.

Case Management Society of America. (2009). What is a case manager? Retrieved from: http://www.cmsa.org/Home/CMSA/WhatisaCaseManager/tabid/224/Default.aspx.

Clark, P., Cott, C., & Drinka, T. (2007). Theory and practice in interprofessional ethics: A framework for understanding ethical issues in health care teams. *Journal of Interprofessional Care*, 21(6), 591–603.

Coleman, K., Austin, B. T., Brach, C., & Wagner, E. H. (2009). Evidence on the chronic care model in the new millennium. *Health Affairs (Millwood)*, 28(1), 75–85.

Cooke, L., Gemmill, R., & Grant, M. (2008). Advance practice nurses core competencies: A framework for developing and testing an advanced practice nurse discharge intervention. *Clinical Nurse Specialist*, 22(5), 218–225.

Cott, C., Falter, L., Gignac, M., & Badley, E. (2008). Helping networks in community home care for the elderly: Types of team. *Canadian Journal of Nursing Research*, 40(1), 18–37.

Crabtree, B., Nutting, P., Miller, W., Stange, K., Stewart, E., & Jaen, C. R. (2010). Summary of the national demonstration project and recommendations for the patient-centered medical home. *Annals of Family Medicine*, 8(Suppl. 1), 580–590.

Cramm, J., & Nieboer, A. (2011). Professional views on interprofessional stroke team functioning. *International Journal of Integrated Care*, 11(25), 1–8.

D'Amour, D., & Oandasan, I. (2005). Interprofessionality as the field of interprofessional practice and interprofessional education: An emerging concept. *Journal of Interprofessional Care*, 19(Suppl 1), 8–20.

Engebretson, J., Mahoney, J., & Carlson, E. (2008). Cultural competence in the era of evidence-based practice. *Journal of Professional Nursing*, 24, 172–178.

Ferrer, R., & Gill, J. (2013). Editorial: Shared decision making, contextualized. *Annals of Family Medicine*, 11(4), 303–305.

Gallagher, L., Truglio-Londrigan, M., & Levin, R. (2009). Partnership for healthy living: An action research project. *Nursing Research*, 16(2), 7–29.

Gardner, D. (2005). Ten lessons in collaboration. *Online Journal of Issues in Nursing*, 10(1), 2.

Ginter, P., Duncan, W. J., & Swayne, L. (2013). *Strategic management of health care organizations* (7th ed.). San Francisco: Jossey-Bass.

Glasgow, R., Goldstein, M., & Kaplan-Liss, E. (2008). Chapter 5: Introduction to the principles of health behavior change. In S. Woolf, & S. Jonas (Eds.), *Health promotion and disease prevention* (2nd ed.) (pp. 129–147). Philadelphia, PA: Lippincott Wilkins.

Goodman, T. (2014). Guest Editorial: The future of nursing: An opportunity for advocacy. *Association of Operating Room Nurses Journal*, 99(6), 668–670.

Grumbach, K., & Bodenheimer, T. (2002). A primary care home for Americans: Putting the house in order. *Journal of the American Medical Association*, 288(7), 889–893.

Guilliford, M., Naithani, S., & Morgan, M. (2006). What is "continuity of care"? *Journal of Health Services Research & Policy*, 11(4), 248–250.

Haggerty, J. L., Pineault, R., Beaulieu, M., Brunelle, Y., Gauthier, J., Goulet, F., et al. (2008). Practice features associated with patient reported accessibility, continuity, and coordination of primary health care. *Annals of Family Medicine*, 6(2), 116–123.

Haggerty, J. L., Reid, P. J., Freeman, G. K., Starfield, B. H., Adair, C. E., & McKendry, R. (2003). Continuity of care: A multidisciplinary review. *British Medical Journal*, 327, 1219–1221.

Haggerty, J. L., Roberge, D., Freeman, G. K., & Beaulieu, C. (2013). Experienced continuity of care when patients see multiple clinicians: A qualitative metasummary. *Annals of Family Medicine*, 11(3), 262–271.

Hall, P. (2005). Interprofessional teamwork: Professional cultures as barriers. *Journal of Interprofessional Care*, 19(Suppl. 1), 188–196.

Havens, D., Vasey, J., Gittell, J., & Lin, W. (2010). Relational coordination among nurses and other providers: Impact on the equality of patient care. *Nursing Management*, 18(8), 926–937.

Institute of Medicine (IOM). (2003). *The future of the public's health in the 21st century*. Washington, DC: National Academies Press.

Institute of Medicine (IOM). (2012). *Primary care and public health: Exploring integration to improve population health*. Washington, DC: National Academy Press.

Joseph, M. J. (2014). *Center for Health Improvement, Primary Care Coalition of Montgomery County*. Maryland: Unpublished manuscript.

Keeling, A., & Lewenson, S. (2013). A nursing historical perspective on the medical home: Impact on health care policy. *Nursing Outlook*, 61, 360–366.

Kleinman, A. (1988). *The illness narratives: Suffering, healing, and the human condition*. New York: Basic Books.

Kripalani, S., LeFevre, F., Phillips, C., Williams, M. V., Basaviah, P., & Baker, D. W. (2007). Deficits in communication and information transfer between hospital-based and primary care physicians: Implications for patient safety and continuity of care. *Journal of the American Medical Association*, 297(8), 831–841.

Lidskog, M., Lofmark, A., & Ahlstrom, G. (2007). Interprofessional education on a training ward for older people: Students conceptions of nurses, occupational therapists and social workers. *Journal of Interprofessional Care*, 21(4), 387–399.

McAllister, M., Dunn, G., Payne, K., Davies, L., & Todd, C. (2012). Patient empowerment: The need to consider it as a measurable patient-reported outcome for chronic conditions. *BMC Health Services Research*, 12, 157.

Mitchell, P., Wynia, M., Golden, R., McNellis, B., Okun, S., Webb, E. C., et al. (2012). *Core principles & values of effective team-based health care*. Washington, DC: Discussion Paper. Institute of Medicine. www.iom.edu/tbc.

Mosser, G., & Begun, J. (2014). *Teamwork in health care*. New York, NY: McGraw Hill.

Muir, J. C. (2008). Team, diversity and building communities. *Journal of Palliative Medicine*, 11(1), 5–7.

Nazareth, I., Jones, L., Irving, A., Aslett, H., Ramsay, A., Richardson, A., et al. (2008). Perceived concepts of care in people with colorectal and breast cancer—a qualitative case study analysis. *European Journal of Cancer Care*, 17, 569–577.

Porter-O'Grady, T. (2014). From tradition to transformation: A revolutionary moment for nursing in age of reform. *Nurse Lead*, 12(1), 65–69.

Paquette-Warren, J., Roberts, E., Fournie, M., Tyler, M., Brown, J., & Harris, S. (2014). Improving chronic care through continuing education of interprofessional primary care teams: A process evaluation. *Journal of Interprofessional Care*, 28(3), 232–238.

Ploeg, J., Hayward, L., Woodward, C., & Johnston, R. (2008). A case study of a Canadian homelessness intervention programme for elderly people. *Health & Social Care Community*, 16(6), 593–605.

Pontin, D., & Lewis, M. (2008). Maintaining the continuity of care in community children's nursing caseloads in a service for children with life-limiting, life-threatening or chronic health conditions: A qualitative analysis. *Journal of Clinical Nursing*, 18, 1199–1206.

Renholm, M., Suominen, T., Puukka, P., & Leino-Kilpi, H. (2016). Nurses' perceptions of patient care continuity in day surgery. *Journal of Perianesthesia Nursing*, 1(10).

Rhudy, L., Holland, D., & Bowles, K. (2010). Illuminating hospital discharge planning: Staff nurse decision making. *Applied Nursing Research*, 23(4), 198–206.

San Martin-Rodriguez, L., D'Amour, D., & Leduc, N. (2008). Outcomes of interprofessional collaboration of hospitalized cancer patient. *Cancer Nursing*, 31(2), E18–E27.

Saultz, J., & Albedaiwi, W. (2004). Interpersonal continuity of care and patient satisfaction: A critical review. *Annals of Family Medicine*, 2(5), 445–451.

Schneller, E., & Epstein, K. (2006). The hospitalist movement in the United States; agency and common agency issues. *Health Care Management Review*, 31(4), 308–316.

Schultz, K. (2009). Strategies to enhance teaching about continuity of care. *Canadian Family Physician*, 56, 666–668.

Shepperd, S., Lannin, N., Clemson, L., McCluskey, A., Cameron, I. D., & Barras, S. L. (2013). Discharge planning from hospital to home. *Cochrane Database of Systematic Review*, 1: CD000313.

Sparbel, K., & Anderson, M. A. (2000). Integrated literature review of continuity of care: Part 1, conceptual issues. *Journal of School Nursing*, 32(1), 17–24.

Stans, S. E., Stevens, J. A., & Beurskens, A. J. (2013). Interprofessional practice in primary care: Development of a tailored process model. *Journal of Multidisciplinary Healthcare*, 6, 139–147.

Starfield, B., & Horder, J. (2007). Interpersonal continuity: Old and new perspectives. *British Journal of General Practice*, 57(540), 527–529.

The Joint Commission. (2013). *Comprehensive accreditation manual for hospitals: The official handbook (CAMH)*. Oakbrook Terrace, IL: Joint Commission on Accreditation of Health Care Organizations.

Thomas, D. (2009). Case management for chronic conditions. *Nursing Management, 15*(10), 22–27.

Van Servellen, G., Fongwa, M., & Mockus D'Errico, E. (2006). Continuity of care and quality care outcomes for people experiencing chronic conditions: A literature review. *Nursing and Health Sciences, 8*, 185–195.

Von Bultzingslowen, I., Eliasson, G., Sarvimaki, A., Mattsson, B., & Hjortdahl, P. (2006). Patients' views on interpersonal continuity based on four core foundations. *Family Practice, 23*(2), 210–219.

Wagner, E., Austin, B., Davis, C., Hindmarsh, M., Schaerer, J., & Bonomi, A. (2001). Improving chronic illness care: Translating evidence into action. *Health Affairs, 20*(6), 64–78.

Walker, J. S., & Shutte, K. M. (2004). Practice and process in wraparound teamwork. *Journal of Emotional and Behavioral Disorders, 12*(3), 182–192.

Weinberg, D., Lusenhop, R. W., Gittell, G., & Kautz, C. M. (2007). Coordination between formal providers and informal caregivers. *Health Care Management Review, 32*(2), 140–149.

Wierdsma, A., Mulder, C., de Vries, S., & Sytema, S. (2009). Reconstructing continuity of care in mental health services: A multilevel conceptual framework. *Journal of Health Services Research & Policy, 14*, 52–57.

Woodward, J., Rice, E. (2015). Case management. *Nursing Clinics of North America, 50*, 109–121.

World Health Organization (WHO). (2002). *Innovative care for chronic conditions: Building blocks for action*. Geneva, Switzerland: Author.

Wright, J., Doherty, M., & Dumas, L. (2009). Caregiver burden: Three voices-three realities. *Nursing Clinics of North America, 44*, 209–221.

Yang, Y. T., & Meiners, M. (2014). Care coordination and the expansion of nursing scopes of practice. *Journal of Law, Medicine & Ethics, 42*(1), 93–103.

e-Documentation in Health Information Technology Systems

Kathleen Underman Boggs

OBJECTIVES

At the end of the chapter, the reader will be able to:

1. Identify purposes for documentation.
2. Discuss electronic health records (EHRs) and computerized provider order entry (CPOE) systems as part of larger electronic health information technology (HIT) systems, evaluating whether "meaningful use" requirements have improved care quality.
3. Draw conclusions as to how use of electronic longitudinal plans of care (LPC), decision support, CPOE, and other aspects of HIT systems improves patient and safety outcomes.
4. Identify business and legal aspects of documenting in electronic records.

Two key elements of collaborative work are communication and documentation (Chao, 2016).

The process of obtaining, organizing, and conveying patient health information to others in print or electronic format is referred to as **documentation.** Fig. 25.1 illustrates the purposes of electronic documentation, especially in terms of improved communication and evidence gathered from aggregated electronic health records (EHRs) to establish "best practice" interventions for quality improvement, a Quality and Safety Education for Nurses (QSEN) competency.

The process of interdisciplinary communication has been increasingly integrated into EHRs as the method nurses use to document outcomes of care given. However, EHRs are only a component of the larger **health information technology** (HIT) system (Rodrigues, Compte, & Diez, 2016). Use of **computerized provider order entry** (CPOE) systems are also described in this chapter. Your use of EHR technology to communicate and manage patient information is a skill specifically cited as part of QSEN's informatics competency. Regulatory and ethical implications of documentation will also be described in this chapter, concluding with a brief discussion of coding and nursing taxonomies. New technology and devices for medical communication at the point of care, clinical decision support systems (CDSSs), remote monitoring, secure messaging, and telehealth are discussed in Chapter 26.

BASIC CONCEPTS

Computerized Health Information Technology Systems

Computers make information more accessible to all who are involved, including your patient. Globally, governments and professional organizations believe computerized systems not only improve the quality of health care but will also eventually reduce its cost. The goal is to use HIT to improve population health outcomes and health care quality (US Department of Health and Human Services, n.d.). HIT is potentially making care safer by engaging patients as partners in their health care, promoting better communication, and increasing use of preventive practices and evidence-based "best practices" (Dolin, Goodrich, & Kallem, 2014). How does this affect you? Use of HIT skills is an expectation at the beginning staff nurse job level. Studies show EHR use skills can be successfully integrated into simulations labs teaching these skills (Georges, Drahnak, Schroeder, & Katrancha, 2016). Your ability to use information technology is among items tested on licensure exams (Bowling, 2016).

Meaningful Use

Adoption of HIT creates an interactive computerized information and communication system. Far more complex

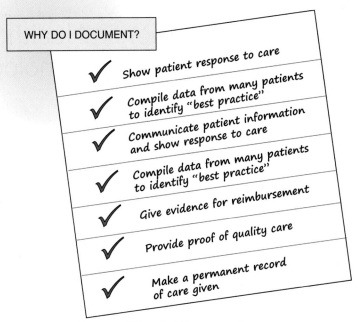

WHY DO I DOCUMENT?

✓ Show patient response to care

✓ Compile data from many patients to identify "best practice"

✓ Communicate patient information and show response to care

✓ Compile data from many patients to identify "best practice"

✓ Give evidence for reimbursement

✓ Provide proof of quality care

✓ Make a permanent record of care given

Fig. 25.1 Why Do I Document?

than just putting existing paper documentation on a computer, HIT systems are designed to support the multiple *information needs* required by today's complex patient care; provide you and others on the health team with *clinical decision support*; and achieve safer care for your patient.

In the United States, the Centers for Medicare and Medicaid Services (CMS) have specified EHR components required for use by providers and agencies who serve their patients. Crucial "meaningful use" information is listed in Table 25.1. In addition to using EHRs, providers must submit electronic patient data to government agencies, as well as share data across agencies, to demonstrate quality outcomes and to facilitate care coordination. "Meaningful use" requires that patients can view their records. This is an example of how new regulations directly impact the way you document.

The authors use the term *EHR* in this book, although electronic records are also known as electronic patient records, person-centered health records, or **electronic medical records** (Fig. 25.2). Most of these terms initially applied to computerized records within a provider's office or agency. Currently there are many different versions of electronic systems in use, *lacking **interoperability*** (cross compatibility). Ideally, EHRs have portability and can

follow your patient to other providers or specialists, or other hospitals, nursing homes, and so forth. Technology exists for secure storage on supercomputers in "the cloud," which would allow anytime, anywhere remote access by multiple providers (with patient permission). Although this chapter focuses on the communication aspect of HIT systems, it should also be mentioned that there are business, financial, and legal aspects. For example, HIT provides the agency with the data necessary for billing without extra effort to providers (Michel-Verkerke, Stegwee, & Spil, 2015), as well as establishing legal records.

Three Keys to Electronic Records

The three keys to electronic records are **interoperability**, **portability**, and **ease of use**.

Interoperability (Interagency Accessibility)

Exchanging health information among agencies is critical to smoothly delivering comprehensive patient-centered care. Interoperability means disparate systems can "talk to each other" to share patient information. This is essential if we are to reduce costs by eliminating redundancy. For example, when your patient's laboratory results or imaging files are available to multiple providers, unnecessary

TABLE 25.1   Components of an Electronic Health Information Technology System in Our Journey to Consumer-Driven Health Care

Mandatory (Required by CMS under its "meaningful use" criteria)	Desirable (Some of which must be chosen to be used)
An integrated, accessible electronic repository of patient data with easy access by a variety of health care providers for exchange of information. Contains and records changes in: Updated problem list Hx; Dx; VS; PE data Medication list Allergy list (crosschecks for drug-drug-allergy problems and sends alerts to providers) Imaging files with real-time access at the point of care	EHR system needs ease of access, perhaps by use of templates that the provider checks or customizes/modifies, e.g., a box is checked when an ECG was done and results are checked "normal" or "abnormal." Information is accessed before and after each task, with nurse documenting not only care given but progress toward goals. EHR can be remotely accessed by providers who can work from anywhere at any time. HIT system has financial tools, as well as clinical tools, e.g., it is able to generate newest ICD codes, do billing information, schedule appointments, etc. Incorporates accommodations to improve work flow and thus increase productivity. Ease of access allows provider to access many screen files with one login.
Has clinical decision support capabilities. Incorporates standard "evidence-based best practice" protocols that monitor your care and send you prompts if care is not recorded.	Sends alerts to providers
Uses CPOE	
Reports quality outcome measures to the government (CMS); public health agencies; state or local governmental agencies while safeguarding privacy/HIPAA requirements	Each year the percentage of total patients for whom your agency must submit reportable information increases.
Required use of EHRs also mandates capability to generate written prescriptions to avoid handwriting errors	May electronically send prescriptions to preferred pharmacy
On request can provide patient with clinical summaries: copies of records, laboratory findings, discharge instructions, educational resources, forms for advanced directives, etc.	Patient may not have access to all levels of information. Has online portals to access their information. Sends electronic reminders or alerts to patients
Provides summary of care at each point of transition, and for referrals	
Aggregates data	

CMS, Center for Medicare and Medicaid Services; *CPOE*, computerized physician/provider order entry; *Dx*, diagnosis; *ECG*, electrocardiogram; *EHR*, electronic health record; *HIPAA*, Health Insurance Portability and Accountability Act; *HIT*, health information technology; *Hx*, history; *ICD*, International Statistical Classification of Diseases and Related Health Problems; *PE*, physical examination; *VS*, vital signs. (Adapted from multiple sources including HealthIT.gov, accessed August 19, 2017.)

repetition of tests or procedures can be eliminated and costs reduced. However, incompatibility of software or privacy regulations can interfere with the communication of information. Although interoperability across agencies and providers has been a major goal for several years, exchanging records among systems remains a big barrier (Butler, 2017).

Governments, the health care industry, and the insurance industry are working to enable different systems to exchange information—to "talk" to each other. In the US Office of the National Coordinator for HIT, a certification process was created to harmonize EHR products for better interoperability. Not only must EHRs be integrated in multiple departments such as pharmacy, radiology, physical therapy, and nursing, they need to be accessible across agencies, as in the Levine case example. Some states are transitioning to statewide EHR systems such as Arkansas' SHARE system.

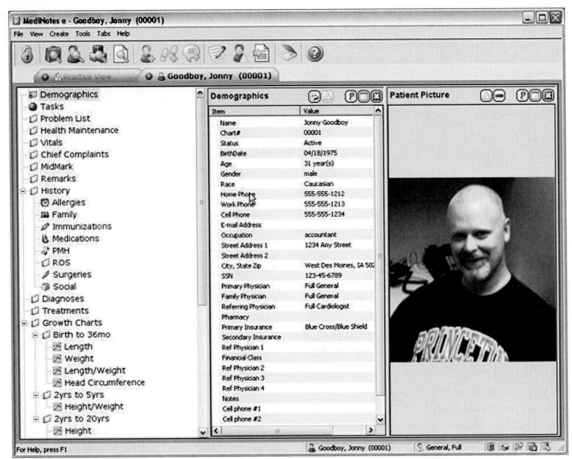

Fig. 25.2 Example of an Electronic Health Record. (Courtesy MediNotes Corporation.)

Mrs. Levine Case

Mrs. Levine's laboratory results can be directly entered into her primary provider's EHR by an outside laboratory and then accessed by you, the nurse, from your specialty outpatient clinic. With interoperability, information flows to providers as needed, allowing seamless transitions. With interoperability we can have anytime, anywhere access of health care records using remote devices. Using her home computer, Mrs. Levine can access her provider's portal to read case notes and look at her lab test results, scheduling another appointment if needed.

Portability

Electronic records are more durable than paper charting and are portable. They are easily transferable. For example, the Veterans Administration record system is fully integrated with the Department of Defense. Therefore, if a soldier is wounded abroad, diagnosed and treated, shipped home, and eventually discharged, records are seamlessly available to Vetrans Administration doctors. Consider another example: you celebrate graduation by traveling across the country on vacation. If you are in a car accident and are admitted to an emergency department (ED), your records stored "in the cloud" are potentially available to the ED physician via the internet. At the very least, you can carry them with you on a flash drive or CD.

Ease of Access

Ease of access ideally means access at the point of care or remotely using various digital devices. While maintaining record security, patients can give permission for access by multiple caregivers for anytime, anywhere communication. However, several studies show this multiple access generates large records which may not easily allow access to specific data of immediate interest to the nurse. In addition, printed copy can be voluminous (Braaf, Riley, & Manias, 2015; Chao, 2016). This 24/7 access from remote devices has markedly changed the way health care is practiced. Through use of internet **portals,** patients can also access some of their health information.

HIT system barriers currently include cost, incompatible hardware and software, government privacy regulations, and most importantly, the great difficulty in keeping stored data secure. Individual related barriers include a tendency to delay entry of salient information until the end of day, which impedes the intended improved communication channel of shared view of a patient's condition across many providers (Chao, 2016).

DOCUMENTING PATIENT INFORMATION IN ELECTRONIC RECORDS

HIT systems thoroughly compile records of patient health care. Yet, the effects on nurse-patient communication during the process of entering data into electronic records are less well known. DeSimone (2016) cites a large nurse survey which found that 92% of hospital nurses were dissatisfied with their agency system.

Advantages to Electronic Health Records
Improved Information Flow
A comprehensive computer information system changes the way information flows through the health care delivery system. Communication is streamlined rapidly. HIT can simultaneously communicate to doctors, nurses, patient, and families, and across agency departments. Continue to follow the Levine case:

Continuation of the Levine Case Example
Mrs. Levine develops trouble breathing. She is admitted via the emergency department (ED) to a medical unit at General Hospital at 11 a.m. with a diagnosis of congestive heart failure. Her ED physician had accessed her prior electronic health record (EHR), updated information, and documented his notes and her electrocardiogram (ECG) results. The ED nurse documented medications and treatments given. The health information technology (HIT) system flags her own physician, who comes in to examine her and enters diagnostic and treatment orders using a computerized provider order entry (CPOE) system. He does not need to repeat the ECG, because the system already contains these data. These orders are simultaneously and instantly transmitted to the pharmacy, the laboratory, and radiology, as well as to you, the nurse assigned on her unit.

IMPROVED COMPLETENESS OF NURSING DOCUMENTATION

Evidence shows EHR use results in more complete records (Agency for Healthcare Quality and Research [AHRQ], 2017). A multisite study ranked problem completeness at 90% (Wright et al., 2015). This may be due to e-prompts to nurses about including certain data; the features which download data such as vital signs automatically; the format which includes check-off boxes; the drop-down menu boxes; and the electronically generated standard interventions for each diagnosis (see Fig. 25.2). The Joint Commission (TJC) cautions us to be aware of patient safety risks evolving from use of technology (TJC, 2016). We need to communicate care our patient received. Timely and accurate documentation of care given is crucial to providing team members with the information they need to make informed decisions. The primary purpose of documentation is to maintain an exchange of information about the patient among all care providers *including staff nurses*. Documentation in EHRs supports the continuity, quality, and safety of your care. Quality documentation not only improves communication about the admitting diagnosis but also may increase recognition of comorbid conditions that can then also be treated (Towers, 2013).

Is it possible to fully document all nursing care given? Lack of visibility seems to be a recurring theme. Nurses report that the individualized care they give their patients is not visible in the format demanded by the computer, especially when a checklist format is used for care. Consequently, some nurses are said to rely on "informal" communication passed along during change of shift, as well as the information on the patient's EHR. Records that are inaccurate, incomplete, or not reinforced verbally compromise clinical decisions and quality of care reporting. So we need to communicate current condition information and response to treatment both in the record and verbally.

PARTNERING WITH PATIENTS IN DOCUMENTING

Studies repeatedly show that when patients are actively involved in decision making about their health, they manage their illnesses better, complying with treatment protocols. In accord with making patients active partners in their health care, new "meaningful use" regulations require that they have access to some areas of their EHRs, allowing them to look at information or even possibly add additional data as needed. For example, Kaiser Permanente's nearly 9 million members can access their immunization records at anytime from anywhere. We have the technology by which the patient can communicate home health–monitored data such as blood pressure, glucose level, weight, and so forth, to the primary provider's office electronically. In fact, some systems automatically input these data. Thus the provider is immediately aware of significant changes. Use of biosensors to transmit patient generated data via internet portals will be further described in Chapter 26.

Essentials of Nursing Documentation

Our documentation is guided by accreditation standards, third-party payers, and the legal system. Every health care agency has its own version of what constitutes complete clinical documentation. Medicare has published guidelines for primary providers saying documentation should include a patient history (a database that often includes a summary list of health problems and needs); physical examination findings; a description of the presenting problem; and rationales for decision making, counseling, and coordination of care in a patient-centered care plan. Nursing documentation contains a daily record of patient progress and evaluation of outcomes. Daily records may include flow sheets, nursing notes, intake and output forms, and medication records. Some data, such as vital signs, are automatically recorded into the EHR.

Clarity

Information should flow in an efficient manner so all members of the team have access to current data, so they are able to do ongoing evaluations of treatment outcomes. Such improvements in communication lead to improved outcomes for patients. Try thinking of it this way: every task sequence you perform requires you to access data before and after completion to maintain continuity. As you chart continually, entering information into the system, communication among the health team is improved. In one example, nurses in a study by Nemeth et al. (2007) accessed current laboratory test results at the point of care, allowing them to discuss changes in care during home visits. A specific example might be instant access to laboratory results on blood clotting time, allowing you to contact the physician for a change in anticoagulation medication levels while you are still at your patient's home.

Clear documentation means using **standardized terms** that are understood by every member of the health team. Documentation of care must be accurate. For example, you are expected to document the presence on admission of catheters and intravenous lines, as well as facts about the status of any decubitus (bed sore).

Efficiency

Access time to records should be enhanced using HIT systems. For example, when using paper files, it took a lengthy time to do audits for agency quality assurance (QA) or by insurance companies verifying reimbursement.

Some literature suggests that nurses feel caught between the demands for meeting all their patient care needs and the agency requirements for complete documentation. However, the majority of evidence shows that EHRs actually save time, allowing staff nurses more time at the bedside, especially when devices for charting are at the bedside (Yee et al., 2012). The potential impact of EHRs on nursing efficiency is measured by a reduction in the amount of time you spend doing activities other than direct nursing care of your patient. Concerns about documentation time may be alleviated as eventually "natural language" computers are able to use voice entry rather than typed data entry. Computerization improves the efficiency and quality of charting, by prompting for information needed, while eliminating duplication. For example, instead of re-questioning patients about health history, this information is already available on their EHR. Efficiency is increased because providers all across the agency have immediate access to information. The literature lists HIT benefits that improve nursing efficiency in other "downstream" ways beyond what is apparent in documentation activities, such as medication record resolution, automatic medication calculations, automatic downloading of bedside monitoring records, automated nursing discharge summaries, and so forth. Capability to document your care from your patient's bedside or home is known as "**point of care.**"

Safety

As discussed in Chapter 2, HIT systems have made care safer. HIT systems force standardization of nursing terminology, eliminate use of inappropriate abbreviations, and avoid problems of illegibility. Errors are prevented because assistance is given with drug calculations, as well as assistance with decision support such as checking drug incompatibility, allergies, and so on. Studies of the medication process show errors or potential errors cut by half (Radley et al., 2013) and errors in labeling lab specimens cut by two-thirds (Rouse, 2017).

ENHANCED QUALITY OF CARE

There are many secondary uses of data contained in patient records. When masses of data are analyzed, information is generated to add to our knowledge of what care measures lead to improved and effective nursing "best practice" care (American Nurses Association [ANA], 2017b).

Documentation to demonstrate quality assurance. Health care has shifted to emphasize measurement of quality outcome indicators. Financial incentives reward evidence of clinical quality rather than volume (Dolin et al., 2014). The United States (AHRQ, n.d.) has adopted a National Quality Strategy outlining three aims: better health care; healthier people; and more affordable care.

Reviews are done to determine the extent to which evidence-based care standards are being met. Ongoing reviews of care are done by internal agency review committees, as well as external audits by entities such as insurance companies or government regulatory bodies, such as those associated with the CMS. Assessments as to quality of care are based on what was documented and coded. Data are examined to see whether the care listed is in compliance with quality and safety guidelines and established standards of care. Clear documentation also provides evidence of effective care and outcomes during accreditation reviews. Evidence is slowly accumulating that shows HIT systems can make health care more patient-centered, promote better coordination of care, and make communication more effective.

Health outcomes. Computerized systems offer ease of access to **aggregate** information from many patients for reports and disease surveillance and to research "best practice" nursing care. Aggregated information from a number of records can be analyzed to determine patient health outcomes. For example, information about the number of postoperative infections that have occurred on your unit can be obtained. Or you may want to find out how many diabetic patients in your primary care practice failed to return for follow-up teaching and then generate a list for call-backs for more education. HIT systems can be used to obtain reports about predictors of patient outcomes in home health care. For example, you can easily get information identifying the most effective specific nursing interventions to establish "best practice" and identify other interventions that need to be changed. In a study examining nurse adherence to clinical guidelines, results showed significant correlation with improved diabetic foot care (Rolley, 2012). By combining data, nurses identify better treatment methods and evaluate the outcomes of their interventions on groups of patients.

Timely feedback from data compilation organizations can help you to improve your practice. As an example, participation in centralized disease registries can give real-time feedback to providers, and participants in the National Cancer Data System can receive electronic "alerts" if best practice care is not started within a certain time frame.

Epidemiological data. Combining data from many care recipients quickly can speed identification of adverse outcomes. Public health agencies analyze information to identify disease trends to generate epidemiological information. One example would be when a government agency such as the Centers for Disease Control analyzes the spread of influenza across the world. In another example, Kaiser Permanente was able to analyze information from 1.3 million patients

receiving Vioxx to identify potential harm from this medication, which led to its removal from the market.

Use of Computerized Provider Entry Systems

Computerized provider order entry (CPOE) refers to that part of HIT in which providers such as physicians, physician assistants, nurse practitioners, or sometimes staff nurses directly enter their orders for diagnosis or treatment, which then transmits the order directly to the recipient responsible for carrying out that order, such as the pharmacy, the laboratory, or radiology. At a minimum, this aspect of the system ensures that orders are complete, use standard terms, and are available in a legible format. However, this system not only processes an order, it cross compares it with data in the patient's EHR such as whether the patient is allergic to this newly ordered medication or has a potential for a drug-drug adverse interaction or whether the dose or route ordered exceeds standard guidelines for safety. CPOE may also check for errors of omission. For example, it would give a prompt about a need to also order a laboratory test to verify acceptable blood level of the new medication. CPOE systems are usually paired with computer-assisted **clinical decision support systems** (CDSSs), which are discussed in Chapter 26.

Outcomes for use of computerized provider entry. Evidence is beginning to suggest that use of these systems improve the appropriateness of orders, positively affect communication, and improve patient outcomes, particularly by reducing adverse drug events and even increasing compliance (AHRQ, PSNet). CPOE is one of thirty "safe practices for better health care" recommended by AHRQ and the National Quality Forum. However, there is still some potential for error, such as entering data on the wrong patient. We still need to use critical thinking skills to evaluate for safe practice, especially in the area of medication administration.

Other Formats for Documenting Nursing Care

Use of structured documentation has been found to be associated with more complete nursing records, better continuity of care, more meaningful nursing data, and perhaps better patient outcomes. In charting electronically, the nurse can call up a template to record today's data.

Flow sheets or checklists. Electronic charting can use **flow sheets** with predefined progress parameters based on written standards with preprinted categories of information. They contain daily assessments of normal findings. For example, in assessing lung sounds, the nurse needs to merely indicate "clear" if that information is normal. Deviations from norm must be completely documented. By marking a flow sheet or checklist, you are saying all care was performed according to existing agency protocols.

Plan of Care

Nursing care plans are still valued by nursing instructors as a tool for student learning. However, in the age of electronic records in hospitals, clinics, and long-term care facilities, the traditional nursing care plans for each patient are being replaced by electronic **longitudinal plans of care (LPCs)**. Clinical pathways stating daily patient goals have mostly either been incorporated into the EHR or been replaced by electronic prompts.

ELECTRONIC LONGITUDINAL PLANS OF CARE

In an effort to reduce regulations for hospitals in the United States, CMS recommends that nurses coordinate care through use of interdisciplinary care plans (replacing nursing care plans). The US Department of Health and Human Services, the national HIT office, and CMS issued a single plan of care format to assist in communication, coordination, and continuity. The plan of care needs to be accessible to all providers across all settings (Cipriano et al., 2013). Data from every discipline on the health care team are used to develop a single individualized interdisciplinary plan of care that sets mutual goals for each patient's progress and is documented by the nurse and other team members daily. The LPC must harmonize data requirements for home care, long-term care, and acute and postacute care; this is the patient-centered LPC.

Standards: Ethical, Regulatory, and Professional

Standards of documentation must meet the requirements of government, health care agency, professional standards of practice, the use of electronic medical records, and storage of personal health information in computer databases has refocused attention on the issues of ethics, security, privacy, and confidentiality that are described earlier in this book. For example, a nurse in one unit of a hospital who accesses the electronic medical record of a patient who is in another unit and for whom the nurse has no responsibilities for care is violating confidentiality. Ethical professional practice requires that you do not allow others to use your access log on. Other ethical issues with electronically generated care plans and standard orders center on how to determine who is responsible for the computer-generated care decisions.

Confidentiality and Privacy

As discussed in Chapter 3, **confidentiality** is the act of limiting disclosure of private matters appropriately, maintaining the trust that an individual has placed in an agent entrusted with private matters. In the United States, most states have laws that grant the patient ownership rights to the information contained in their health record. Electronic storage and transmission of medical records have sparked intense scrutiny over privacy protection. Many breaches have been reported in popular media. More than 70% of consumers have expressed concerns that their personal health records stored in an EHR with internet connections will not remain private, and 89% say they withhold health information (Gordon, 2017). Indeed, experts say a breach of your health records is not a matter of whether but is a matter of when.

Ethical and legal parameters limit when you can share patient information. When computers are located at the bedside, the screen displays information to anyone who stops by the bedside. You need to be alert to this potential privacy violation. Violations of confidentiality because of unauthorized access or distribution of sensitive health information can have severe consequences for patients. It may lead to discrimination at the workplace, loss of job opportunities, or disqualification for health insurance. Personal information in health records such as social security numbers, home address, etc. can be used in identity theft. Issues of privacy will dominate how nurses and other health care providers address clinical documentation in the years ahead. Currently, a **personal medical identification number** is used on patient records. Hardware safeguards such as workstation security, keyed lock hard drives, and automatic log-offs are used in addition to user identification and passwords to prevent unauthorized access. Some advocate that individuals be able to choose how much of their information is shared and be notified when their information is accessed. In the United States, federal law now requires patients be notified in the event of a breach of their EHR. Authorization is not needed in situations concerning the public's health, criminal, or legal matters. Refer to Chapter 3 for federal medical record privacy regulations (Health Insurance Portability and Accountability Act [HIPAA]).

Legal Aspects of Charting

Management literature emphasizes the need for quicker documentation that still reflects the nursing process. At the same time, documentation must be legally sound. The legal assumption is that the care was not given unless it is documented in the record, which is a legal document, even though it is digital (Merriweather, 2017). Malpractice settlements have approached the multimillion-dollar mark for individuals whose charts failed to document safe, effective care.

"If it was not charted, it was not done." This statement stems from a legal case (*Kolesar v. Jeffries*) heard before Canada's Supreme Court, in which a nurse failed to document the care of a patient on a Stryker frame before he died. Because the purpose of the medical record is to list care given and outcomes, any information that is clinically significant must be included. Aside from issues of legal liability, third-party reimbursement depends on accurate recording of care given. Major insurance companies audit records and contest any charges that are not documented. Every nurse should anticipate having their patients' records subpoenaed at some time during their nursing career (refer to Box 25.1 for recommendations).

Any method of documentation that provides comprehensive, factual information is legally acceptable. This includes graphs and checklists. By signing a protocol, check sheet, pathway, and so forth, you are documenting that

---

BOX 25.1   Tips for Electronic Health Record Use Which Promotes a Culture of Patient Safety

Do

Change your electronic health record (EHR) password frequently

Enter notes in "real time" as much as possible (chart promptly)

Maintain confidentiality (e.g., enter data in way that visitors cannot see)
Verbalize a summary of what you enter at the bedside, so patient can validate
Explain to patient the e-documentation process, letting them know they can ask questions as you enter data
Review or read back crucial data you have entered
Make eye contact periodically

Document progress: all changes in patient condition, any bizarre behavior
Verbally reinforce crucial info with staff, even though you entered it into patient's record
Participate in all offered e-training updates
Correct errors per agency protocol, usually by adding addendum to your notes, listing correct info with explanation

Do Not

Avoid sharing your EHR password
Do not rush: ask for administrative time for data entry
Do not rush when typing data.
Avoid short cuts such as "copy and paste"
Avoid saving all charting until end of shift. Do not make "untimely" entries (after another shift has charted)
Do not just rely on the "sleep" screen
Avoid the "cut and paste" that is a common data entry work-around

Try not to depersonalize, by ignoring patient as you type
Do not fail to record any ordered care which is omitted and who was notified
Do not let confusing information in the record stand unremarked

Avoid using "soft" or "hard" delete

DEVELOPING AN EVIDENCE-BASED PRACTICE
Health communication literature frequently alludes to the effects use of computers has on nurse-patient-family interactions. One common theme: does documenting patient information on computers interfere with our interpersonal relationship with our patient? Mayor and Bietti (2017) examined 40 journal articles describing nurse-patient conversations.

Results: Despite our avowal of patient-centered care, their analysis reveals interaction asymmetry, with nurses dominating the flow of communication. Nurses were found to exert control over most of the progress of an interaction, including setting the topic of conversation. Patient participation in health care centers showed nurse-directed communications focusing on collection of clinical information. However, the opposite was found when the interaction occurred in the patient's own home. Very rel-

evant for our increased use of technology-mediated interactions, the authors concluded that technology limits the possibilities for interactions with patients.

Implications for Your Clinical Practice: If the patient's EHR prompts you with a set checklist of needed information, how could you heighten the patient's participation? Mayor and Bietti recommend that nurses compiling patient-generated information into a computerized health record first encourage the patient to tell his or her entire story, before using the computer tool to record data. Others have suggested allowing the patient to see what you are typing, using this as a conversation booster. What suggestions might realistically work considering the workload demands made on many nurses? "Natural language" data entry/recording is replacing manual typing. This may facilitate patient contact.

From Mayor, E., & Bietti, L. (2017). Ethnomethodological studies of nurse-patient and nurse-relative interactions: A scoping review. *International Journal of Nursing Studies, 70,* 46–57.

every step was performed. If a protocol exists in a health care agency, you are legally responsible for carrying it out.

Accountability

We in health care will increasingly focus on measures that matter. HIT allows us to develop data for multiple levels of accountability, including for individual nurses, units, or agencies. There is a move to make health care outcomes more transparent to consumers. For example, some hospital websites now post their infection rates. Just as there are websites that post customer evaluations of individual hotels, there are sites such as CMC's site www.hospitalcompare.com that post patient comments about their care and their caregivers by name.

APPLICATIONS

Computer Literacy

One of the QSEN competencies expected of the new graduate is ability to use **informatics.** To practice nursing in coming years, you will need to continually upgrade your technology skills. As students, you learn skills such as data entry, data transmission, word processing, internet accessing, spreadsheet entry, and use of standard language and codes describing practice. Will voice recognition software for clinical documentation make documentation easier for nurses?

Communicating Medical Orders
Written Orders

Nurses are required to question orders that they do not understand or those that seem to them to be unsafe. Failure to do so puts the nurse at *legal risk*. "Just following orders" is not an acceptable excuse. Conversely, nurses can be held liable if they arbitrarily decide not to follow a legitimate order, such as choosing to withhold ordered pain medication. Reasons for such a decision would have to be explicitly documented. With computerization, it is possible to have standing orders, such as for administering vaccines. The computer is programmed to recognize the absence of a vaccination and then to automatically write an order for a nurse to administer. What might the legal implications be?

Persons who are licensed or certified by appropriate government agencies to conduct medical treatment acts include physicians, advance practice nurses, and physician assistants. In the United States, these providers have their own state prescribing numbers and must abide by government rules and restrictions. To prescribe controlled substances, they must also have a Drug Enforcement Agency (DEA) number. Nurse practitioners may choose not to apply for a DEA number. Consult your agency policy regarding who is allowed to write orders for the nurse to carry out.

Although electronic anytime, anywhere digital access should have replaced older communication, you may need to consider some other routes.

Faxed Orders. The physician or nurse practitioner may choose to send a faxed order. Because this is a form of written order, it has been shown to decrease the number of errors that occur when transcribing verbal or telephone orders. However, there is the risk for violating confidentiality when faxing health-related information.

Verbal Orders

Often, a change in condition requires the nurse to text or telephone the primary physician or hospital staff resident to obtain new orders. Most primary providers work in group practices, so it is necessary to determine who is "on call" or who is covering your patient when the primary provider is unavailable. It may be necessary to call for new orders if there is a significant change in the physical or mental condition as noted by vital signs, laboratory value reports, treatment or medication reactions, or response failure. Before calling for verbal orders, access the EHR and familiarize yourself with current vital signs, medications, infusions, and other relevant data. Read Chapter 2 on using the SBAR (situation, background, assessment, recommendation) format to communicate with doctors.

Charting for Others. It is not acceptable to chart for others. Reflect on what you would do in the following case if you were called by Juanita Diaz, RN.

Diaz Case Example

Juanita Diaz worked the day shift. At 6 p.m. she calls you and says she forgot to chart Mr. Reft's preoperative enema. She asks you to chart the procedure and his response to it. Can you just add it to your notes? In court, this would be portrayed as an inaccuracy. The correct solution is to add an addendum to your EHR notes, "1800: Nurse Juanita Diaz called and reported..."

WORKLOAD AND WORK-AROUNDS

Nurses are trained as problem solvers. They are constantly tinkering to improve. In their review of multiple studies, Ranji, Rennke, and Watcher (2013) suggest that some nurses perceive adverse impact on their workload and on their ability to care for their patients. Nurses carry heavy workloads and do not like technology that disrupts or adds to their work flow. For example, "alarm fatigue" was described in Chapter 2.

To avoid burden and allow for task completion, some nurses create shortcuts to bypass aspects of the computerized system, known as "work-arounds." This raises safety concerns and may alter a system that is designed to improve safety and make it less safe (Finkel & Galvin, 2017). Report system problems and errors so we can work together to create a safer system. Barnsteiner (2017) urges us to come to work each day seeking ways to improve the system.

Documenting on a Patient's Health Record

Documenting electronically requires learning the specific system at your agency. There is a learning curve; that is, initially it may take longer, but as you become familiar with each agency system, EHRs should increase your nursing efficiency. Electronic charting for nurses usually combines dropdown boxes with forced choice pick lists with free text boxes for narrative information. Keep in mind the need to use standardized terminology and, where possible, to use checklists. These allow for combining information into large data sets to examine outcomes for the purpose of establishing "best practices."

Although it is recognized that for some, entry of e-data takes longer, it is a safety issue (Finkel & Galvin, 2017). Refer to Box 25.1 for some tips. You are encouraged to document completely, to use the narrative section to describe changes in your patient's outcomes. Remember that free text boxes may have word count limits. In addition, narrative comments may provide needed detail, but they may also perpetuate the electronic invisibility of nursing unless information can be captured into categories. Tips for efficient documentation include not repeating checklist information, use of proofreading narrative comments, checking all numbers to detect transpositions, and avoiding abbreviations.

Keeping the Interpersonal While Doing Computerized Charting

Nurses have also reported reservations about unintended effects on their communication with patients. Although some individuals complain, most have adapted to providers who spend time not making eye contact or pausing the dialog because they are busy typing data into the EHR. According to HealthIT, 74% of patients report that EHRs have enhanced their care. How would you manage communication rapport during an interview, when the HIT system keeps prompting you to obtain data?

Make documenting at the bedside warmer in a human relation sense. If your patient seems to be bothered by the lack of interpersonal contact while you are busy typing on the bedside computer, what steps could you take? One suggestion is to face the computer terminal toward the patient, so you do not turn your back while typing information. Some nurses comment aloud about the general information they are inputting, stopping every minute or so to make eye contact with their patient. Asking for information and then typing it in may make them realize they are actively contributing to their EHR information. In addition, explaining about how these entries are keeping the team aware of updated information about the patient's condition may help them to value this process.

Coding

Coding allows nursing information to be easily communicated and extracted from EHRs for the purpose of compiling information to make cross-comparisons: evaluations, audits, research, or develop standards of care. A prerequisite for this was to move nursing terminology to a standard taxonomy. It is crucial to nursing that nursing terminologies become embedded into EHRs, both to improve communication between nurses, such as at change of shift, and to allow data to be extracted to describe nursing care (Fig. 25.3).

Coding Nursing Practice Provides Information:

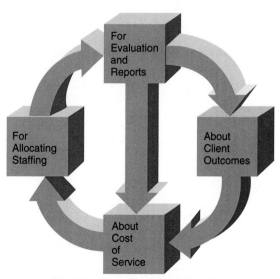

For
Evaluation
and
Reports

About
Client
Outcomes

For
Allocating
Staffing

About
Cost
of
Service

Fig. 25.3 Coding in Nursing Practice.

Classification of Care: Use of Standardized Terminologies and Taxonomies

The nursing profession was very active in developing standardized terminology, an essential element of EHRs. The International Council of Nurses (ICN) developed a unified nursing language system, the International Classification for Nursing Practice (ICNP). As nurses, our goal is to classify the care provided and document outcomes of care, to effectively communicate. Global adoption requires adequate translation into local languages, a difficult task (Hou, Chang, Chan, & Dykes, 2013).

In the past, nursing has been unable to describe the units of care and its effect on patient outcome or to establish a cost for its contributions to patient care. Nowhere on one's hospital bill does the cost of our nursing care appear. It traditionally has been part of the "room charge." Our goal in developing standardized terminology and classification codes is not only to improve communication, but to make nursing practice visible within (computerized) health information systems and to assist in establishing evidence-based nursing practice.

In home health records, nurses most often document nursing problems or diagnoses related to the medical diagnosis, but some report they actually spend most of their care in patient teaching. How can this be reflected in the EHR?

Taxonomies: Standardized Language Terminology in Nursing

The ANA recognizes a number of different taxonomies for describing nursing care, based on specific criteria. Because no one system meets the needs of nurses in all areas of practice, technological applications are needed to communicate across classification systems (see Table 25.2).

Taxonomy is defined as a hierarchical method of classifying a vocabulary of items according to certain rules. For example, the Bloom taxonomy is used to categorize the cognitive levels of some of the end of chapter discussion questions in this book. Various taxonomies have been developed to be used in communication and comparisons across health care settings and providers, insurers and payers, and policy makers who set priorities and allocate resources. The North American Nursing Diagnosis Association International (NANDA-I) is the best researched and most widely implemented nursing classification internationally. The N3 terminologies (NANDA-I, Nursing Interventions Classification [NIC], and Nursing Outcomes Classification [NOC]), used together to plan and document nursing care, are sometimes referred to as **NNN.** Their use creates a systematic schema for implementing the nursing process. Other nursing coding systems include the Omaha System designed for use in the community (Simulation Exercise 25.1).

TABLE 25.2   N3: Example of Linkages of North American Nursing Diagnosis Association, Nursing Interventions Classification, and Nursing Outcomes Classification

Nursing Diagnosis	Nursing Outcome (Rate Each Indicator on 1–5 Scale)	Nursing Interventions for Management of Long-term Pain
Chronic pain (domain: perceived health V)	Pain control—1605	*Assessment:*
Defining characteristics:	*Indicators:*	• Have patient assess pain at least daily using a 0-10 scale [zero is no pain ranging to 10 the worst ever].
• Sudden or slow onset	Recognizes pain onset— 160502	• Have patient record this daily pain rating in a log or diary, which can be submitted to nurse electronically, using patient portal.
• Consistent or reoccurring	Uses analgesics as recommended—160505	*Nursing activities for pain management:*
• Duration >6 months	Uses diary to monitor symptoms over time—160510	• Determine impact of pain on quality of daily life.
	Reports symptom changes to provider—160513	• Evaluate objective and subjective evidence to determine effectiveness of pain control measures
	Reports pain controlled— 160511	• Help patient administer analgesics as prescribed
		• Teach nonpharmocologic pain control measures such as heat/cold applications; massage; biofeedback; electronic stimulation with TENS unit; use of guided imagery, music therapy, therapeutic touch, etc.
		• Use pain control measures before pain escalates
		• Promote adequate rest
		• Have patient download and use APPS for pain management

Modified from Bulechek, G. M., Butcher, H. K., & Dochterman, J. (McCloskey). (2008). *Nursing classification (NIC)* (5th ed.). St. Louis, MO: Mosby/Elsevier; Johnson, M., Bulechek, G., Dochterman, J. M., et al. (2001). *Nursing diagnosis, outcomes, and interventions: NANDA, NOC, and NIC linkages.* St. Louis, MO: Mosby; Moorhead, M., Johnson, M., Maas, M., & Swanson, E. (2008). *Nursing outcomes classification (NOC)* (4th ed.). St. Louis, MO: Mosby/Elsevier.

SIMULATION EXERCISE 25.1   Application of Nursing Intervention Classification Finding

Purpose:

To make use of Nursing Interventions Classification (NIC) meaningful taxonomy.

Procedure:

Consider the following finding from Dochterman's (2005) study, then answer the questions.

On day 3 of hospitalization, nurses averaged four intravenous therapy interventions for patclients with a diagnosis of hip fracture but averaged only two interventions for (oral) fluid management.

1. How could you use this information to justify the need for skilled nursing care?
2. Suppose data showed that by day 6, skilled care activities had been cut in half. How might the nurse manager readjust the patclient assignment for her nurse aides?

On day 3, patclients with hip fractures received three times as many nursing interventions encouraging proper coughing as were made for patclients with congestive heart failure.

1. Speculate about why there was this difference.
2. Suppose hospital units with more nursing interventions to encourage coughing were shown to have greatly decreased rates of patclients with pneumonia complications. Could this information be used to justify a better nurse-to-patient ratio?

From Dochterman, J., Titler, M., Wang, J., Reed, D., Pettit, D., Mathew-Wilson, M., et al. (2005). Describing use of nursing interventions for three groups of patients. *Journal of Nursing Scholarship, 37*(1), 57–66.

Advantages and Disadvantages of Nursing Classification Systems

Nursing classification systems provide a standard and common language for nursing care so that nursing contributions to patient care become visible, promote "best practices," and define professional practice. ANA says that standards for terminology are an essential requirement for a computer-based patient record (ANA, 2017a); however, nursing classifications have not been incorporated into most agency's electronic clinical records.

Other Coding Systems in Health Care

The National Library of Medicine maintains a meta-the-saurus for a unified medical language. Because of the complexity of health care and the variety of providers involved, multiple medical classification systems have emerged. Often providers use several in combination. Examples of common medical classification and coding systems include 10th revision of the International Statistical Classification of Diseases and Related Health Problems (ICD-10) codes for medical diagnoses by body system; ICD-10-PCS codes for medical procedures; and the fifth edition of the *Diagnostic and Statistical Manual of Mental Disorders* (DSM-5) diagnoses for psychiatric conditions. Health Care Financing Administration's (HCFA) Outcome and Assessment Information Set (OASIS) assessment for the purpose of describing home care patients, developing outcome benchmarks, and providing feedback regarding quality of care to home health agencies. The OASIS assessment is required for home health agencies to receive reimbursement for the care provided to Medicare recipients. To learn more, visit HCFA's Medicare website (www.medicare.gov/).

SUMMARY

This chapter focuses on electronic documentation of care in the nurse-patient relationship. Documentation refers to the process of obtaining, organizing, and conveying information to others in the patient record. The broad aspects of health information systems, as well as the nurse's role in using EHRs, were discussed. Emphasis on the EHR's role in reducing redundancy, improving efficiency, reducing cost, decreasing errors, and improving compliance with standards of practice was stressed. The many secondary uses of compilations of electronic records for generation of knowledge were described, especially those which identify which nursing care practices produce "best" patient outcomes. Classification systems such as ICD-10 coding and NANDA, NIC, NOC were briefly described. Chapter 26 discusses eMobile technology that can facilitate communication among health care workers, increase patient education and increased engagement, and assist the providers of health care with decision making.

ETHICAL DILEMMA: What Would You Do?

A coworker mentions that a staff nurse you both know, Alice Jarvis, RN, has been admitted to the medical floor for some strange symptoms and that her laboratory results have just been posted in her electronic health record (EHR), showing she is positive for hepatitis C, among other things.

1. Identify at least two alternative ways to deal with this ethical dilemma. (What response would you make to your coworker who retrieved information from the computerized system? What else might you do?)
2. What ethical principle can you cite to support each answer?

From Sonya R. Hardin, RN, PhD, CCRN.

DISCUSSION QUESTIONS

1. Explain why "use of technologies to assist in effective communication in a variety of health care settings" is listed as an expected nurse competency by QSEN and other nursing organizations.

2. Documentation is an important aspect in your nursing. Of the reasons to document, determine the one of greatest concern to the novice nurse. Defend your selection.

REFERENCES

Agency for Healthcare Quality and Research (AHRQ). (n.d.). *PSNet: Patient safety network. Patient safety primer: Computerized provider order entry.* Retrieved from: http://psnet.ahrq.gov/Primers. [then click on 'Computerized Privider Order Entry']. (Accessed 10/1/18).

Agency for Healthcare Quality and Research (AHRQ). (2017). *Teams, TeamSTEPPs and team structures: Models for functional collaboration.* Webinar.

American Nurses Association (ANA). (2017a). *Electronic personal health record: ANA position statement.* Retrieved from: http://nursingworld.org/MainMenuCategories/Policy-Advocacy/Positions-and-Resolutions/ANAPositionStatements/.

American Nurses Association (ANA). (2017b). *Electronic health record: ANA position statement (approved 2009, copyright 2017)* Silver Spring, MD: Author. Retrieved from: http://nursingworld.org/MainMenuCategories/Policy-Advocacy/Positions-and-Resolutions/ANAPositionStatements/.

Barnsteiner, J. (2017, May 29). Chicago: Opening remarks at QSEN National Conference.

Bowling, A. M. (2016). Incorporating electronic documentation into beginning nursing courses facilitates safe nursing practice. *Teaching and Learning in Nursing, 11,* 204–208.

Braaf, S., Riley, R., & Manias, E. (2015). Failures in communication through documents and documentation across the perioperative pathway. *Journal of Clinical Nursing, 24,* 1874–1884.

Butler, M. (2017). Making HIPAA work for consumers. *Journal of AHIMA, 88*(3), 14–17.

Chao, C. (2016). The impact of electronic health records on collaborative work routines: A narrative network analysis. *International Journal of Medical Informatics, 82,* 418–426.

Cipriano, P. F., Bowles, K., Dailey, M., Dykes, P., Lamb, G., & Naylor, M. (2013). The importance of health information technology in care coordination and transitional care. *Nursing Outlook, 61,* 475–489.

CMS. (n.d.). Center for Medicare and Medicaid Services. Retrieved from: www.cms.gov/.

Dochterman, J., Titler, M., Wang, J., Reed, D., Pettit, D., & Mathew-Wilson, M., et al. (2005). Describing use of nursing interventions for three groups of patients. *Journal of Nursing Scholarship, 37*(1), 57–66.

DeSimone, D. M. (2016). *EHRs, communication and litigation: The high cost of all 3.* Oklahoma Nurse.

Dolin, R. H., Goodrich, K., & Kallem, C. (2014). Getting the standard: EHR quality reporting rises in prominence due to meaningful use. *Journal of AHIMA, 85*(1), 42–48.

Finkel, N., & Galvin, H. (2017). EHRs: Medication decision support for inpatient medicine. *Hospital Medicine Clinics, 6*(2), 204–215.

Georges, N. M., Drahnak, D. M., Schroeder, D. L., & Katrancha, E. D. (2016). Enhancing prelicensure nursing students' use of an EHR. *Clinical Simulation in Nursing, 12,* 152–158.

Gordon, L. T. (2017). Connecting consumers to their health information. *Journal of AHIMA, 88*(3), 13.

HealthIT. (n.d.). Retrieved from: www.HealthIT.gov/topic/health-it-basics/benefits/ehrs. (Accessed 10/1/18).

Hou, I., Chang, P., Chan, H., & Dykes, P. C. (2013). A modified Delphi translation strategy and challenges of international classification for nursing practice. *International Journal of Medical Informatics, 82,* 418–426.

Mayor, E., & Bietti, L. (2017). Ethnomethodilogical studies of nurse-patient and nurse-relative interactions: a scoping review. *International Journal of Nursing Studies, 70,* 40–57.

Merriweather, K. (2017). CDI in the outpatient setting: Finding the hidden gems of opportunity for improvement. *Journal of AHIMA, 88*(7), 48–51.

Michel-Verkerke, M. B., Stegwee, R. A., & Spil, T. (2015). The six P's of the next step in electronic patient records in the Netherlands. *Health Policy and Technology, 4,* 137–143.

Nemeth, L. S., Wessell, A. M., Jenkins, R. G., Nietert, P. J., Liszka, H. A., & Ornstein, S. M. (2007). Strategies to accelerate translation of research into primary care with practices using electronic medical records. *Journal of Nursing Care Quality, 22*(4), 343–349.

QSEN Institute. (n.d.). Quality and safety education for nurses. Retrieved from: www.QSEN.org/. (Accessed 10/1/18).

Radley, D. C., Wasserman, M. R., Olso, L., Shoemaker, S. J., Spranca, M. D., & Bradshaw, B. (2013). Reduction in medication errors in hospitals due to adoption of computerized provider order entry systems. *Journal of the American Medical Informatics Association, 20*, 470–476.

Ranji, S. R., Rennke, S., & Watcher, R. M. (2013). Chapter 41: Computerized provider order entry with clinical decision support systems: A brief update review. In Health Care Safer Making (Ed.), *An updated critical analysis of the evidence for patient safety practices*. Evidence Report/Technology Assessment No. 211. Rockville, MD: Agency for Healthcare Quality and Research (AHRQ). Retrieved from: http://www.ahrq.gov/research/findings/evidence-based-reports/ptsafetyuptp.html. (Accessed 10/1/18).

Rolley, J. X. (2012). Three-year follow-up after introduction of Canadian best practice guidelines for asthma and footcare in diabetes suggests that monitoring of nursing care indicators using electronic documentation system improves sustained implementation. *Evidence-Based Nursing, 15*(1), 5–6.

Rouse, T. (2017). *Poster presentation: Patient identification and specimen labeling at the bedside: Unit 1B Collaborative Council in Action*. Cleveland, OH: TeamSTEPPS National Conference. June 18.

The Joint Commission (TJC). (2016). *Sentinel alert event, #54: Safe use of HIT*. Retrieved from: www.jointcommission.org/assests/1/6/SEA_54_HIT_4_26_16.pdf. [search sentinel event alert #54: HIT]. (Accessed 10/1/18).

Towers, A. (2013). Clinical documentation improvement—A physician perspective. *Journal of AHIMA, 84*(7), 34–43.

US Department of Health and Human Services. (n.d.). *Healthy people 2020. Health communication and health information technology*. Retrieved from: www.healthypeople.gov/2020/topicsobjectives2020/. [search 'health communication and health technology']. (Accessed 10/1/18).

Wright, A., McCoy, A. B., Hickman, T., & Hilaire, D. S., et al. (2015). DProblem list completeness in electronic health records: a milti-site study and assessment of success factors. *International Journal of Medical Informatics, 84*, 784–790.

Yee, T., Needleman, J., Pearson, M., Parkerton, P., Parkerton, M., & Wolstein, J. (2012). The influences of integrated EMRs and computerized nurses' notes on nurses' time spent in documentation. *Computers, Informatics, Nursing, 30*(6), 287–292.

m-Health and Communication Technology

Kathleen Underman Boggs

OBJECTIVES

At the end of the chapter, the reader will be able to:

1. Evaluate use of mobile-Health technology applications and their effects on nurse-patient communication.
2. Discuss the advantages and disadvantages of various technologies for continual communication at point of care, as well as anytime, anywhere access.
3. Describe nurse advantages in using clinical guidelines and clinical decision support systems with regard to increasing efficiency in delivery of safe, quality health care.
4. Analyze strengths and weaknesses of various health technologies in improving communications and facilitating patient self-management.

Advances in technology continue to revolutionize health care through digital communication. This chapter will focus on use of mobile internet access devices (called "smart" devices) as an essential nursing competency. We have entered a new era in which smart phone applications with biomedical sensors are becoming widely used by patients to communicate with health providers (Topol, 2015). Nurses are playing a part in changing the focus from illness care to health care. We employ the latest in technology to communicate with other providers and with patients. "Smart" devices such as portable laptops and tablets are used at the point of care, be it hospital bedside or in our patient's home. Mobile devices such as tablets and smart phones are becoming indispensable for engaging our patients in their own health care. We communicate with patients for health care, health promotion, to support their self-management, and to connect them to e-support groups. Mobile devices and voice-activated systems allow continual **real-time interactive communication** of information, customized clinical decision making, and **decentralized, remote access** to information at the point of care. Technology enhances our work flow through expanded use of devices which input data automatically, provide "alerts," and enable us to give remote care via telehealth. Since our focus is nurse communication, we describe some e-Mobile technologies. We also discuss technology

support for safe practice through access to computerized clinical decision support systems (CDSSs), secure messaging, remote monitoring, and use of internet-based clinical practice guidelines.

BASIC CONCEPTS

Competency Expectations

As discussed in Chapter 25, nursing organizations advocate informatics proficiency for student nurses to promote safe, high-quality care. Novice nurses are expected to be proficient in the use of digital technologies for communication and for information management (American Academy of Colleges of Nursing [AACN]; Institute of Medicine [formerly IOM, now NASEM] competency; QSEN Prelicensure Competency). In addition to the electronic health records (EHRs), technology management includes monitoring systems, medication systems, and continual updating on new technologies associated with our care. Electronic compilation of patient outcome data should lead us to distill "best practice" to make better decisions. We are expected to integrate patient and caregiver into care. Another expected outcome of improved communication is decreases in health care costs over the long term. These rapidly evolving technologies offer new ways to deliver health care.

m-Health

The term mobile health care (**m-Health**) can mean the use of any wireless device and its downloaded health-related applications (**apps**). These use the internet and are independent of location.

Internet Use. Globally, the majority of the world's 7 billion people have access to internet devices, with nearly 5 billion subscribers (Bautista & Lin, 2016). By 2020 it is anticipated there will be 200 billion "smart" devices in use. More than two thirds of Americans use smart phones, including more than 75% of teenagers (Lusk, 2017; Powell, Chen, & Thammachart, 2017). *Healthy People 2020's* goals stated technology be used to improve health quality and improve communication to achieve health equity. New technologies such as m-Health foster "anywhere, anytime" communication with access to health providers and health information.

Communication Facilitation

Evidence shows that technologies facilitate our communication and teamwork to provide more effective, safe care. Ideally, we work to establish **fully integrated computerized systems** that share information across the entire health care system. Globally, care focus is shifting toward engaging persons in their own care (Anwar, Joshi, & Tan, 2015). Technology helps us shift from providing just "sick" care to a "preventative" mode.

Handheld internet devices are small enough to be easily carried. Their internet access is termed "wireless." Decentralized access to information and ability to document your care at your patient's location are referred to as **"point-of-care"** capability. You can use your smart phone or tablet to access nursing information databases to obtain evidence-based clinical care interventions. You document at the "point of care" either at your patients' bedsides or in their homes, as in the Sulif case.

Mrs. Sulif Case

Sam Esteves, RN, is employed by Medical Center on a medical unit. This hospital is part of a large health care system of primary care offices, clinics, laboratories, nursing homes, and three hospitals, all of which use the fully integrated computer system affectionately termed "Simon." Sam is notified at 0800 that his new patient, Mrs. Sulif, is in admissions getting her bar-coded name bracelet with her photo image affixed to it. In admissions she is entering her own history information into a "Simon"-affiliated tablet which has also scanned and uploaded her history from her own smart card into her EHR. Dietary is flagged because she has nut allergies. Preadmission laboratory results are already in her EHR,

having been uploaded by a lab tech, who notes the system has flagged her low hematocrit results and sent an "alert" to Sam and her admitting physician's office. Sam is also advised as to her need for handicapped-accessible equipment. On the unit by 0845, a robot has delivered equipment to the room while Sam has summoned a patient care technician by text to help lift Mrs. Sulif into bed wearing linen stored right in her room (refer to Transforming Care at the Bedside [TCAB]). Sam reviews the reason for admission, discusses her history with Mrs. Sulif, and enters additional information at the bedside using his tablet, correcting some minor misinformation. Dr. Chi, the intensivist physician, arrives to examine her. Dr. Chi enters his orders into the computerized provider order entry (CPOE) system, which simultaneously notifies the lab and pharmacy. Sam then prints out bar-coded labels with Mrs. Sulif's identity number, sending off urine for analysis. He then checks for robot delivery of her STAT meds, which he administers after scanning her name band and double verifying her name orally. Sam uses his tablet to find the latest clinical guidelines associated with Mrs. Sulif's diagnosis.

1. How is the care described so far both safe and efficient?
2. What additional steps could make care safer or more efficient?
3. When it is time for her discharge and follow-up by a home health nurse, what other communication should occur?

Technology continues to drive major shifts in our nursing practice and communication methods. e-Mobile devices promote greater patient control of their own care, potentially improving health outcomes. Patients are using more technology **apps** (application programs) on their mobile devices to communicate and to actively participate in their own care. As nurses, what interventions can we adopt to increase patient engagement?

m-Health technologies useful in patient education, self-monitoring, and support are expanding rapidly.

Decentralized Access: Technology for Communicating at the Point of Care

Nurses believe that technology should be designed to reduce the burden associated with work flows in documentation, medication administration, communication, orders, and obtaining equipment and supplies. Nurses also say it is essential to have smart, portable, point-of-care devices to document and transmit information. But this technology must be user friendly, function well, and not add to existing workload or nurses will be dissatisfied. For technology to be effective and congruent with nursing expectations, nurses need to seek input into software design (Zadvinskis, Chipps, & Yen, 2014). If use is cumbersome, nurses will devise work-arounds so they can complete their assigned care in a timely manner. Some work-arounds are potentially unsafe, as described in Chapter 2.

"Smart" devices allow nurses decentralized access to patient records, incorporating point-of-care information and documentation. Mobile wireless devices allow continual use of updated information and reference material at any patient location. Communication in a timely manner is a standard of effective communication. Communication in "real time" is the hallmark of bedside nursing in the age of technology. Refer to Fig. 26.1. With fiscal cutbacks, fewer nurses per patient, and increased acuity of conditions, use of technology can enhance our **critical thinking**, **clinical decision making**, and **delivery of safe, efficient care** (HealthIT.gov, n.d.).

Information Collection. Information can be stored and sent to your agency computer or directly to a printer. You can update your patient's records including history, your assessment, the problem list, or other data and nursing notes. Your wireless device can also be used to track

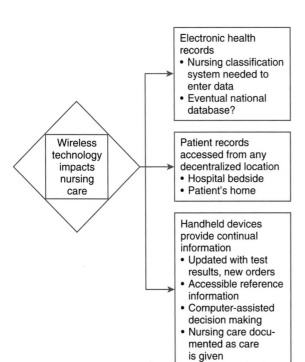

Fig. 26.1 Health Information Technology: Wireless Technology Impacts Nursing Care.

information such as a patient's medications and dosages or laboratory test results in a flow sheet format. For example, a nurse practitioner using a handheld device can call up previous prescriptions, renew them at a touch, record this new information in the agency server, correctly calculate the dosage of a new medication, write the order, and send this prescription to the patient's pharmacy instantly—all without writing anything on paper.

m-Health Devices
Cellular Telephones
Ordinary cell phones can be used to locate clinicians or verify and clarify information. While some agencies ban them perhaps fearing non-job-related distraction, others are issuing mobile phones to staff nurses so they can directly contact physicians or hospital departments from the bedside, give condition updates, or obtain orders.

Smart phones
Smart phones represent the convergence of cellular phones and complex computers. In addition to making calls, these devices have other functions useful to nurses. They enable you to download and access information resources; use health care apps; provide internet access to patient information (new laboratory results or physician orders); and do instant messaging (IM). Some downloaded apps provide alerts by beeping when there are new orders or newly available test results. In addition to housing downloaded reference programs, smart phones may even have computer-assisted decision support systems. For example, downloadable apps such as Epocrates (www.epocrates.com), a free drug information program, not only provide drug information but when you type in patient information such as age, weight, and diagnosis, they provide you with guidelines for correct dosage, contraindications, and side effects. New information alerts are sent to your device in a timely manner. Guidelines for best practice can also be downloaded.

Tablets and Laptop Computers
Laptop computers are more powerful than tablets, yet both are still small and portable enough to be taken into the patient's hospital room or home. Uses of tablets to chart and to transmit and receive data are described throughout this book. Try Simulation Exercise 26.1.

Smart Cards
Until we achieve total interoperability between EHR systems all of a patient's history can be carried on a **smart card** or a flash drive. When this patient is admitted to a hospital with a fully integrated computer information system, the

patient's data may be scanned into the electronic record. This can aid safe care. For example, an allergy to aspirin can be part of the information carried by your patient. When the patient travels outside the system, this information could be scanned into the new system's records.

Mobile Biomedical Sensors

Topol writes that biomedical sensors interfacing with smart phones are changing communication (2015). Sensors can be part of the smart phone or interfaced as an attachment. Some sensors are worn on your body (such as Apple Watch) or even ingested or implanted into your body. Using these in conjunction with smart phones, patients in the community monitor their own health data and communicate this data to health providers (or to their computers). Examples include measurement of heart rate or blood pressure, blood glucose or oxygenation, lung function or eye pressure. Other sensors can obtain and transmit ultrasounds, image organs, or obtain electrocardiograms. Sensors can be embedded into medication as "smart pills" (Proteus sensors) that track ingestion of prescribed medication (Reporting live from your stomach, 2017). Algorithms, designed to manage big data, receive and analyze this data. What roles do you see evolving for nurse-patient communication as all this data accumulates? (Fig. 26.2).

Enhanced Work Flow

Remote Site Monitoring, Diagnosis, Treatment, and Communication

Technological innovations can help make our care more efficient. Formerly, staff nurses in hospitals spent less than 40% of their day in actual patient care and spent at least 25% of their time walking to answer phones, obtain charts, gather supplies, locate other staff, and so on. Nurses now use new technology systems to improve their work flow and allow them more time at the bedside! Remote-site patient self-monitoring of disease and treatment progress can allow more timely early interventions. Technology innovations are coming so fast the authors cannot be all inclusive. The following sections describe some examples of health care technology related to nurse-patient communication.

Hand-Free Communication

Voice-Activated Communication. Voice communication systems use wearable, hands-free devices that use the existing wireless network to support instant voice communication and messaging among staff within an agency. The nurse wears a small, lightweight badge that permits one-button voice access to other users of the system. It also will connect to the telephone system. One example is **Vocera**. It is said to reduce the time for key communications, such as looking for the medication keys, looking for others (a 45% reduction), paging doctors, or walking to the nursing station telephone (a 25% reduction). Nurses report that voice-activated communication results in fewer interruptions, promotes better continuity of care, and improves their work flow.

In-hospital biomedical monitoring.

When the point of care is at the hospital bedside, several of the technologies already mentioned, such as noninvasive automatic recording of vital signs, wireless telemetry, or the use of "smart" beds with sensors, automatically transmit and upload data into the patient's EHR. In another example, telemetry sensors might monitor information such as whether nurses wash hands. Or you might receive a signal if a patient falls and does not get up.

Care in the Community

E-Visits and Telehome Health Care. Wireless technology extends into the patient's home, helping achieve a Healthy People 2020 goal to increase the proportion of people who communicate with their health care providers over the internet (Healthy People, 2020, HC/HIT-5-2). **E-visits** offer opportunities for diagnosis, treatment, and monitoring of patient status via internet portals. This makes care more affordable and convenient. A patient may use intelligent vital monitoring products to obtain updates such as blood pressure, blood glucose levels, or current electrocardiogram strips. Your patient then transmits this information to you, which you can assess without having to make a home visit. E-visits are offered by numerous health systems and are reimbursable by some insurance companies. Studies show positive outcomes including major reductions in hospital admissions and in the number of actual home visits required.

Radio Frequency Identity Smart Technology. Information can also be communicated to providers via data transmitted by **radio frequency identity (RFID)**

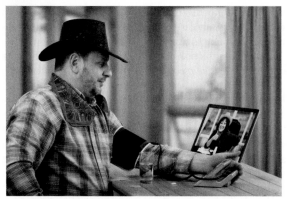

Fig. 26.2 Cowboy Takes His Own Blood Pressure On-line. (Copyright © verbaska_studio/iStock/Thinkstock.)

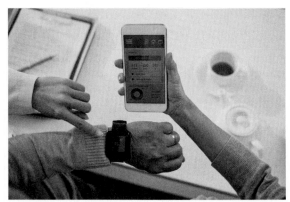

Fig. 26.3 Phone Screen and Smart Watch With health Data. (Copyright © DragonImages/iStock/Thinkstock.)

chips or sensors inside our identification cards that we wear or have implanted. If we need to locate a member of our team, such sensors assist in tracking that doctor or other team member. Lots of us have chips implanted into our pets so they can be located if lost. Is it ethical to implant similar devices into Alzheimer patients or others who are unable to function without supervision? Families are using sensors (tiles or chips) at home to monitor for potential problems (such as a serious fall) or a health crisis (such as an epileptic seizure).

Staff nurses walk hundreds of miles a year trying to locate and gather equipment and supplies they need to carry out their bedside care. RFID technology could instantly locate equipment, such as a needed infusion pump stored in the supply room. Perhaps robots will then deliver needed supplies to you! In a large review of this topic, Ajami and Rajabzadeh (2013) concluded that RFID technology needs to be integrated into an agency's health information technology (HIT) to best reduce clinical and medication errors.

Computer-Mediated Communication in the Community
Telehealth
Telehealth, also called telemedicine, telenursing, or eHealth (in England), is changing the way health care is delivered. Use is exploding due to new technology combined with patient demand for easy access, efficient care (deShazo & Parker, 2017; Olson & Thomas, 2017). Telehealth is a general term for any real-time interactive use of the internet for delivery of health care or diagnosing and treating illnesses across a distance. It needs high-definition visual and audio two-way communication, allowing the telehealth nurse to see, monitor, and

remotely interact with patients using their own devices (American Telemedicine Organization, n.d.). Advanced Practice Nurses can monitor diagnostic and lab tests and assess for physiological changes remotely even for patients requiring intensive care. For the nurse using telehealth, clinical skill expertise and communication skills are indispensable (Kleinpell, Barden, Rincon, McCarthy, & Zapatochny Rufo, 2016; Van Houwelingen, Moerman, Ettema, Kort, & Ten Cate, 2016).

Information is exchanged across geographic distances and is often used for specialist consultations. The consultant can manipulate ophthalmoscope or stethoscope attachments to assess retinas or breath sounds. Use of this communication technology is becoming commonplace. Studies tend to show telehealth decision making and diagnosing improves health outcomes with no difference between face-to-face encounters and remote intervention (Raskas, Gali, Schinasi, & Vyas, 2017a, 2017b). Telehealth originated at health facilities, but now telehealth often originates from the patient's home using cameras in smart phones (Fig. 26.3). Refer to the case of Mr. Dakota.

Mr. Dakota Case
Jim Dakota, age 69 years, runs Eagleview, a bed and breakfast business in rural South Dakota. He recently was discharged after bowel surgery in a hospital 3 hr away. Instead of closing his business and traveling 3 hr to the medical center, he is able to self-manage his wound healing by taking "selfie" photos of his wound to send to his nurse, allowing her to provide guidance and monitor for complications remotely.

Home-Based Telehealth Monitoring Unit

Outcomes of Telehealth Use. Although results are mixed, more studies show use of this technology reduces hospitalizations, increases quality of care and patient satisfaction, decreases emergency department visits, and decreases health care costs. Not to mention eliminating the extensive travel costs to patients. Use barriers are legal and financial. Barriers include privacy concerns, interstate licensure or insurance coverage, and problems with insurance reimbursement (Wakefield, 2017).

Computerized Clinical Decision Support Systems

Decision Support System Information to Assist Critical Thinking and Decision Making

An important asset of HIT adoption is the provision of computerized **clinical decision support systems (CDSS)**. CDSSs are cloud-based information programs designed to assist your decision-making (Lugtenberg, Weenink, van der Weijden, Westert, & Kool, 2015). You input your patient information and the database provides you with patient-specific care guidelines. By doing so, they enhance the quality of your care as well as its safety. CDSS is often integrated with order entry systems in the hospital, but versions can be available to nurses working in the community. Key CDSS issues are speed and ease of access. CDSSs are useful but, of course, do not take the place of your own clinical critical thinking. The following case about Mrs. Sanchez is an example of how this technology is designed to assist us to deliver better and safer nursing care more efficiently.

Case Example: Mrs. Sanchez Case

Gail Myer, RN, is assigned to Mrs. Sanchez as one of her eight patients on an obstetrical unit. Mrs. Sanchez is in preterm labor. Gail's clinical decision support system (CDSS) automatically lists desired patient outcomes based on her work assignment, lists "best practice" interventions, and then gives real-time feedback about outcomes. Her tablet receives electronic prompts to assist in clinical decision making. For example, the hospital's CDSS program calculates expected delivery date for Mrs. Sanchez and supplies the correct dose of the prescribed medication based on her weight. It alerts Gail if the prescribed dose she intends to administer exceeds maximum standard safety margins, and also cross-checks this new drug for potential drug interactions with the drugs Mrs. Sanchez is already taking. It pops up a screening tool for Gail to use to assess Mrs. Sanchez's current status and then alerts Gail if she should forget to document today's results.

The more sophisticated CDSS systems give interactive advice after comparing entries of your data with a computerized knowledge base. The information offered to you is personalized to your patient's condition (filtered) and is offered at appropriate times in your workday.

Since the National Academies of Science, Engineering and Medicine [formerly IOM] and the Canadian Institutes of Health Research began advocating CDSS programs or supporting research into CDSS effect on patient care, the suggested types of data in the CDSS system have come to include:

- Diagnosis and care information displays with care management priorities listed
- A method for communication, that is, for order entry and for entering data (system offers prompts so you enter complete data; offers smart or model forms)
- Automatic checks for drug-drug, drug-allergy, and drug-formulary interactions
- Ability to send reminders to patients according to their stated preference
- Medication reconciliations and summary of care at transitions of patient care
- Ability to send electronic alerts or prompts if problems occur or you have not acknowledged receipt of information, such as the patient's laboratory test results

The hardware can be a computer terminal on your hospital unit or wireless handheld device. A software database can be information residing in the agency server or a central repository such as a disease registry or government database.

For the nurse, some CDSS software can generate specific information for your particular patient, including assessment guidelines and forms, analyses of their laboratory test results, and use of best practice protocols to make specific recommendations for safe care. Ideally, this is integrated into the EHR system your agency is using. Ease of use is crucial. Studies continue to show that the majority of time, staff nurses still prefer to rely on colleagues to validate their decisions.

Based on input about your patient's current condition, the CDSS is programmed to provide you with appropriate reminders or prompts. For example, after you complete care for your first assigned patient, specific information is presented to you if you have not yet documented a needed intervention. This assists you in preventing treatment errors or omissions and helps improve your documentation. Blaser et al. (2007) demonstrated that their CDSS could speed up the time to intervention. More timely interventions should lead to fewer patient complications. Our central focus remains patient-centered care, so we include our patient's preferences in our clinical decisions.

Outcomes of Computerized Clinical Decision Support Systems

CDSS technology is slowly being adopted. Early systems were stand-alone, but technology is rapidly advancing, leading to more user-friendly systems integrated into HIT to provide timely, relevant content. Because the system stores your information about your activity, you can, for example, obtain reports about your overall compliance with standards of care or provide data for research.

In Chapter 2 we noted that IOM attributed over 70% of health care errors to poor communication. Constant improvements to our electronic health care technologies are geared to improving the flow of communication, increasing safety, and improving the quality of our care. As an example, Fogel (2013) reported critically ill patients had significantly better blood glucose control when providers used a CDSS. In fact, reviewers who analyzed more than 15,000 articles concluded that the evidence is *strong* that CDSS use effectively improves health outcomes on a range of measures for patients in diverse settings (Agency for Healthcare Research and Quality [AHRQ], 2012).

Alerts. The literature shows mixed results when reminders or alerts are sent. Nurses have been found to be more likely to chart when an electronic reminder is received. Patients respond positively to reminders such as texts and to CDSS coaching about their self-care.

Clinical Practice Guidelines: Access to Online Information

By standardizing interventions based on outcome evidence, practice guidelines promote quality and safety. Nurses have the opportunity to search databases when they need information, using computers or smart phones. Clinical practice guidelines need to be easily accessible, usable in your daily practice, with content from trusted, credible sources. Clinical guideline databases should allow input from you about your patient, and then provide customized clinical decision guidance. Clinical databases have been systematically developed to provide appropriate care recommendations for your patient's specific diagnoses based on available research evidence.

Apps for Health Care Provider

Apps useful to nurses are accessible in iOS and Android operating systems. Among many free, downloadable apps and guides for care, one example is *The Guide to Clinical Preventive Services.* You can search by age, sex, and risk factors (US Preventive Services Task Force: www.epss.ahrq.gov). Many other protocols are available from AHRQ (www.ahrq.gov), from professional organizations such as the American Nurses Association (ANA) (www.nursingworld.com/ce), and from free or subscribed databases such as Mosby's Nursing Consult where you click on the diagnosis of interest. Many national and regional nurse associations also have or soon will have such databases. There are multiple private for-profit companies that would also supply you with such information for a subscription fee. Most hospitals and larger agencies have resident experts, such as medical librarians or clinical nurse specialists, to help staff nurses access information about evidence-based care guidelines.

Disease-Specific Apps. One example of such an app is mySugr, designed for providers caring for patients with diabetes mellitus. This app is rated as being very useful by Krauskopf (2017). It can be accessed at https://mysugr.com/apps or via your app store.

Patient Engagement

Governments as well as health care executives state that involving patients more actively in their own health care is a priority (AHIMA, 2017). In the United States, one of the CMC Stage 2 Meaningful Use Criteria is to promote "more patient-controlled data." Use of newer technologies can foster this goal of greater patient engagement. In addition to use of e-mail, texting, and internet e-referrals, patients can use "portals" or personal health records, allowing them to use HIPPA-secure platforms to communicate with nurses and physicians in order to gain information, make appointments, or view their records (including lab test results).

e-Mobile Nurse-Patient Health Care Communication. Mobile technology has not only changed the way we document, it now provides communication resources which we can use for patient education. This information can be specifically tailored for each individual patient.

To review technologies involved in nurse-patient communication, we mention the following:

E-mail. E-mail can be a convenient, rapid, inexpensive method of communicating between providers and patients. Yet, while most patients express a desire to communicate with their health care providers via e-mail, not all providers choose to do so, citing concerns about confidentiality, malpractice, and time factors. Read the case about Ms. Trooper.

Case Example: Trooper Case

Ms. Trooper RN, an office nurse, uses e-mail for posting test results, providing prescription refills or health reminders, and doing follow-ups. For example, she tracks the response of patients who are on new medication, instead of waiting until their next office appointment.

The American Medical Association (AMA) guidelines (2004) suggest that electronic or paper copies be made of e-mail messages sent to patients.

Texting: Secure Instant Messaging. Text IM is commonly used in daily life. **Secure IMs** can be used to improve communications between members of the health team or between patients and providers. For example, you want to request an additional pain medication from the resident on call. (You recognize, however, that you are not supposed to accept texted orders back.) IM can be used by patients to communicate self-monitored information to their care provider. In the above case, Ms. Trooper could text reminders to monitor blood glucose today to her patient.

Technology for Patient Health Self-Management

e-Mobile Health Apps for Patients. Digital devices are perfect for anytime, anywhere learning. Because tablets and smart phones have mobility, available health apps have become common (Cho, 2016). They provide effective communication at minimal cost. Try downloading one app for monitoring your diet, or share information about how your wearable device monitors your exercise.

Patient Disease Management: Gaining Information. Online learning has been found to be as effective as traditional learning. Most people have searched the internet for health information, using one of the many consumer health information sites. There is strong potential for improved health learning associated with interactive computer teaching programs.

Patient Disease Management: Recording Data. Active participation is said to increase the likelihood of producing positive health outcomes. Surveys show consumers hold positive attitudes toward use of technology including m-Health apps. Patients can use apps to record glucose levels, dietary intake, sleep deprivation, etc. The Agency for Healthcare Research and Quality's analysis of 146 studies of the impact of computer health modules on outcomes found that these programs succeeded in engaging patient attention, but more significantly they improved health (AHRQ, 2009). Just as studies have documented positive health outcomes after telephone support from nurses, contact with providers using interactive computer programs for health education or to provide answers to illness-related questions lead to positive health outcomes.

Lifestyle Management. Just as many of us use wearable devices like Fitbit or Applewatch to encourage exercise, devices and web sites increase patient knowledge about health promotion. Information about health conditions has been shown to positively impact outcomes. Nurses should recommend reliable internet sites to patents, helping them avoid disinformation.

Other Technology for Assisting Patients in Self-Management
Portal Technology to Assist Patients to Communicate and to Self-Manage

Portals are HIPPA-secure software gateways interfacing with a patient's EHR information, giving providers and patients a shared view of that patient's health. Portals can be "view only" or they can be "interactive." Patients have continuous *access to their health information*, such as immunizations or lab results.

More sophisticated interactive portals allow the patient to pay bills, to record and share results of their home monitoring, to access the status of their insurance claims, and to schedule appointments. They also provide a mechanism for secure texting between patient and providers, and for downloading personalized health information or requesting prescription refills. Studies report highest patient use occurs in viewing lab tests, making appointments, and viewing visit summaries. Providers use portals to send reminders about appointments. They are important for care coordination and allow us to give self-management support to patients (AHRQ, 2017). Insurance and pharmaceutical companies have portals that provide consumer and health care provider access to drug information. Patients sign on and click on various menu bars to access some areas of their EHRs or to access customized educational information (Nambisan, 2017). Some services provide access to physicians or nurses to answer questions or even make diagnoses when the patient first answers a series of questions about their condition. Potentially their care provider could make a diagnosis, order treatment, write a progress note in the EHR, and reply to the patient, as in the Mr. Williams case. This not only decreases use of staff time to answer phone calls and so on, but it also records that this patient accessed and received certain information (HealthIT.gov, n.d.).

Case Example: Mr. Williams: Portals and e-Visits

Mr. Williams is traveling on an important business trip. Having ignored a random area of numbness and itching across his chest and back for several days, he now notices a linear blistering rash forming across the right side of his trunk. Recalling the Herpes Zoster vaccination TV commercials, he suspects shingles. He accesses his primary provider's interactive patient portal and because he has completed a check-up within the last 12 months, the e-visit feature is unlocked and available for certain complaints, including rashes. Selecting the option to initiate an e-visit related to the

Continued

topic of rashes, the software prompts him to provide the necessary relevant information, including a digital "selfie" photo that he uploads from his smart phone. Mr. Williams is able to add free text comments to request his prescription be sent to an alternative pharmacy at his current travel location. Mr. Williams receives an email confirming the suspicion of shingles, followed by a text notifying him that his prescription is ready for pick up at the preferred destination.

___Contributed by Laura Holbrook, MSN, RN, 2017

Public Portals. Other portals are open to the public and allow consumers to anonymously rate hospitals and individual care providers by name, such as the Hospital Compare web site (www.medicare.gov-/hospitalcompare; or www.medicare.gov/doctorcompare).

Personal Health Records

The literature speaks of portals and personal health records [PHRs] somewhat similarly. PHRs are records of one's health history which the patient maintains, entering data to provide a lifelong medical history compellation, able to be accessed by all providers. This system allows patients to control their own data and is said to assist them in self-management (Laugesen & Hassanein, 2017). PHRs are seen as a tool to overcome the fragmentation of information that occurs when a patient is seen by multiple providers and agencies. They were intended to be a centralized source for self-management, to provide communication tools similar to portals for making appointments, receiving reminders for prescription refill, and decision-support tools. To be effective and to appeal to users they need to be a seamless component of the patient's EHR, perhaps in the form of a compatible app.

Nursing Outcomes of m-Health Technology Use

For nurses, technology is said to improve work flow, provide safer care, provide automatic monitoring and documentation of some patient data, allow more nurse independence, and improve communications among team members. Acute care providers quickly adopted wireless devices at the bedside for communication. Evidence is mixed about the effects of technology. There is an expectation that it will decrease long-term costs. Generally, it seems to improve the flow of communications. But some negative outcomes include perceptions that electronic communication damages the team interpersonal relationships (Wu et al., 2011). This may decrease as "natural language" computers that recognize vocal data entry become more widely used. Does new technology assist or impede work flow? Evidence is mixed.

Nurses are assuming increased responsibilities for interpretation of transmitted data and for instituting interventions.

Patient-Nurse Communication Outcomes

Few studies are available showing effects of technology on nurse-patient communication. Generally, care may be less labor intensive and easier if delivered remotely via smart phones to patients. Technology is said to facilitate self-monitoring, improve self-management, improve cognitive functioning, reduce time spent in physician offices, provide needed information, provide support, decrease rehospitalization, increase markers of quality of life, and improve timely communication with health providers. Smart phone apps are effective methods for teaching preventive care. In an example, apps such as "Call the Shots" or texting reminders

---

DEVELOPING AN EVIDENCE-BASED PRACTICE: TELE-HEALTH OUTCOMES This article contains evidence mapped systematic reviews of 58 studies from over 1000 articles describing key characteristics of telehealth use to inform practice, policy, and research decisions.

Results:
Overall, use of telehealth technology produced positive health improvements when used for patient monitoring for several chronic conditions such as cardiovascular or respiratory disease, as well as for delivering psychotherapy. The most consistent benefit across studies was when telehealth was used for communication and counseling for patients with chronic conditions. Authors suggest the next step is to broaden research to decrease barriers to this method of delivering health care.

Application to Your Practice:
Consider opportunities for using technology to reach off-site patients. How can technology help your practice? QSEN defines evidence-based practice (EBP) as "integrating the best current evidence with clinical expertise and patient/family preferences and values for delivery of optimal health care" (www.qsen.org). Try using one or more apps to find EBP guidelines and then mark which of your next interventions are evidence-based. Some suggested sites are:
National Guideline Clearinghouse (NCG): www.guideline.gov
Skyscape Medical Library: www.skyscape.com
Electronic preventive services selector (ePSS): http://epss.ahrq.gov/PDA/index.jsp

From Totten, A. M., Womack, D. M., Eden, K. B., McDonagh, M. S., Griffin, J. C., Grusing, S., et al. Telehealth: Mapping the evidence for patient outcomes from systematic reviews. AHRQ Publ No.16-EHC034-EF, June 2016.

have been shown to increase compliance with immunization (Peck, 2014). It may be the preferred modality for some.

APPLICATIONS

Technology Use

Technology cannot replace your accumulated knowledge and expertise in making a decision, but it can provide supplementary tools to help make these decisions. Competency in HIT use has broadly been cited by national nursing organizations, accrediting agencies, government agencies, and policy organizations as an essential of basic nursing practice. Use of informatics is a QSEN expected competency for new nurse graduates. Under this competency, *knowledge* objectives include ability to identify information available in a common database to support care. *Skills* include ability to respond appropriately to clinical decision-making supports and alerts. We are expected to demonstrate an *attitude,* which values use of technology for making decisions, preventing errors, and coordinating care.

In addition to employers, regulatory agencies, professional agencies, and academic agencies, we, as professional nurses, are each responsible for maintaining this competency (American Nurses Association [ANA], 2008).

Standards of care are applicable to electronic nursing just as to bedside care. General standards are discussed in Chapter 2. More specific standards may be available from nursing organizations such as ANA or the American Academy of Ambulatory Care Nursing.

In electronic care, as in all our care, we need to be aware of our patient's preferences. For example, maybe only one-third of our patients will say they prefer digital reminders be sent to them.

Point of Care

Wireless entry of data at the point of care can increase your access to and use of evidence-based resources in your practice. If smart phones are used for personal business, as well as in work situations, secure separate e-mail and/or messaging accounts would be needed. Handheld devices at point of care provide timely access to patient information, are convenient, and are cost-effective in the long run. Their prompts should help you provide safer, more comprehensive care.

Device Use Guidelines

Infection Control

Prevention of device contamination is a concern. When we are giving hands-on care or setting our device down in a patient's space, we need to avoid contamination by disinfecting before and after. Some suggest using an inexpensive

plastic bag to encase our device. Certainly, hand hygiene is crucial. Some reports describe use of hand hygiene sensors. In studies, an amazing 40% to 70% of providers failed to disinfect, although the known presence of sensors does improve compliance (Miskelly, 2013).

Electronic Mail Guidelines

Guidelines are available for physician use of e-mail to communicate with patients (AMA, 2004); these guidelines are also appropriate for nurses. No one knows how many nurses are accustomed to using wireless technology devices in their care of patients. Better guidelines for their use in giving care still need to be developed.

Smart Phone Use Guidelines

Although just about every nursing student has seen or used a wireless device, not everyone has used them as an aid to giving patient care. There are still hospitals that prohibit nurses from using cell phones, even though studies show these devices can save time, decrease errors, and simplify information retrieval at the point of care. Ethically, you do not use electronic devices in your workplace for personal, nonprofessional use. All information needs to be Health Insurance Portability and Accountability Act (HIPAA) secure.

Texting and e-Messaging Personal Use Guidelines

In the work environment, electronic provider–patient IM can be used to communicate simple data. Both telephone and IM have been shown to be as effective as in-person education for patients with chronic conditions. Texts are used to remind patients of appointments, services, or to take a medication or perform self-monitoring care. This may promote better quality care and improved patient utilization. The Joint Commission (TJC) continues to say "it is NOT acceptable for the physician or licensed independent practitioner to text orders for patients to the hospital…" (TJC, 2011). The rationale is that you cannot verify who is actually sending the order. How is this different from faxed orders or verbal orders?

Multiple articles in the literature describe the efficacy of using personalized IM for helping patients manage their conditions, as illustrated in the Ryan case.

Case Example: Nurse Ryan Case

Mr. Simpson, 47 years, is newly diagnosed with hypertension. He is taking a new medication and texts his self-monitored blood pressure readings daily to Ms. Ryan RN, his nurse. She could text message a reminder to take his evening dose. Next, she texts

Continued

a reminder to Ms. Sweet, an elderly diabetic patient who has forgotten to submit her blood glucose level this morning, However, there are concerns about violations of patient privacy. See Social Media Guidelines listed in Chapter 3. Other concerns involve threats to safety. When an incoming message distracts a nurse during a crucial procedure, this distraction could potentially contribute to making an error (Shaw & Abbott, 2017).

Use of Social Media

Social media sites are powerful communication platforms, using the internet-based venues to communicate, strengthen interpersonal relationships, and even disseminate information for education. Social media and portable devices with downloadable apps are revolutionizing our communication with patients. Social media sites provide opportunities for obtaining information to make more educated health choices and obtain input from supportive "friends." Unfortunately there is a lot of incorrect information also available. Use of social media may improve our nursing practice by increasing our access to information and support.

Guidelines for nurse use of social media were discussed in Chapter 3. According to the National Council of State Boards of Nursing (NCSBN) and HIPAA, nurses breach patient privacy and HIPPA rules when they post photos or videos or comment about patients. We differentiate between the general open-to-all social sites, such as Twitter, from secure sites with restricted access, such as those created by hospitals as internal professional staff social networks.

Clinical Decision Support System Use

While use of CDSSs never eliminates the need for us to think critically, such systems are another tool to help us manage our nursing care. Use of CDSSs allows you to align your clinical decisions for your specific patient with best practice guidelines, as in the case of Ms. Esteves.

Case Example: Ms. Esteves case

As the staff nurse in the CCU unit, you sign on to the Esteves electronic record. The CDSS offers you a reminder (alert) about a medication order. You are given information about possible harmful interactions with other medications she is already taking. This CDSS "reminder" then gives you a suggestion to obtain a lab INR result prior to considering giving this med. Thus, the CDSS is integrated with your work flow, giving you suggestions about interventions based on researched best practice. Perhaps the CDSS next reminds you

that later meds be held since Ms. Esteves has an NPO (nothing by mouth) order beginning at midnight. It might offer you a suggested alternative if you fail to document this intervention.

In another example, nurses working with pediatric cancer patients have long used calculators to determine correct fractional dosage based on the child's weight. Now instead, they can use this automated support system because it automatically predetermines the correct doses.

Clinical Decision Support System Concerns

Alarm Fatigue. A common problem is that the CDSS might send you so many alerts that you ignore them. **Alarm fatigue** is a commonly reported problem. This is particularly true for drug-drug interactions. Studies suggest that as many as 90% of alarm alerts are overridden. Customizing alerts to your patient assignment or gradating the warning into low-priority (warning but no alarm) and high-priority (audible alarm) might overcome this. More studies are needed to examine effects of CDSS on communication, but data suggest a positive effect. In Canada, nurses use mobile devices to access the Registered Nurses' Association of Ontario best-practice guidelines to receive timely information specific to their assigned patients. Try Simulation Exercise 26.2 to explore usability.

Cost and Ease of Use. Cost and ease of use are the main concerns in adopting this technology.

Application of Clinical Guidelines to Practice Integration into your workflow and relevance to your care are two serious concerns. Access at the point of care to databases containing evidence-based guidelines for care means you have resources specifically tailored to suggest interventions for a specific patient.

SIMULATION EXERCISE 26.2   Critique of an Internet Nursing Resource Database

Purpose:
To encourage students to gain familiarity with internet resources.

Procedure:
As an out-of-class assignment, access any nursing resource database, preferably using a smart phone or tablet. Many sites are listed in the online references.

Reflective Analysis and Discussion:
1. Discuss results, listing sites you think useful.
2. Evaluate each web site's credibility for professional use.

Criteria for Downloadable Clinical Practice Guidelines
- They are evidence-based.
- They are easily accessible on your wireless device.
- They allow you to enter patient data to customize the interventions (data from EHR).
- They contain hotlinks to allow you to obtain and print more information.

m-Health: Technology for Patient Engagement
Use of Health and Lifestyle Monitoring Apps

This chapter describes possible app uses, but, of course, use of apps is not quite as easy as it sounds, requiring devices, science-based programs, and use skills. Would you recommend consumers owning smart phones download some of the many apps that assist them in tracking their self-assessment? For example, should a diabetic patient try using Glucose Buddy (an iPhone app) that allows them to enter glucose testing results and record carbohydrate consumption and other parameters? Or maybe uChek, which is a digital log of

---

BOX 26.1 Use of m-Health Devices (Wireless, Wi-Fi-Enabled, Handheld Devices)

Advantages
- Improve the flow of communication, as well as work flow
- Easily portable; can be used at the point of care (patient's bedside, in the home, etc.)
- Quick charting when nurse enters information by tapping menu selections
- Can contain reference resources about treatment, for medication dosage, and so forth, if uploaded
- Assists with customized decision making, reminders about standards of care, sends alerts
- Instant communication (e.g., nurse is signaled by beep regarding receipt of new information)
- Provide quick access to patient records
- Provide patients with self-management tools
- Build support networks
- Provide a method of connecting with hard-to-reach patients

Disadvantages
- Possible threats to patient's legal privacy rights
- Nurse does not have a printed copy of information (until downloaded to agency printer)
- Small screen does not allow view of entire page of information
- Technical problem may result in dysfunction and/or downtime

---

urinalysis testing results with data entered using the smart phone camera to record urine dipstick results? What factors would you consider before making this recommendation? Wearable devices, such as smart watches, make wellness and diagnostic apps even easier to use (Box 26.1).

Outcomes of m-HEALTH
Cyber Health Education for Health Promotion

There is considerable evidence about the efficacy of providing health care education and information online. See Chapter 14 for discussion of health promotion concepts.

Post Discharge Patient Education. New technology increases our options for providing needed information. One hospital example would be unit-owned tablets containing disease management information in skill-based learning modules which are lent to patients. Similar modules could be provided after discharge. Use of national web-site-based modules would eliminate the need for each agency to develop their own programs.

Disease Management and Follow-Up. Health information about controlling their chronic disease conditions can be provided to patients effectively, quickly, and inexpensively via the internet. Nurse-provided information, often to their mobile device, allows patients to make better self-management decisions, such as reminding a diabetic patient to submit a1c results this week. Actively engaging and giving decision support is another way to provide patient-centered care, shifting the focus to self-care in their own home. One problem for patients accessing internet health information is that not all online information is accurate or easy for the user to verify in measurable *outcomes.* Internet-based education programs have been shown to lead to better understanding and to greater disease control. See Chapter 15 for health teaching concepts.

In the United States, documentation of each patient education session must contain:
- The topic discussed
- The time spent
- Your mutual behavioral goal
- Your assessment of patient's readiness to learn
- Your observations about the patient's level of understanding of his or her disease

Patient Alert Notifications

Using the internet, you can send electronic alerts to your patients who need medication renewals, screening examinations, or other health services. A 2009 Kaiser Permanente study showed a marked decrease in primary care office visits after implementation of an electronic system with intensive provider-patient communication via a secure internet portal. According to Kaiser, 85% of users report that being able to communicate electronically with their physicians improved their ability to manage their own health. Nearly all health care organizations have their own sites. Just as agency sites might provide health information with hyperlinks embedded to access general information, portals give providers a two-way communication highway, as in Anna Smith's case.

Anna Smith Case Example: Management of a Teen With Asthma

Anna, age 14, has asthma. Her treatment regimen significantly improved as technology became available to facilitate communication in several ways. Anna uses smart devices with mobile apps for both her preventive maintenance and rescue medications as well as her peak flow meter. Bluetooth technology allows her inhalers to be paired with her smart phone for administration tracking. She can receive an alert if she forgets a routine dose. The frequency of use of rescue doses is also tracked. Her app automatically sends compiled information to her care provider and parents regarding treatments used and peak flow meter readings, and provides urgent alerts when an increase in rescue inhaler use or marked decrease in forced exhale volume is detected. When paired with a wearable smart device, this app can also integrate biometric data such as heart rate and episodes of waking in the night. By trending data, this individualized app can facilitate communication, improve treatment effectiveness, and prevent hospitalizations related to unrecognized asthma exacerbations.

Contributed by Laura Holbrook, BSN, RN, 2017

Group E-support

Chat Rooms. Computers are used to mediate support groups for families and patients with various health problems. These formal internet groups provide information, but they also importantly have been shown to provide improved social support for those who are ill. Studies show group participants report decreased stress, less depression, increased quality of life, and improved ability to manage their disease condition. The chat rooms are usually synchronous, in real time, providing immediate feedback. Usually discussion forums are asynchronous with time delays between postings and responses, allowing for more reflection before posting. More studies are needed before we can specify the needed frequency, duration, or quality of content for optimal support.

Caregivers. Caregivers of people with chronic conditions can use internet support groups, chat rooms, e-mail, or direct communication with care providers to gain support. Nurses can gain insight and better understand the "lived experiences" of their patients by participating in these internet opportunities. Internet or telephone support has been shown to be a cost-effective method for improving functioning and quality of life for patients with chronic conditions, and similar beneficial effects in nurse-caregiver relationship support are occurring (Solli, Hvaloik, Bjork, & Helleso, 2015). Do you believe chat rooms can improve nurse–patient communication?

Outcomes

One goal of *Healthy People 2020* is an increase in the proportion of persons who use electronic personal health management tools. Early evidence shows use of devices, portals, and apps results in improved health outcomes (AHRQ, 2017). For example, in the Loyola study of alcohol-dependent veterans, use of a mobile compatible site resulted in a 63% decrease in hospitalizations (Lusk, 2017). But more data are needed, especially on long-term effects.

Nurses can recommend sites, preferably interactive ones, on the internet that patients can use to have a positive impact on their health. Laptops, notebooks, and smart phones can be used for anywhere, anytime learning. Online learning has been repeatedly shown to be as effective or superior to traditional forms of learning. Have you used podcasts or webinars?

Issues

The main concerns with technology are interoperability and security. Other things to consider:

Access. Cautions or barriers to application of new technologies include user resistance and literacy issues. The transition to use of eHealth technology in nursing implies a learning curve. Some providers cite problems such as the time involved in learning how to use, cost, equipment design limitations, access issues, interference with work flow, and fears about losing handheld devices. In all cases, our communication needs to be tailored to the needs and literacy level of our patient.

Competency. For nurses, rapid advances in technology mean we need to continuously transform the way we communicate. For patients, new technology offers tools to become more engaged in self-management of their own health. Information needs to be in a context which they understand. Emerging are verbal avatars, graphics, or video-based formats which provide this context (Morrow, Hasegawa-Johnson, Huang, & Schuh, 2017).

Guidelines for professional relationships apply to use of electronic media. Caution is advised in communicating with patients outside the professional relationship. Online contact with former patients blurs the relationship boundary.

Costs. Major costs are involved in developing and obtaining software and hardware. A big consideration for providers is cost recovery. How will patients be billed for the time physicians, nurses, dieticians, therapists, etc., devote to interacting with patients using internet modalities?

Liability Issues. Use of the internet presents many questions about how to maximize its communication potential with an increasingly diverse population. Liability and regulatory statutes are outdated. For example, if transmission (and treatment) crosses state lines, in which region does the provider need to be licensed? If malpractice occurs, in which region or state would legal action occur?

Privacy and Security Issues. Separate organizations providing care to the same patient need to share information securely. Any information you learn during the course of treatment must be safeguarded. With any computer use, we are concerned about maintaining *security*. Many surveys of consumer concerns cite breach of privacy as their biggest concern. As HIT systems become more sophisticated and accessibility is a top priority, mechanisms and regulations to ensure privacy become more complex. As m-Health devices, wearable devices, and implanted devices interconnect on the internet, there is potential for harm from unintended or malicious actors. Major breaches of health care databases have occurred and attempts are likely to increase since these datasets are worth millions to thieves (Williams, 2017).

Security experts recommend data encryption and always using a required login password, which is changed frequently. Refer to Chapter 3 for discussion of HIPAA privacy rules. This is why you have sign-on pass codes for portable computer terminals or automatic screen saver modes to darken screens, preventing visitors from reading records.

Professionally, you are bound by laws for privacy protection. Except for sharing information with other health team members, a nurse can reveal patient information only in very limited, specific situations: when failure to disclose would result in significant harm or when legally required to do so. One example would be if you recognize signs of physical abuse in a child. Refer to Table 26.1 for a useful guideline. NCSBN states that in the majority of times, complaints result in disciplinary action by licensure agencies.

Ethically, rules for disclosure are less concrete, but an example might be a patient who tells you he is going to commit suicide or murder. In professional relationships, patients are usually advised upfront that such comments are not bound by rules of confidentially. Reflect on the Ethical Dilemma box at the end of this chapter.

SUMMARY

Mobile health (m-Health) is an emerging force transforming the way nurses communicate with other professionals, patients, and data. Technology provides nurses with new tools to deliver nursing at the patient's point of care. Handheld and wearable devices and use of portals provide patients with easy access to communicate with health care professionals. It is anticipated that use of HIT will improve the quality of care, giving us new ways to partner with our patients to educate them and actively manage their own care.

ETHICAL DILEMMA: What Would You Do?
One of the staff nurses you work with "friends" you on Facebook allowing you to read postings sent to her by a student nurse assigned to her unit. The student has posted information about a 17-year-old former patient who threatens to commit suicide. You do not personally know either the student nurse or the patient.

1. Since this information is openly available on the internet, what ethical responsibility do you have to intervene?
2. Did the student nurse violate the patient's legal right to privacy?
3. If you were the student, what steps would you take as soon as you receive this information?

DISCUSSION QUESTIONS

1. Social media sites have become a prominent component of our society. Identify any future professional uses for social media that you can envision.
2. AHRQ sites described in this chapter could provide you with useful information. Argue for or against use, including ease of access and whether they should implement periodic emails or tweets.
3. Construct a set of criteria for determining if web sites are providing reliable information for your clinical practice.

REFERENCES

Agency for Healthcare Research and Quality (AHRQ). (2009). Impact of consumer health informatics applications. Evidence Report, Publication No.10–E019. Retrieved from: www.ahrq.gov/professionals/clinicians-providers/guidelines-recommendations.index.html. (Accessed 10/2/18).

Agency for Healthcare Research and Quality (AHRQ). (n.d.). *Questions to ask your doctor: Questions are the answer: Your health depends on good communication.* Retrieved from: www.ahrq.gov/questionsaretheanswer. (Accessed 10/2/18).

Agency for Healthcare Research and Quality (AHRQ). (2012). *Healthcare decision-making.* Publication No.12-E0001-EF. Retrieved from: www.ahrq.gov/research/findings/evidence-based-reports/er203-abstract.html. (Accessed 10/2/18).

Agency for Healthcare Research and Quality (AHRQ). (2017). *A national web conference on effective design and use of patient portals and their impact on patient-centered care.* Retrieved from: www.ahrq.gov/.

AHIMA. (2017). In brief. *Journal of AHIMA, 88*(3), 9.

Ajami, S., & Rajabzadeh, A. (2013). Radio frequency identification (RFID) technology and patient safety. *Journal of Research in Medical Science, 18*(9), 809–813.

American Academy of Colleges of Nursing (AACN). *The essentials of baccalaureate education for professional nursing practice.* Washington, DC: Author.

American Medical Association (AMA). (2004). Guidelines for physician patient electronic communication. Report in response to AMA Resolution 810(A-99) bot2a00.rtf. Retrieved from: www.ama-assn.org.

American Nurses Association (ANA). (2008). *Position statement 'professional role competence'.* Retrieved from: www.nursingworld/professionalcompetencies. (Accessed 10/2/18).

American Telemedicine Organization. (n.d.). Retrieved from: www.Americantelemed.org/[type 'telemedicine' into the search box]. (Accessed 10/2/18).

Anwar, M., Joshi, J., & Tan, J. (2015). Anytime, anywhere access to secure, privacy-aware health care services: Issues, approaches and challenges. *Health Policy and Technology, 4,* 299–311.

Bautista, J. R., & Lin, T. T. C. (2016). Sociotechnical analysis of nurses' use of personal mobile phones at work. *International Journal of Medical Informatics, 95,* 71–80.

Blaser, R., Schnabel, M., Biber, C., Bäumlein, M., Heger, O., Beyer, M., et al. (2007). Improving pathway compliance and clinician performance by using information technology. *International Journal of Medical Informatics, 76,* 151–156.

Cho, J. (2016). The impact of post-adoption beliefs on the continued use of health Apps. *International Journal of Medical Informatics, 87,* 75–83.

deShazo, R. D., & Parker, A. B. (2017). Lessons learned from Mississippi's telehealth approach to health disparities. *The American Journal of Medicine, 130,* 403–408.

Fogel, S. L. (2013). Effects of computerized decision support systems on blood glucose regulation in critically ill surgical patients. *Journal of the American College of Surgeons, 216*(4), 1–2.

HealthIT.gov. (n.d.). *Benefits of EHRs: Patient participation.* Retrieved from: www.healthit.gov/providers-professionals/patient-participation/.

Healthy People, 2020. U.S. Department of Health and Human Services. Retrieved from: www.Healthypeople.gov/2020/.

Kleinpell, R., Barden, C., Rincon, T., McCarthy, M., & Zapatochny Rufo, R. J. (2016). Assessing the impact of telemedicine on nursing care in Intensive Care Units. *American Journal of Critical Care, 25*(1), e14–e20.

Krauskopf, P. B. (2017). Review of American Diabetes Association Diabetic Care standards and mySugr mobile App. *International Journal of Nursing Practice, 13*(3), e159–e160.

Laugesen, J., & Hassanein, K. (2017). Adoption of personal health records by chronic disease patients: A research model and an empirical study. *Computers in Human Behavior, 66,* 256–272.

Lugtenberg, M., Weenink, J., van der Weijden, T., Westert, G. P., & Kool, R. B. (2015). Implementation of multiple-domaign covering computerized decision support systems in primary care: A focus group study on perceived barriers. *BMC Medical Informatics and Decision Making, 15,* 1–11.

Lusk, K. (2017). HIM using mHealth to teach patients why and how to access health records. *Journal of AHIMA, 88*(3), 30–31.

Miskelly, F. (2013). Application of a novel smart-sensor technology to achieve accurate hand hygiene monitoring and sustained compliance, without disruption to work flow. *American Journal of Infection Control, 41*(6), 1–2.

Morrow, D., Hasegawa-Johnson, M., Huang, T., & Schuh, W. (2017). A multidisciplinary approach to designing and evaluating electronic medical record portal messages that support patient self-care. *Journal of Biomedical Informatics,* e1–e16. https://doi.org/10.1016/j.2017.03.015.

Olson, C. A., & Thomas, J. F. (2017). Telehealth: No longer an idea for the future. *Advances in Pediatrics, 64,* 347–370.

Peck, J. L. (2014). Smartphone preventive healthcare: Parental use of an immunization reminder system. *Journal of Pediatric Health Care, 28*(1), 35–42.

Powell, A. C., Chen, M., & Thammachart, C. (2017). The economic benefit on mobile Apps for mental health and telepsychiatry services when used by adolescents. *Child & Adolescent Psychiatric Clinics of North America, 26,* 125–133.

QSEN. (n.d.). Retrieved from: www.QSEN.org/Pre-licensurecompetency. (Accessed 10/2/18).

Raskas, M. D., Gali, K., Schinasi, D. A., & Vyas, S. (2017a). Reporting live from your stomach. *Journal of AHIMA, 88*(8), 56.

Raskas, M. D., Gali, K., Schinasi, D. A., & Vyas, S. (2017b). Telemedicine and pediatric urgent care: A vision into the future. *Clinical Pediatric Emergency Medicine, 18*(1), 24–31.

Shaw, P. A., & Abbott, M. (2017). Distracted nursing: Strategies to teach nursing students about mobile devices. *Nurse Educator, 42*(4), 203.

Solli, H., Hvaloik, S., Bjork, I. T., & Helleso, R. (2015). Characteristics of the relationship that develops from nurses-caregiver communication during telehealth. *Journal of Clinical Nursing, 24,* 1995–2001.

The Joint Commission (TJC). (2011). *Standards FAQ details: Texting orders.* http://www.jointcommission.org/standards_information/standards.aspx. (Accessed 10/2/18).

Topol, E. (2015). *The patient will see you now.* New York: Basic Books.

US Department of Health and Human Services. (n.d.) *Healthy People 2020. Health Communication and Health Technology.* Retrieved from: www.healthypeople.gov/2020/topicsobjectives2020/overview.aspx?topicid=18 [type your topic into the search box]. (Accessed 10/2/18).

Van Houwelingen, C. T. M., Moerman, A. H., Ettema, R. G. A., Kort, H. S., & Ten Cate, O. (2016). Competence required for nursing telehealth activities: A Delphi study. *Nurse Education Today, 39,* 50–62.

Wakefield, B. (2017). Telemonitoring improves diabetes control but more work is needed. *Evidence-Based Nursing, 20*(1), 18.

Williams, P. A. H. (2017). Standards for safety, security and interoperatability of medical devices in an integrated health environment. *Journal of AHIMA, 88*(4), 32–35.

Wu, R., Rossos, P., Quan, S., Reeves, S., Lo, V., Wong, B., et al. (2011). An evaluation of the use of smart phones to communicate between clinicians: a mixed-methods study. *Journal of Medical Internet Research, 13*(3), e59.

Zadvinskis, I. M., Chipps, E., & Yen, P. (2014). Exploring nurses' confirmed expectations regarding health IT: A phenomenological study. *International Journal of Medical Informatics, 83*(2), 89–98.

GLOSSARY

A

Accommodation   A desire to smooth over a conflict through cooperative but nonassertive responses.

Acculturation   Describes how a person from a different culture initially learns the behavior norms and values of the dominant culture and begins to adopt its behaviors and language patterns.

Active listening   A communication skill embodying listening with full attention on the patient for the purpose of developing and understanding collaboratively constructed meanings.

Acute grief   Refers to somatic distress that occurs in waves with feelings of tightness in the throat, shortness of breath, an empty feeling in the abdomen, a sense of heaviness and lack of muscular power, and intense mental pain.

Acute stress   Intense anxiety that disables the individual.

Advance directive   A legal document, executed by a competent individual or legal proxy, specifically identifying individual preferences for level of treatment at end of life, should patient become unable to make valid decisions at that time.

Advanced practice nurses   Registered nurses with a baccalaureate degree in nursing and an advanced degree in a selected clinical specialty with relevant clinical experience.

Advocacy   Interceding or acting on behalf of patients to provide the highest quality of care obtainable.

Affective domain   The learning domain concerned with emotional attitudes related to acceptance, compliance, and taking personal responsibility for health care.

Ageism   Discrimination against older adults based on their age.

Aggregated data   Compilation of multiple bits of factual information into large groupings allowing analysis.

Aggressive behavior   A response in which the individual acts to defend self, deflecting the emotional impact of personal attack, with an extreme reaction.

Andragogy   Art and science of helping adults learn.

Anticipatory grief   An emotional response that occurs before the actual death around a family member with a degenerative or terminal disorder.

Anticipatory guidance   A proactive provider strategy of sharing information to help patients cope effectively with stressful situations, thereby reducing unnecessary stress.

Anxiety   A vague, persistent feeling of impending doom.

Aphasia   A neurological linguistic deficit that is most commonly associated with neurological trauma to the brain.

Apraxia   The loss of ability or the inability to take purposeful action even when the muscles, senses, and vocabulary seem intact.

Art of nursing   A seamless interactive process in which nurses blend their knowledge, skills, and scientific understandings with their individualized knowledge of each patient as a unique human being.

Assertive behavior   Setting goals, acting on those goals in a clear, consistent manner, and taking responsibility for the consequences of those actions.

Authenticity   The capacity to be true to one's personality, spirit, and character interacting within the nurse-patient relationship.

Authoritarian Group Leadership   A leadership style in which leaders take full responsibility for group direction and control group interaction.

Autonomy   The individual's right to self-determination.

B

Beneficence   Ethical principle guiding decisions, based on doing the greatest good for the greatest number and avoiding malfeasance.

Behavioral emergency   Refers to crisis escalation to the point that the situation requires immediate intervention to avoid injury or death.

Best practice   Nursing interventions derived from research evidence demonstrating successful outcome for patient.

Biofeedback   Immediate and continuous information about a person's physiological responses; auditory and visual signals that increase one's response to external events.

Body image   The physical dimension of self-concept.

Body language (also kinesics)   Involving the conscious or unconscious body positioning or actions of the communicator.

Boundaries   Represent invisible structures imposed by legal, ethical, and professional standards of nursing that respect nurse and patient rights and protect the functional integrity of their relationship.

Boundary violations   Violation of distance within a professional relationship interaction which can represent a conflict of interest and may be harmful to the goals of the therapeutic relationship.

Brief   Oral statement of roles and responsibilities prior to activity.

Burnout   A state of fatigue or frustration brought about by devotion to a cause, way of life, or relationship that failed to produce an expected reward.

C

Callouts   The team reviews the situation aloud.

Caring   An intentional human action characterized by commitment and a sufficient level of knowledge and skill to allow the nurse to support the basic integrity of the client.

Case finding   Proactive strategy to identify individuals at high risk.

Case management   A collaborative process of assessment, planning, facilitation, and advocacy for options and services to meet an individual's health needs that is used to promote quality cost-effective outcomes.

Catastrophic reactions   Emotional overreactions to situations that look like temper tantrums; can occur with dementia.

Chronic health conditions   Refers to health problems that require ongoing self-management over a period of years or decades.

Chronic sorrow A normal grief response associated with an ongoing living loss that is permanent, progressive, recurring, and cyclic in nature.

Circular questions Questions that focus on family interrelationships and the effect of a serious health alteration on individual family members and the equilibrium of the family system.

Civil laws Developed through court decisions, which are created through precedents rather than written statutes.

Clarification A therapeutic active listening strategy designed to aid in understanding communication by asking for more information or for elaboration on a point.

Clinical Decision Support System (CDSS) Software programs that input specific information about a patient, analyze it, and make recommendations for care based on best practice outcomes as established by research.

Clinical practice guidelines Protocols listing standardized recommended care.

Clinical preceptor A formal relationship with an experienced nurse, chosen for clinical competence, who supports, guides, and evaluates student clinical competence.

Close-ended questions Question format which requires a yes or no or single-phase response; they are used in emergency situations to quickly gather information.

Cloud Supercomputers storing health data that can be accessed remotely by a variety of providers with patient permission.

Coaching A teaching strategy that provides information and support, teaching self-management and problem-solving skills to patients and families experiencing unfamiliar tasks and procedures.

Coding systems Alphanumeric assigned to label each type of health care intervention, making computerization possible.

Cognition Refers to the thinking processes people use to make sense of their perceptions.

Cognitive dissonance The holding of two or more conflicting values at the same time.

Cognitive distortions Faulty or negative thinking that causes a person to interpret neutral situations in an unrealistic, exaggerated, or negative way.

Cognitive restructuring Changing beliefs to make them more positive.

Cohesion (group) An essential curative factor in therapeutic groups defined as the value a group holds for its members and underscores the level of member commitment to the group.

Collaborative (interprofessional) health care team A health care team refers to a coordinated group of professionals with complementary skills, all of whom are valued and share goals and accountability for goal achievement.

Commendations The practice of noticing, drawing forth, and highlighting previously unobserved, forgotten, or unspoken family strengths, competencies, or resources.

Communication A combination of verbal and nonverbal behaviors integrated for the purpose of sharing information that is timely, accurate, complete, unambiguous, and is understood by the receiver.

Communication disability Any impairment in body structure or function that interferes with communication.

Community Any group of citizens that have either a geographic, population-based, or self-defined relationship and whose health may be improved by a health promotion approach.

Compassion fatigue A syndrome associated with serious spiritual, physical, and emotional depletion related to caring for those who are seriously ill.

Compassionate witnessing Defined as noticing and feeling empathy for others, which helps to support and broaden one's perspective.

Competency A set of knowledge, skills, and attitudes.

Complicated grieving Represents a form of grief, distinguished by being unusually intense, significantly longer in duration, and emotionally incapacitating.

Computerized provider entry systems (CPOE) Part of the health information system which allows providers to order tests and treatments.

Confidentiality The respect for another's privacy that involves holding and not divulging information given in confidence except in case of suspected abuse, commission of a crime, or threat of harm to self or others.

Connotation A more personalized meaning of the word or phrase.

Continuity of care Describes a multidimensional longitudinal construct in health care, which emphasizes seamless provision and coordination of patient-centered quality care across clinical settings.

Coping Any response to external life strains that serves to prevent, avoid, or control emotional distress.

Countertransference Feelings representing unconscious attitudes or exaggerated feelings a nurse may develop toward a patient.

Crisis A crisis describes a stressful life event, which overwhelms an individual's ability to cope effectively in the face of a perceived challenge or threat.

Crisis de-escalation The process for defusing and resolving a crisis.

Crisis intervention The systematic application of problem-solving techniques, based on crisis theory, designed to help the individual move through the crisis process as swiftly and painlessly as possible with a return to their pre-crisis functional level.

Crisis state An acute normal human response to severely abnormal circumstances; it is not a mental illness.

Critical incident debriefing Strategy used to help a group of people who have witnessed or experienced a mass trauma crisis event externalize and process its meaning.

Critical thinking An analytical process in which you purposefully use specific thinking skills to make complex clinical decisions.

Cultural competence A set of cultural behaviors and attitudes integrated into the practice methods of a system, agency, or its professionals, which enables them to work effectively in cross-cultural situations.

Cultural diversity Variations among cultural groups.

Cultural relativism The belief that each culture is unique and should be judged only based on its own values and standards.

Culture A complex social concept that encompasses the entirety of socially transmitted communication styles, family customs, political systems, and ethnic identity held by a particular group of people.

C.U.S. A communication tool used by team members to promote safe care; I am Concerned; I am Uncomfortable; this is a Safety issue.

D

Debrief   A short meeting after an event to review the incident.

Decentralized access   Use of internet devices to view or document health information.

Delegation   The transfer of responsibility for the performance of an activity from one individual to another while retaining accountability for the outcome.

Democratic group leadership   A group leadership style in which the leader involves members in active open discussion and shared decision making.

Denial   An unconscious refusal to allow painful facts, feelings, and perceptions into conscious awareness.

Denotation   The generalized meaning assigned to a word.

Deontological model (duty-based model)   A duty-based model for making ethical decisions.

Dependent nursing interventions   Interventions that require an oral or a written order from a physician to implement.

Discharge planning   A process of concentration, coordination, and technology integration, through the cooperation of health care professionals, patients, and their families, to ensure that all patients receive continuing care after being discharged.

Discipline of nursing   Nursing is a "practice" discipline, which combines specialized knowledge and skills with prudent clinical judgment to meet patient, family, and community health care needs.

Discrimination   A legal statute refers to actions in which a person is denied a legitimate opportunity offered to others because of prejudice.

Disease prevention   A concept concerned with identifying modifiable risk and protective factors associated with diseases and disorders.

Disenfranchised grieving   Feelings of loss experienced by a nurse following death of patient.

Disruptive behavior   Conduct that interferes with safe care by negatively affecting the ability of the team to work together, such as bullying, harassment, blaming, etc.

Distress   A negative stress causes a higher level of anxiety and is perceived as exceeding the person's coping abilities.

Documentation   The process of obtaining, organizing, and conveying health information to others in print or electronic format.

Dysfunctional conflict   Conflict in which information is withheld, feelings are expressed too strongly, the problem is obscured by a double message, or feelings are denied or projected onto others.

E

Ecomap   A sociogram illustrating the shared relationships between family members and the external environment.

Ego defense mechanisms   Conscious and unconscious coping methods used by people to protect themselves by changing the meaning of a situation in their minds.

Ego integrity   Relates to the capacity to look back on your life with satisfaction and few regrets.

Electronic health record (EHR) [also electronic medical record]   Various types of computerized health records.

Empathy   The ability to be sensitive to and communicate understanding of the patient's feelings.

Empowerment   Helping a person become a self-advocate; an interpersonal process of providing the appropriate tools, resources, and environment to build, develop, and increase the ability of others to set and reach goals.

Environment   The internal and external context of an individual, as affected by their health care situation.

Ethical dilemma (also moral dilemma)   The conflict of two or more moral issues; a situation in which there are two or more conflicting ways of looking at a situation.

E-prescribing   Prescriptions typed into the health record and transmitted as hardcopy and electronically.

Ethnicity   Personal awareness of a shared cultural heritage with others based on common racial, geographic, ancestral, religious, or historical bonds.

Ethnocentrism   The belief that one's own culture should be the norm and has the right to impose its standards of "correct" behavior and values on another because it is better or more enlightened than others.

Eustress   A short-term mild level of stress.

Evidence-based nursing practice   Implementing nursing interventions which are based on sound clinical research and professional judgment in real-time situations.

F

Familismo   Refers to having a strong family loyalty with corresponding responsibilities for ensuring the family stability; particularly strong value in Hispanic/Latino communities.

Family   A self-identified group of two more or individuals whose association is characterized by special terms, who may or may not be related by bloodlines or law, but who function in such a way that they consider themselves to be a family.

Family projection process   An unconscious casting of unresolved family emotional issues or attributes of people from the past onto a child.

Feedback   A message given by the nurse to the patient in response to a message or observed behavior.

Flow sheets   Charting patient's status information in preprinted categories of information.

Focused questions   Inquiries that require more than a yes/no one-word response to a specific discussion topic.

Functional status   A broad range of purposeful abilities related to physical health maintenance, role performance, cognitive or intellectual abilities, social activities, and level of emotional functioning.

G

General Adaptive Syndrome (GAS)   A physiological response to stress.

Genogram   A standardized set of connections to graphically record basic information about family members and their relationships over three generations.

"Good" death   A death that is free from unavoidable distress and suffering for patients, families, and caregivers; in general accord with patients and families' wishes; and reasonably consistent with clinical, cultural, and ethical standards.

Grief   Represents a holistic, adaptive process that a person goes through following a significant loss.

Group dynamics   Communication processes and behaviors occurring during the life of the group.

Group norms   Refer to the unwritten behavioral rules of conduct expected of group members. Norms can be universal (present in all groups) and group specific referring to those constructed by group members.

Group process   Refers to the structural development of small group relationships (forming, storming, performing, and adjourning).

Group think   Occurs when the approval of other group members becomes so important that group members support a decision they fundamentally do not agree with, just for the sake of harmony.

H

Handheld wireless communication devices   Any small portable computer that uses the internet to transmit information, such as tablets, smart phones, etc.

Handoffs (also handovers)   Transfer process taking place when patients are reassigned to another team of health care providers.

Health   A multidimensional concept having physical, psychological, sociocultural, developmental, and spiritual characteristics that is used to describe an individual's state of well-being and level of functioning.

Health care team   A health care team refers to a coordinated group of professionals with complementary skills who collaborate to give care and are mutually committed to specific performance goals, with shared accountability for goal achievement.

Health disparity   A particular type of health difference that is closely linked with social, economic, and/or environmental disadvantage.

Health information technology (HIT)   An electronic interactive system designed to support the multiple information needs required by today's complex health care.

Health Insurance Portability and Accountability Act (HIPAA)   In the United States, federal privacy standards enacted in 2003 designed to protect an individual's health records and other health information.

Health literacy   The degree to which people have the capacity to obtain, process, and understand basic health information and services needed to make appropriate health decisions.

Health promotion   An educational support process that enables people to take control over their health.

Health teaching   A specialized form of teaching, defined as focused, creative, interpersonal interventions which provide information, emotional support, and health-related skill training.

Homeostasis (also dynamic equilibrium)   A person's sense of personal security and balance.

Hospitalist   A physician or nurse practitioner employed by the hospital to clinically manage a patient's medical care; this provider assumes *full* responsibility for coordinating care.

Huddle   Brief, informal health team gathering to review a course of action.

Human rights-based ethical decision model   Based on the belief that each person has basic rights.

I

Identity   An internal construct about one's abilities, self-image, characteristics.

Independent nursing interventions   Interventions that nurses can provide without a physician's order or direction from another health professional.

Inference   An educated guess about the meaning of a behavior or statement.

Informational continuity   Refers to data exchanges between providers, provider systems, and patients for the purpose of providing coordinated care.

Informed consent   A focused communication process in which a clinician discloses all relevant information related to a procedure or treatment, with full opportunity for dialogue, questions, and expressions of concern, prior to asking for the patient's signed permission.

Interagency accessibility   Transmission and availability of patient information across departments in a health care agency.

Intercultural communication   Conversations between people from different cultures that embrace differences in perceptions, language, and nonverbal behaviors, and recognition of different interpretative contexts.

Interpersonal competence   The ability to interpret the content of a message from the point of view of each of the participants and the ability to use language and nonverbal behaviors to achieve the goals of the interaction.

Interprofessional education   Learning experiences when two or more professions interact to improve collaboration and the quality of care.

Interprofessional health team   See PPC.

Intrapersonal communication   Takes place within the self in the form of inner thoughts; beliefs are colored by feelings and influence behavior.

J

Just culture   A work environment in which staff are empowered to safely speak about their safety concerns.

Justice   Ethical principle guiding decision making. Justice is actually a legal term; however, in ethics it refers to being fair or impartial.

L

Laissez-faire group leadership style   A disengaged form of leadership style in which the leader avoids decision making and is minimally available to group members.

Leadership   Refers to interpersonal influence that is exercised in situations and directed through the communication process toward attainment of a specified goal or goals.

Learning readiness   A person's mind-set and openness to engage in a learning or counseling process for the purpose of adopting new behaviors.

Lifestyle   Patterns of choices made from the alternatives that are available to people.

Linear communication model   Consists of sender, message, receiver, channel, and context.

Longitudinal plan of care (LPC)   Electronic multidisciplinary care plan used across sites to improve continuity of care.

M

Magnet recognition program   A unique national program that recognizes quality patient care and nursing excellence in health care institutions and agencies by identifying them as work environments that act as a "magnet" for professional nurses desiring to work there because of their excellence.

Management continuity   Management strategy of developing pathways and aligning resources to encourage timely effective information flow between all entities involved in facilitating patient-centered care.

Medical home A medical home is a place that serves as a central first contact point in primary care and provides regular, accessible, comprehensive primary care services for designated patients and families within a single familiar setting.

Mentoring A special type of informal professional relationship in which an experienced nurse or clinician (mentor) assumes a role responsibility for guiding the professional growth and advancement of a less-experienced person (protégé).

Message Consists of the transmitted verbal or nonverbal expression of thoughts and feelings.

Message competency The ability to use language and nonverbal behaviors strategically in the intervention phase of the nursing process to achieve the goals of the interaction.

Metacommunication A broad term which describes all the verbal and nonverbal factors used to enhance or negate the meaning of words.

Metaparadigm The four core nursing concepts: person, environment, health, nursing.

m-Health Refers to use of wireless mobile devices in health care.

Mindfulness Refers to awareness within the present moment, especially regarding safety issues.

Minimal cues The simple, encouraging phrases, body actions, or words that communicate interest and encourage patients to continue with their story.

Modeling A behavioral strategy that describes learning by observing another person performing a behavior.

Moral distress A feeling that occurs when one knows what is "right" but feels bound to do otherwise because of legal or institutional constraints.

Moral uncertainty A difficulty in deciding which moral rules (e.g., values or beliefs) apply to a given situation.

Motivation The forces that activate behavior and direct it toward one goal instead of another.

Multigenerational transmission The emotional transmission of behavioral patterns, roles, and communication response styles from generation to generation.

Mutuality An agreement on problems and the means for resolving them; a commitment by both parties to enhance well-being.

N

NNN Abbreviation designating the combination of North American Nursing Diagnosis Association (NANDA), Nursing Interventions Classification (NIC), and Nursing Outcomes Classification (NOC).

Noise Noise factors refer to *any* distraction that interferes with one's ability to pay full attention to the discussion.

Nonmaleficence Avoiding actions that bring harm to another person.

Nonverbal communication Refers to physical expressions and behaviors not expressed in words, which help clinicians understand the emotional meanings of messages.

North American Nursing Diagnosis Association International (NANDA-I) A professional organization of registered nurses that promotes accepted nursing diagnoses.

Nuclear family emotional system The way family members relate to one another within their immediate family when stressed.

Nurse Practice Acts Legal documents that communicate professional nursing's scope of practice, and outline nurses' rights, responsibilities, and licensing requirements in providing health care.

Nursing Interventions Classification (NIC) A standardized language describing direct and indirect care that nurses perform. NIC and Nursing Outcomes Classification (NOC) attempt to quantify nursing care so that it becomes visible and defines professional practice.

Nursing Outcomes Classification (NOC) The measure of how nursing care affects client outcomes. NOC and Nursing Interventions Classifications (NIC) attempt to quantify nursing care so that it becomes visible and defines professional practice.

Nursing process Embodies five phases in health care delivery: assessment, problem identification/diagnosis, planning, implementation, and outcome evaluation.

O

Open-ended questions A question format designed to help individuals express health problems and needs in their own words. Open-ended questions are open to interpretation and cannot be answered by yes, no, or another one-word response.

P

Palliative care A philosophy of care aimed at primarily relieving symptoms associated with terminal illness and providing support for seriously ill patients and their families.

Paralanguage The oral delivery of a verbal message expressed through tone of voice and inflection, sighing, or crying.

Paraphrasing Transforming the patient's words into the nurse's words while keeping the meaning intact.

Patient-centered care (PCC) model Clinical collaborative team partnership with patients, according to their preferences, needs, and values.

Patient education A set of planned educational activities, resulting in changes in health-related behaviors and attitudes as well as knowledge.

Patterns of knowing Multiple integrated knowledge data patterns—empirical, personal, aesthetic, ethical—that nurses use to provide effective, efficient, and compassionate care based on patient needs, individuality, complexity, and situational contexts.

Pedagogy The processes used to help one learn.

Perception A cognitive process by which a person transforms external sensory data into personalized images of reality.

Personal medical identification number A unique series of digits assigned to each individual, used by every health agent and agency. (This would replace use of identifying numbers such as American social security numbers, which were not intended to be used for health care.)

Personal space The invisible and changing boundary around an individual that provides a sense of comfort and protection to a person and that is defined by past experiences and culture.

Point of care Whatever location the nurse is in to provide care to the client, whether at the bedside in the hospital room, in an outpatient clinic, or even in the patient's own home.

Point-of-care information Health information updated via wireless internet devices at any location.

Portals See WEB portals.

Possible selves Used to explain the future-oriented component of self-concept.

Prejudices Stereotypes based on strong emotions.

Premack principle Term used in behavior modification to choose reinforcers that have meaning and value to the individual learner.

Presbycusis Decrease in hearing associated with aging.

Presbyopia Decrease in visual adjustments associated with aging.

Primary care Refers to a wide range of integrated ambulatory health care services delivered in community-based settings.

Primary prevention Actions taken to preclude illness or to prevent the natural course of illness from occurring; strategies target modifiable risk factors with health education to promote a healthy lifestyle.

Privacy The right to have control over personal information, whereas confidentiality refers to the obligation not to divulge anything said in a nurse–patient relationship.

Problem-focused coping Task-oriented stress-coping strategies.

Problem-oriented record (POR) Part of the medical record listing identified patient health problems [diagnoses].

Professional boundaries The invisible structures imposed by legal, ethical, and professional standards of nursing that respect nurse and patient rights and protect the functional integrity of their alliance.

Professional communication An interactive process to help individuals achieve health goals.

Professional standards A competent level of professional knowledge, skills, and attitudes needed to provide quality, safe care.

Protective factors Behavioral activities or conditions delay the emergence of chronic disease or lessen its impact.

Proxemics The study of an individual's use of space.

Psychomotor domain Domain of learning focused on learning a skill through hands-on practice.

Q

QSEN Quality and Safety Education for Nurses (QSEN) nursing competencies considered fundamental to providing safe, high-quality patient-centered care and team collaboration in clinical practice.

QSEN competencies (Quality and Safety Education for Nurses) Clinical practice behaviors (attitudes, knowledge, and skills) expected of nurses, as defined by the QSEN organization.

Quality improvement (QI) The combined efforts of health care professionals, patients and their families, researchers, payers, planners, and educators—to make changes resulting in better clinical outcomes (health) care and system performance.

Quality of life A personal experience of subjective well-being and general satisfaction with life that includes, but is not limited to, physical health.

R

Radio frequency identity chips (RFID) Small embedded computerized chips that can be located remotely.

Reflection A listening response focused on the emotional implications of a message used to help patients clarify important feelings related to message content.

Reframing Changing the frame in which a person perceives events in order to change the meaning.

Reinforcement Refers to establishing consequences for performing targeted behaviors; positive reinforcement increases the probability of a response, and negative reinforcement decreases the probability of a response.

Relational continuity A shared enterprise of therapeutic care delivery relationships across multiple systems, characterized by patient centeredness, collaboration, and coordination.

Resilience Strength and stability during change and stressful life events with rapid recovery from adversity.

Role A multidimensional psychosocial concept defined as a traditional pattern of behavior and self-expression, performed by or expected of an individual within a given society.

S

Safety The minimization of risk of harm; the avoidance of adverse outcomes or injuries stemming from the health care process.

SBAR (situation, background, assessment, recommendation) A standardized communication tool.

Scope of practice A broad term referring to the legal and ethical boundaries of practice for professional nurses defined in written statutes.

Secondary prevention Interventions designed to promote early diagnosis of symptoms through health screening or timely treatment after the onset of the disease, thus minimizing their effects on a person's life.

Self-awareness An intrapersonal process in which a nurse reflects on how their own feelings and beliefs influence professional behaviors.

Self-concept A term describing peoples' complex understanding of their cultural heritage, their environment, their upbringing and education, their basic personality traits, and cumulative life experiences.

Self-differentiation A person's capacity to define him- or herself within the family system as an individual having legitimate needs and wants.

Self-efficacy A term which refers to a person's perceptual belief about their capability to perform tasks and execute courses of action successfully.

Self-esteem The emotional degree to which people approve of themselves in relation to others and the environment.

Self-reflection Developing mindfulness of personal behaviors and values, which allows nurses to recognize the effects their words and behaviors have on the communication process.

Self-talk A cognitive process people can use to lessen cognitive distortions.

Sentinel event A life changing health care occurrence; The Joint Commission specifically uses this term to refer to serious errors in health care which harm patients.

Shaping The reinforcement of target behaviors.

Social cognitive competency The ability to interpret message content within interactions from the point of view of each of the participants.

Social determinants of health A term used to identify a wide range of contextual factors influencing the health and well-being of individuals and communities.

Social support A person's social network connections available to assist them.

Societal emotional process Parallels that Bowen found between the family system and the emotional system operating at the institutional level in society.

Spirituality A unified concept, closely linked to a person's worldview, providing a foundation for a personal belief system about the nature of God or a Higher Power, moral-ethical conduct, and reality.

Standardized communication tools Uniformly used formats for communication of patient information among all care providers, such as the SBAR tool.

Statutory laws Legislated laws.

Stereotyping The process of attributing characteristics to a group of people as though all persons in the identified group possessed them.

Stress A natural physiological, psychological, and spiritual response to the presence of a stressor.

Stressor A demand, situation, internal stimulus, or circumstance that threatens a person's personal security or self-integrity.

Subculture A smaller group of people living within the dominant culture who have adopted a cultural lifestyle distinct from that of the mainstream population.

Subsystems Member unit relationships within the family such as spousal, sibling, and child-parent subsystems.

Summarization An active listening skill used to pull several ideas and feelings together, either from one interaction or a series of interactions, into a few succinct sentences.

Sundowning Episodic agitated behavior occurring later in the day in those suffering from dementia.

T

Taxonomy A hierarchical method of classifying vocabulary.

TCAB An acronym for the program Transforming Care At the Bedside, which empowers nurses to make changes that improve patient safety.

Teach-back method A teaching strategy used in patient education to evaluate and verify their understanding of health teaching; their ability to repeat a demonstration of requisite knowledge and skills.

Team-based principles Group collaboration by all professionals giving care to a patient which includes shared goals, clear roles, mutual trust, and effective communication.

TeamSTEPPS A program (Team Strategies and Tools to Enhance Performance and Patient Safety) which emphasizes improving outcomes by improving communication.

Telehealth Any use of Internet-transmitted visualization for health care diagnosis or treatment. Also known as telemedicine, telenursing, eHealth.

Tertiary prevention Rehabilitation strategies designed to minimize the handicapping effects of a disease or injury once it occurs.

Therapeutic communication A goal-directed form of communication used in health care to achieve objectives that promote patient health and well-being.

Therapeutic relationship A professional alliance in which the nurse and patient join for a defined period to achieve health-related treatment goals.

Timeout A communication tool used by teams to stop and review a situation.

Transactional communication models Communication models that employ systems concepts to describe communication context, feedback loops, and validation; each person influences the other and is both a sender and receiver simultaneously within the interaction.

Transference Projecting irrational attitudes and feelings from the past onto people in the present.

Transitional care A set of actions designed to ensure the coordination and continuity of health care as patients transfer between different locations or different levels of care within the same location.

Triage A term used to describe how health workers sort out the severity of multiple patient needs and determine the priority of treatments in a crisis situation.

Triangles A defensive way of reducing, neutralizing, or defusing heightened anxiety between two family members by drawing a third person or object into the relationship.

Trust A dynamic relational process, involving perceptions of reliance reflecting the deepest needs and vulnerabilities of individuals.

Two challenge rule A safety communication tool in which a team member states their concern twice.

U

Uniform standards Guidelines of accepted practice.

Utilitarian or goal-based model A framework for making ethical decisions in which the rights of the patient and the duties of the nurse are determined by what will achieve maximum welfare or overall good.

V

Validation A focused form of feedback involving verbal and nonverbal confirmation that both participants have the same basic understanding of a message. Feedback loops validate information or allow the human system to correct its original information.

Values A set of personal beliefs and attitudes about truth, beauty, and the worth of any thought, object, or behavior. Attitudes, beliefs, feelings, worries, or convictions that have not been clearly established are called value indicators.

Values acquisitions The conscious assumption of a new value.

Values clarification A process that encourages one to clarify one's own values by sorting them through, analyzing them, and setting priorities.

Violence A health emergency, which can create a critical challenge to the safety, well-being, and health of patients, staff, or others in their immediate environment.

W

Web portal An agency web site that provides opportunities for consumers to use hyperlinks to access a variety of information, receive cyber support, make appointments, pay bills, etc.

Well-being A person's subjective experience of satisfaction about his or her life related to six personal dimensions: intellectual, physical, emotional, social, occupational, and spiritual.

Wisdom The virtue associated with Erikson's final stage of ego development represents an integrated system of "knowing" about the meaning and conduct of life.

Work-arounds Use of nonapproved shortcuts in giving health care.

Worldview The way people tend to look out upon their world or their universe to form a picture or value stance about life or the world around them.

INDEX

Note: Page numbers followed by "f" indicate figures, "t" indicate tables, "b" indicate boxes..